DRUG THERAPY
AND
NURSING CARE

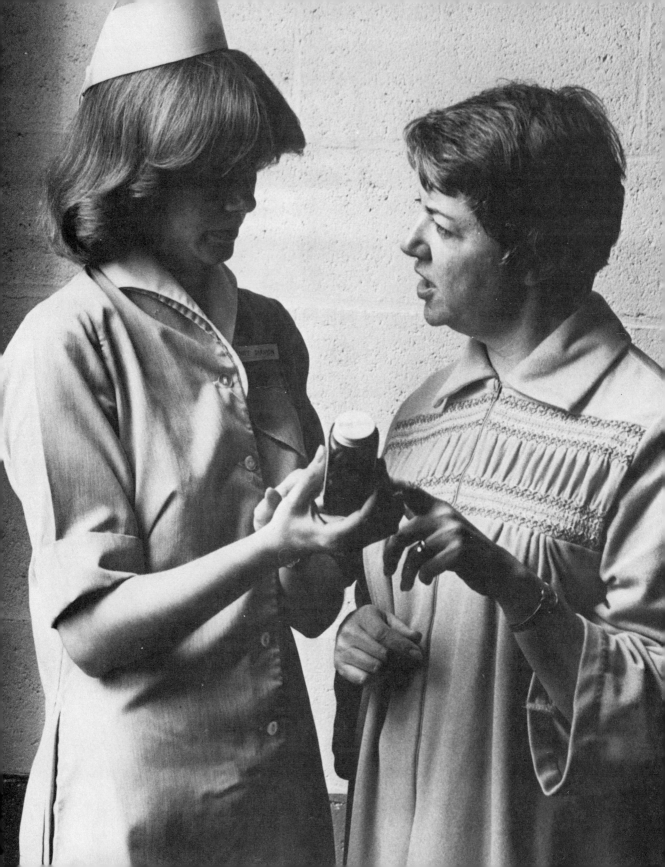

DRUG THERAPY
AND
NURSING CARE

By

Marjorie P. Johns, R.N., M.S.

ASSOCIATE PROFESSOR OF NURSING

Northeastern University
College of Nursing
Boston, Massachusetts

IN CONSULTATION WITH

O. James Inashima, Ph.D.

PROFESSOR OF PHARMACY AND PHARMACOLOGY
Northeastern University
College of Pharmacy and Allied Health Professions
Boston, Massachusetts

MACMILLAN PUBLISHING CO., INC.
NEW YORK

COLLIER MACMILLAN PUBLISHERS
LONDON

Copyright © 1979, Marjorie P. Johns
PRINTED IN THE UNITED STATES OF AMERICA

Macmillan Publishing Co., Inc.
866 Third Avenue, New York, New York 10022
Collier Macmillan Canada, Ltd.

Library of Congress Cataloging in Publication Data

Johns, Marjorie P.   (date)
  Drug therapy and nursing care.

  Bibliography: p.
  Includes index.
  1. Chemotherapy. 2. Nursing. I. Title.
[DNLM: 1. Drug therapy—Nursing texts.
2. Nursing care. 3. Pharmacology—Nursing texts.
QV4.3. J65d]
RM262.J64   615′.58′024613   78–17822
ISBN 0–02–360800–5

Cover illustration and frontispiece:
Courtesy, Northeastern University College
of Nursing, Boston, Massachusetts

Printing: 1 2 3 4 5 6 7 8   Year: 9 0 1 2 3 4 5

Preface

Drug therapy is an integral part of many plans for health maintenance. The focus of this textbook is on the contribution that drugs make to the resolution of physiologic or emotional problems of patients. The approach that is employed allows the study of drug effects and mechanisms of action without extensive consideration of the multifaceted nonpharmacologic treatment of specific disease entities.

An understanding of the biopsychosocial factors that affect drug therapy requires an appreciation of fundamental concepts from the basic sciences. The chapter content presentation provides a review of the relevant physiologic and pathophysiologic correlations that are required for the study of the drugs that are included in the chapter. The text presents essential basic content about drugs in current use and integrates pharmacology with nursing care. It also includes data that can be utilized for identifying, analyzing, and interpreting the needs of patients when the nurse is implementing comprehensive, individualized plans in clinical situations. Nursing measures are interwoven throughout the presentations of *therapy considerations*. Guidelines for assessment, planning care, and counseling of patients are presented in the sections entitled Nursing Intervention, which are highlighted by an orange tint to connote their importance to drug therapy and to facilitate referral to the guidelines when planning nursing care. The guidelines are intended to provide information that can be utilized to promote optimal care and maintain patient compliance with the drug therapy plan.

The primary goal of this book is to prepare the nurse to utilize independent and interdependent modes of action in contributing to the effectiveness of drug therapy plans in varied health care settings. A broad understanding of the effects of drugs on body systems allows nursing intervention that includes preplanning for the protection of patients' health status and for recognizing the implications of status changes that occur when patients are receiving drugs for the treatment of health problems.

The emphasis of the pharmacologic content is on the common drugs in current use; less commonly used drugs generally are compared with the prototype. The nonproprietary, or generic, names of the drugs are employed in the discussions of drug therapy. The proprietary, or trade, names are indicated parenthetically in SMALL CAPITAL LETTERS at least once for each drug. In the introductory chapters (Chapters 1 through 6), drugs are designated in a similar manner. The inclusion of specific drugs in the early chapters is intended to provide a more extensive frame of reference for the student who reviews the content for a deeper understanding of a problem encountered in the clinical setting.

The suggested additional readings, which are included at the end of each chapter, provide detailed data from clinical studies of drug therapy regimens and current information about drug therapy in clinical situations. A listing of pharmacology textbooks that provide comprehensive information about varied aspects of drug therapy is included in the back matter (see Table of Contents).

In general the term *patient* is used in the text to indicate a recipient of therapy in a hospital setting. The words *person* or *individual* generally indicate an ambulatory, or infrequently supervised, recipient of drugs.

The term *counseling* has been selected in preference to the terms instruction or teaching. Counseling is viewed as more accurately describing the interactive role of the nurse in explaining the drug therapy regimen and in preparing the person to assume responsibility for using the drug in the unsupervised home situation.

In the selection of content for this textbook, the

author was guided by responses to a questionnaire that was sent by Macmillan Publishing Co., Inc., to all associate-degree, diploma, and baccalaureate nursing programs in the United States. The hundreds of faculty responses indicated the desirability of having a pharmacology textbook that emphasized the effects of drugs on physiologic processes, drug therapy, and nursing intervention. Most of the faculty also mentioned that such a text should include legal aspects of drug administration, drug standards, tables that summarize dosages, and review questions at the end of the chapters. Each of the suggestions has been implemented in the preparation of this textbook. Many of the respondents to the questionnaire also indicated the desirability of having a pharmacology workbook that utilized a realistic clinical case study approach to the study of drug therapy. As a result, *Case Studies in Drug Therapy* by Johns, Brogan, Lynch, and Marchessault (Macmillan, 1979) has been prepared for use with this and other pharmacology textbooks.

The author is grateful to Professor O. James Inashima, whose meticulous attention to the pharmacology content of *Drug Therapy and Nursing Care* was invaluable in the preparation of the specific material related to pharmaceutical preparations and dosages. The author also is deeply grateful to Professor Anne Marie Brogan, who generously reviewed all of the content and offered constructive criticism and suggestions. A debt of gratitude is owed to Joan Carolyn Zulch, medical editor of Macmillan Publishing Co., Inc., whose encouragement, patience, and editorial expertise facilitated completion of the text. The author gratefully acknowledges the assistance of the staff in the Office of Learning Resources at Northeastern University, who provided the specialized photographs for inclusion in the book.

The sincere interest and enthusiasm of innumerable students and faculty have been a source of joy and stimulation during the preparation of the manuscript. The author is sincerely grateful for the thoughtful suggestions and enthusiastic response of students and faculty to requests for realistic clinical data and photographs to demonstrate concepts within the text. The nursing students' continual quest for information that is required to improve patient care provided the initial impetus for the preparation of this textbook, and an ongoing evaluation of their learning needs assisted the author in the selection of content that is relevant to the nurse member of the health team.

Marjorie P. Johns

Contents

UNIT

General Aspects of Drug Therapy   1

UNIT

Drugs Used to Maintain Hemodynamic Equilibrium   89

UNIT

Drugs Used to Maintain Cellular Reproduction
and the Integrity of Tissues   257

IV
UNIT

Drugs Used to Maintain Gas Exchange and Removal of Toxicants and Wastes   425

V
UNIT

Drugs Used to Maintain Rest, Activity, and Emotional Equilibrium   481

VI
UNIT

Drugs Used to Maintain Nutritional Balance   617

General Aspects of Drug Therapy

1

Implementing Drug Therapy Plans

Treatment with medication makes a significant contribution to the well-being and health maintenance of the general population, and there are hundreds of drugs and combinations of drugs available for use. Drug therapy is an integral part of the care plan for acutely ill patients, and drugs are the most frequently prescribed therapy for the posthospital period. It would be a difficult task to find a home without a variety of preparations stored for treatment of common health problems. The frequency with which prescription and over-the-counter (O.T.C.) drugs are employed and the availability of information about drugs in the news media have had a noticeable effect on public awareness of drug action.

HEALTH TEAM PLANNING

Professional health team members are responsible for planning and implementing drug therapy plans that are safe and effective and can be properly utilized by the patient. A prerequisite for planning is that the professionals have comprehensive data about the patient's health problem, the characteristics of the drugs, and the contribution drug therapy will make to the total care plan for the patient. It is possible to define the probable biochemical or physiologic action of

drugs employed for therapy, but those effects must be considered with an understanding that drug action is influenced by variations in individual responses to drugs and knowledge of the pathophysiologic processes that can modify responses.

Physician, nurse, and pharmacist each has a particular area of expertise to contribute to planning and evaluating the patient's drug regimen. Legal definitions separate those functions that are unique for each professional group: the physician prescribes and may administer drugs; the nurse administers drugs; and the pharmacist prepares and dispenses drugs. The shared aspects of each professional's involvement in the drug therapy plan are *monitoring the patient's responses and evaluating the effectiveness of therapy*. The multiplicity of drugs employed in therapy and the potential for adverse effects and drug interactions make it useful to have clinical pharmacists, who have special knowledge of the properties of pharmaceuticals, as members of the health team. Working together, the professional team members formulate plans that include *measures to protect the patient's resources, support the action of the drug being given, make optimal use of restored function effected by the drug, and prepare the patient for maintenance of the drug regimen.*

3

NURSING ROLES

Nurses have a dynamic and active role in implementing and evaluating drug therapy plans. Professional nurses have been prime movers in the evolutionary process that has expanded their activities from administrators of prescribed drugs to include all aspects of drug therapy. The modern nurse participates as an informed observer and collaborates with the physician and pharmacist in evaluating the effectiveness of drug therapy plans.

Communication is a key element in accumulating and validating data that can be utilized for planning and modifying patient care strategies. Nurses can contribute to health team planning by communicating relevant data from round-the-clock surveillance of the patient and evaluation of progress or problems occurring during therapy. As communicators, nurses share information with team members and utilize diverse communication media to improve patient understanding and acceptance of the drug regimen. Nurses have innumerable opportunities to interpret the therapeutic plan to patients and to prepare them to participate as contributing members of the health team. The input from patients combined with assessment of knowledgeable professionals provides the data required for planning optimum care. An explicit description of areas of competence that the modern nurse contributes to planning drug therapy includes *surveillant, data gatherer, patient advocate,* and *information disseminator.*

Nurses contribute directly to the patient's progress by administering drugs, monitoring their effects, and preparing the patient to assume responsibility for those functions when his health status permits. The process includes many challenging opportunities for utilizing abilities to synthesize information and to analyze problems in patient care situations. Viewing nursing function in this broader dimension places the focus on health problem resolution rather than on the limited function of drug administration.

The Modern Patient

Social changes within the past decade have provided the impetus for developments within the nursing profession that facilitated and stimulated change in functional modes. A timely societal factor that strongly influenced the expansion of the nursing role was the philosophic change that modified the patient role definition from passive recipient to involved consumer. Modern legal interpretation of the patient's rights requires that the individual have sufficient information to allow an intelligent choice between treatment, no treatment, or alternative treatment methods. The patient must be informed of the risks involved, the alternatives, and the possible outcomes of all forms of therapy offered, and consent must be obtained before services are rendered.

The patient seeking therapy for resolution of a health problem has the right to information about predictable actions and adverse effects of drugs prescribed so he can participate as an informed member of the health team planning the therapeutic program. When a drug initially is prescribed, the physician may tell the patient about the planned effect and adverse effects that may occur. It is the shared responsibility of the physician, nurse, and pharmacist to define whether the patient has sufficient information to assure safe use and continuance of therapy when the individual is to assume responsibility for taking the drugs at home.

The patient often can provide information about the effects of drugs taken, and the individual's input about personal physiologic patterns and responses adds another dimension to the data available for evaluating the effectiveness of the therapeutic plan. The patient may provide clues that help in identification of problems before they are obvious by objective assessment measures.

Nursing Care Guides

Nurses who actively participate as members of the health team have frequent opportunities to examine alternative care plans, and the experience enables them to create nursing plans adapted to the changing needs of the patients they serve. Assessment and teaching guides, or protocols, are developed when nurses find approaches that are effective in assisting patients with varying health problems to progress toward optimum achievable objectives. In contrast to traditional directives for care, modern guides are nonformularized outlines allowing individualization of approaches in their implementation. The process in the broadest sense is consistently moving professional nursing practice toward the goal of *expanding and improving health care.*

Knowledge Required

Professional nurses must have a broad theoretic background to prepare for informed participation as contributing members of the team implementing drug therapy plans. The necessary knowledge base includes:

1. Predictable effects of drugs on physiologic and emotional problems.
2. Commonalities and variations between the actions of drugs employed for comparable therapeutic effect.
3. Adverse effects and interactions of drugs commonly occurring during drug therapy.
4. Biopsychosocial factors influencing drug therapy plans.

Preparation for the continually expanding role in implementing drug therapy plans begins with study of the scientific foundations of drug therapy and of drug administration procedures. Basic knowledge of drug actions, adverse effects, and interactions is expanded each time the nurse assumes responsibility for administering drugs and monitoring the effectiveness of drug therapy. Clinical experiences provide opportunity for comparisons between responses of individuals by careful analysis of the differences in therapeutic plans for an increasing number of patients. Each experience provides a vivid recall pattern that is useful in subsequent patient care situations.

Whenever the nurse assumes responsibility for patient care, it is important that each aspect of the therapeutic program be understood, and drug therapy is an integral part of most patient care

plans. To meet the commitment to understanding drugs, the nurse must know the actions of the drugs and the rationale for giving the drugs to the particular patient. In addition to knowing the planned therapeutic outcome, the nurse must define the factors to be monitored to assess progress and to determine end points of therapy. When expected physiologic outcomes do not ensue, discussion of the problem with the health team members may allow adjusting dosage, discontinuing the drug, or replacing it with another more effective drug.

The broad responsibilities that are an integral part of the nursing role require continual study to maintain competency in implementing drug therapy plans. Enrichment or expansion of knowledge about drugs is easier if drugs are viewed in groups having commonalities of action because the process allows building on previous knowledge rather than approaching new drugs as novel or separate entities differing entirely from older prototypes.

NURSING ACTIVITIES

An organized system for data gathering and assessment of the data assures inclusiveness of plans implemented and provides base lines for evaluating or auditing the effectiveness of care. Therapy and nursing intervention are comprehensive integrated approaches directed at restoration or maintenance of optimum health status. In any health care setting, patient care involves assessing the patient's status, coordinating therapeutic procedures, planning nursing care, monitoring progress, and preparing the individual for unsupervised ambulatory care or preparing a significant other person to assume responsibility for the patient's care.

Nurse involvement in patient teaching has contributed to the increase in guides for conducting these patient learning experiences. Teaching modules are gradually being produced by nurses for use by staff responsible for preparing the patient for diagnostic procedures or surgery or for home care. The modules vary from simple outlines to audiovisual programs prepared by nurses specifically for the needs of particular groups of patients within the agency.

Each nurse-patient contact provides an opportunity to interview, observe, and examine the individual for indicators of health status. Some of the data that are appropriate to establishing base lines for assessing progress of the drug therapy regimen, and problems the individual has encountered with maintenance of that regimen, may be obtained from existing medical or nursing histories, or from other data in the clinical record. In the absence of background data, the onus is on the nurse to obtain the data required to objectively evaluate the individual's status.

Initial Status Evaluation

Complex biopsychosocial factors affect continuance of health care maintenance regimens. In each nurse-patient contact, the nurse has an opportunity to interview, observe, and examine the individual for indicators of health status. The base-line data are essential for defining the problems the individual has experienced with maintaining previous drug therapy plans and for assessing progress of the ongoing therapy regimen.

Patient Involvement. A crucial factor, basic to any plan requiring behavioral change, is the individual's perception of the problem and its effect on personally valued patterns of living. During the patient's interview, astute "on-the-spot" analysis of verbal and nonverbal clues allows immediate inquiry by the nurse and additional specific input from the patient about the problems. A clear understanding of the patient's perception of the functional problems, and the factors contributing to them, serves as a base line for planning measures to assist the individual in resolution of those problems.

Planning Nursing Intervention

Each dimension of the patient's care can be analyzed, and an outline for planning each aspect of care then can be established. The process yields separate inclusive guides that can be merged to formulate a comprehensive and meaningful plan

for care. The following outline provides a guide for implementing nursing aspects of drug therapy plans:

I. Establish base lines for assessing drug effect on the individual's problem.
   A. Obtain the patient's statement of the problem and its effect on his ability to function (i.e., abilities, limitations).
   B. Obtain information about psychosocial factors affecting resolution of the problem (i.e., health history, health care practices, previous problems with drugs, compliance to prescribed therapies).
   C. Examine the patient for evidence of the problem.
   D. Obtain relevant data from members of the health team and from the clinical record.
II. Plan measures for maximizing drug effect and for monitoring the patient's progress.
   A. Establish an individualized plan for taking prescribed medications.
   B. Involve the patient (and family) in implementation of the drug therapy plan (i.e., clarify roles, health care goals).
   C. Employ, or clarify for the patient, measures that support drug action.
   D. Establish a plan for purposeful observation of drug effects (i.e., surveillance intervals and methods).
   E. Share observations of drug effect with health team members evaluating the plan.
III. Prepare the individual for assessing progress of the drug therapy plan.
   A. Review with the patient (and family member) the plan for drug therapy.
      1. Plan the specific pharmacotherapeutic plan within the individual's pattern of living.
      2. Provide specific written instructions for use at home.
   B. Explain common adverse effects and factors that may change drug requirements.
   C. Describe the plan for scheduled follow-up care and the interim problems (i.e., new symptoms) requiring physician contact.
   D. Reassess the individual's readiness to

maintain the drug therapy plan and future instructional needs.

The broad outline provides an approach that assures inclusion of vital dimensions of the drug therapy plan, and it retains focus on the individual and his involvement throughout the period of therapy. Each aspect of the guide can be expanded to include the specific items relevant to a patient with a particular physiologic or emotional problem. For example, Item I. C. would be expanded to include specific examination of the patient for signs of excess tissue fluid in extremities, periorbital and sacral areas, lungs, or peritoneal cavity when the patient is receiving a diuretic for control of fluid accumulation. When the patient has a problem requiring use of a bronchodilator, the item would be expanded to include specific examination for evidence of abnormal breathing patterns and interference with gas exchange.

Drug therapy is part of an overall plan for control of health problems, and discussion of the drug regimen with the patient involves explaining related aspects of the plan for improving health or preventing illness. For example, discussion of measures to maximize the effectiveness of diuretic drug therapy (Item II. D.) would naturally include explanation of the relationship of sodium intake and activity modification to the control of edema.

Preplanning guides provide base-line data and directions for surveillance procedures. The process allows anticipation and prevention of predictable problems before they adversely affect the patient's progress. The preplanning guides also allow determination of therapy progression, and it is easier for the patient to accept severe restriction if there is a predictable end point beyond which limitations will be lessened. Interpretation of progress and clarification of changes that are implemented can facilitate the patient's understanding and acceptance of therapy.

Patient Teaching

Behavioral modification is the distinct goal of teaching. To reach the goal, the individual who must change is the natural focus of all activities. When the "should system" representing the values of the nurse is used didactically to instruct the individual, there may be an indication of assent and in some instances the patient may rigidly follow the directives. Strict adherence to rules set forth interferes with autonomy, and the confines of a set of standards leaves the individual without a flexible guide for managing the complex and diverse problems that arise in life situations.

Preplanned periods of instruction that allow joint problem solving and establishing of goals acceptable to the individual can lead to a higher level of compliance with the planned therapeutic regimen. In this frame of reference, teaching is more than telling, and the nurse assumes the richer role of the teacher as a facilitator of learning.

Patient Motivation. Patient teaching is a collaborative effort involving various health team members, and it may include family members or significant others in the individual's community system who can assist with accomplishing behavioral modification. Motivation is a key factor in the learning process, and all efforts are directed at patient involvement in the process. In addition to the individual's predisposition to learn, reception of the information is affected by level of intelligence, attitudes, and ethnic or religious beliefs. Much of the information required for determining the level of readiness of the patient can be obtained in the course of periodic contact prior to planned instruction. The individual's self-image, role perception, and scope of interest in community events can provide clues to measures that can be employed to move the individual forward.

Patient Involvement. Patients learn when they are actively involved in the process in diverse ways. Many individuals will remain passive and receive instruction without inquiry. The nurse presenting the information can indicate that questions are invited and encouraged by accepting and responding to each query in a manner that shows respect for the sincerity of the inquirer. Allowing time for questions is part of the process of setting

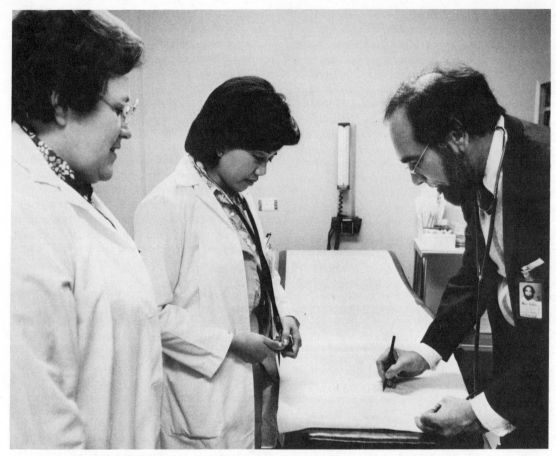

Fig. 1–1. Information sharing between health team members maintains the reliability and consistency of the data presented to the patient. (Courtesy, Beth Israel Hospital, Boston.)

the environment for learning. An informal, relaxed manner and focus on the individual by consistent eye contact communicate concern with the worth and needs of the individual during the period of instruction. Selection of the environment depends on the situation, but some privacy in the instruction session will prevent interruptions and their natural disruption in thought patterns and will allow the individual to present problems of a personal and confidential nature. The opportunity for the patient to solve problems

related to personal situations can provide the challenge that raises the level of motivation and consequently increases involvement with the therapy plan. Ideas presented to the individual should be within a familiar frame of reference so the new idea can be related to personal life situations.

Learning results in behavioral changes, and the process can be frustrating and even painful. The nurse may provide the initial impetus and proceed based on cues obtained in the nurse-patient discussion, but motivation for behavioral change is

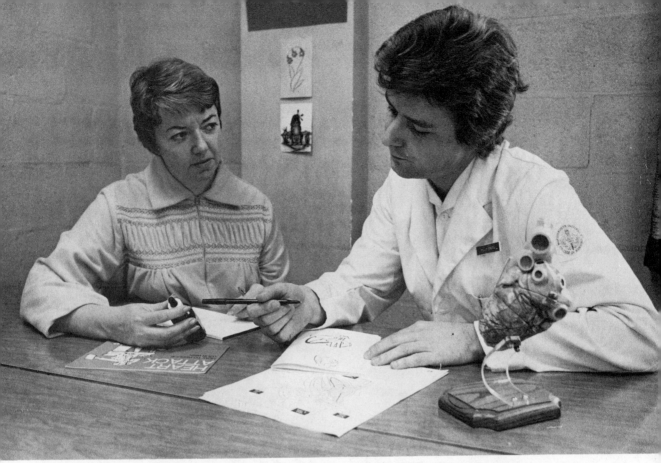

Fig. 1–2. Anatomic models and simple illustrations of anatomic relationships facilitate the nurse's explanation of the health problem to the patient. (Courtesy, Northeastern University College of Nursing, Boston.)

within the learner, who makes the final decision to accept or reject some or all aspects of therapy.

Planning the Presentation. Timing and environment are important factors in patient instruction. It would be ludicrous to instruct the individual in an intensive care situation about all details of therapy, since the complex plan probably will be revised during the recovery phase of illness. It is equally inappropriate to attempt to teach a highly anxious individual until measures are taken to modify anxiety and increase readiness for learning.

Patient instruction is seldom a solo effort. The patient benefits when information sharing between health team members maintains reliability and consistency in the data provided to the patient

(Fig. 1–1). From the patient's point of view, changes in therapy consequent to difference in health status can cause frustration, fear, and lowering of confidence in the competence of health professionals. In the hospital situation, opportunities occur to present information, to explain aspects of the therapy plan on a continuing basis, and to provide for reinforcement of learning. An essential element in planning for posthospital maintenance of the drug therapy plan is provision of a specified time period for discussion of the plan within the context of the patient's living patterns.

Learning Progression. Preinstruction evaluation involves definition of clues indicating the individual's informational needs. The extent and

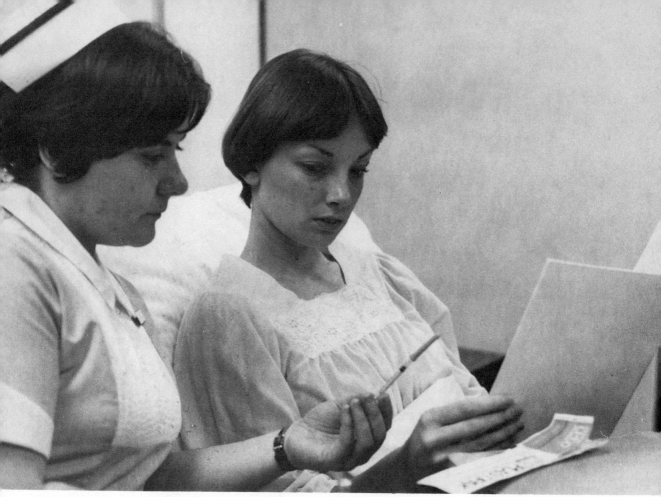

Fig. 1–3. Early involvement of the patient in discussion of the drug therapy plan allows introduction of instructional materials in small packets. The person has an opportunity to inquire about details and to assimilate the information during the interaction with the nurse. (Courtesy, Niagara College of Applied Arts and Technology, The Mack Centre of Nursing Education, Welland, Ontario.)

accuracy of knowledge about the disease, drugs, and therapeutic plans influence the starting point for teaching, after which it is possible to introduce information and to proceed as the individual's assimilation of data and ability to use the concepts in self-identified situations are tested by encouraging the feedback of examples of ways therapy will be managed within daily living patterns.

Visual Aids. Written instructions must be inclusive to assure that the individual has a reference source. For example, a form (i.e., a 5 × 8″ file card) can be prepared with a sample of the drug taped on it, a caption stating the name of the drug, a concise legend describing the effect of the drug on the patient's problem, adverse reactions, problems requiring notification of the physician, dosage schedule, exact hours, and special instructions for taking the medication.

It is useful to prepare simple outlines with terminology at the sixth- or seventh-grade reading level if standardized instructions are prepared for distribution to patients. Many individuals need concrete examples and written information, and only about one fourth of the population has a high-level ability to conceptualize. Simple illustrations of anatomic relationships will be understood better than verbal descriptions when the individual is dependent on concrete references for learning (Fig. 1–2). Many patients benefit from taking written notes of suggestions presented during discussion periods. Clarification of unclear terms or of misinformation about aspects of the therapeutic program can be accomplished during informal discussion with the individual or with small groups of patients with comparable problems and therapeutic plans.

Reinforcement of Learning. Involvement of the patient in the therapeutic plan while in a supervised setting allows opportunity for introduction of content in manageable packets and opportunity to modify approaches to teaching and to discuss possible alternatives suited to the patient's living patterns (Fig. 1–3). When procedural aspects of medication preparation or administration are practiced under supervision, the patient's confidence and ability to personally manage the therapy are increased. Reinforcement opportunities occur when the patient practices any skill in a supervised situation (Fig. 1–4). The frustrations identified in the guided experiences allow revision while the same failures or challenges may cause discontinuance of therapy when the unsupervised ambulatory patient experiences them. The positive feedback from succeeding or from the praise of the nurse can contribute to the patient's motivation to learn. Gradual attainment of autonomy may itself reward the patient who learns aspects of care required by therapy. Periodic reassessment of performance allows an opportunity to reinforce learning and sustain motivation.

Monitoring Drug Effects

The specific measures for monitoring the progress or emerging problems of any individual receiving drugs relate to the action of the particular drug and to the individual's specific problem. In the intensive care situation, graphic records or flow charts provide vivid illustrations of interrelated aspects of therapy and changes occurring at closely spaced intervals, but in most clinical situations vital signs are recorded on graphic charts and other assessments are recorded in narrative form on the patient's record.

Therapeutic Effect. Plans for surveillance are comprehensive approaches based on knowledge of the patient's problem, drug action, adverse effects, and possible drug interactions. An important and often neglected aspect of monitoring is the positive effect of the drug on the patient's problem. Lessening of physiologic or emotional problems deserves equal attention with the occurrence of new problems. The desired changes reflect success of the plan. Positive indicators of drug effect provide guidelines for lessening drug dosage or limitations imposed on the patient, and they show progress toward the end points of intensive therapy.

When patients are receiving drugs for control of pain, nursing judgments are required before implementing prescriptions for drugs to be given "as the occasion arises," or p.r.n. Assessment of factors contributing to the patient's discomfort allows modification of unnecessary stimuli and enhances the effect of the pain-relieving drug. Subsequent monitoring of the onset, duration, and quality of pain relief provides a guide to therapeutic effectiveness.

Adverse Effects. Occurrence of adverse reactions may be identified by unexplained new symptoms or flare-up of old symptoms. The patient's vague complaints of discomfort, or changes in blood pressure, temperature, plasma values, and other vital parameters without apparent reason may be the first clues to emerging problems. Most adverse effects are minor gastrointestinal disturbances, but diverse body systems are involved in the very common adverse drug reactions such as rashes, itching, drowsiness, insomnia, and headache. When a new drug is added to the therapeutic regimen or when a drug is withdrawn, it is important to plan closely scheduled observations for changes in status. Any change is significant when the individual is receiving several drugs concurrently because there are many potential drug interactions.

Drug Interactions. There are numerous guides showing theoretic or possible drug interactions, and it is difficult to screen out those with clinical

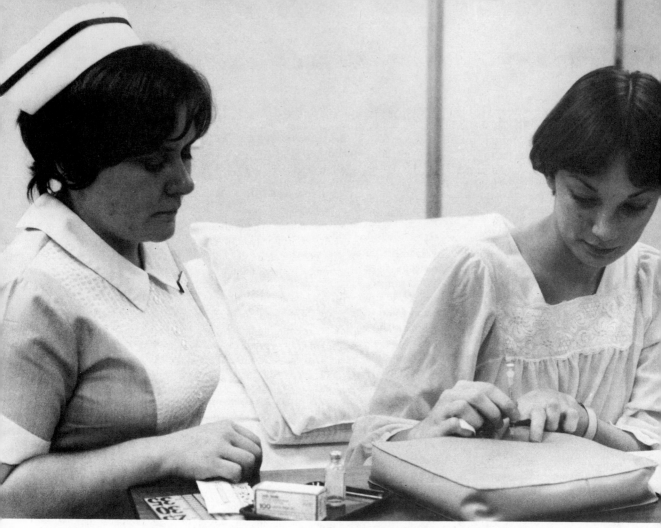

Fig. 1–4. The patient can acquire skill in management of complex procedures when opportunity is provided for supervised practice that is guided by the nurse. (Courtesy, Niagara College of Applied Arts and Technology, The Mack Centre of Nursing Education, Welland, Ontario.)

significance. Drug therapy may be affected by drugs that have properties causing interaction with other drugs. The interactions are classified as resulting from similar or opposing pharmacodynamic actions; stimulation or inhibition of drug metabolism; alteration of absorption, excretion, electrolyte levels, or volume of distribution; competition for protein-binding sites; or interaction at receptor sites of drug action. It is impossible to memorize all the potential drug interactions, but it is possible to provide a safeguard during drug

therapy by using the available literature and consulting with informed resource persons to obtain reliable and relevant information.

Individual Responses. Multiple biopsychosocial factors affect drug therapy. The patient's perception of need for a drug or factors in the immediate environment may influence demands for medication, the therapeutic effect of drugs administered, or compliance with the drug therapy plan.

Additional Readings

Aspinwall, Mary Jo: Nursing diagnosis—the weak link. *Nurs. Outlook,* **24**:433, July, 1976.

Hallburg, Jeanne C.: The teaching of aged adults. *J. Gerontol. Nurs.,* **2**:13, May, June, 1976.

Johns, Marjorie P.: The nurse and drug surveillance. *Drug Information J.,* **9**:75, April–September, 1976.

Murray, Ruth, and Zentner, Judith: Guidelines for more effective health teaching. *Nursing '76,* **6**:44, February, 1976.

Redman, Barbara K.: *The Process of Patient Teaching in Nursing,* 3rd ed. The C. V. Mosby Company, St. Louis, 1976.

Riley-Kesler, Arlene: Pitfalls to avoid in interviewing outpatients. *Nursing '77,* **7**:70, September, 1977.

Winslow, Elizabeth Hahn: The role of the nurse in patient education. *Nurs. Clin. North Am.,* **11**:213, June, 1976.

2

Psychosocial Factors Affecting Drug Therapy

Through varying communication media, consumers receive information about health problems that previously was available only to select members of the professional community. There are problems intrinsic in the modern patterns of widely disseminated general information about drugs, diseases, and therapeutic procedures. In addition to the "half-truth" there are variations in interpretation and application of information by individuals with divergent physical, educational, cultural, or social backgrounds. The composite picture is one of a population with preconceived ideas about health care based on partial information, misinformation, or bias.

Barriers must be overcome whenever a patient is required to change lifelong behavior patterns by maintaining a therapeutic regimen for control of a health problem. The nurse, as the most consistently available professional, has an opportunity to know the individual and the subsystems that constitute his world or community system. Interaction with the patient allows opportunity to become familiar with the interface of biopsychosocial factors impinging on the individual.

As surveillant, the nurse can recognize and analyze the subtle signs of therapeutic effect or adverse effects of drugs. Frequent contact with the patient and awareness of usual behavioral patterns sensitize the nurse to nonverbal or verbal indicators of status changes. A patient's preliminary interpretation of a changing condition may lead him to view the emerging problem as a threat to clinical progress or discharge from the hospital, and he may hesitate to discuss it with the physician. The nurse can explore and analyze the clues with the patient's assistance and consider their relevance to drug action or to other factors in the patient's environment. For example, when a patient becomes dizzy while dressing and assembling his belongings before leaving the hospital, his preliminary interpretation may be related to failure of some aspect of the therapy. The nurse viewing the situation and putting the relevant factors in the context of activities in which the patient has been involved immediately previous to the episode can separate the single incident from the overall progress of therapy. The incident can be a basis for discussing the advisability of spacing and modifying the pace of necessary activities in the immediate posthospital period.

Much valuable information can be obtained when taking the nursing history. The patient's general health status and health practices may provide clues to the depth of concern about factors contributing to health maintenance. The data also provide base-line information against which to evaluate progress during therapy. When inquiring about previous health problems, the nurse should elicit information about previous medication-taking practices, patterns for scheduling medications at home, and problems precipitated by the drugs. The foregoing data can provide guides to planning administration of drugs while the patient is hospitalized, but the most important use of the assessment data may be for identification of factors influencing drug taking and as predictor of continuance of therapy in the post-hospital period. Realistic teaching is based on knowledge of the patient's life-style and usual behavior patterns.

ATTITUDES AND BELIEFS

Attitude changes are difficult to accomplish, and they are affected by the individual's perceptions of the health problem and of the sick role. When the patient's life-style conflicts with therapy goals, he will change or ignore the medical regimen rather than allow it to threaten or change familiar life patterns.

The common belief that use of medication weakens the body or causes the body to become dependent on the drugs makes it difficult to implement programs for asymptomatic patients. That belief also is a problem when attempting to institute prophylactic use of drugs. For example, many individuals view nitroglycerin, which is used in treatment of angina pectoris, as bits of TNT, or dynamite, and that perception carries with it a view that taking the drug prophylactically, before exercise induces pain, will weaken the heart and that the drug won't work when needed for pain control. Those individuals will use one dose when acute pain occurs but will hesitate to take a second or third tablet as prescribed to control anginal pain. They also will avoid taking the drug prophylactically as instructed previous to strenuous activity to decrease the incidence of pain.

It is difficult to convince an individual with an asymptomatic health problem to follow the prophylactic use of drugs for prevention of acute attacks or to decrease risk factors. Weight control, cessation of smoking, activity limitation, and drug taking may be perceived as requiring sick role behavior from a patient who doesn't feel sick. Emotional resistance is seen as rationalization about the disease and drug therapy regimen requirements. Denial or resistance may cause the individual to consult several physicians until one is found who will lessen restrictions or who agrees with the individual's personal diagnosis. Long-term therapy can be viewed by the patient as loss of control over one's own life, and the rejection of a prescribed drug therapy regimen may be a means of remaining in control.

Cultural concepts and traditions influence the individual's perception of drug therapy. Although the American "drug culture" has received much notoriety, a deeply ingrained attitude remains against taking medication when no problem is evident. It also is common practice to hold back before seeking medical advice to see if the problem will decrease or disappear and to avoid "unnecessary costs." In the interval before seeking medical assistance, the individual attempts to identify cause-effect relationships, to make a preliminary diagnosis of the problem, and to use familiar remedies to alleviate the problem.

Ethnic groups have deeply rooted beliefs that may affect their ability to accept prescribed therapy. For example, Puerto Ricans classify diseases or illnesses as *caliente* (hot) or *frio* (cold), and the Chinese perceive illness as imbalance between *yin* energy forces (cold air) and *yang* energy forces (hot air). Individuals will not take prescribed medication that is perceived as causing imbalance, but they may be encouraged to take drugs with vehicles perceived as maintaining balance.

Therapy that considers the individual's beliefs will succeed but that in contradiction will fail. In instances where drug therapy will be affected by cultural patterns, it is important to ascertain the beliefs and other life activities (i.e., food and fluid intake patterns) that may influence therapy. By careful analysis of the patient's perception of how therapy can support or be merged with the existing belief system, it is often possible to find methods of instituting therapy without compromising the beliefs of ethnic groups.

The problems are complex, but unless the attitudes are changed the patient will completely or partially neglect to follow the prescribed regimen. A preliminary step is to identify the patient's perceptions. Once the problems are identified, strategies can be gradually and tactfully implemented. Flexibility is a key factor in the process of guiding the patient toward attitude change and consequently leading to health practices acceptable to the individual.

An individual who has experienced and solved a problem can be an excellent teacher of small groups of patients requiring assistance with changing attitudes about a similar problem. A respected authority figure also may be effective in gradually moving the individual toward behavioral change. Patients often seem enthralled with advice based on the personal testimonials of relatives or friends, and it may be possible to capitalize on this when an informed individual is available.

COMPLIANCE

It is estimated that more than 50 percent of patients with chronic health problems fail to follow the prescribed pharmacotherapeutic plan when they are responsible for self-care. Compliance with the prescribed therapeutic regimen is an important consideration in planning measures to move the patient toward optimum health. More than three quarters of the drugs consumed are self-administered by individuals in ambulatory settings. A well-planned drug regimen loses its purpose if not adhered to by the unsupervised ambulatory patient. The noncompliance problem is expensive, wasteful, and frustrating because there is little that health professionals can accomplish without the cooperation of the patient.

The individual's compliance with previous therapeutic plans or personal standards of health care maintenance may provide indicators of the probability of consistent drug use when the patient assumes responsibility for a drug therapy plan, but only a selected few patients can be

specifically identified as potential noncompliers. Angry, dissatisfied patients or alcoholics constitute a minority segment of the population who predictably will ignore or compromise the prescribed regimen. Noncompliance occurs in all socioeconomic groups, all types of individuals, and all types of patient care settings. There seem to be no discernible differences between patients who comply and those who fail to comply with all aspects of the prescribed plan. The complexity of the phenomenon is evident when considering inconsistencies in behavior: the same patients may comply at one time or with some aspects of their plan and default at another time.

Community clinics find that the "no-show" rate for appointments compares with the 50 percent noncompliance rate for adherence to a planned therapeutic drug regimen. Appointment keeping is higher during the acute phase of illness when the patient has symptoms (80 percent), but falls to 50 percent when the patient becomes asymptomatic and falls 10 percent lower when long-term therapy is required. The asymptomatic individual has difficulty accepting the concept of taking drugs when the immediate benefit is not apparent and discontinuing therapy does not cause acute or discernible disease symptoms.

The idealistic belief of health professionals that health is a right of all citizens leads to the expectation that patients will take advantage of all advice, counsel, and therapy available to them. That unrealistic expectation can lead to overestimation of patient compliance. Evidence that there is need for improving the compliance to drug therapy by unsupervised ambulatory patients is found in the following: one third of patients always take prescribed medications, one third sometimes take them, and one third never take prescribed medications. In the ambulatory setting, the patient is the final decision maker; compliance or noncompliance to a drug therapy program is in the hands of the individual.

Reasons for Noncompliance

In addition to problems related to attitudes about therapy, professionals, and drug taking, individuals may be partial or complete defaulters because of factors in their daily living patterns that contribute to forgetting. Lack of information or confusing directions for taking the drugs may cloud the individual's perception of the importance of the medications to health problem control. It seems natural that the rush of the average household may cause enough confusion in the early-morning hours to cause forgetting, but the problem may be minimized if the individual is highly motivated by clearly understanding the relationship of the drug to health maintenance.

The individual who has inadequate information about the drug and its relationship to resolution of his health problem has a low-level commitment to maintaining therapy. Noncompliance with prescribed drug therapy plans can be viewed in the context of medication errors resulting from *omission, inaccurate knowledge,* or *self-medication* because individuals are taking the drugs incorrectly or not at all. Errors in drug use may occur as the individual omits one or more doses of the drug, takes the drug twice because previous use is forgotten, or doubles the dosage in an attempt to increase the therapeutic effect.

Omission of Drugs

Almost half of the individuals found to be defaulters inadvertently or knowingly omit one or more doses of the drug or voluntarily discontinue therapy before the planned program is completed. Discontinuance of therapy is a common problem. It is estimated that 80 percent of the individuals receiving a prescription for a ten-day course of penicillin for control of streptococcal throat infection stop taking the drug when the pain and swelling subside enough to allow eating and return to life activities. Many individuals will hoard the remaining drug and use it at a future time when a similar infection occurs. In addition to the possible resurgence of the initial streptococcal infection, the self-therapy presents a problem in diagnosis when the individual seeks therapy for a subsequent streptococcal throat infection. The absence of growth in cultures is an enigma when a patient has obvious symptoms unless the individual admits to taking the drug stored from a supply prescribed for a previous infection.

Inaccurate Knowledge

Many factors influence the individual's acquisition of necessary information about the drugs he is expected to take on a regularly scheduled basis. An obvious problem is that busy physicians or personnel in an active clinic situation may give information without sufficient focus on the individual to determine whether the data are received and understood. Patients are hesitant to impose on individuals who are obviously rushing to care for large numbers of patients, and many individuals will show signs of assent and understanding rather than admit they are unable to comprehend. Anxiety, educational limits, and language barriers are among the factors that interfere with reception of instructions.

Many individuals can describe the effect of the drugs on symptoms previously bothering them, but they are unable to describe in realistic terms the effects on the disease process. The implications of the knowledge deficit are clearer when viewing the absence of understanding in relation to an integrated plan for control of a health problem. For example, the individual with congestive heart failure is expected to maintain dietary restrictions for weight and sodium intake control, monitor fluid accumulation, and modify activity to allow rest periods after strenuous activity in addition to taking digitalis and diuretics on a carefully planned schedule. Unless the interrelationship of each component of therapy is clear to the individual, infraction or default in one or more aspects of the plan can occur.

There may be considerable variation in the details of information about the therapeutic plan that make an impression on the patient. For example, individuals receiving oral anticoagulants seem to understand general aspects of drug action and can reiterate the evidence of bleeding they should look for; yet few patients know they should notify the physician of evidence of bleeding before continuing drug therapy. The situation with anticoagulants is unique because most patients do not know the adverse effects of drugs they are receiving.

Termination of Therapy

Individuals who are diagnosed as having a health problem in the course of a routine examination (i.e., hypertension, diabetes) may have difficulty accepting restrictions and drugs required for treatment. When an individual is asymptomatic, it is very difficult to convince him that he must follow a prescribed therapeutic regimen that interferes with established living patterns. For example, a middle-aged woman had a frightening episode of pounding headache after an emotionally traumatic incident and the physician she consulted diagnosed the problem as related to hypertension. An antihypertensive drug and tranquilizer were prescribed. Within two days the woman felt better and discontinued the medications and canceled the appointment for further evaluation.

The same resentment and resistance can occur when an individual with a chronic health problem becomes asymptomatic. Patients often discontinue taking medications, without informing their physician, if an adverse effect occurs. For example, the drugs prescribed for a middle-aged man after recovery from an acute cardiac problem were digitalis, warfarin, phenytoin, aldactone, furosemide, and potassium chloride. He stopped taking aldactone because he had soreness in his breasts, and he discontinued taking furosemide and potassium chloride because he became nauseated. The alteration of the drug therapy plan was made without consulting the physician. The man was admitted to a hospital in cardiogenic shock with acidosis, and he had serious uncontrollable arrhythmias for two days. He discontinued aldactone, furosemide, and potassium chloride and accurately related the adverse effects to the particular drugs capable of causing the problems. His actions indicated insufficient knowledge of the effects of the drugs on his cardiac problem.

Each of the examples illustrates the problem of omission by discontinuation of therapy, but it is difficult to assess how much of each situation was related to incomplete or inaccurate knowledge. Probably each individual received sufficient information about the relationship of drug therapy to the disease process, but emotional, environmental, or personal factors at the time of instruction interfered with reception of the data.

Self-medication

Individuals have a heritage of knowledge about common health problems like the common cold, constipation, and nausea and how to control them with trusted folk remedies or familiar and time-tested medicines. Problems arise when they seek to accelerate recovery or progress by adding such drugs to the medicines prescribed for control of a health problem being treated by a physician. The added drugs may render useless, inhibit, or intensify the action of the prescribed drugs. Individuals with more than one health problem may be treated by two or more physicians, and neglecting to indicate what drugs other physicians are prescribing may lead to overlap in the medication regimen. In addition to the possible medication errors occurring when taking several drugs, overdosage or drug interactions may occur when the individual takes drugs prescribed independently by more than one physician.

IMPROVING COMPLIANCE

Health team members responsible for planning and supervising maintenance of drug therapy can play a vital role in reducing the noncompliance percentage by personalized instruction concerning the relationship of drug action to the patient's health status. In several studies of patients with hypertension, community clinic personnel who provided consistent contact with the same staff and conducted a personalized follow-up by telephoning individuals remiss in keeping appointments reduced the noncompliance rate to 25 percent of their patients.

Therapy Relief

Long-term therapy requires continued involvement of the patient with measures that interfere with life patterns, and the process often causes periods of noncompliance. Short periods of relief from rigid requirements of therapy are sometimes possible, and the "vacation" allows relief of the monotony of continued restrictions. For example, the psychiatrist may allow the patient to take tranquilizers on weekdays and to omit the drugs on the weekend.

Individualized Instruction

Noncompliance is a problem in short-term therapy as well as in long-term therapy of chronic health problems, and it is important that instructions be explicit when any patient is expected to take medications without supervision. Passive patients may ask few questions, and anxious patients or parents of small children may ask numerous questions about therapy outcomes. With all patients, it is important to provide opportunity for clarification of the aspects of therapy that are of concern to them before moving forward to discussion of the prescribed drugs.

Drugs are effective only when they are taken. When the patient is responsible for self-administration of drugs, safety in use in increased if the individual understands the reason the drug is being employed, specific schedules for taking the drug, predictable effects of the drug, and adverse reactions that may occur.

When feasible, the patient should assume full responsibility for the drug therapy plan at home, and specific knowledge about the drugs is a prerequisite for fulfilling that role. Inclusion of a family member in discussion of the drug therapy plan tends to increase the patient's motivation, and it affords an opportunity for clarification of information within the context of normal household activity patterns. It is important to preplan the presentation of data to assure inclusiveness of the information and to provide opportunity during the discussion for clarification of unclear points.

Explanations of the relationship of the drug to the patient's problem should be simplified to fit into the individual's frame of reference and intellectual level. Lists of specific problems may be confusing and frightening to the patient, but careful wording of the presentation and use of realistic examples fitting the individual's experiential reference patterns allow the problems to be discussed in a less threatening manner. The discussion will be meaningful to the patient when adverse reactions are presented with suggestions for immediate or emergency control while emphasizing the reporting of relevant problems to the physician promptly. The approach allows the patient to provide input about measures he previously has found effective for comparable problems and provides opportunity for discussion of the relevance of those practices to the present situation. Recommendations for physician contact have greater meaning to the patient when presented in the context of the probability that the physician will prescribe measures for control of the problem, lower drug dosage, or change the drug to one that does not cause the adverse reaction.

Planning Schedules

Preplanning of schedules for drug use with the patient contributes to the probability that the prescribed dosage will be consistently taken. Specific guides for recording dosage taken are discussed with the patient, and the interchange should include a reminder of the necessity for getting a refill of prescriptions before the supply is depleted to allow continuance of therapy without interruption (Fig. 2–1). The need for specificity in directions is evident in findings indicating that individuals take medications on a regular schedule around the clock when they are prescribed for use every four hours as needed. Detailed planning with the patient may lessen the common problems of dosage omission and the patient's subsequent dosage doubling at a later time to correct the deficit.

Guides for the patient to use should be prepared for resolution of the predictable problems the individual will encounter in scheduling drug taking at home. One patient may manage his plan by simply marking a calendar after taking the drug, while another individual may require sev-

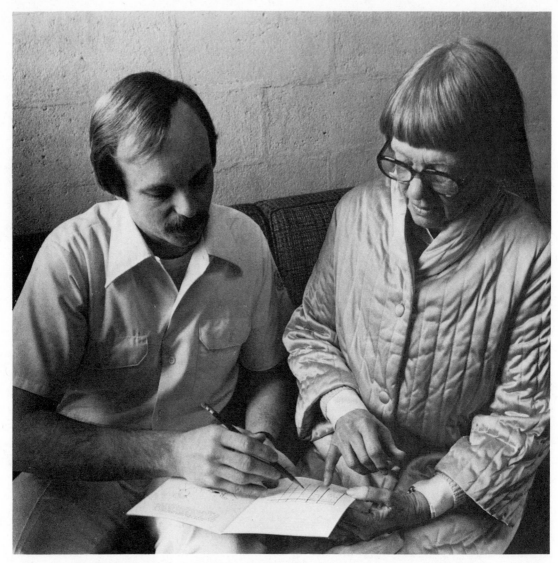

Fig. 2–1. Errors in drug taking may be reduced when the nurse and the patient preplan the schedules for taking the drugs. Specific guides for recording the doses that are taken can assist the patient in maintaining the therapy plan. (Courtesy, Northeastern University College of Nursing, Boston.)

eral mechanisms to maintain the schedule. The latter individual may benefit from a specially constructed calendar format providing time blocks for check-off after each drug is taken. When patients require additional reminders, it often helps to have the schedule correlated with major daily events (i.e., mealtime, bedtime) or to place the container of drugs adjacent to the bathroom sink or on the table so they will remember to take the drug. When the latter suggestion is implemented, it is mandatory that they be cautioned against leaving drugs within the reach of children who may enter the household. Once the importance of reminding mechanisms is discussed, some creative individuals prepare ingenious measures for their personal use.

Specific scheduling directions are important for maintenance of therapeutic plasma levels of many drugs, and patients, parents of young children, or others responsible for administering drugs must comprehend how and when to administer the drug before contact is terminated. For example, when an antibiotic is prescribed for administration every six hours, discussion of the schedule with the parent can minimize disruption of household schedules and provide several hours of undisturbed sleep for the parent and child. It is important also to state straightforwardly that the drug must be taken for the prescribed time period. The point can be reinforced in a meaningful manner by explaining that the exuberance of the child that predictably will occur after a few days of therapy does not justify terminating drug use. Discussion of this period with the parent allows introduction of the concept that the child can feel better although the offending organisms are not completely eradicated.

Follow-up Instruction

Clinic personnel or the visiting nurse in the community has an opportunity to reinforce initial teaching and to implement measures to remotivate or assist the patient with maintenance of the therapeutic program. Many of the patients with chronic health problems are elderly, and they often are being treated concurrently for several health problems. The frustration of maintaining complex schedules for diet and activity modification and having several drugs with varying prescribed schedules contributes to the incidence of medication errors and noncompliance. Written instructions that include a concise statement of drug action, adverse effects, instructions for use, and schedules for taking the drugs provide a ready reference for the individual to use at home.

Follow-up visits to the clinic or office provide opportunity to take a 24-hour medication history, to reinforce previous instruction, and to inquire about progress and problems (Fig. 2–2). Provocative questioning may yield information that otherwise would not surface. Concern is communicated when the focus is on the patient's expectations about the therapeutic plan, his worries, and his need for further clarification or assistance.

Noncompliance Monitoring

Patients frequently are instructed to bring records of drug taking and their medication bottles to the clinic or office when they return for follow-up care. Counting tablets remaining in the bottles should indicate whether omission has occurred, but patients learn to remove "extra" tablets from the containers. The most important aspect of bringing the medications to the office is the opportunity to review knowledge about the schedules, to check that the medications are in the correct containers, and to correct labels when time schedules are changed.

Monitoring of plasma or serum levels may be planned to determine the effectiveness of therapy, and in some instances the same procedures can be employed to monitor compliance with the planned program. Blood levels of drugs (i.e., theophylline, phenytoin, digitalis glycosides) are compared with that status of the patient, and the findings guide dosage regulation. Urine monitoring (i.e., in methadone clinic patients) and analysis of salivary content of drugs, which has an essentially constant ratio with plasma level (i.e., digoxin, lithium carbonate, phenytoin, theophylline), are indirect, noninvasive procedures for monitoring effectiveness of therapy and compliance with therapy. To assure monitoring of drug distribution after absorption, the blood, urine, or saliva sample is obtained 8 to 24 hours after the daily dose has been taken by the individual.

Maintaining Therapy Goals

Potentially serious problems can occur when the individual omits medication, alters the drug

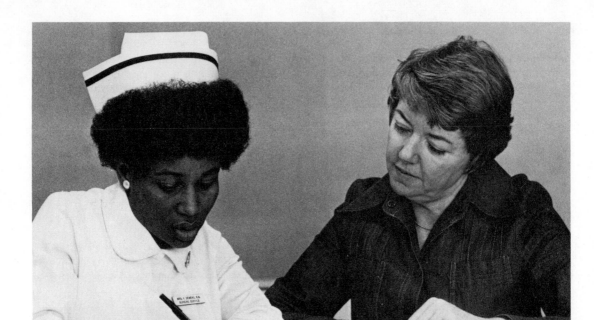

Fig. 2–2. The patient's clinic visit provides an opportunity for the nurse to take a medication history and to reinforce instructions about the therapy plan. (Courtesy, Northeastern University College of Nursing, Boston.)

regimen, or adds to the drug therapy plan by taking nonprescribed drugs. Prevention of medication problems begins with initiation of therapy and continues throughout the period of drug therapy. Consistent patient-centered discussions may lessen the occurrence of problems that have dangerous consequences for the patient or conflict with the goals of therapy.

Additional Readings

Brink, Pamela J.: *Transcultural Nursing: A Book of Readings*. Prentice-Hall, Inc., Englewood Cliffs, N.J., 1976.

Eddy, Lyndall, and Westbrook, Linda: Multidisciplinary retrospective patient care audit. *Am. J. Nurs.*, **75:**961, June, 1975.

Freis, Edward D: *The Modern Management of Hypertension*. Veterans Administration, Washington, D.C., 1973.

Gray, T. Kenny: Endpoints of therapy: a vital concept in surveillance and drug records. *J. Clin. Pharmacol.*, **15:**221, April, 1975.

Gulko, Candace S., and Butherus, Constance: Toward better patient teaching. *Nurses' Drug Alert*, **1:**49, March, 1977.

Joubert, Pieter, and Lasagna, Louis: Patient package inserts II. Toward a rational patient package insert. *Clin. Pharmacol. Ther.*, **18:**663, December, 1975.

Lamy, Peter P., and Vestal, Robert E.: Drug prescribing for the elderly. *Hosp. Pract.*, **11**:111, January, 1976.

Leininger, Madeleine: Cultural diversities of health and nursing care. *Nurs. Clin. North Am.*, **12**:5, March, 1977.

Lima, J.; Nazarian, L.; Charney, E.; and Lahti, C.: Compliance with short-term antimicrobial therapy. *Pediatrics*, **57**:383, March, 1976.

Matthews, Daryl: The noncompliant patient. *Primary Care*, **2**:289, June, 1975.

Orque, Modesta S.: Health care for minority clients. *Nurs. Outlook*, **24**:313, May, 1976.

Parker, William R.: Medication histories. *Am. J. Nurs.*, **76**:1969, December, 1976.

Podell, Richard N., and Gary, Louis R.: Compliance: a problem in medical management. *Am. Fam. Physician*, **13**:74, April, 1976.

Reidenberg, Marcus M.: Patient compliance, patient education and ego defense. *Hosp. Pharmacy*, **10**:168, 1975.

Rosenstock, Irwin M.: Patients' compliance with health regimens. *J.A.M.A.*, **234**:402, October 27, 1975.

Schwartz, Doris: Safe self-medication for elderly outpatients. *Am. J. Nurs.*, **75**:1808, October, 1975.

Shields, Eldonna Marie: Introduction to drug therapy for older adults. *J. Gerontol. Nurs.*, **1**:8, March–April, 1975.

Weiner, Bruce: 10 ways to boost patient compliance with therapy regimens. *Pharmacy Times*, **42**:34, June, 1976.

3

Drug Administration

Drug therapy is a dynamic field that expands as scientific data become available. At the beginning of the twentieth century there were only eight reliable and effective pharmacologic preparations (aspirin, digitalis, diphtheria antitoxin, ether, morphine, quinine, and rabies and smallpox vaccines), and the situation remained stable until World War II when the number of drugs manufactured proliferated rapidly. New drugs, new forms of older drugs, and drug combinations are continually being produced and older drugs are discarded in preference for newer forms. A new drug may be used only five years before it is replaced by another drug that is more effective or safer for treatment of a particular health problem.

Administration of drugs and surveillance of patients' status during this era of polypharmacy require gathering and retention of extensive information about drugs. It is possible only to store detailed data about those drugs commonly encountered. Basic study of drugs provides the baseline knowledge of prototypes that can be expanded as clinical experiences broaden knowledge

about the drugs or other drugs having commonalities with the prototype. A card file or categorized note-taking system facilitates review of data and provides an accurate reference source if the content is updated as new information about drugs becomes available.

In this chapter some of the variables affecting drug administration to patients of differing ages will be presented. Additional data about drug action appear with the presentation of Dosage-Response Relationships (Chapter 5) and Adverse Drug Reactions (Chapter 6) and in discussion of specific drugs in chapters throughout the text.

INFORMATION SOURCES

Drug information systems vary in clinical settings, but all agencies have some references readily available on the units and in their libraries. In hospital settings, a pharmacy committee prepares and periodically updates a formulary that includes the drugs available from the hospital pharmacy and a description of the forms in which it is dispensed within the agency. The individual hospital formulary also includes the usual dosage range for drugs administered by enteral or parenteral routes. The formulary is distributed to each physician on the staff and copies are available for use on the patient units.

Many hospital pharmacy committees also publish drug information bulletins that include descriptions of drugs in common use. Pharmacy staff members are willing consultants and they can provide valuable information about drugs when the data are difficult to find in available reference sources.

Drug Information Publications

There is an increasing trend toward providing a copy of the two-volume publication of the American Society of Hospital Pharmacists, the *American Hospital Formulary Service* (AHFS), on each patient unit. The publication provides a series of monographs describing the drug, pharmacodynamic aspects, contraindications, uses, and dosage. The monographs represent an unbiased and authoritative résumé of data prepared by pharmacists and represents their experiences and analyses of drug studies. The volumes are in loose-leaf format, allowing insertion of quarterly supplements provided by the AHFS for updating information about older drugs or about new drugs released by the FDA for clinical therapy.

The *Physicians' Desk Reference* (PDR), frequently available on patient units, provides information about single drugs or drug combinations prepared by manufacturers. The descriptions are prepared by the drug companies and their product advertisements constitute the text of the one-volume publication. Comparable data prepared by the manufacturers can be found packaged with vials, ampules, and sometimes with capsules dispensed from the pharmacy.

Nurse-Oriented References

Both the AHFS and the PDR are written for use by physicians, and the nurse must supplement the information with data about approaches to patient care during drug therapy. There is a need for expansion of nurse-oriented drug information materials that provide guidelines for assessing drug effect on common physiologic problems. Nursing teams sometimes prepare card files or assemble reference notebooks that include articles about drug action and guides for assessment of patient progress and socioeconomic or legal issues influencing drug usage.

Interest in drugs has led to numerous clinical conferences about drugs. There are often clinical presentations, or grand rounds, which are open to all health team members interested in drug therapy and other aspects of therapeutic plans.

DRUG SOURCES AND FORMS

The drugs prepared by manufacturers in units for convenience of administration are prepared by a variety of methods from the following source materials:

Sources

1. *Active constituents of plants,* which include alkaloids, glycosides, gums, resins, tannins, waxes, volatile or fixed oils.
2. *Animal sources of biologic products,* which include enzymes, bile salts, sera, vaccines, antitoxins, toxoids, hormones.
3. *Minerals,* which include iron, iodine, epsom salts.
4. *Chemicals,* which are the source for most new drugs completely synthesized from basic chemicals and semisynthetic drugs made with chemicals obtained from plants and animals (i.e., steroids).

Forms

1. Solid forms (capsules, tablets, troches).
2. Liquid forms, which include solutions (waters, true solutions, syrups), aqueous suspensions

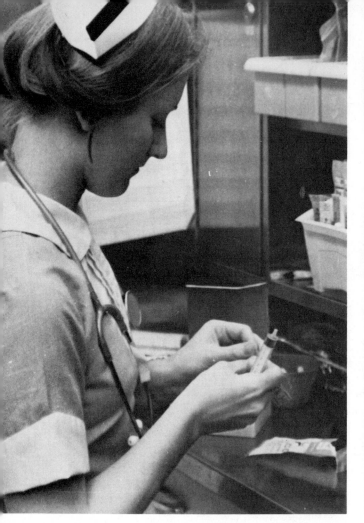
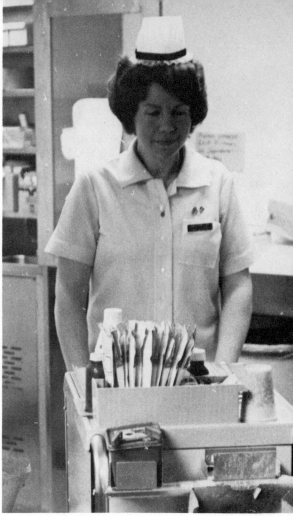

A   B

Fig. 3–1. *A*. The medication storage area contains a variety of drug preparations. The oral or parenteral drugs for each patient may be prepared at a central location. *B*. A mobile medication cart also may be used by the nurse to dispense drugs at the bedside. (*A* and *B* courtesy, Lynn Hospital School of Nursing, Lynn, Massachusetts.)

(mixtures, emulsions, magmas, gels), spirits, elixirs, tinctures, fluidextracts, extracts.

3. Ointments, pastes, lotions, suppositories, powders.

The medication cabinet or closet on a hospital unit contains drugs in a variety of forms for administration to patients (Fig. 3–1). Reserve supplies or stock drugs to be adminstered internally (i.e., capsules, extended-release capsules, tablets, enteric-coated tablets, extended-release tablets, troches, pills, and liquid chemical preparations) are separated from drugs applied topically (i.e.,

liniments, lotions, creams, ointments, pastes). Drugs for parenteral administration (ampules, vials, prefilled cartridges, and intravenous solution bottles) usually are stored apart from the frequently used oral forms of drugs. A small refrigerator is part of the standard equipment because some drugs (i.e., suppositories, insulin, biologic preparations) require cold storage to protect against deterioration.

The modern trend toward a unit dose system provides drugs in dosage-prescribed containers clearly identified as belonging to the individual

Table 3–1.

Common Latin Terms, Abbreviations, and Interpretation

Latin Term	Abbreviation	Meaning
ad libitum	ad lib	freely
alternis horis	alt	every other hour
ana	aa	of each
ante cibum	a.c.	before meals
auris	a	ear
bis in die	b.i.d.	twice a day
capsula	cap.	capsule
cibus	cib./c.	food, meal
compositus	co./comp	compound
cum	$\bar{c}$	with
dies	d.	a day
gramme	gm	gram
granum	gr	grain
gutta	gtt	drop
hora	h.	hour
hora somni	h.s.	just before sleep
ibidem	ibid.	in the same place
injectio	inj.	an injection
jentaculum	jentac.	breakfast
minimum	m.	a mimum
nocte	noct.	at night
oculo dextro	O.D.	in the right eye
oculo sinistro	O.S.	in the left eye
oculo utro	O.U.	in each eye
omni hora	omn. hor.	every hour
per os	p.o.	by mouth
post cibum	p.c.	after meals
prandium	prand.	dinner
pro re nata	p.r.n.	as occasion arises
quantum sufficiat	q.s.	a sufficient quantity
quaque	qq.	each or every
quaque die	qd	every day (once/day)
quaque six hora	q6h	every six hours
quater in die	q.i.d.	four times a day
semissem	ss.	one-half
signa	Sig.	write, label
sine	$\bar{s}$	without
si opus sit	s.o.s.	if needed
statim	stat	immediately
sume	sum.	take
ter in die	t.i.d.	three times a day
unguentum	ung.	ointment

patient. There is a separate container for each patient on the unit. The modern system gradually is replacing bulk storage of drugs on hospital units.

DRUG PRESCRIPTIONS

In the hospital setting, the only drugs the patient receives are those prescribed by the physician. The directions for the individual's drug therapy are usually included in the overall prescription for therapy found in a "Doctor's Order Book" or on sheets bearing the same designation and found in the individual's clinical record. All prescriptions must include the patient's full name, date written, name and dosage of the drug, and the method and frequency of administration above the signature of the prescribing physician. The same data are included on the individual prescription form that patients receive in clinics or private settings for filling at a local pharmacy. Symbols derived from Latin words are used in prescribing drugs, and the common terms appear in Table 3–1.

The nurse is legally responsible for accuracy in administration of prescribed drugs; therefore, the prescription must be inclusive. When aspects of the prescription are unclear or absent, the physician is contacted for clarification or additional details. Nurses, or specifically trained staff members, may transcribe prescriptions to a graphic guide for drug adminstration, which becomes the frame of reference for those preparing medications for the patient. Checking the transcribed listing against the original prescription assures accuracy when preparing the patient's medications from the listing. The precaution is an added protection that the traditional directive for administering drugs is followed: give the right medication to the right patient at the right time in the right dose and by the right route using the right technique (Fig. 3–2).

DOSAGE EQUIVALENTS

The metric system for measurement is used almost universally. The United States has adopted the metric system and gradually is moving toward implementation of the system common to all other nations. The metric system is based on the decimal system and has for its units the *gram* (weight), *liter* (volume), and *meter* (linear). Prefixes are used to designate subdivisions or

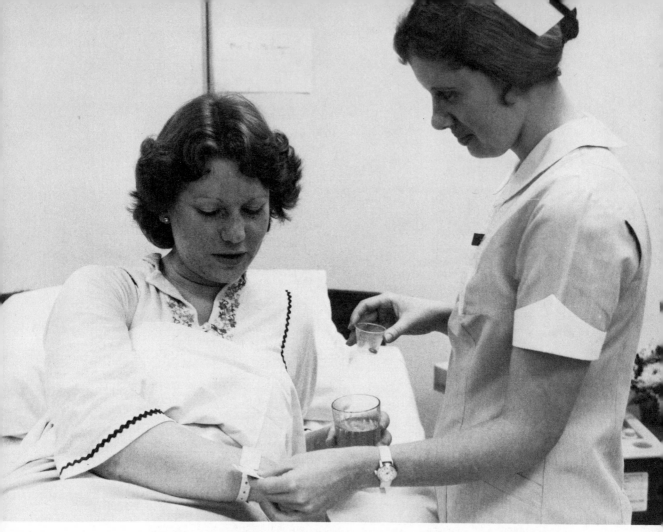

Fig. 3–2. Safe practice in the administration of medications includes identification of the patient before administration of the drug. The interaction also provides an opportunity for the patient to identify the drug and to discuss its action with the nurse. (Courtesy, Niagara College of Applied Arts and Technology, The Mack Centre of Nursing Education, Welland, Ontario.)

multiples of the units of the metric system. For example:

Designation			Factor	
1 kilogram (kg)	=	10^3	1000	gm
1 hectogram (hg)	=	10^2	100	gm
1 dekagram (dg)	=	10^1	10	gm
1 gram (gm)	=		1	gm
1 decigram (dg)	=	10^{-1}	0.1	gm
1 centigram (cg)	=	10^{-2}	0.01	gm
1 milligram (mg)	=	10^{-3}	0.001	gm

Metric System Conversions

Drugs are generally prescribed and dispensed in dosage representing the metric system, but there are instances where physicians educated under the apothecary system use those gradations in dosage designation. Conversion to the metric system can be accomplished readily by using the major gradations of the apothecary system shown in Table 3–2. Round figures are used to define approximate equivalents in translating dosages from one system to the other.

Table 3–2.
Metric Doses with Approximate Apothecary Equivalents

Weights	
Metric	Approximate Apothecary Equivalent
30 gram	1 ounce
1 gram	15 grains
60 milligrams	1 grain
Liquids	
Metric	Approximate Apothecary Equivalent
1000 milliliter	1 quart
500 milliliter	1 pint
30 milliliter	1 fluidounce
4 milliliter	1 fluid drachm
1 milliliter*	15 minims

* A cubic centimeter (cc) is the approximate equivalent of a milliliter (ml).

Conversions in the Home

Household equivalents are sometimes required when describing dosage to patients, but care must be taken to encourage use of standard measuring devices. A measuring teaspoon holds 5 ml of liquid, but a teaspoon used for meal service may hold from 4 to 7 ml. Calibrated droppers or 30-ml-sized glass or disposable measuring cups may be obtained at pharmacies when measuring devices are not available to the individual.

Linear Conversions

Additional conversions may be required until conversion to the metric system is completed. For example, metric measurements are referred to in medical literature, and it may be necessary to convert to the familiar measurement by inches to visualize the description. There are approximately 2.5 cm in 1 in., and 39.37 in. equal 1 meter.

Weight Conversions

Conversion may be required also when drugs are described as a given amount per kilogram of body weight. Most scales currently employed for weighing patients use the pound unit. Because there are 2.2 kg/pound, the conversion can be made by dividing the weight in pounds by 2.2.

Temperature Scale Conversions

In many clinical settings body temperature is defined by the Celsius scale in contrast to the former use of Fahrenheit calibration. In the interval until the change is accepted by the general population and thermometers are available only in Celsius scales, it is possible to convert from one scale to the other by using the formula

$$(°\text{Fahrenheit}) - 32 = 1.8 \ (°\text{Celsius})$$

DOSAGE CALCULATION

After the prescription and the planned dosage schedule are verified, locating the drug allows preliminary determination of the quantity of capsules, tablets, or liquid that will be required to provide the presecribed dose. Parenteral drug administration often requires calculation of fractional dosage. It is expected that the calculation of a divided dosage done by one nurse will be checked by another nurse before the drug is administered (Fig. 3–3).

In pediatric settings it often is necessary to calculate divided dosage. Concern with safety in preparation of drugs (i.e., insulin, digitalis, narcotics) has led to establishment of criteria that are consistently followed by nurses preparing drugs. When fractional dosages are required, both the calculation of the dosage and the amount of drug actually prepared for administration are checked by a second nurse before the drug is given to a child.

Oral drugs come in a variety of dosages, and it is seldom necessary to divide a tablet to attain the prescribed amount of drug for administration. Calculation of dosage may be required when a liquid oral dosage form is substituted for a solid form. For example, the patient receiving phenytoin capsules providing 300 mg of drug will be given phenytoin suspension if a nasogastric tube is inserted. The suspension is available in 125 mg/5 ml. The patient will require 12 ml of phenytoin suspension to provide the 300 mg of phenytoin that was given in the oral capsules.

Dosages differ between forms of the same drug prepared for administration by oral and parenteral routes and the drugs are not generally inter-

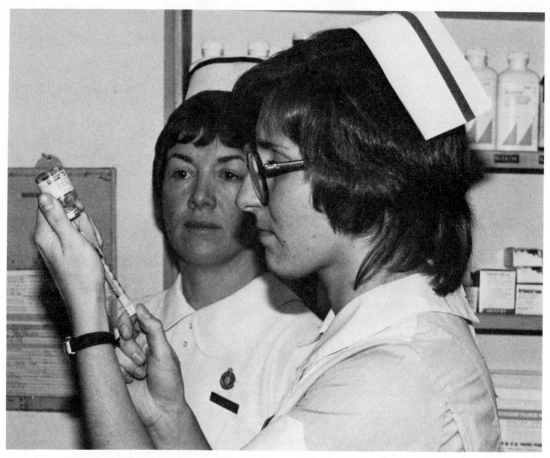

Fig. 3–3. The calculation and preparation of divided dosages are checked by a second nurse during preparation of parenteral drugs. That practice is followed by nurses to protect against medication errors. (Courtesy, Saint Catharines General Hospital, Ontario.)

changeable. Bioequivalence may be different between dosage forms of a drug (i.e., oral tablet and oral liquid) even though they are given by the same route. Unless the bioequivalence of the products is known, it is necessary to consult with the pharmacist prior to calculating the dosage of an alternate form of the drug.

PREPARING THE DRUG

Nursing departments in hospitals prepare and periodically revise detailed procedures for admin-

istration of medications using the methods established for general use on all units. Medication errors are reported and the situations are meticulously analyzed in an attempt to find measures to avert the problem. Most errors represent neglect of one or more aspects of safe procedure.

The practice of reading labels three times (when removing the drug from the medicine cabinet shelf, before removing the required dosage from the container, and before replacing the drug on the shelf) is a precautionary measure planned to prevent medication error (Fig. 3–4). It is dif-

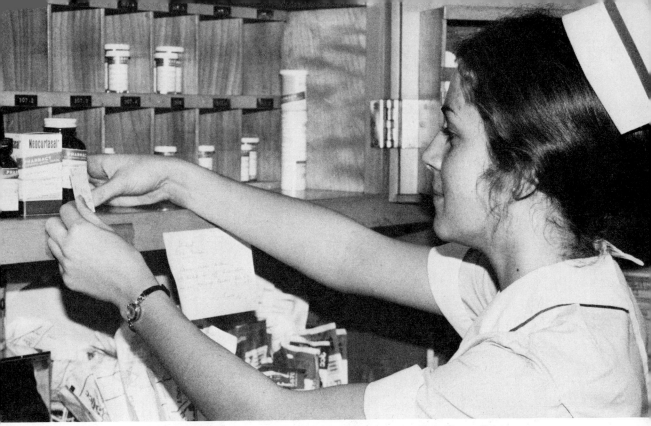

Fig. 3–4. Safe practice in the preparation of a patient's drugs includes reading the label before removing the drug from the storage area, before removing the required dosage from the container, and before replacing the drug on the storage shelf. (Courtesy, Saint Catharines General Hospital, Ontario.)

ficult to retain a focus on the procedure without being distracted by the activities of a busy unit, but interruptions cause enough disruption of function to allow errors to occur.

Care in preparation of accurate dosage is essential when drugs are administered by all routes. An emetic, a lavage, or an antidote may be administered to lessen adverse reactions by slowing drug absorption from the stomach or intestine when an individual receives an incorrect drug dosage by the oral route. Absorption and distribution of a drug administered into tissues in an extremity can be delayed when an adverse reaction occurs by using ice to cause venous constriction or by applying a tourniquet above the injection site. Intravenous administration disseminates the drug throughout the body, and attempts to slow or halt circulating drug action require the use of parenteral drugs that neutralize or inactivate the drug before it becomes sequestered in tissues. The

foregoing procedures are frightening and uncomfortable for the patient, and prevention of error by attention to details protects the individual from unnecessary trauma.

Cleanliness, caution, and concentration are important elements in the medication procedure. Medicines need not be touched if solid forms are moved from the bottle to the inverted cap and then to the cup that will be carried to the patient's bedside (Fig. 3–5). In addition to protecting the patient's tablet or capsule from contact with skin oils and contamination by skin bacteria, the practice allows return of extra tablets to the storage supply bottle in an unchanged state.

Crushed tablets or the contents of capsules may be sprinkled on puréed fruit to facilitate administration to children or adults who have difficulty swallowing solid forms of drugs. Care must be taken to assure that the patient takes all of the prepared formulation to assure that the prescribed

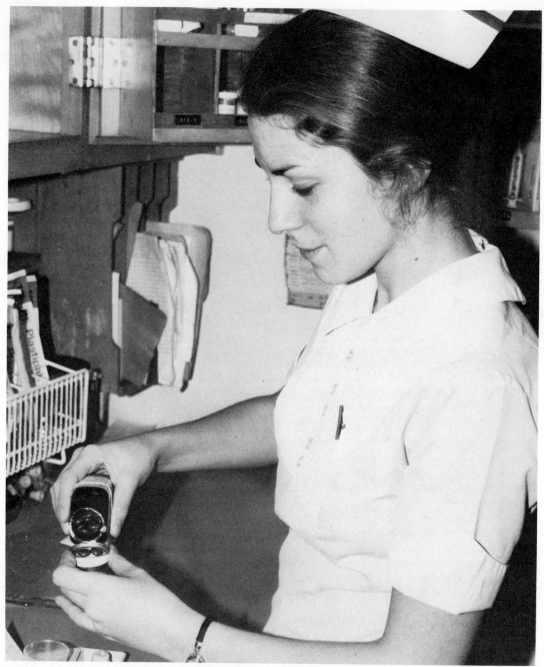

Fig. 3–5. Dropping the tablets into the bottlecap during the measurement process allows the return of extra tablets to the bottle because they are uncontaminated by contact with the nurse's hands or equipment in the environment. (Courtesy, Saint Catharines General Hospital, Ontario.)

amount of drug is ingested. It is advisable to mix the drug in a small amount of fruit and provide additional unaltered puréed fruit after the drug preparation is taken.

Many drugs are available in liquid forms (solutions, syrups, elixirs, emulsions) that facilitate administration to children and adults who have difficulty swallowing solid forms. Liquid forms also increase the probability that the drug will be swallowed rather than sequestered in the cheek pouch by patients who resist taking medication.

When suspensions are utilized, the bottle must be shaken vigorously to assure that the drug content of the suspension is evenly distributed in the bottle. Proper agitation of the suspension assures that the first patient to receive a prescribed amount of drug receives the same dosage as the last patient when the amount of suspension administered from the container is the same. Oral suspensions (i.e., emulsions, magmas, gels) are not refrigerated because cold storage causes aggregation of molecules and retards absorption.

Competence Requirements

Safety in administration begins with the initial receipt of the prescription and continues through each step of the preparation procedure to the time when the drug is administered to the patient (Fig. 3–6). In addition to the expectation that the nurse will follow safe practices in preparing the drug, the nurse also is legally responsible for using discretion in drug administration. Legal requirements for competence in nursing intervention necessitate assessment of the patient's status before administering the drug to ascertain that *the prescribed dosage is within the safe range for the individual; the patient's physiologic or emotional status indicates that the drug is required; coexisting physiologic problems or concurrent therapies do not contraindicate administration of the drug to the patient; records of drug administration and patient responses are maintained.*

ORAL DRUG ADMINISTRATION

Most of the drugs given orally are intended for intestinal (enteral) absorption, but tablets, solu-

tions, or powders may be given orally for effect on, or absorption by, mucous membranes. The patient requires instructions to assure appropriate use of tablets for sublingual dissolution, solutions for gargles or mouth rinses, or powders for insufflation.

Oral Membrane Absorption

Administration of tablets into the mouth for absorption by sublingual or buccal tissues bypasses the dissolution-absorption barriers affecting drug availability from the gastrointestinal tract. The oral, or percutaneous, route allows absorption of tablets by lipid membranes and provides a noninvasive method of administering drugs (i.e., progesterone) that would be destroyed by proteolytic enzymes in the gastrointestinal tract. The drugs are rapidly absorbed and they travel with venous blood to target sites without passing through hepatic biotransformation sites.

Gastrointestinal Factors

Ease of administration makes pills, tablets, or capsules the most desirable forms for systemic use, but local factors in the stomach or intestine affect dissolution or absorption of oral drugs. Alternate routes must be employed for hormones and other protein drugs because gastric acidity and proteolytic enzyme action in the stomach and intestine alter protein compounds, and the intestinal mucoprotein barrier to absorption decreases drug transport across membranes of the digestive tract.

Gastric Irritation. Administration of drugs with food or an antacid may decrease gastric irritation, but its effect on dissolution or absorption of some drugs must be considered. The patient's complaints of indigestion or nausea may be the first indicators of gastric irritation. Persistent nausea or vomiting may be controlled by antiemetics, and timing of their administration to precede drug administration may allow continuance of drug therapy. When patients vomit after

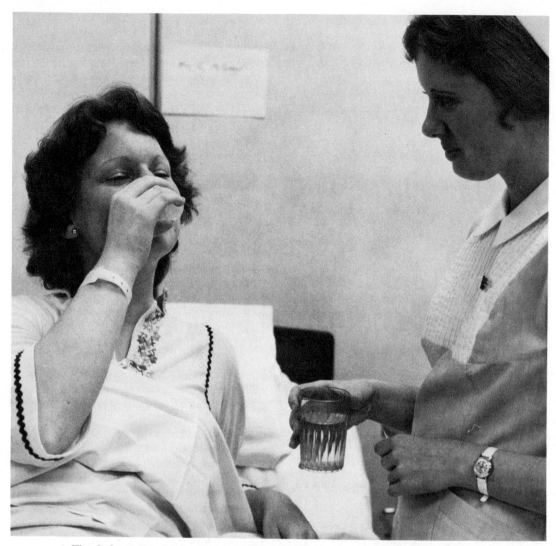

Fig. 3–6.   Safety in drug administration includes remaining with the patient until the drug is ingested. The use of fluids after the tablets assures their travel to the stomach. (Courtesy, Niagara College of Applied Arts and Technology, The Mack Centre of Nursing Education, Welland, Ontario.)

taking drugs, the vomitus should be examined for drug content and the time lapse between drug administration and emesis should be reported to the physician. The practice allows consideration of replacement of lost drug when maintenance of plasma concentrations is essential for control of the patient's health problem. Alternate routes may be required for administration of drugs when nausea or vomiting is persistent. Conversely, parenteral administration may be discontinued in favor of oral administration when the patient's status improves.

Enteric-Coated Tablets. Many drugs are irritating to the gastric mucosa, and nausea or vomiting may occur during therapy. Some drugs are available in forms that lessen gastric irritation by preventing drug liberation in the stomach. Enteric-coated tablets (E.C.T.) have an acid-resistant casing that remains intact until the tablet reaches the alkaline content of the intestine. Patients should be told not to chew or crush the tablets because it destroys the protective coating and drug is liberated in the stomach. Aspirin is an example of a drug available in an enteric-coated form, and it is available also with an antacid, or buffer, and in suppository form. Enteric dissolution of enteric coating varies in individuals and the feces should be examined after the first four or five doses to ascertain that intact tablets are not being excreted.

Select Contraindications. In select situations the composition of a drug contraindicates its use for specific patient problems. Syrups (i.e., cough syrups) provide glucose and the carbohydrate content must be considered when patients with diabetes mellitus receive serial doses of the drug. Drugs with a high sodium content (i.e., sodium bicarbonate, sodium penicillin) are contraindicated for patients on sodium intake restriction, and alternate drugs or drug forms (i.e., potassium penicillin) are usually prescribed. It is necessary also to consider the alcohol content of elixirs, tinctures, or fluidextracts before administering drugs to the patient who is an alcoholic on voluntary maintenance therapy for control of the problem. Although most alcoholics taking disulfiram for abstinence therapy will refuse alcohol-containing fluids, inadvertent administration can precipitate the same symptoms occurring when the patient drinks an alcoholic beverage: violent vomiting and circulatory collapse.

PARENTERAL DRUG ADMINISTRATION

Drugs may be given by the subcutaneous (SC), intramuscular (IM), or intravenous (IV) routes. The decision of the physician to prescribe a particular injection method for administration of the drug is based on the status of the patient, rapidity of action desired, and the effect of the chemical preparation on tissues. Many drugs that are available in forms for oral administration are manufactured in forms that are employed for parenteral injection when the patient is unable to take drugs by mouth.

Delayed Absorption Preparations

Drug diluents may contain retardants added to lengthen the time span for release of the drug component of the preparation from depot sites. Delayed absorption decreases the need for frequent injections while assuring the availability of circulating drug at therapeutic concentrations. For example, the action span of regular insulin injection is six hours, but addition of protamine and zinc to the insulin injection preparation increases the therapeutic action time of the hormone to 36 hours. An increase in therapeutic action time to approximately 18 hours occurs when globin zinc is added to insulin injection.

Colloids, oils, metals, and vasoconstrictors are additives that retard absorption of intramuscular solutions, or a local anesthetic may be added to decrease pain at the injection site. The additives limit use of the preparations to intramuscular injection, and a form without additives would be used for intravenous administration. The package inserts supplied by the manufacturers and the labels on drug vials provide useful information about solvents, dilution, routes of administration, and incompatibility with other drugs and product additives.

Tissue Mass Assessment

Drug absorption from the injection site is dependent on arterial circulation to the site and venous circulation from the area. When examination of the tissues reveals that there is insufficient mass or that the tissues are edematous, alternate sites must be used for injections. The dorsogluteal muscle is most frequently employed for intramuscular injections; it is important to review anatomic landmarks (i.e., routes of nerves, arteries, and veins) when less familiar sites are selected for injections. The poorly developed gluteus muscles in infants and the proximity of the sciatic nerve to the usual injection point make it necessary to use alternate sites for administration of drug into their muscle tissues. The anterior or lateral thigh is usualy employed when injecting drug into muscle tissues of children under two years old. These sites have sufficient muscle mass and the limb can be restrained more securely during administration.

Site Alternation

Alternation of administration sites lessens the patient's discomfort and lessens tissue trauma when frequent subcutaneous or intramuscular injections are necessary. Although patients feel the discomfort in areas frequently injected, they are not a reliable source of information about the particular site that was used for a previous injection. Preparation of a graphic form that allows checking off the site when drug is administered provides a reference source for each nurse giving injections to the patient. Placement of the graphic form at the patient's bedside assures that it is available when positioning the patient for the injection.

Patient Involvement

The patient may remain a passive recipient and can be protected from viewing the equipment employed when injections are being given for short time periods. The individual who is to assume responsibility for self-administration is gradually introduced to steps involved in the procedure of medication injection and allowed supervised practice to assure safe practices in injecting the drug.

Subcutaneous Administration

The subcutaneous tissues are employed for administration of small volumes of drugs (less than 2 ml) that are highly soluble and nonirritating to tissues. The needle must pass through epidermis and dermis to reach subcutaneous adipose tissue.

Drug Injection. Thin patients may have insufficient subcutaneous tissue on the arms to allow injections, and alternate injection sites should be employed. Subcutaneous tissues may be reached by using a small-bore needle (i.e., 26 gauge) and inserting one that is 1/2 in. in length at an angle of 90 degrees or one that is 5/8 in. long at a 45-degree angle into a cushion of tissue held between the thumb and forefinger (Fig. 3–7). When heparin is administered, a hematoma may result from massage of the tissues, but gentle massage following injection of most other drugs distributes the solution and consequently capillary absorption is facilitated.

Site Alternation. Subcutaneous injections can be rotated between sites on the right and left anterior thighs, the right and left buttocks, the right and left lower abdomen, and the right and left arms when frequent injections are required by the patient. The patient is instructed to use a similar rotation pattern when being taught to administer subcutaneous drugs (i.e., insulin).

Intramuscular Administration

Drugs injected into intramuscular tissues are absorbed fairly rapidly, and solutions that are potentially irritating or painful can be tolerated better by muscle tissues than by subcutaneous tissues. The maximum amount of drug injected into the gluteal muscle mass is 5 ml because larger quantities of fluid cause stretching and distortion at the site occupied by the drug, and abscess formation or scarring can occur. The maximum amount of solution injected into small muscles is 3 ml. Tissue trauma consequent to frequent intramuscular injections may elevate serum creatinine phosphokinase (CPK) levels.

Muscle Mass Assessment. The length of the needle or the depth of insertion depends on the tissue mass of the individual. Muscle layers are readily accessible in lean patients, but obese patients have quantities of adipose tissue between the surface tissues and muscle layers. A longer needle is required to reach the muscle tissue in

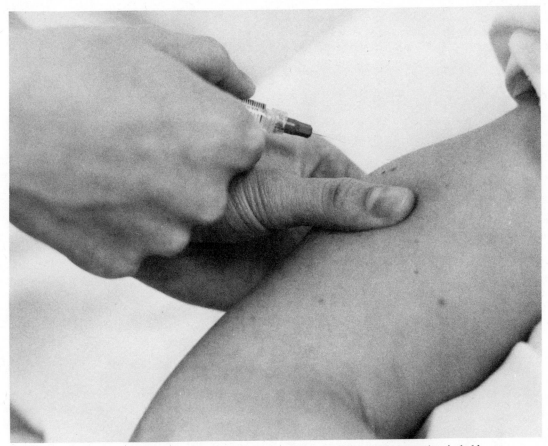

Fig. 3–7. The subcutaneous injection is made into a cushion of tissue that is held between the thumb and the forefinger. The use of an alcohol sponge to gently massage the site after the injection increases absorption of the drug. (Courtesy, Niagara College of Applied Arts and Technology, The Mack Centre of Nursing Education, Welland, Ontario.)

obese patients, otherwise the injection is administered subcutaneously rather than intramuscularly. In addition to muscle mass, peripheral circulation should be evaluated when preparing to administer drugs into the muscles of the thigh. Elderly patients often have some deterioration of the thigh muscles, and their common problems with both arterial and venous circulation in the lower extremities may make it necessary to avoid those sites in an injection rotation plan.

Muscle Relaxation. The patient's discomfort and tissue trauma are lessened by positioning him to improve relaxation of the muscle to be injected. When the muscle is tense, there is resistance to needle insertion, and tissue trauma and stimulation of nerve endings along the injection tract cause pain or discomfort. Positioning contributes to the relaxation of muscle. For example, the gluteus maximus relaxes when the femur is internally rotated, and asking the patient to lie

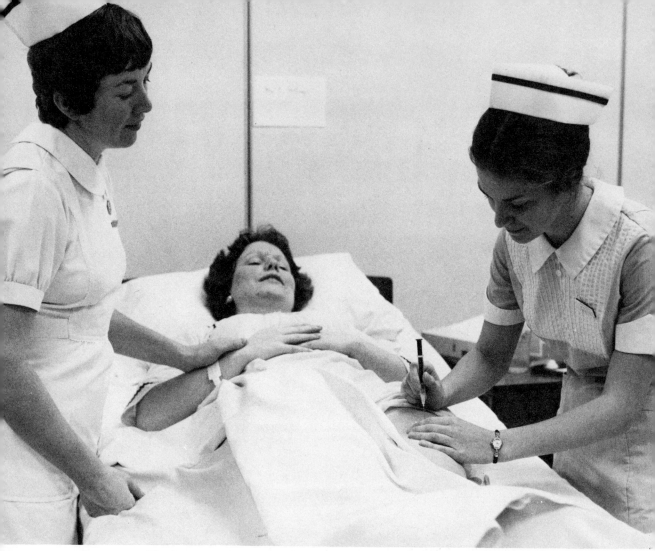

Fig. 3–8. The intramuscular injection is given after the patient has been positioned to relax the muscle. After cleansing of the skin, the skin is held taut and the injection is made with a forward thrust into the musculature. (Courtesy, Niagara College of Applied Arts and Technology, The Mack Centre of Nursing Education, Welland, Ontario.)

prone with the feet pointed inward provides the relaxation required for injection into the dorsogluteal site. It is sometimes useful to involve the patient in distracting activity (i.e., breathing deeply, wiggling the toes) when the anxiety level is high.

Drug Injection. Careful preplanning can allow the drug to be injected before the individual has time to become highly anxious about the in-

jection. After the injection site is located, the skin is cleaned, and with the tissues held taut, the needle is held close to the skin surface and inserted with one forward thrust (Fig. 3–8). During aspiration and administration of the drug, the needle must remain steady in the site to prevent tissue trauma. Releasing traction on tissues after removal of the needle seals the injection tract and consequently drug does not seep back to irritate tissues along the tract.

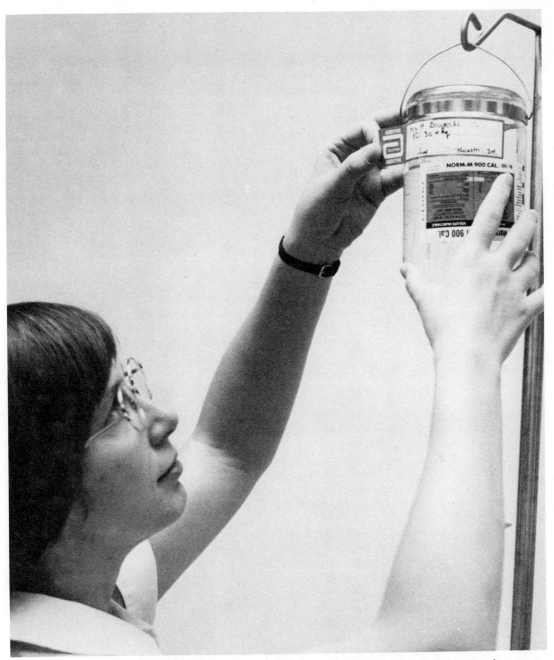

Fig. 3–9. A label is placed on the intravenous solution bottle after the drug is added. The label clearly identifies the drug that was added. The amount of the drug, the time, and the initials of the nurse who made the addition are written on the label. (Courtesy, Niagara College of Applied Arts and Technology, The Mack Centre of Nursing Education, Welland, Ontario.)

Some drugs are especially irritating to tissues (i.e., chlorpromazine), and drug adhering to the outside of the needle after aspiration of the drug from an ampule or vial can irritate the injection tract tissues. Wiping the needle with a sterile gauze pad or placing a new needle on the syringe after the drug is withdrawn from the ampule or vial lessens irritation of tissues when the injection is administered.

Site Alternation. Intramuscular injections may be rotated between the right and left anterior lateral thighs, the right and left buttocks, and the right and left deltoid muscles when the patient is receiving frequent intramuscular injections. The deltoid muscles are the least preferred sites, and they are included only when multiple injections at frequent intervals are required by the individual.

Intravenous Administration

The intravenous route frequently is employed for administration of drugs to acutely ill patients, and it is the route required for therapeutic effect of some drugs. Drug effects generally are immediate because the solution travels rapidly with circulating blood to tissue sites throughout the body.

Many different solutions are used for intravenous therapy, but drugs are added only to isotonic saline or to 5 percent dextrose in water. The reason for caution in selection of the fluid vehicle for administration is that complex electrolyte solutions increase the hazard of incompatibilities. Extensive guides are prepared by pharmacy committees in clinical agencies to provide a ready reference for preparation of drugs for intravenous administration. Minimum and maximum dilutions and known incompatibilities are described on the package inserts supplied by manufacturers with most of the drugs administered intravenously. Most hospitals have specialists, or IV nurses, who assume responsibility for preparing drug solutions and inserting the needle into the vein. Their expertise in venipuncture lessens vein trauma and increases the probability that mixtures of intravenous solution are compatible.

A drug label is attached to the bottle at the time the drug is added to the solution. The label contains the name of the drug and the time and date of reconstitution (Fig. 3–9).

Maintaining Sterility. Since intravenous solutions contain sufficient nutrients to support bacterial growth, aseptic practices are important when the continuity of a running IV is interrupted for the addition of drugs (Fig. 3–10). Ideally, intravenous bottles would be opened only in an aseptic environment, but in reality they are opened for addition of drugs in a clean area apart from the patient's room where airborne organisms are in abundance. There is a trend toward preparation of intravenous solutions with additives in hospital pharmacies where sterile procedures can be consistently followed.

Monitoring During IV Therapy. The nurse attending the patient throughout the period when the intravenous is in place is responsible for monitoring the flow rate and the integrity and patency of the system and vein into which the fluid is flowing (Fig. 3–11). The site of injection is examined periodically for evidence of tissue fluid and tenderness. The patient's complaints of discomfort may provide a clue that the drug is irritating the intima of the vein; slowing of the solution flow rate may relieve the problem. Continued discomfort may necessitate administration of a more dilute solution or removal of the needle from the irritated site.

There is usually a routine for changing the intravenous needle or catheter (i.e., every three days), and the specific schedule is based on attempts to prevent phlebitis. When the needle is inserted, the date and time are written on the tape with a ballpoint pen as a reminder, when the scheduled time period has elapsed, that the needle should be removed.

Bolus Drug Administration. Intravenously administered drug is diluted in the circulating blood, and the rate of infusion is calculated to allow hemodilution and to deliver adequate amounts of the drug to target sites for therapeutic effect.

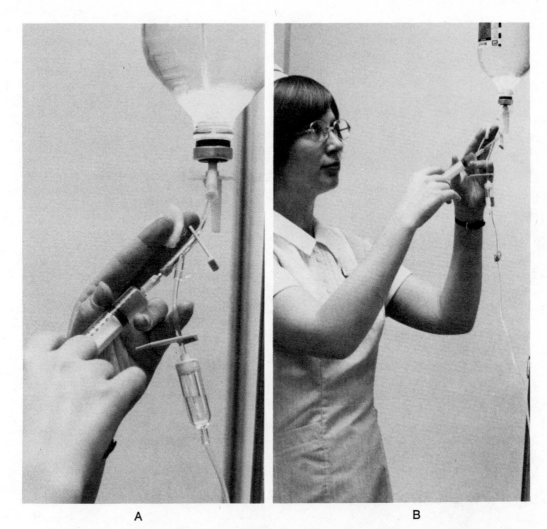

A   B

Fig. 3–10. *A*. The additive connector on the intravenous tubing makes it possible to maintain sterility during the introduction of medication into the tubing of a running intravenous solution. The rubber diaphragm is cleansed with an alcohol sponge before the needle is inserted. *B*. The mixing of the drug with the total intravenous solution is observed during the slow injection of the additive. (Courtesy, Niagara College of Applied Arts and Technology, The Mack Centre of Nursing Education, Welland, Ontario.)

When intravenous drugs are given in a large single dose, or bolus, the process is described as an "IV push." Bolus drug injection provides rapid distribution to tissues and attainment of effective drug levels. The minimum time required for hemodilution of drugs is one minute, and administration time for a bolus of drug must be slow enough to allow drug dilution in circulating fluids. Rapid administration may cause adverse effects related to properties of the drug.

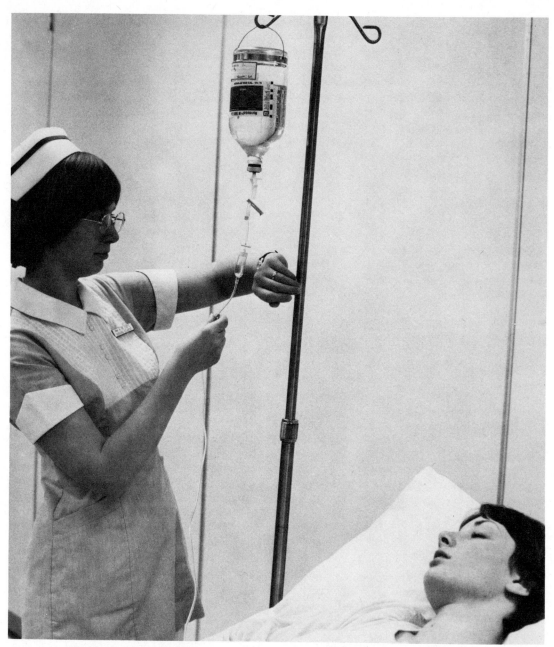

Fig. 3–11. The nurse who is caring for the patient is responsible for periodically monitoring the rate of the intravenous flow and for maintaining it at the precalculated rate for infusion of the solution. (Courtesy, Niagara College of Applied Arts and Technology, The Mack Centre of Nursing Education, Welland, Ontario.)

Titrating Fluid Flow Rate. Some of the drugs that are administered by intravenous infusion are regulated, or titrated, against the planned physiologic response occurring consequent to administration. Use of a minidrip flow chamber (60 drops/ml) allows fine control of the amount of drug being administered. Placement of a second set of clamps on the tubing provides additional protection against inadvertent rapid infusion of the drug. Graphic records of the amount of drug being administered and tabulation of the physiologic responses are useful to team members responsible for modification of the intravenous flow rate.

Titration of intravenous infusion is dependent on calculation of the dilution of the drug and the rate of flow. For example, when 1 mg of epinephrine hydrochloride is diluted in 250 ml of solution and the minidrip equipment dispenses 60 drops/ml, there will be 1000 mcg in 15,000 drops, or 1 mcg in 15 drops. At an infusion rate of 15 drops/minute, the patient will be receiving 1 mcg/minute. Planned periods for recording exact drug dosage and changes in physiologic status (i.e., blood pressure, heart rate) provide evidence of drug effect on the target tissues and allow maintenance of circulating drug levels at the safe therapeutic range. Rapid calculation of the amount being delivered is time consuming in an acute care situation, and it is helpful if a conversion guide is placed with the graphic guide used to monitor drug administration (Table 3–3).

TOPICAL ADMINISTRATION

Drugs containing ointments, lotions, creams, or solutions may be applied for local treatment of superficial tissues (i.e., skin, mucous membranes, eyes), and a few pastes (i.e., digoxin paste, nitroglycerin paste) are applied for slow absorption and sustained therapeutic effect. Characteristics of the medication or of the tissues may allow drug absorption into the capillary bed and consequent distribution in the circulation.

Repeated applications of drugs that are intended for topical effect but are absorbed to a significant degree may raise plasma concentrations sufficiently to cause adverse drug reactions (i.e., side effects, toxic effects, allergic reactions, or sensitization). For example, gamma benzene hexachloride (KWELL) is frequently applied to the scalp of children with pediculosis. The drug is a chlorinated hydrocarbon with lethal effects on nits and adult tinea capitis, and a single treatment may eliminate the parasites. When repeated treatment is required, a four-to-five-day time lapse is recommended because the drug can be absorbed through the superficial tissues. Absorption and distribution occurring with frequent or copious application without shampooing can raise circulating drug levels and produce neurotoxic effects (i.e., convulsions). Whenever drugs are applied topically, it is important to ascertain the absorption potential and the characteristics of the tissues at the site of application (i.e., highly vascular, inflamed) that may accelerate absorption.

ADMINISTERING DRUGS TO CHILDREN

Concurrent with societal changes that moved adult patients from passive recipients of therapy to active participants in planning and implementing

Table 3–3.

Guide for Conversion of Drops to Drug Dosage

Drug Solution: 1 mg epinephrine hydrochloride in 250 ml isotonic sodium chloride solution.*

Drops/minute		Drug/minute
15 gtts	=	1 mcg/minute
14 gtts	=	0.93 mcg/minute
13 gtts	=	0.87 mcg/minute
12 gtts	=	0.8 mcg/minute
11 gtts	=	0.73 mcg/minute
10 gtts	=	0.67 mcg/minute
9 gtts	=	0.6 mcg/minute
8 gtts	=	0.53 mcg/minute
7 gtts	=	0.47 mcg/minute
6 gtts	=	0.4 mcg/minute
5 gtts	=	0.33 mcg/minute
4 gtts	=	0.27 mcg/minute
3 gtts	=	0.2 mcg/minute
2 gtts	=	0.13 mcg/minute
1 gtts	=	0.07 mcg/minute

* Microdrip (60 gtts/ml).

their therapy regimen, children have been gradually changed from rebellious recipients of drugs to decision makers in planning drug therapy. It may be necessary to place a liquid formulation in the mouth of an infant and use a measure encouraging swallowing (i.e., gently massaging the nose or throat), but most children accept medication better when they are allowed choice based on individual preferences.

Base Lines for Assessment

Nursing intervention is directed at decreasing the psychologic and physiologic trauma of drug taking. Knowledge of development stages facilitates assessment of the developmental tasks that have been accomplished by the child, and individualized plans can be made after compilation of the data. Parents can supply information, and the examples of behavioral responses, attitudes, and general disposition are invaluable guides in planning measures for the child's care.

Time spent in playing with the child or providing physical care allows opportunity to determine responses to the environment and allows the child to establish a relationship with the nurse. The situation is an active process in which each is observing the other for indicators of acceptance. It is important to recognize that children are highly intuitive and "read" responses to their behavior as accepting or rejecting with a fairly high degree of accuracy.

Individual Preferences

When alternatives can be offered in the procedure for taking drugs (i.e., taking a soft drink after a liquid or tablet), the child can be encouraged to select favored ways to make the process easier. The reasoning ability of the child affects the level of decision making, and there are usually aspects of drug taking that are open to modification to meet the child's suggestions. The aspect not open to change, taking the medication, is stated forthrightly as a task the child must accomplish. Honest statements, and discussion based

on the child's level of understanding, should include accurate descriptions of drug administration.

Oral Drug Palatability

Oral drugs may be given in the form of flavored liquids or tablets crushed and disguised by placing the drug in puréed fruit. Tasting the mixture can assure that it is palatable, because the child may acquire an aversion to the puréed fruit or other substance used to disguise the drug. Milk should never be used as a vehicle for administration of drugs. A straw is required when administering liquid iron preparations, to prevent staining of teeth, but drinking other liquid medications through a straw is fun for most children.

Whenever possible, the taking of drugs should be kept to a brief experience in the child's day. It may be possible to administer medicines to the child involved in play or watching TV cartoons with minimal interruption in concentration and prompt return to the activity.

Parenteral Drug Administration

Injections hurt! This fact should not be minimized and injections should not be described as less uncomfortable for the recipient than is realistic. Supervised injections into a doll or other object may help the child work through the basic fear about unknown aspects of the injection. Protective restraint may be required, and the child may be helped to view even that traumatic procedure by discussion, in terms he can understand, of the need for injecting the drug safely. After an episode of resistive behavior or crying, the child will perceive continued love and acceptance if he is assured that he did the best he could, and the situation then is set aside in preference for more pleasurable activities.

It is upsetting to the parents of an infant to view an intravenous being administered into a scalp vein of their child. They can accept the situation better if they are informed about the need for the intravenous drug before they approach the nursery.

Pediatric nurses find that intravenous drug infusions are tolerated better by children when the bottle is screened from their view while remaining within the line of vision of nurses in the area. Nurses have reported a lower incidence of nausea during anticancer drug therapy when the children are protected from the continual visual reminder that the solution is running.

ADMINISTERING DRUGS TO ELDERLY PATIENTS

The normal aging process causes changes in many body systems, and elderly patients often have multiple diseases necessitating use of several drugs. It is estimated that the elderly consume one fourth of all drugs used by the general population. Problems occurring consequent to the polypharmacy of geriatric patients are evident when viewing the fact that 90 percent of the elderly experience adverse reactions to drugs.

Biologic aging influences physiologic responses to drugs. Dissolution and absorption of oral drugs may be adversely affected by decreased motility of the esophagus, stomach, and intestines and decreased production of saliva and digestive enzymes; the biotransformation of drugs may be slowed by decreased activity of hepatic enzymes; excretion of drugs may be lessened by the 50 percent reduction in blood flow through the kidneys and the decreased renal tubule function common in elderly patients. The complex physiologic changes have a negative effect on drug availability and they also increase the probability that drug cumulation will occur.

Diminished Reserves

The elderly have a lower reserve capacity in organ systems and ability to adapt to stress is lessened. More time is required for equilibrium of the cardiovascular system after activity, and the pulse and blood pressure remain elevated longer than they would in younger people. Administration of some drugs (i.e., digitalis, antihypertensives) requires taking the pulse or blood pressure prior to giving the drug; the reading will be falsely high if the individual has just completed a strenuous activity (i.e., a difficult bowel movement).

Stressor Tolerance

Abnormalities in elderly patients also occur as a consequence of the stress induced by intensive therapy. For example, an 85-year-old woman was receiving maximum dosage of an antiarrhythmic drug intravenously for control of an abnormal heart rhythm, and she was on a cardiac monitor. The arrhythmia rate increased, but the physician removed the intravenous, detached the monitor leads, and prescribed rest. There was a prompt decrease in the abnormal heart rhythm as the stressful situation was eliminated.

The unfamiliar, often bustling activity of a hospital unit can cause psychologic recession in elderly during illness, and the demands placed on the patient by complex tasks or routines slow action and reaction speed. The procedure of administrating medications may be time consuming, but the individual should be allowed time to take the drug without being pressured to rush and without being fed the drug. Sitting at the bedside communicates that the nurse has time to remain until the drug is taken and allows opportunity to provide gentle reminders that there is a task to be accomplished, taking the medication. Edentulous patients or those with ill-fitting dentures have difficulty swallowing tablets. Use of liquid forms or crushing tablets and mixing with puréed fruit makes swallowing easier.

Base Line Assessment

It is important to evaluate the status of the individual elderly patient and to obtain information from family and friends about preillness abilities and limitations before relating all problems to the aging process. There is considerable variability in abilities, and nursing intervention should be planned on the basis of assessment of the individual. Base-line data about the patient provide a guide to assessment of adverse effects that otherwise might be considered as deterioration. For example, cumulation of sedatives may cause persistent drowsiness, and only comparison with the pretreatment status will provide clues indicating that the problem is related to the drug rather than to decreased central nervous system activity consequent to the aging process.

Additional Readings

Geolot, Denise H., and McKinney, Nancy P.: Administering parenteral drugs. *Am. J. Nurs.*, **75**:788, May, 1975.

Lamy, Peter P., and Vestal, Robert E.: Drug prescribing for the elderly. *Hosp. Pract.*, **11**:111, January, 1976.

Lang, Susan Havens; Zawacki, Ann M.; and Johnson, Jean J.: Reducing discomfort from I.M. injections. *Am. J. Nurs.*, **76**:800, May, 1976.

Ormond, Elizabeth A. R., and Caulfield, Colleen: A practical guide to giving oral medications to young children. *Am. J. Maternal Child Nurs.*, **1**:320, September/October, 1976.

Ungvarski, Peter J.: Parenteral therapy. *Am. J. Nurs.*, **76**:1974, December, 1976.

Vidt, Donald G.: Use and abuse of intravenous solutions. *J. A. M. A.*, **232**:533, May 5, 1975.

4

Drug Safety, Efficacy, and Distribution Controls

LEGAL REGULATON OF DRUG DISTRIBUTION

Widely publicized information about the withdrawal of some commonly used food additives and drugs from the market has increased public consciousness of the surveillance activities of the federal Food and Drug Administration (FDA) of the Department of Health Education and Welfare. The first federal legislation regulating the quality of medicines was enacted by passage of the Pure Food and Drug Act of 1906. The legislation that provides the authority for present FDA action is the federal Food, Drug, and Cosmetic Act, enacted in 1938. One of the premises of the statute was that drug trials be conducted in animals to determine toxicity before the product could be marketed. The Drug Amendments of 1962 (Kefauver-Harris Act) empowered the FDA to regulate procedures for testing drugs in humans. Congress presently is considering legislation (i.e., Drug Regulation Reform Act of 1978) that will decrease the time required for initial investigative studies and thereby shorten the time required for release of a new drug.

The aim of legislation is protection of the pub-
lic against fraudulent claims about drug action and to provide for the enforcement of standards for drug manufacture and distribution. The statutes require that the FDA obtain substantial evidence that drugs approved by the agency for marketing are safe, effective for the purposes claimed, and properly packaged and labeled. Substantial evidence has been interpreted as adequate and well-controlled investigations, including clinical investigations, by experts qualified to evaluate the effectiveness the drug is purported to have under the conditions of use recommended on the labels and in the advertisements.

Legal requirement of substantial objective scientific evidence before the release of the drug for marketing is the basis of the stringent FDA criteria for conducting trials in animals to determine the toxicity and efficacy and for presenting all available data at the time that the manufacturer submits an Investigational New Drug (IND) application to the FDA for approval of clinical trials in humans. At the termination of the trials when the manufacturer files a New Drug Application (NDA), all data from the animal and human studies are submitted to the FDA. Experts examine reports of the study methodology and the data obtained from clinical trials. Data must show safety, therapeutic effectiveness, and a low incidence of adverse effects before the drug is released for marketing.

CLINICAL DRUG TRIALS

Drug trials are a frequent occurrence in clinical settings as health professionals seek to improve patient care. Studies are conducted to validate the safety, action, and efficacy of new drugs or drugs that have been prescribed on an .empiric basis over many years, or they may be planned to evaluate new uses for a drug previously employed to control another unrelated health problem. Each planned clinical study has a clearly defined protocol including statements of the purpose, scope of the study, and the problems described as *intercurrent medical events,* which constitute criteria for removal of the patients from the study sample.

Study Phases

Human drug studies are conducted in three phases. *Phase I trials* are conducted after the safe and effective levels of the drug are determined from trials in animals. The sample population is given the drug at a low dosage level, which is gradually increased to that producing an optimal therapeutic effect. Surveillance measures are planned for assessing the status of the patient at frequent intervals during the clinical trial period. When the study data reveal that the drug is safe and effective for humans with a particular medical problem, the scope of the trials is expanded to include more individuals. In *phase II trials* the drug is compared for safety and efficacy with other drugs commonly employed for control of the particular health problem that is the planned therapeutic goal for the study drug. *Phase III trials* may be regional or interagency studies to assure the inclusion of large numbers of individuals with the problem being studied. In phase III studies, the drug is evaluated for an acceptable low incidence of adverse effects by tabulation of their occurrence in the large sample population.

Study Format

Each patient who is invited to participate in the study is informed of the purpose of the trials, and their inclusion in the study is planned when written consent has been obtained. An essential element in consent is that the patient has been sufficiently informed of any inherent risks to allow the consent decision to be made intelligently.

Specifically identified research staff retain control of the investigational drug in the clinical setting where the study is conducted. Patients who have consented to participate in the trials are assigned by random placement to either a treated group, which receives the drug, or a control group, which receives a placebo or inactive compound in the form of a tablet or liquid similar in physical appearance to the study drug. To assure the objectivity and reliability of the data obtained from the study, a double-blind approach is commonly employed. Neither researchers, health team members, nor patients know whether the particular tablet or liquid is the drug or the placebo. The pharmacist maintains the master code and prepares the drug for each of the patients in the study population. Labels of drug bottles or vials are marked with coded numbers rather than drug names and the directions for administration to both the treated and control groups are comparable. The code assignment is "broken" only when complications, or intercurrent medical events, necessitate that the patient be removed from the study sample; otherwise the code remains secure until the trial is completed.

Administration of Study Drugs

Members of the research team may assume the responsibility for administration of the study drug and for monitoring changes in the patient's status during the study period. Under those circumstances, it is the responsibility of the nurse to report to the research team any changes occurring between observation periods. When the nurse is the drug administrator, the legal requirement for informed participation applies: the nurse must know the safe dosage range, action, adverse effects, and expected therapeutic outcome for the drug. A written or verbal summary of the study and a description of the drug can be obtained from the physician who is designated as responsible for the clinical study.

Ongoing Drug Evaluation

Surveillance of patients in the study population produces copious amounts of data related to the drug action and the adverse drug reactions, and the FDA release of the drug for marketing depends on the reports of the studies. The drug is released for treatment of the problem studied in the clinical trials, and use of the drug for control of a different problem requires additional clinical trials.

Clinical drug trials represent the continuing search for drugs that are safe and effective in control of health problems and have minimal disruptive effects on noninvolved body systems. The clinical trials provide base-line information that is expanded each time the drug is employed after it is released by the FDA. Widespread use of the drug provides a very large sample population, and previously unrecognized problems of allergic or adverse responses may be identified in the expanded population. Each time a health team member identifies and records an observation of a drug effect or an adverse effect on the individual's clinical record, the information provides additional data about responses to the drug (Fig. 4–1). The increasing use of computers for tabulating problems and observations should provide retrievable data that can be used in the future to identify patterns and configurations in a patient's responses to particular drugs.

As the most consistently available observers, nurses can make a meaningful contribution to drug research. Whenever a patient is receiving a drug, the nurse's observations of the drug effect are important in evaluation of the progress of the drug regimen. A high level of objectivity and astute patient assessment are particularly important during clinical drug trials because data obtained from the study sample may lead to the availability of a drug that can control one of the many frustrating health problems occurring in the general population.

DRUG NOMENCLATURE

The 1962 Drug Amendments to the federal Food, Drug, and Cosmetic Act required that each drug have only one established nonproprietary name. In 1964 the United States Adopted Names (USAN) Council was organized to select appropriate nonproprietary names for drugs. The USAN Council is sponsored by the American Medical Association, the United States Pharmacopeial Convention, Inc., and the American Pharmaceutical Association. A member of the FDA sits on the Council.

A new drug that is developed in a pharmaceutical laboratory has an identification number and a name designating the chemical composition. The drug manufacturer and the USAN Council negotiate for a nonproprietary name during the premarket phase of drug testing when the manufacturer files an application for an Investigational New Drug with the FDA. A nonproprietary name is assigned to the drug before it is released by the FDA for clinical use. The manufacturer selects and registers a unique trade, or proprietary, name for the product that is prepared in its laboratories, and a similar nonproprietary drug may be produced by several drug companies under different trade names. At the time of general clinical availability, a drug has a chemical name (which is seldom referred to in clinical practice), a nonproprietary name, and one or more trade names. Although the word *generic* would, by definition of the term, refer to the origin or chemical composition of a drug, common usage has led to the interchange of *generic* for *nonproprietary* when referring to the name of a drug.

Nonproprietary names coined by the USAN Council are similar for the groups of drugs that are related both chemically and pharmacologically. Use of an identifying stem, which often appears as a suffix within the name, helps to link the drug to its chemical relatives and gives some hint to the pharmacologic properties. For example, thiazide is the identifying suffix in the names

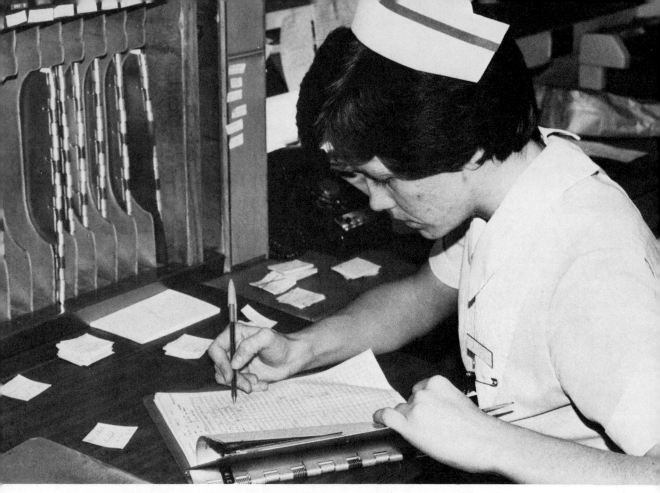

Fig. 4–1. Recording the administration of the drug in the patient's clinical record is a standard part of the drug administration procedure. The nurse's comments about the patient's progress and the effects of the drugs are essential in the evaluation of the drug therapy plan. The data also contribute to long-range drug research. (Courtesy, Saint Catharines General Hospital, Ontario.)

of a large group of diuretics (i.e., benzthiazide, chlorothiazide, flumethiazide, polythiazide) that are similar chemically and generally act at common sites in the nephron.

The Council selects names that combine usefulness and simplicity in addition to being adequately distinctive to prevent confusion among drugs in the same series. Other than the identifying stem, the name distinguishes the particular drug, and the nonstem portion is an identifying characteristic without relevance to how it differs from others within the particular drug grouping. In some instances, the complex older names of drugs have been changed (i.e., diphenylhydantoin was renamed phenytoin), and the newer designa-

tion usually retains sufficient resemblance to the former name to allow identification by professionals who have been familiar with the older name for many years.

The Council recommends new names to the FDA, and when approved the official name appears in the Federal Register. When the drug is released for clinical use for a specific therapeutic purpose, the name appears in subsequent revisions of the *United States Pharmacopeia* (USP) or the *National Formulary* (NF).

Physicians employ both nonproprietary and proprietary names when prescribing drugs, but in clinic and hospital settings the nonproprietary name is generally employed when prescribing. In clinical agencies, drugs are purchased from manufacturers on a competitive cost basis, and the drugs are dispensed from the pharmacy to meet the prescription requirements for a drug described by either its nonproprietary or proprietary name. Because of the similarity in the sound or the appearance of the complex nonproprietary names of drugs, it is important to check the names carefully before administering a drug to assure that the correct drug is given to the patient. Although the drug language is difficult, use of the terminology provides a common frame of reference and facilitates understanding of drugs as relatives of others within groupings having a similar mode of action.

OFFICIAL DRUG STANDARDS

National and international publications provide official standards for the compounding and therapeutic use of drugs. The drug compendia provide data about the drug source, properties, purity assay, storage, efficacy in therapy, administration, and dosage range. In the United States the official compendia are the *United States Pharmacopeia* (USP), which provides standards for single drugs, and the *National Formulary* (NF), which provides standards for drug compounds. Drug manufacturers or pharmacists compounding the drugs are required to conform to the official standards for the drugs, which are based on the chemical or bioassay of content.

The *Pharmacopoeia Internationalis* (PhI), prepared by a committee of the World Health Organization, has been translated into many languages. The published standards can be adopted by any country as its authority, but many countries publish a separate national compendium. The international publication has provided guidelines that gradually are unifying the drug standards in national pharmacopeias. A liberal exchange occurs between the national official groups and the international committee. For example, the USAN Council submits projected new names to the committee for critical review in an attempt to avoid duplication in names selected for drugs prepared in the United States.

Some countries employ more than one official

publication in defining standards for the drugs utilized within the country. For example, the *British Pharmacopoeia* (BP) provides standards for the drugs manufactured or compounded by the pharmacists in Canada, but the USP or NF is employed as the reference source for criteria about those drugs imported from the United States.

FDA Controls

The law places under FDA control any drug employed for the treatment of disease or intended to affect the structure or function of the body. Drugs must conform with the standards of potency established by chemical or biologic assay, which require that a specified amount of the drug elicit a specific response. The FDA conducts periodic tests of marketed drugs, and those found to be subpotent, impure, or ineffective are removed from the market. For example, studies of serum drug levels indicated that there was a wide variation in the bioavailability of digoxin from oral tablets. Products manufactured by different companies included fillers and additives that influenced the dissolution rate and the amount of drug absorbed from the intestine. The FDA action in response to the problem was based on concern that the low dissolution rates decreased the therapeutic effectiveness and that the high dissolution rates increased the hazard of toxic effects in individuals taking the products from different manufacturers at the same recommended dosage. In 1974 the FDA established a certification program involving the use of the USP digoxin dissolution rate standard (55 to 95 percent dissolution in one hour) for testing each batch of digoxin before it is marketed. The standards necessitated the reformulation of 7 to 8 percent of the digoxin products previously marketed. A similar certification program, which was established for oral digitoxin in 1977, affected approximately 50 percent of the marketed digitoxin products.

Regulations for labeling drug containers require that the printed information specify the ingredients, accepted therapeutic use, and warnings about situations in which the drug may be hazardous to health. When preparations contain a narcotic, hypnotic agent, or habit forming substances, or any derivative with similar properties, the label must include a warning that the drug may be habit forming. Descriptive literature must clearly identify the diseases or conditions in which use of the drug is contraindicated. Regulations also require that disclaimers be included for those situations that have not been studied to determine safety or efficacy (i.e., dosages for children; use in pregnancy).

There are legal requirements for the packaging of drugs to prevent accidental ingestion of hazardous substances by children. Regulations provide the criteria for varying types of unit packaging, which require manual maneuvers to release more than one dose and child-resistant safety caps on all oral prescription drugs and compounds containing aspirin. Nitroglycerin can be dispensed in its original, sealed packet because individuals with angina pectoris require the drug for emergency use. Conventional packaging can be requested by the consumer when opening of the safety container presents a problem for the individual.

NARCOTIC REGULATIONS

Federal, state, and local laws control the distribution and sale of narcotics. Although state and federal laws are generally similar, each state has its own controlled-substances laws. Whichever law (state or federal) is more stringent supersedes the other. Variations between state laws make it necessary to be informed about the regulations in the state in which one is practicing. Drug traffic in the United States is controlled primarily by federal regulations. Standards of purity and the regulation of sales and dispensing of opium and coca leaves originated with the enactment of the *Harrison Narcotic Act of 1914*. In addition to internal controls, the United States has a number of treaties that control international production and distribution of narcotics.

Comprehensive Drug Abuse Prevention and Control Act of 1970 replaced all previous federal legislation controlling narcotics and other dangerous drugs. The specific intent of the law *is to provide increased research into, and prevention of, drug abuse and drug dependence; to provide for treatment and rehabilitation of drug abusers and drug-dependent persons; and to strengthen existing law enforcement authority in the field of drug abuse.* The statute assigns responsibility for annual updating of controlled substances to the secretary of the Department of Health, Education, and Welfare. Broad statutory responsibility for the surveillance and control of traffic in drugs was delegated to the *Drug Enforcement Administration* (DEA) of the Department of Justice when that agency was established in 1973. The DEA resulted from a merger of the Bureau of Narcotics and Dangerous Drugs, Office for Drug Abuse Law Enforcement, Office of National Narcotic Intelligence, those elements of the Bureau of Customs that had drug investigative responsibilities, and those functions of the Office of Science and Technology that were related to drug enforcement.

Controlled Substances

The law provides guidelines for designation of a drug as a controlled substance. The criteria stated in the statute for placement of a drug in one of the five schedules of controlled substances are:

Schedule I

(A) The drug or other substance has a high potential for abuse.

(B) The drug or other substance has no currently accepted medical use in treatment in the United States.

(C) There is a lack of accepted safety for use of the drug or other substance under medical supervision.

Examples:

Acetorphine	Lysergide (LSD)
Bufotenine	Marihuana
Diacetylmorphine (heroin)	Mescaline
	Peyote
Dimethyltryptamine (DMT)	Tetrahydrocannabinols (THC)
Ketobemidone	

Schedule II

(A) The drug or other substance has a high potential for abuse.

(B) The drug or other substance has a currently accepted medical use in treatment in the United States or a currently accepted medical use with severe restrictions.

(C) Abuse of the drug or other substances may lead to severe psychologic or physical dependence.

Examples:

Narcotic

Anileridine	Meperidine
Cocaine	Methadone
Codeine	Morphine
Diprenorphine	Opium
Etorphine	Oxymorphone
hydrochloride	Piminodine
Hydromorpohone	

Nonnarcotic

Amobarbital	Amphetamine
Methaqualone	Dextroamphetamine
Pentobarbital	Methamphetamine
Secobarbital	

Schedule III

(A) The drug or other substance has a potential for abuse less than the drugs or other substances in schedules I and II.

(B) The drug or other substance has a currently accepted medical use in treatment in the United States.

(C) Abuse of the drug or other substance may lead to moderate or low physical dependence or high psychologic dependence.

Examples:

Narcotic

Hydrocodone
Paregoric

Narcotic-Containing Compounds or Mixtures

ASA compound with codeine
Empirin compound with codeine
Hycodan
Phenaphen with codeine
Tylenol with codeine

Nonnarcotic

Aprobarbital	Chlorhexidol
Butabarbital	Glutethimide
Methyprylon	

Schedule IV

(A) The drug or other substance has a low potential for abuse relative to the drugs or other substances in schedule III.

(B) The drug or other substance has a currently accepted medical use in treatment in the United States.

(C) Abuse of the drug or other substance may lead to limited physical dependence or psychologic dependence relative to the drugs or other substances in schedule III.

Examples:

Barbital	Mephobarbital
Chloral betaine	Meprobamate
Chloral hydrate	Methohexital
Ethchlorvynol	Paraldehyde
Ethinamate	Phenobarbital
	Propoxyphene

Schedule V

(A) The drug or other substance has a low potential for abuse relative to the drugs or other substances in schedule IV.

(B) The drug or other substance has a currently accepted medical use in treatment in the United States.

(C) Abuse of the drug or other substance may lead to limited physical dependence or psychologic dependence relative to the drugs or other substances in schedule IV.

Examples:

Narcotic-Containing Compounds or Mixtures

Cheracol with codeine	Lomotil
Elixir terpin hydrate	Robitussin-AC
with codeine	

The law requires that physicians or other dispensers of drugs be registered with the DEA. Regulations for prescription writing by physicians, dentists, veterinarians, and selected designated registered practitioners require that the prescription be dated and that it bear the full name and address of the patient and the name, address, and registration number of the practitioner.

A prescription for a drug in schedule II cannot be refilled, and the written prescription must be presented to the pharmacist within five days of the date of issue if it is to be filled. Some states limit the quantity that can be prescribed and dispensed to a 30-day supply of the drug.

Prescriptions for drugs in schedules III and IV may be refilled (if so authorized by the prescribing practitioner) up to five times. Filling or refilling of a prescription is limited to a six-month period as determined by the date on which the prescription was written. A record of refills is maintained on the reverse side of the prescription, and the data include the date, amount of drug dispensed, and the initials of the pharmacist.

Drugs in schedule V are essentially codeine-containing cough syrups that may be dispensed when a prescription is presented. In some states schedule V drugs may be sold over the counter by the pharmacist. Over-the-counter sales may require the signature of the purchaser.

Any agent holding controlled substances (i.e., a clinical nursing unit) provided by the registered dispenser (i.e., the hospital pharmacist) is charged with the responsibility for maintaining security measures to protect against illicit distribution of the drugs. The drugs are kept in a locked cabinet and access is controlled by the designation of authorized individuals who are allowed to obtain the key.

Controlled Substance Records

Record keeping in clinical settings provides a detailed description of narcotic distribution to patients. Nurses record the amount of the drug in the container before removal of the prescribed dose, time and the amount of the drug removed for administration, name of the patient receiving the drug, and amount of drug remaining in the container after removal of the dosage. When the narcotic supplies are checked at the end of each tour of duty, any discrepancies are brought to the attention of the staff on duty during the previous time period, and they are required to account for the missing drug. It often happens that the drug was administered to a patient by a nurse who failed to record the removal of the drug dose from the supply in the cabinet.

Close monitoring of all controlled substances by nurses assures that the distribution of drugs provided by the registered dispenser is carefully controlled in the clinical setting. Replacement of narcotic supplies by the pharmacists is dependent on submitting an accurate record for the drug previously dispensed to the clinical unit.

Additional Readings

Azarnoff, Daniel L.; Abrams, William B.; Cuttner, Janet; Hervitt, William L.; and Hailman, Harold F.: Panel 3: phase III investigations. *Clin. Pharmacol. Ther.,* **18:**650, November, 1975.

Blackwell, Barry; Stolley, Paul D.; Buncher, Ralph; Klimt, Christian R.; Temple, Robert; Venn, Dorian; and Wardell, William M.: Panel 4: phase IV investigations. *Clin. Pharmacol. Ther.,* **18:**653, November, 1975.

Byar, David P.; Simon, Richard M.; Friedewald, William T.; Schlesselman, James J.; DeMets, David L.; Ellenberg, Jonas H.; Gail, Mitchell H.; and Ware, James J.: Randomized clinical trials. *N. Engl. J. Med.,* **295:**74, July 8, 1976.

Crout, J. Richard: Clinical trials of drugs from the viewpoint of the food and drug administration. *Clin. Pharmacol. Ther.,* **18:**634, November, 1975.

Fink, Joseph L., III: Interdisciplinary health care. *Am. J. Pharm.,* **147:**45, March–April, 1975.

Goldberg, Leon I.; Besselaar, G. Hein; Arnold, John D.; Lemberger, Louis; Mitchell, Jerry R.; and Whitsett, Thomas L.: Panel I: phase I investigations. *Clin. Pharmacol. Ther.,* **18:**643, November, 1975.

Hollister, Leo E.; Martz, Bill L.; Carr, Edward A.; Cohn, Howard D.; Crout, J. Richard; and Levine, Jerome: Panel 2: phase II investigations. *Clin. Pharmacol. Ther.*, **18:**647, November, 1975.

Jerome, Joseph B., and Sagan, Pamela: The USAN nomenclature system. *J.A.M.A.,* **232:**294, April 21, 1975.

Jick, Hershel: The discovery of drug-induced illness. *N. Engl. J. Med.,* **296:**481, March 3, 1977.

5

Dosage-Response Relationships

The amount of drug prescribed is based on an established range for dosage and is intended to maintain an adequate drug level for treatment of the patient's problem. Drug dosage is prescribed at varying levels within the established range. The dosage for a particular patient may be at or above the minimum dosage level, or it may be at or below the maximum dosage level of the therapeutic range. When there are pathophysiologic changes that affect the rate of drug metabolism or excretion, the dosage may be below or above the usual range. Acute treatment of a life-threatening situation may necessitate use of a dosage that exceeds the usual limits of minimal effective to maximal levels. The minimum and maximum dosage levels represent the safe dosage range. When drugs are prescribed at levels above that range, careful consideration is given to the risk to benefit factors in the individual situation.

Therapeutic Index

The therapeutic index (TI) is based on the dosage of a drug that is lethal in 50 percent of animals tested (LD50), and the dosage required to produce a specified intensity of effect in 50 percent of humans tested (ED50). The therapeutic index is obtained by the following formula:

$$TI = \frac{LD50}{ED50}$$

Lethal dose-response curves are plotted during studies of drug effect in animals. Both human and animal studies provide the data for plotting the therapeutic dose-response curves. For example, studies have shown that the commonly prescribed preoperative drug, *atropine sulfate* 0.6 mg, has a therapeutic effect by blocking the activity of the parasympathetic nervous system. The drug action lessens secretions and produces a desirable decrease in motility of the gastrointestinal tract. At a dosage range of 2 to 6 mg, atropine sulfate produces adverse, or toxic, reactions manifested as skin flushing, rapid pulse and respiration rate, restlessness, hallucinations, and disorientation. Animal studies showed the LD50 to be about 10 mg. The TI of atropine sulfate is approximately 16, which is sufficiently high to allow safe administration. Although adverse effects may occur at three to ten times the 0.6-mg dosage level, it is estimated that 16 times that dosage can cause death. When studies show that a drug has a TI below 2.0, the risk is considered too grave for the use of the drug in humans.

Surveillance Plans. Many drugs have a high therapeutic index and concern about adverse drug reactions and lethal effects with those drugs is negligible. Administration of drugs with a low therapeutic index, however, requires continual monitoring and close supervision of the dosage and the patient's response to the drug. For example, antineoplastic drugs have a low therapeutic index, and the patient may receive a high dosage of the drugs while in the hospital. Surveillance plans include closely spaced observations and laboratory tests to monitor the effects of the drugs on the normal susceptible body tissues as well as on the rapidly proliferating cancer tissue. The surveillance plan allows careful analysis of the risk to benefit effects of the drugs.

The therapeutic index and the severity of adverse effects are guides for the physician in the selection of an appropriate drug and its dosage for the patient's particular problem. The amount of drug required to produce an effect or an adverse reaction varies with the individual and the method of administration; therefore, careful observation of the patient is necessary at initiation of drug therapy and at regularly scheduled intervals during therapy.

Patient Instruction. The patient who is to assume responsibility for taking drugs with a low therapeutic index at home (i.e., antiarrhythmics, anticoagulants, antineoplastics, digitalis glycosides, insulin, oral hypoglycemics) needs specific instructions about the disease process and the method of taking the drug; guides for monitoring drug effect; instruction about problems to be reported to the physician; and appointments for regularly scheduled follow-up evaluation of therapy. The patient, or a responsible family member, can safely continue the therapeutic drug regimen when the person has sufficient information about the therapy to allow for assessing progress and identifying problems related to the disease and the drug therapy.

Serum Assay. Periodic assay of serum, plasma, or blood concentrations of potent drugs with a narrow margin of safety (i.e., digoxin)

provides data for fine regulation of dosage. The laboratory analysis also allows measurement of safe and effective dosage when other medical problems mask the usual parameters employed to evaluate the patient's status. When intensive therapy with drugs at high dosage is required for critically ill patients, the monitoring of the blood drug levels concurrent with measurement of the associated physiologic effects allows continual dosage adjustments when the patient's status changes. The monitoring plan allows attainment of an optimal therapeutic effect while minimizing the adverse effects of the drugs.

Individual Variables

Physical condition, age, sex, weight, height, and body build are considered by the physician in the selection of drugs and their dosage. Genetic and environmental factors also affect the responses to drugs, but these variables are more difficult to predict. Physiologic factors affect the consideration of specific dosage levels for individuals requiring therapy. For example, immaturity of hepatic and renal systems in the newborn and the possibility of some deterioration of the same organs in elderly or debilitated patients necessitate careful consideration of the implications of decreased drug metabolism on the dosage required to attain and maintain effective and safe drug levels in the patient. Many factors affect the effectiveness and safety of a drug, and continual assessment of the relationship of the dosage to physiologic changes is necessary throughout the period of therapy.

Body build, weight, and height are important determinants of therapeutic dosage, since the distribution of drug in the body depends on the relationship of drug to tissue mass. To obtain the same therapeutic effect, the muscular athlete may require more drug than the thin individual. Calculations based on body weight are done on the basis of actual weight. When patients are obese or have large amounts of extracellular fluid, the dosage is based on the calculated ideal weight for size, bone structure, and age. Lean body weight also must be considered in calculations of dosage for drugs that are widely distributed in muscle tissues (i.e., digoxin).

Pediatric Dosage Calculation

The prescribed drug dosage for an infant or a child may be based on calculation of the amount recommended as milligrams per kilogram of body weight (mg/kg BW). The prescribed dosage may be compared, before administration, with the normal dosage range for infants or children when information about pediatric dosage is available in the literature.

The therapeutic dosage for adults also can be used as a guide for calculation of the probable dosage for children. There are traditionally used guides for estimation of pediatric dosage:

Clark's rule for estimation of dosage based on child's weight:

$$\frac{\text{Weight (in pounds)}}{150} \times \text{Adult dose} = \text{Child's approximate dose}$$

Clark's rule for estimation of dosage based on body surface area:

$$\frac{\text{Body surface area (in M}^2)}{1.73} \times \text{Adult dose} = \text{Child's approximate dose}$$

Young's rule for estimation of dosage based on child's age:

$$\frac{\text{Age (in years)}}{\text{Age} + 12} \times \text{Adult dose} = \text{Child's approximate dose}$$

Guides for conversion of the adult dosage provide only base lines. There are many variables in the individual pediatric situation and in the characteristics of specific drugs that influence the physician's decision to prescribe a particular dosage. The guidelines assist the nurse in determining the general dosage range. The data are useful for making a judgment about dose safety before admininstering a drug to a child. None of the guides for pediatric dosage calculation described above provides an accurate dosage level for drugs to which children are highly sensitive (i.e., opiates). The dosage for those drugs should be committed to memory when caring for children.

Basic Terminology

Pharmacology is the science that involves all aspects of drug knowledge. It includes the biologic action of chemicals and the study of their source, structure, function, action, and interactions. The subdivisions of the science that are relevant to nurses in studying drug therapy include:

Pharmacodynamics, which deals with the biochemical and physiologic effects of drugs and their mechanisms of action on healthy, living tissue.

Pharmacokinetics, which deals with analysis of the concentration–time course of drugs that is influenced by absorption, distribution, metabolism, and excretion variables affecting their biologic effects.

Pharmacotherapeutics, which deals with the use of drugs in the prevention and treatment of disease and the prevention of pregnancy.

Pharmacy, which deals with the standardization, preparation of dose forms, efficacy, safety, utilization, and delivery of drugs.

There are many specific terms generally employed to describe drug action, but the basic definitions for the words *chemotherapy, drug, and receptor* provide a frame of reference for approaching further discussion:

Chemotherapy describes the use of drugs to control or destroy invading organisms (i.e., bacteria) or abnormal tissue (i.e., cancer cells).

Drug designates a chemical agent that interacts with living systems and is employed to prevent, diagnose, or treat a medical problem.

Receptor sites are tissue areas where union or a reaction between a drug and a cellular constituent produces a tissue response.

Drug Therapy

Plans for control of disease often include prescriptions for several drugs. Knowledge of the pharmacodynamic action and elementary pharmacokinetics of each drug is important for implementing the pharmacotherapeutic plan. Throughout the text the actions, effects, and interactions of drugs are presented in the context of functional problems. In clinical situations, patients often have multiple functional problems, and the drugs employed for control of each problem contribute to the total body response to therapy. Prescription of several drugs for one patient is called *polypharmacy,* and it has been estimated that the average hospitalized patient receives at least six drugs concurrently. The use of multiple drugs can confuse the analysis of individual drug action. The practice also increases the hazard of adverse reactions and drug interactions because most drugs have secondary effects in addition to their primary action.

Drugs are prescribed for a particular planned effect on target tissues, and drugs entering the systemic circulation produce responses by interacting with body tissues or with other molecules present in the internal environment. There is seldom a purely specific drug–target tissue relationship without concurrent effects on other body processes. Drugs produce no original physiologic effects, but they modify physiologic activity. Drugs can *replace, interrupt,* or *potentiate* physiologic processes. Examples of the use of drugs to affect physiologic function are seen in the use of insulin to *replace* deficient endogenous supplies of the hormone required for glucose utilization in diabetes; narcotic analgesics *interrupt* nerve transmission and decrease pain perception; administration of thiazide diuretics *potentiates* the hypotensive effects of antihypertensive drugs.

DOSAGE-CONCENTRATION FACTORS

Therapeutic effectiveness is dependent on active drug molecules reaching the target site for activity at a concentration high enough to achieve the intended response. Drug *dosage, absorption, distribution, biotransformation,* and *excretion* affect the onset, duration, and intensity of drug action after administration.

Biologic Half-Life

Each drug has a characteristic rate at which it is absorbed, metabolized, and excreted, and the processes are reflected in blood levels, which show a rise in the drug content to a therapeutic concentration, attainment of a peak level, and gradual decline to a minimum therapeutic concentration (Fig. 5–1).

The biologic half-life ($t1/2$) is the time period in which the peak drug level is reduced by one half through metabolism or elimination (Fig. 5–2). Graphic representations of time-concentration curves can be employed to calculate the biologic half-life of a drug. When metabolism or elimination of the drug is accelerated, the $t1/2$ is shortened. When hepatic dysfunction interferes with drug metabolism or renal dysfunction interferes with elimination (Fig. 5–3), the $t1/2$ is lengthened. The half-life is a measurement used to reflect the rate of drug disappearance.

Time-concentration data provide information about the duration of biologic availability of drugs, and these data can be employed to attain optimal drug therapy regimens adjusted to individual variables. The shortened time span of therapeutic plasma concentration levels occurring with accelerated drug metabolism or elimination may result in an absence of clinical improvement in the patient. With knowledge of the pharmacokinetics of the drug, the physician can adjust the dosage to the level required to attain the desired therapeutic response. Excess prolongation of the time span of drug concentrations in the plasma allows cumulation and consequently increases the potential for toxic drug reactions. Decreased dosage and less frequent administration may be required to avert problems associated with high plasma drug levels when hepatic or renal function is impaired.

The normal biologic half-life has been defined for many drugs, and the data allow optimal spacing of dose frequency for attaining an effective duration of plasma concentrations. For example, the anticonvulsant drug *phenytoin sodium* has a slower absorption and distribution rate than other forms of phenytoin. It has a biologic half-life of

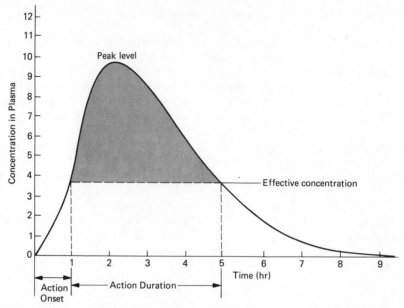

Fig. 5–1. Plasma drug levels provide data showing the time-concentration factors indicating the period of therapeutic effectiveness. The diagram above shows that one hour after administration drug absorption has raised the plasma levels to the effective concentration and the plasma drug content remains above that level for four hours.

20 hours and effective levels lasting 12 or more hours. After definition of the half-life, the dosage regimen was adjusted to a once-a-day schedule that provided equal or better seizure control than the former twice-a-day dosage method. The change also provided better patient acceptance and compliance with the therapeutic plan for seizure control.

A plateau, or steady state, of drug concentration is attained when a drug is repetitively administered by any route. Steady-state serum concentration for a continuous intravenous infusion is reached when the rate of infusion equals the rate of drug elimination. When it is desirable to attain a steady-state serum concentration of drug in a short time span, a loading dose may be prescribed. The initial dosage may be double the amount prescribed for regularly scheduled administration (i.e., sulfonamides), or the dosage may be higher in the first two or three days of therapy (i.e., digitalis glycosides). The procedure

raises the peak plasma concentration level and prolongs the drug disappearance curve so more drug is available in the plasma at the time of subsequent drug administration.

Most orally administered drugs achieve peak plasma concentration levels in one to two hours, and the plasma levels decline to an ineffective concentration within three to four hours. It is important, when planning to monitor a patient's response to a drug, to consider not only the effect of a single dose, but also the cumulative effect of repeated doses on the steady-state plasma concentration. It is estimated that it takes about seven and one-half half-lives before a drug is completely removed from the body.

DRUG ABSORPTION

The route of drug administration is a primary factor affecting absorption, distribution, and onset of pharmacologic action. Drugs administered by

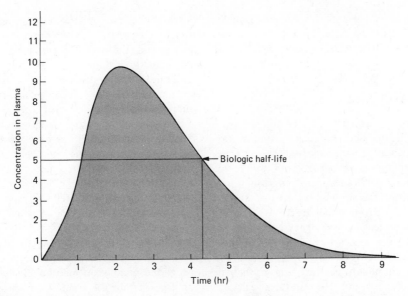

Fig. 5–2. The biologic half-life (t1/2) of a drug is based on the drug disappearance curve, which shows the concentration gradually reduced to one half of the peak level in 4.25 hours.

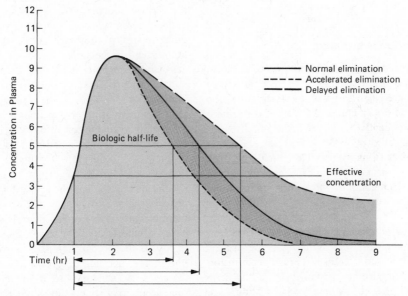

Fig. 5–3. The duration of therapeutic action is shorter when metabolism or elimination is accelerated, and the duration is longer when those processes are slowed by hepatic or renal pathology.

any except the intravenous route must reach the circulating fluids to be disseminated to the widely distributed tissue receptor sites that are the targets for drug action.

Oral Drug Absorption

Drugs may be placed under the tongue (sublingual) or in the buccal pouch for absorption from the mucous membranes of the oral mucosa. Rapid absorption of the drug from the highly vascular lipid membranes provides drug effect without awaiting the slower processes of absorption from the gastrointestinal tract. Acceleration of therapeutic effect at tissue sites occurs consequent to drug delivery with the venous blood to receptor sites. Direct venous transport avoids first-pass biotransformation of the drug at hepatic sites. For example, a nitroglycerin tablet can provide relief of pain for the patient with angina pectoris within two minutes after the tablet is placed under the tongue. If nitroglycerin were taken orally, the drug would be inactivated at hepatic sites and there would be no therapeutic effect.

Gastrointestinal Absorption

There are drugs administered orally for local action within the gastrointestinal tract, but most oral agents are given to provide a systemic effect. Although the oral method is the most convenient and most frequently employed route for drug administration, absorption from the gastrointestinal tract is subject to many variables, including drug dissolution, gastric emptying rate, gastrointestinal motility, and interaction with gastric or intestinal contents.

Membrane Transport. Most drugs are absorbed from the gastrointestinal tract by passive diffusion or by active transport. Passive diffusion is the more important mechanism, and the drug moves from the gut, where concentrations are high, to the plasma, where drug concentration is negligible. Passive diffusion continues down the concentration gradient until equilibrium is estab-

lished. Other factors affecting transfer include the weight, size, and lipid solubility of the drug molecules, and the blood flow, surface area, and permeability of the mucosa.

Drugs must be absorbed across the lipoprotein membranes of the gastrointestinal tract, which share the characteristic structure of other body membranes: lipids 40 percent; protein 50 percent; carbohydrate 10 percent of the mass by weight. The membranes are permeable to nonionized lipid-soluble substances, but ionized substances are poorly absorbed. Most free drug forms are lipid soluble and readily move across the lipid-containing cells of the intestinal mucosa.

Dissolution Factors. Absorption from the digestive tract is dependent on the solubility of the drug, and dissolution may be affected by the pH of fluids within the tract. Many drugs are weak acids (i.e., barbiturates, clofibrate, penicillin, phenylbutazone, sulfonamides, phenytoin, warfarin), and they tend to be nonpolar (nonionized and lipid soluble) in the acidic environment of the stomach. The weak acids may be absorbed from the gastric mucosa. Weak bases (i.e., amphetamines, antihistamines, erythromycin, guanethidine, opiates, phenothiazines, tricyclic antidepressants) tend to be polar (ionized) in the gastric acid, and absorption is delayed until they become nonpolar in the alkaline secretions of the small intestine.

Drugs in solution at the time of administration are readily available for absorption, but gelatinous capsules must be softened and tablets must be disintegrated to liberate the drug content. Dissolution of solid forms of drugs breaks them into smaller molecules, which accelerates diffusion and provides more surface area for drug action when the molecules arrive at receptor sites. Some drugs have an enteric coating, which maintains the integrity of the preparation thus preventing liberation of the irritating drug until the tablet reaches the intestine. Dissolution of the enteric coating can occur if the pH of stomach contents is changed by concurrent administration of oral antacids, and nausea and vomiting may occur consequent to gastric irritation.

Gastric Emptying. Most drugs are poorly absorbed from the stomach; so the rate of gastric emptying determines the rate at which drugs are delivered to the sites of maximal absorption in the small intestine. The very large surface area provided by the capillary-rich villi of the small intestine speeds the absorption of the drug molecules.

Slowing of gastric emptying by concurrent administration of food delays passage of drug into the small intestine. Most drugs are administered between meals to assure prompt passage to absorption sites in the intestinal tract, but drugs that are irritating to the gastric mucosa may be administered with a snack to decrease the incidence of nausea or vomiting consequent to local irritation.

Gastric Interactions. Concurrent use of foods with drugs requires consideration of the effect that delayed or decreased absorption may have on the maintenance of therapeutic drug levels in the plasma. Tetracycline absorption can be negligible when it is administered with food, or with drugs containing calcium, magnesium, aluminum, sodium bicarbonate (i.e., antacids), or iron compounds because the chemicals bind tetracycline and form insoluble complexes that remain in the intestine and are eliminated with the feces.

Gastric Metabolism. Metabolism of some drugs (i.e., levodopa, penicillin, phenobarbital) begins in the stomach and delayed gastric emptying may allow near-complete metabolism of the weak acids before the drug moves into the intestine. For example, phenobarbital metabolism in the stomach may lessen the amount of active drug available for absorption from the intestine and negate the planned hypnotic effect of the drug.

Intestinal Absorption. Some drugs are dependent on the presence of food to assure their absorption, but they constitute a small group of drugs. For example, absorption of the antifungal drug *griseofulvin* is enhanced when fat-containing foods are present to facilitate transfer of drug molecules across the intestinal membranes. The fat-containing foods increase the output of bile and that is important for the absorption of the fat-soluble drug.

The very rapid intestinal transit of drug molecules that may occur with diarrhea or with the frequent use of cathartics or laxatives may speed the movement of drugs through the intestinal lumen so rapidly that dissolution is incomplete and absorption is limited. The problem could occur with long-acting drugs or timed-release formulations, which have ingredients designed to slow dissolution in the intestinal lumen. Rapid intestinal transit of the formulations allows only negligible amounts to diffuse across the enteric membranes and most of the drug is eliminated intact.

Parenteral Absorption

The physical properties of some drugs prevent their absorption from the gastrointestinal tract, and other drugs (i.e., insulin) are protein products that would be destroyed by proteolytic enzymes, so the drugs must be administered parenterally. The rate of absorption of drugs from intramuscular or subcutaneous injection sites is dependent on the blood supply and the rate of blood flow from the tissues.

Muscle Absorption Variables. Massaging the injection site or exercising the muscle distributes the injected drug in the interstitial fluid and hastens capillary absorption. Lipophilic drug molecules dissolved in interstitial fluid rapidly diffuse through the membranes of capillary endothelial cells. Small molecules of water-soluble drugs diffuse through the pores in the capillary membrane. Although the capillary pores are small, the rapid thermal motion of drug molecules in solution accelerates absorption.

Drugs are more rapidly absorbed from the deltoid mucles, but these sites are generally avoided because they cause the greatest discomfort for the patient receiving intramuscular injections. In females, drug absorption from the gluteus muscle is slow, and the absorption rate is only slightly better in males. When rapid absorption of a drug is desirable, the site of choice is the vastus lateralis or deltoid muscle.

Absorption-Retarding Solvents. Colloidal solutions or suspensions have retardants added to the solution to decrease the rate of absorption from the injection site. For example, *protamine* added to *insulin* decreases the rate of absorption from the depot site and provides the drug by gradually releasing it from the tissues over a longer period of time. Viscous organic solvents (i.e., cottonseed oil, glycerine, polyethylene glycol, sesame oil) release drug very slowly and can provide clinically effective drug levels over weeks or months when the solutions are injected intramuscularly. Water-insoluble suspensions also maintain drug at depot sites for prolonged release. The foregoing mechanisms are useful to decrease the repeated administration of drugs and they can be utilized when the probability that the individual will return for therapy is doubtful. For example, the administration of *benzathine penicillin,* which is a water-insoluble suspension, allows single-injection treatment of gonorrhea.

Tissue Fluid Accumulation. Excessive accumulation of tissue fluid (i.e., edema) decreases drug absorption because there is a greater distance between the pool of the injected drug and the capillaries. Alternate injection sites are employed to assure the absorption of drugs when tissues are edematous. For example, the drug may be administered into the deltoid rather than the gluteal muscle.

Venous Infusion. Injection of drugs into the venous route provides rapid distribution to receptors, and drug may arrive at receptor sites before fractions are metabolized by the liver. The intravenous route is employed as an alternate method of providing drugs for systemic effect when the rate of blood flow from peripheral tissues is decreased (i.e., in shock), and it is the route commonly employed when there is a continuous intravenous infusion inserted for provision of nutrients or fluids. The intravenous route is the most direct and dependable route for the delivery of drugs to effector sites, but it can be the most hazardous route if not controlled properly.

BIOAVAILABILITY

Drugs marketed by manufacturers under their trade name are chemically equivalent to the nonproprietary drug and meet USP, NF, or FDA standards for content of active ingredient, purity, and potency. There can be differences in the absorption, or bioavailability, of oral formulations containing the same quantity of active principles in the drugs produced by more than one pharmaceutical laboratory. The active ingredient is only one factor in bioavailability of the drug for therapeutic effect.

The absorption characteristics of capsules or tablets depend on the size of the particles of the active ingredient and the fillers, binders, coating, stabilizers, or other adjuvants within the formulation. Adequate absorption depends on the way the product is made (i.e., hardness of a tablet), and the differences between proprietary products can affect the plasma levels of the drug and present problems of underdosage, overdosage, or adverse reactions when the products are used interchangeably. When a patient receiving a particular proprietary drug changes to a drug marketed by another company, the same dosage may result in therapeutic failure or cause an unexpected toxicity as a consequence of the differences in bioavailability.

The problem has attracted considerable attention in the health professions, and concerted efforts are being made to find methods for assaying the time course of drug concentration in plasma to define the differences in bioavailability between various formulations of proprietary drugs. Assays of blood samples are employed during intensive therapy of patients receiving *digoxin, gentamicin sulfate,* or *phenytoin,* and the laboratory values provide guides to availability of drug for therapeutic action. The foregoing assays use a method particular to the individual drugs, but methodologies for testing bioavailability of most drugs have not been developed. A stated long-range goal of the FDA is the assurance of therapeutic equivalence of dosage forms of all chemically similar drug products on the market.

DISTRIBUTION

Drugs administered for systemic effect are distributed to their active receptor sites after being absorbed from tissues at the administration site. Drugs that enter the bloodstream may remain free in the serum, or they may become bound to plasma proteins. Only the free fraction of the drug is active. The circulating blood gradually moves the drugs toward tissues or receptor sites where they perform their primary therapeutic function. Varying tissues and receptor sites attract particular compounds, and drugs are chemical molecules with some specificity for selected action sites. Some drugs have a high affinity for particular tissue. For example, barbiturates are avidly taken up and stored in adipose tissues.

The blood supply of the receptors and the rate and concentration of the drug diffused from the capillary bed affect the onset of drug action. The duration of drug action is dependent on the rate at which the circulating drug is metabolized and excreted, and the intensity of response is dependent on the concentration of the free drug at the receptor sites.

Protein Binding

Many drugs are bound to plasma proteins, usually albumin, and the tenacity of protein binding affects the rate of distribution to receptor sites. Only unbound or free drug can diffuse into the tissues because the drug-protein complex is too large to pass the membrane barriers. Protein binding decreases the initial concentration of the drug at the receptor sites but it prolongs the duration of drug action.

Protein binding is a reversible process that provides a circulating reservoir of inactive drug that releases the drug when tissue stores of free drug are low. A sustained therapeutic effect can be maintained by the replenishment of active drug from the protein-binding sites when metabolism or excretion lowers the concentration at receptor sites. Protein binding affects the movement of drugs into all body tissues and body fluids (Fig. 5–4).

Low Albumin Levels. Low levels of plasma albumin (hypoalbuminemia) may require an adjustment in the dosage of a drug that is dependent on protein binding for distribution. In situations where low albumin levels occur secondary to losses from wounds, hepatic damage, or body cavity drainage, intravenous replacement of albumin may provide the necessary vehicle for drug distribution. The problem occurs in postoperative patients who are selectively placed on oral anticoagulant, (i.e., warfarin) therapy for control of clot formation. When the blood samples show hypoalbuminemia, the prothrombin level may remain below the therapeutic level in spite of continued administration of the anticoagulant, and albumin replacement raises and stabilizes the circulating prothrombin level to that required for therapeutic effectiveness.

Binding-Site Competition. In the alkaline environment of plasma, acidic drugs are anionic and they compete for common binding sites on proteins. The drug with a higher affinity can displace another drug that shares a protein-binding site. The process liberates larger amounts of the second drug into the circulation and the additional free drug may produce a higher-level response during therapy. For example, metabolites of the hypnotic drug *chloral hydrate* have a high affinity for albumin and they may displace warfarin from binding sites. High plasma levels of the anticoagulant may cause adverse reactions. The problem may be reflected in laboratory tests (prothrombin time) of warfarin effectiveness in the control of coagulation factors, and the patient's blood levels may be erratic. An elevation above the therapeutic range may be found when blood tests are done in the morning after nights when the patient takes chloral hydrate to induce sleep, but the prothrombin level may be within the normal range

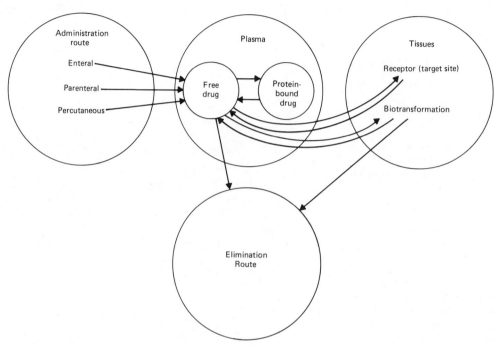

Fig. 5–4. The bioavailability of the absorbed drug is affected by the protein binding, biotransformation, and elimination rate.

when the patient sleeps without taking chloral hydrate. *Aspirin, phenylbutazone,* and *mefanamic acid* also displace coumadin from binding sites when the drugs are used concurrently, and the outcome is a serious potential for hemorrhage when the oral anticoagulant continues to be taken without monitoring of blood levels. In general, binding-site displacement is clinically significant only when drugs are more than 90 percent bound to plasma proteins.

Blood-Brain Barrier

The barrier to the movement of some drugs into brain tissue is known to exist, but poorly understood components of the hypothetic blood-brain barrier selectively allow passage of some drugs while presenting a barrier to other drugs. Capillaries in the central nervous system are en-

veloped in *glial cells* that resist the passage of many drugs, but the glial cells allow movement of some lipid-soluble agents (i.e., barbiturates, general anesthetics). When the meninges are inflamed, the integrity of the barrier is lessened, and many drugs (i.e., antibiotics) that cannot pass through the normal capillary membranes readily cross into the brain tissue.

Placental Passage

A primary concern when drugs are administered to women during pregnancy is the possibility that drugs may cross the placenta and affect the development of the fetus. Drugs with *teratogenic* effects disrupt the biosynthesis of protein or alter metabolism during the early weeks of fetal development and cause death of the fetus. When drugs with teratogenic effects are administered to the mother during the critical third-week-to-third-month period when embryonic cells are proliferating rapidly and organ development is occurring (organogenesis), the drugs may cause multiple anomalies (i.e., cleft palate, transposed or incompletely developed organs). For example, administration of the antineoplastic drug *methotrexate* to the mother during the first trimester of pregnancy may cause abortion, or the term of pregnancy may be completed and the neonate may have cleft palate and skull deformities. The vulnerability of fetal organs to malformation is highest during the days of the gestational period when the various fetal systems develop: nervous system, fifteenth to twenty-fifth days; eyes, twenty-fourth to fortieth days; heart, twenty-fifth to fortieth days; legs, twenty-fourth to thirty-sixth days of gestation.

Warnings against administration of teratogenic, or mutagenic, drugs to women of childbearing years are based on concern that the drugs may affect the fetus at a time when the mother is unaware of her pregnancy. Drugs present in the internal environment may affect the developing fetus from the time of conception until the blastocyst embeds in the placenta. Direct transfer may occur as drugs traverse the placenta to equilibrate with the content in the fetal circulation. The teratogenic effects of most drugs in man have not been adequately studied. The maternal use of drugs should be limited to those that are essential or those adequately tested for use during pregnancy.

Placental Structure.   Throughout pregnancy the placental structure consists of a villi sheath (syncytium) and villi stroma, which drugs circulating in the maternal blood must traverse to reach the fetal blood. In the first 20 weeks of pregnancy, villi have an additional double covering of cell layers, and the added protection resists passage of many drugs that later may move across the placenta. Placental tissue enzymes metabolize some substances (i.e., cholines, catecholamines) and the process affords protection to the fetus by inactivation of some chemicals from the maternal circulation.

Diffusion Rates.   Lipid-soluble drugs traverse the placenta by passive diffusion, which equilibrates the fetal blood drug content with the concentration of the maternal blood. The placenta provides a barrier only to large molecules (molecular weight of 1000). The quantity of the drug reaching the fetus may be small, but the fetal tissue mass is small. The limiting factor in distribution of a drug to the fetus is related to the rate of transfer.

Drug Effect of the Fetus.   The effect of a drug on the fetus correlates with the gestational period in which the mother takes the drug (Table 5–1). The problems are myriad and an inclusive list would include those drugs known to have comparable effects on tissues of adults: *streptomycin* causes nerve damage affecting hearing and the child may have partial deafness when the drug is taken by the mother for control of tuberculosis during pregnancy. *Chlorpromazine* or *thioridazine* may accumulate in fetal melanin-containing eye tissues causing loss of sight. Problems related to maternal drug use may appear in the later years of the child's life. For example, vaginal adenocarcinoma has been identified in young women whose mothers received *diethylstilbestrol* (DES) during pregnancy.

Maternal Instruction.   Precautions against administration of drugs that cross the placenta are necessary throughout pregnancy because fetal enzymatic pathways for biotransformation of drugs are inadequate for metabolism of drugs. The enzyme systems remain immature into the early neonatal period. Pregnant women are instructed to report emerging problems so drugs can be prescribed for them and they are told not to take drugs without consulting the physician. The practice is directed at decreasing the possibility that any drug causing teratogenic, mutagenic, or adverse reactions in the fetus will be taken by pregnant women.

Information Sources.   One of the objectives of drug studies in animals is to identify those drugs that affect the developing fetus. Many drugs have

Table 5–1.
Effects of Drugs on the Fetus During Gestational Periods

Maternal Drug Ingestion	Gestational Period	Effect on Fetus
Androgens, estrogens, oral progestogens	Early pregnancy	Masculinization and labial fusion in females
	Later pregnancy	Clitoral enlargement
Methimazole, potassium iodide, prophylthiouracil	+14 weeks	Goiter, mental retardation
Tetracyclines	2nd and 3rd trimester	Inhibition of bone growth, defects and discoloration of teeth enamel
Heroin	Near term	Addiction (respiratory depression, death)
Chloramphenicol	Near term	"Gray" syndrome (fatal)
Salicylates (excess)	Near term	Bleeding, temporary coagulation defects
Sulfonamides (long acting), vitamin K (large amounts)	Near term	Hyperbilirubinemia, kernicterus
Phenobarbital (excess)	Near term	Bleeding, increased rate of drug metabolism
Lysergide (LSD), chlorpromazine, diphenhydramine, perphenazine	Near term	Chromosomal breaks
Vitamin A (large amounts)	Throughout pregnancy	Cleft palate, eye damage, fusion of fingers and toes
Vitamin D (large amounts)	Throughout pregnancy	Excess blood calcium, mental retardation

been tested, and those with known effects on the fetus are clearly identified on the labels of the drug containers and in all literature describing the drug.

BIOTRANSFORMATION

The rate of metabolism is an important factor in providing the duration and intensity of drug action required for a therapeutic effect. Although drugs may be metabolized in the intestine, lung, kidney, or skin, the liver is the chief organ for biotransformation.

Oral Drug Distribution

Orally administered drugs enter the portal vein after absorption from the gastrointestinal tract. Portal blood passes directly to the liver where it enters the sinusoids of the liver lobules (Fig. 5–5). Some of the drug arriving at hepatic cells is metabolized by hepatic microsomal enzymes. The initial biotransformation of drugs reaching the liver with the portal blood is called "first-pass" metabolism. Blood leaving the liver through the hepatic veins enters the vena cava and follows the same circulatory pathway traveled by parenteral drugs en route to receptor sites. Each time the drug or its metabolites pass through the liver, additional fractions of the drug are transformed. The drug molecules may be converted to active or inactive metabolites.

Hepatic Metabolism

Biotransformation by hepatic microsomal enzymes occurs in two closely interrelated phases.

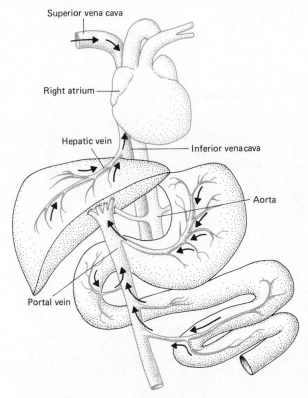

Superior vena cava

Right atrium

Hepatic vein

Inferior vena cava

Aorta

Portal vein

Fig. 5–5. Orally administered drug is absorbed from the small intestine and travels through the small blood vessels to the portal vein en route to the liver biotransformation sites. The hepatic vein carries metabolites to the vena cava. Parenteral drug from the injection sites also travels the vena caval route toward the arterial circulation.

In the first phase of biotransformation, fat-soluble drug metabolites are converted to ionized, water-soluble metabolites. Most drugs are more soluble in lipids than in water and must be metabolized into water-soluble derivatives before they can be excreted. In the second phase of biotransformation an enzyme-catalyzed reaction forms a conjugate that can be excreted.

In the hepatic endoplasmic reticulum the *microsomal enzyme system* alters the drug by *oxidation, reduction, hydrolysis,* or *conjugation*. Oxidation, which occurs in the first phase of biotransformation, is the most common of the metabolic processes. In phase two, inactive metabolites produced by oxidation are coupled with acetic acid, inorganic sulfate, or amino acids, but the most important conjugation process is the enzymatic activity of *glucuronyl transferase,* which conjugates metabolites with carbohydrate to pre-

pare the readily excreted metabolite *glucuronic acid*.

Hepatic dysfunction can interfere with the biotransformation of drugs and unchanged drug or active metabolites remain in the circulation. The retained agents elevate the plasma drug concentration and can cause adverse reactions. Retention of unchanged drug or active metabolites also occurs with renal dysfunction because most drugs are excreted in the urine.

Cumulation

The term *cumulation* describes elevation of circulating drug levels that occurs when metabolism or excretion is delayed. Cumulative drug levels constitute overdosage, and the patient will show the same symptoms as those present when the maximum therapeutic level has been exceeded.

Monitoring of liver and kidney function is important when drugs having a high cumulative potential (i.e., digitalis) are used. Hepatic and renal function as well as serum drug levels is evaluated frequently when the patient is hospitalized for intensive therapy with potent drugs.

Newborn infants have little ability to oxidize drugs, and the duration of drug action may be lengthened considerably. Residual drug acquired from the maternal circulation before severing of the umbilical cord may remain in the bloodstream of the neonate, and immaturity of liver enzyme systems allows the drug to circulate without inactivation. Newborn infants also have a deficiency of glucuronyl transferase, which conjugates metabolites to form glucuronides, and both active and inactive metabolites may remain in the infant's circulation. Coupled with incompletely developed kidney function, drug cumulation may produce toxic effects.

EXCRETION

Drugs are excreted primarily by the kidneys, but free drug or inactive metabolites may be eliminated in breast milk, feces, expired air, or sweat. The drug content of feces usually represents unabsorbed portions of oral drugs, but feces may contain drug metabolites that have passed into the biliary tract from the liver. Enterohepatic recycling of bile returns some drug metabolites to hepatic sites and lessens the amount eliminated by feces.

Elimination in Breast Milk

Any drug, including alcohol, ingested by a nursing mother may enter the breast milk and be administered to the nursing infant. Although amounts of drug obtained may be small, problems can arise from the quantity of drug an infant receives in a 24-hour nursing period. In addition to the undesirability of administering drugs to a healthy infant, the deficient metabolizing system of the neonate allows cumulation of drug and circulating drug concentrations may gradually rise to a hazardous level. The intestine of the newborn also permits passage of undigested macromolecules, and antibiotic passage to the nursing infant may allow sensitization and a consequent allergic reaction to the drugs if they are administered later for control of a health problem.

Renal Excretion

In the normal kidney, protein products do not pass through the membranes of the glomerular capillaries; therefore, only unbound, or free, drug is removed from the circulating fluids by glomerular filtration. Once in the renal tubule, the drug may be reabsorbed and returned to the circulation along with the large number of electrolytes and water reabsorbed in the proximal and distal tubule.

Tubular Reabsorption. The more lipid soluble the drug, the greater is the proportion reabsorbed in the kidney by back diffusion into the tubule cells. The driving force is the concentration gradient produced during reabsorption of water and solutes. The process returns drug metabolites to the circulation, but on each pass through the kidneys, additional fractions pass into the glomerular filtrate and are eliminated.

Tubular Secretion. Protein binding affects renal clearance and can prolong the biologic half-life of a drug. The elimination of bound drug is dependent on tubular secretion. Renal tubular cells secrete free drug by active carrier mechanisms that transport the drug into tubular urine. The process decreases the concentration of free drug in the serum, and the drug is released from binding sites to maintain equilibrium. Free drug then is secreted by the renal tubules, and the process decreases the amount of protein-bound drug in the circulation.

The active carrier mechanisms of the renal tubules are involved in secretion of many naturally occurring compounds. Diverse substances use common carrier systems in the renal tubule, and high levels of metabolic products or drugs competing for the transport mechanisms may exceed the amounts that can be secreted. There is some specificity of the carrier mechanisms, and preferential transport of one substance may block the secretion of a second substance.

Acid Carrier Systems. The tubular active carrier systems that are selective for acid substances transport the metabolic waste uric acid and the drug metabolite glucuronic acid. The acid carrier system can be blocked by transport of any of the acidic drugs (i.e., indomethacin, phenylbutazone, salicylates, sulfonamides, which include probenecid and thiazides). Blocking by one drug can inhibit the secretion of another drug or a metabolic product and raise its plasma concentration. For example, the thiazide diuretics compete with uric acid for transport by the renal tubular cells and the drugs inhibit the secretion of uric acid. During therapy adverse effects (i.e., gout) may occur because circulating uric acid levels become elevated.

Knowledge of the competitive blocking has led to utilization of the process as a therapeutic tool. For example, *probenecid* has been employed to block secretion of penicillin, thereby maintaining higher therapeutic plasma levels of the antibiotic for longer periods of time.

Base Carrier Systems. Naturally occurring bases (i.e., ammonium) are transported by different active transport mechanisms in the renal tubules. The same competition can occur as that found with acid transport mechanisms because the carrier systems also transport drugs and metabolites that are bases.

Urine Acid-Base Modification. The normal acidity of the urine can be modified to change the pH and accelerate elimination of undesirable toxic compounds from the circulation. For example, administration of sodium bicarbonate intravenously to an individual with an overdose of barbiturate or salicylates may accelerate elimination of those weakly acidic drugs. Conversely, acidification of the urine may accelerate elimination of the weak bases amphetamine and quinidine. The process is somewhat inefficient and requires persistent modification of the pH to provide an effective elimination route.

Additional Readings

Blanchard, James: Gastrointestinal absorption 1, mechanisms. *Am. J. Pharm.,* **147:**135, September–October, 1975.

Bossone, M. Christine McDevitt: The Liver: a pharmacologic perspective. *Nurs. Clin. North Am.,* **12:** 291, June, 1977.

Coleman, James H., and Straughn, Art B.: Assurance of drug quality (bioavailability). *Dis. Nerv. Syst.,* **36:**63, February, 1975.

Feldman, Stuart: Drug distribution. *Med. Clin. North Am.,* **58:**917, September, 1974.

Galant, Stanley P.: Biologic and clinical significance of the gut as a barrier to penetration of macromolecules. *Clin. Pediatr.,* **15:**731, August, 1976.

Gibaldi, Milo, and Levy, Gerhard: Pharmacokinetics in clinical practice. *J.A.M.A.,* **235:**1864, April 26, 1976.

————: Pharmacokinetics in clinical practice, 2. Applications. *J.A.M.A.,* **235:**1987, May 3, 1976.

Greenblatt, David J., and Koch-Weser, Jan: Drug therapy: clinical pharmacokinetics. *N. Engl. J. Med.,* **293:**702, October 2, 1975.

————: Drug therapy: clinical pharmacokinetics: *N. Engl. J. Med.,* **293:**964, November 6, 1975.

————: Drug therapy: intramuscular injection of drugs. *N. Engl. J. Med.,* **295:**542, September 2, 1976.

Hussar, Daniel A.: Review of some significant drug interactions. *Pharm. Times,* **41:**46, January, 1975.

Kappas, Attallah, and Alvares, Alvito P.: How the liver metabolizes foreign substances. *Sci. Am.,* **232:** 22, June, 1975.

Koch-Weser, Jan, and Sellers, Edward M.: Drug therapy: binding of drugs to serum albumin. *N. Engl. J. Med.,* **294:**311, February 5, 1976.

————: Drug therapy: binding of drugs to serum albumin. *N. Engl. J. Med.,* **294:**526, March 4, 1976.

Lambert, Martin L., Jr., Drug and diet interactions. *Am. J. Nurs.,* **75:**402, March, 1975.

Lesko, Lawrence J.: The geriatric series, part 1: biopharmaceutical aspects of geriatric pharmacy. *The Apothecary*, **89:** (Reprint), May, 1977.

Milkovich, Lucille, and van den Berg, Bea J.: An evaluation of the teratogenicity of certain antinauseant drugs. *Am. J. Obstet. Gynecol.*, **125:**244, May 15, 1976.

Mudge, Gilbert H.; Silvia, Patricio; and Stibitz, George R.: Renal excretion by non-ionic diffusion. *Med. Clin. North Am.*, **59:**681, May, 1975.

O'Brien, Thomas E.: Excretion of drugs in human milk. *Nurs. Digest*, **3:**23, July–August, 1975.

Prescott, L. F.: Gastrointestinal absorption of drugs. *Med. Clin. North Am.*, **58:**907, September, 1974.

Robinson, Donald S.: Pharmacokinetic mechanisms of drug interactions. *Postgrad. Med.*, **57:**55, February, 1975.

Stortz, Laurie J.: Unprescribed drug products and pregnancy. *J. Gynecol. Nurs.*, **6:**9, August, 1977.

Trottier, Ralph W., Jr.: Teratogenesis—toxicity in utero. *Am. J. Pharm.*, **147:**147, September–October, 1975.

Vukovich, Robert A.; Brannick, Leo J.; Sugerman, Arthur A.; and Neiss, Edward S.: Sex differences in the intramuscular absorption and bioavailability of cephradine. *Clin. Pharmacol. Ther.*, **18:**215, August, 1975.

Wagner, John G.: Drug bioavailability studies. *Hosp. Pract.*, **12:**119, January, 1977.

Wilkinson, Grant R., and Shand, David G.: A physiologic approach to hepatic drug clearance. *Clin. Pharmacol. Ther.*, **18:**377, October, 1975.

6

Adverse Drug Reactions

Therapeutic effectiveness is dependent on sufficient concentration of the drug at an action site to produce a desired response. The time-concentration factors may be altered by a variety of interceding reactions that increase or decrease availability of drug or active metabolites at receptor sites. Adverse drug reactions may be categorized broadly as adverse effects resulting from chemical or pharmacologic properties of a drug, dosage regimen error, allergic reactions, drug-food interaction, or drug-drug interactions.

In some clinical situations it is difficult to assess whether reactions are drug induced or are manifestations of changes in the disease process. To compound the problem of identification, predictable reactions may not appear in all patients because of variations in genetic inheritance.

Most clinical agencies have reporting systems allowing a central committee to monitor problems arising during drug therapy. When the data are analyzed, the results can be used as guides for establishing procedures and practices to lessen the incidence of adverse drug reactions and for planning drug education programs. At the national level, the FDA has established a voluntary adverse drug reaction reporting system, which provides data for analysis through a computer-retrievable system. The *Drug Experience Report*

provides an easy-to-complete profile of the patient's reaction, and it can be expected that analysis of the more than 130,000 reports received each year from physicians throughout the country will yield useful information that can be used in monitoring drug therapy programs.

INDIVIDUAL RESPONSE VARIATION

Variations are seen in the natural responses of individuals to drugs. Natural variations are nebulous and sometimes unpredictable. When a drug is initially administered, a normal therapeutic dosage may elicit a different response in two individuals of similar age and body size. For example, an analgesic may provide pain relief for four hours in one individual and the patient may be relaxed and comfortable, whereas the second individual may have pain relief that seems transient or only partial and the patient may appear restless and uncomfortable after receiving the same dosage.

Individual variation in responses occurs in a relatively normal distribution within the population. Approximately 90 percent of the individuals given a comparable amount of a drug will respond in a similar manner. The foregoing example of two individuals receiving the same analgesic drug to relieve pain represents a normal response and a response at the lower extreme on the distribution curve (Fig. 6–1). Five percent of the population is extremely sensitive, and 5 percent of the population is equally insensitive to the same dosage of drug that produces a given response in 90 percent of the population.

Drug Tolerance

Acquired tolerances to drugs usually occur when a drug has been used by the patient for a long period of time. The individual on long-term therapy may gradually find he is not receiving the same therapeutic effect that previously occurred when taking the drug. Acquired tolerances may occur consequent to alterations in biotransformation, excretion, or sensitivity of organ systems, and the patient requires increased dosage to obtain the therapeutic response attained during the initial days of drug therapy. Interruption of the drug regimen for a short time or interim periods of therapy with another drug may make it possible to reinstitute therapy with the drug at previous dosage levels. *Tachyphylaxis* is the term employed to describe rapidly developing tolerance to a drug.

Idiosyncrasies

Responses to drugs that contrast sharply with those usually observed when the drug is taken are generally described as *idiosyncrasies*. The recipient of the drug reacts in an unusual, or paradoxic, manner when given a drug. For example, when phenobarbital is given to a geriatric patient for its hypnotic effect and sleep induction, the individual may become confused, anxious, hyperactive, or disoriented. Change to a nonbarbiturate hypnotic drug may prevent recurrence of the problem. Some problems previously described as idiosyncrasies have been linked with genetically conditioned enzymatic or receptor responsiveness, which affects the biotransformation or excretion of drugs.

Enzyme Deficiency

Differences in metabolic makeup, which is genetically determined, affect responses to drug therapy. Biotransformation of drugs is dependent on enzymatic action, and genetic errors in enzyme systems may inhibit or accelerate the processes of metabolism. During therapy the individual may have adverse drug reactions significantly different from those occurring in the general population when the same therapeutic dosage is prescribed. Many of the pharmacogenetic problems have been identified retrospectively from data about adverse reactions commonly occurring during drug therapy. The genetic variation is evident only when the individual receives a drug requiring the specific enzymes for biotransformation; otherwise the genetic variation creates no health problems. The discontinuous variation seen in patients' responses to drugs is being studied in an attempt to identify factors that could indicate which individuals have enzyme variations. Identification of those individuals would allow alternate drugs to be administered thereby averting adverse responses.

Acetylating Enzyme Deficiency. One of the common genetic errors involves deficiency of the enzymes that catalyze the acetylation reaction. For example, *isoniazid (INH)* is transformed to

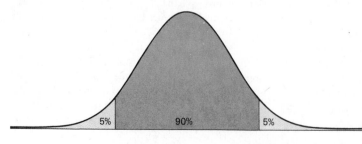

Fig. 6–1. Distribution curve of the responses to drugs shows 10 percent of the population having higher or lower effect from therapeutic drug dosage than 90 percent of the individuals benefiting from the drug.

5%   90%   5%

an inactive metabolite primarily by acetylation, which is dependent on activity of the enzyme *N-acetyl transferase.* The inactive metabolite *acetylisoniazid* is excreted in the urine. Almost 50 percent of the population receiving isoniazid for prophylaxis or treatment of tuberculosis has a deficiency of the acetylating enzyme, and isoniazid is metabolized and excreted more slowly. Individuals with the enzyme deficiency are designated as *slow inactivators* of isoniazid. Higher levels of the drug remain in the body, and interaction of the drug with vitamin B_6 leads to a deficiency of the vitamin and consequent peripheral neuritis. Lowering of the isoniazid dosage and concurrent administration of vitamin B_6, or pyridoxine, prevents neuritis. Because the number of slow inactivators is so high, vitamin B_6 is usually prescribed with isoniazid.

Deficiency of enzymes for acetylation also effects the biotransformation of the antihypertensive drug *hydralazine* and the antiarrhythmic drug *procainamide.* When individuals with deficiency of the acetylating enzymes receive either of the drugs, elevated blood levels of the drug metabolites may precipitate a lupus-like syndrome with rheumatoid arthritis-like symptoms.

G-6-PD Deficiency. The widespread use of *quinine*-related drugs for control of malaria has led to identification of individuals who have a deficiency of *glucose-6-phosphate dehydrogenase* (G-6-PD) in red blood cells. The blood cells of the genetically predisposed individuals are sensitive to concentrations of antimalarial and other oxidant drugs (i.e., synthetic vitamin K, sulfonamides, nitrofurans, sulfones, salicylates, chloramphenicol) that would have no effect on the erythrocytes in other individuals in the general population. G-6-PD in the erythrocytes plays a key role in aerobic metabolism of glucose. When blood cells of the enzyme-deficient individual are exposed to oxidant drugs or their metabolites, essential cell components are oxidized and hemolysis occurs. The inborn error of metabolism appears most frequently in African and Mediterranean populations, but it is present in an estimated 13 percent of black American males. At normal therapeutic dosage range of the drugs, individuals with G-6-PD deficiency may have moderate hemolysis, mild anemia, methemoglobinemia, and hemoglobinuria. Problems may be more severe in Caucasians than in blacks with G-6-PD deficiency, and use of the drugs may cause Caucasian patients to have massive hemolytic reactions.

TOXIC AND SIDE EFFECTS

Any pharmacodynamic event other than the intended action of the drug is a side effect. Any undesirable or "untoward" effect of a drug is an adverse reaction. The chemical and pharmacologic properties of a drug can cause predictable dose-related effects described as toxic effects or as side effects of the drugs. The complexity of actions of drugs can be simplified somewhat by viewing toxic effects in the context of *extension of effects related to the primary use of the drug* and side effects in the context of *effects unrelated to the primary use of the drug.* Although side effects often are undesired responses, there are instances when the side effects are desirable for the individual patient. For example, drowsiness is a side effect of the antihistamines, but the side effect can provide rest for the individual who has a sleep-disturbing allergic cough.

Toxic Effects

Within the category of problems related to the primary use of the drug, or toxic effects, are pathologic extensions of the planned therapeutic effect of the drug. Toxic drug levels may occur as a result of cumulation consequent to slowing of metabolic pathways or excretory mechanisms, or to administration of high dosage of the drug. Elevation of circulating levels of the drug may cause reactions exceeding the planned therapeutic response. For example, digitalis may be prescribed for its effect on the cardiac conduction pathway and myocardial tissue that slows conduction and strengthens cardiac contraction. Excessive slowing of cardiac action (bradycardia, heart block) would be a pathologic extension of the planned therapeutic effect.

Side Effects

Undesired effects other than those related to the primary use of a drug, or side effects, may result from the same mechanism of action on non-target tissues as that on target tissues. For example, atropine sulfate has an acetylcholine-blocking mechanism that is useful when a decrease in secretions is desirable (i.e., preoperatively). Dilation of the pupils is a side effect occurring by the same acetylcholine-blocking action on nontarget tissues.

Side effects also can occur as a result of a drug acting by a mechanism unrelated to the action on target tissues. For example, the nausea that occurs with high blood levels of digitalis is unrelated to the primary therapeutic action of the cardiac glycoside. Nausea occurs secondary to digitalis action at the vomiting center in the medulla, and it can occur when circulating drug reaches that site.

There are many mechanisms by which the chemical properties of drugs can cause side effects; some of the problems can be related to irritation of the tissues at the site of administration. For example, the most common side effects of drugs are gastrointestinal disturbances occurring consequent to tissue irritation when drugs are administered by the oral route.

There are few drugs administered for systemic therapy that act specifically on a particular problem without having some effect on other body systems. Lists of known side effects can be memorized, but viewing the adverse drug reactions in the framework of cause-effect relationships facilitates the understanding and recall of responses to drugs. Nausea, vomiting, dry mouth, blurred vision, diarrhea, and constipation are seemingly unrelated problems frequently described as side effects occurring with drugs, but in many instances the symptoms occur as a consequence of drug effects on the autonomic nervous system. When viewed in the context of chemical properties of drugs and their effect on physiologic processes, there is greater unity in the information gathered, and there is a broader base line for planning relevant surveillance measures.

Parasympathetic Nerve Stimulation Effects. Numerous drugs are employed to control the diverse problems related to autonomic nervous system function, and there also are many drugs with chemical properties that produce autonomic nerve responses unrelated to the planned action of the drugs. When the primary action of a drug is stimulation of parasympathetic nervous system activity, it is referred to as a *cholinergic* drug because physiologic responses result from tissue responses to the neurotransmitter *acetylcholine* (Fig. 6–2). The drugs also are referred to as *parasympathomimetic* drugs.

Several drugs are employed for stimulation of visceral activity controlled by the parasympathetic nervous system. It can be predicted that the drug used for control of cholinergic activity at a specific site will have effects on other receptor sites where acetylcholine is the neurotransmitter. For example, use of a cholinergic drug for stimulation of bladder motility to lessen urinary retention in the postoperative patient may precipitate symptoms consequent to stimulation of parasympathetic nerve responses at other sites (i.e., nausea, vomiting, abdominal cramps, diarrhea, excess salivation, nasal stuffiness, and pupil constriction). Consideration of the problems as related to stimulation of parasympathetic nervous system activity provides an "alert" system for planning surveillance procedures whenever drugs with cholinergic properties are employed for therapy.

Interpretation of observations is an essential element in monitoring a patient's progress. When the patient complains of nasal stuffiness and states his personal diagnosis as the onset of a cold, sharing information about drug action can clarify the problem for him and lessen concern that an intercurrent illness is forthcoming.

Parasympathetic Nerve Blocking Effects. Many drugs are available for use as cholinergic-blocking (parasympatholytic) agents, and many drugs have anticholinergic properties that can

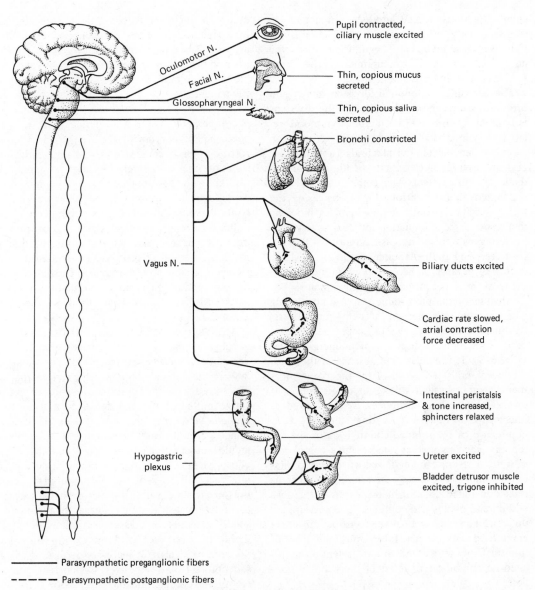

Pupil contracted,
ciliary muscle excited

Thin, copious mucus
secreted

Thin, copious saliva
secreted

Bronchi constricted

Biliary ducts excited

Cardiac rate slowed,
atrial contraction
force decreased

Intestinal peristalsis
& tone increased,
sphincters relaxed

Ureter excited

Bladder detrusor muscle
excited, trigone inhibited

Oculomotor N.

Facial N.

Glossopharyngeal N.

Vagus N.

Hypogastric
plexus

———— Parasympathetic preganglionic fibers

– – – – – Parasympathetic postganglionic fibers

Fig. 6–2. Schematic diagram of the parasympathetic division of the autonomic
nervous system and the effect of nerve stimulation on organ function.

produce side effects while the drugs are being employed for control of physiologic or emotional
problems (i.e., antihistamines; the phenothiazine
group of tranquilizers; the antiarrhythmic drugs
procainamide and quinidine; the tricyclic group

of antidepressants). Although the parasympathetic and sympathetic divisions of the autonomic
nervous system may act reciprocally in control of
organ function, there is generally dominance of
one division in maintaining physiologic equilib-

rium. The division that produces an active response usually predominates (i.e., vasoconstriction over vasodilation). The division producing an active response also predominates when both systems are stimulated simultaneously.

The alternate autonomic division may gain prominence in control when one of the divisions is blocked by drugs. For example, symptoms related to sympathetic nervous system activity can emerge when belladonna alkaloids (anticholinergic) are used to block activity of the parasympathetic nervous system. The belladonna alkaloids are employed for control of gastric spasm, and their pharmacodynamic action involves blocking the response to stimulation by the parasympathetic nerves controlling gastric motility. The patient receiving the belladonna alkaloids will have decreased parasympathetic responses, and sympathetic nervous system activity predominates.

Analysis of the predictable responses occurring when sympathetic nervous system control predominates provides guides to problems that may occur with repeated use of anticholinergic drugs (Fig. 6–3). It is evident that absence of the natural "feed-and-breed" control by the parasympathetic nervous system will result in disruption of several normal body processes. When viewed as interrelated problems occurring consequent to dominance of the sympathetic division of the autonomic nervous system, the patient's complaints of blurred vision can be viewed as related to dilation of pupils; dryness of the mouth and nose as related to constriction of blood vessels in the nose and parotid glands and consequent decreased production of mucus and saliva; constipation as related to decreased peristalsis and inhibition of intestinal sphincters; and urinary retention as related to inhibition of bladder muscle contraction.

The analysis of problems requires knowledge of the primary functions of the parasympathetic and sympathetic divisions of the autonomic nervous system, and it facilitates understanding of the myriad of problems occurring because of chemical properties of many drugs. When any drug is employed for blocking of cholinergic activity or when a drug has anticholinergic properties in addition to the primary constituents, repeated use may lead to symptoms of decreased cholinergic activity. When more than one drug with anticholinergic properties is given concurrently, cholinergic blockade may cause more severe problems for the patient.

Sympathetic Nerve Stimulation Effects. Epinephrine and norepinephrine are the primary neurotransmitter hormones of the sympathetic division of the autonomic nervous system. The well-known "fight-or-flight" mechanisms occur consequent to release of the neurotransmitters from nerve endings and from the adrenal medulla. In several clinical situations the neurotransmitter levels are elevated by administration of drugs for control of problems consequent to deficiency of endogenous hormone (i.e., shock states) or to provide high levels of circulating hormone to control acute physiologic problems (i.e., anaphylaxis).

The neurotransmitter receptors at tissue sites affected by the sympathetic nervous system are described as *adrenergic* receptors. The name relates to the adrenal medulla, which originally was discovered to be the source of the adrenergic neurotransmitters. Drugs are described as *sympathomimetic* when they are employed to supply additional hormone and surveillance is planned to include observations for excess sympathetic nervous system activity. For example, closely spaced intervals will be required for monitoring blood pressure when exogenous norepinephrine (levarterenol bitartrate) is administered to a patient in shock to assure that vasoconstriction provides a therapeutic response without raising the blood pressure to levels that increase the hazard of vessel rupture (toxic response). Concurrent drug effect on the cardiac rate and contraction force may produce side effects evident as tachycardia and arrhythmias as the rate and force of contraction increase.

Receptors of the sympathetic nervous system are described as *alpha-adrenergic receptors* or *beta-adrenergic receptors,* and the characteristics of the receptor govern whether it will respond to a particular natural or synthetic sympathetic stim-

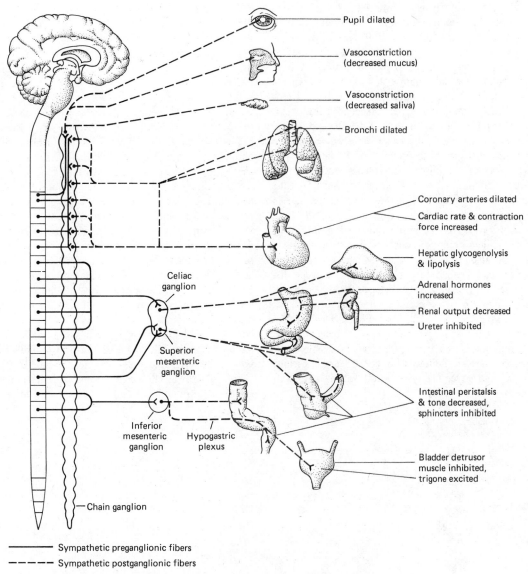

Fig. 6–3. Schematic diagram of the sympathetic division of the autonomic nervous system and the effect of nerve stimulation on organ function.

ulation. Beta-adrenergic receptors are subclassified as beta$_1$ or beta$_2$ receptors. Stimulation of beta$_1$ receptors causes cardioacceleration, and stimulation of beta$_2$ receptors causes bronchodilation.

Norepinephrine released from sympathetic nerve endings primarily excites the alpha-adrenergic receptors, but it may have minor stimulatory effects on beta-adrenergic receptors. Epinephrine excites both types of receptors almost equally.

Physiologic activity is maintained by the natural endogenous supplies of both hormones, which transmit impulses from nerves to tissues and elicit a specific response.

Drugs with differing chemical structures may be employed to stimulate either alpha or beta receptors. Some organs have alpha and beta receptors, and stimulation of each receptor may produce opposite effects or it may produce the same effect. For example, arteries have alpha receptors and stimulation causes constriction of the artery whereas stimulation of the arterial beta receptors causes dilation (Fig. 6–4). Stimulation of either alpha or beta receptors in intestinal tissues causes relaxation.

When drugs are administered for stimulation of particular adrenergic receptors, concurrent effects will be evident in organs having the same receptors. The predictability of problems can be increased by recognizing the responses that can occur when alpha receptors are stimulated at tissue sites: arteries constrict; pupils dilate; intestines relax; piloerector muscles contract; veins constrict. Stimulation of beta receptors causes cardioacceleration: arteries dilate; bronchi dilate; intestines relax; and glycogenolysis and lipolysis occur in the liver.

Sympathetic Nerve Blocking Effects. Drugs may be employed for varying approaches to counteracting the vasoconstricting effects of norepinephrine in patients with hypertension. Several of the antihypertensive drugs commonly employed for control of severe hypertension act by blocking release of the neurotransmitter at ganglionic sites. The neurotransmitter relaying stimuli to the postganglionic fibers of the sympathetic nerve is acetylcholine (Fig. 6–5). When drugs are employed to interfere with acetylcholine at ganglionic sites, concurrent action at other sites of neurotransmitter activity causes side effects. Because the neurotransmitter of the preganglionic and postganglionic sites of the parasympathetic nervous system is acetylcholine, side effects of the drugs will be evidenced by decreased parasympathetic nervous system function. The side effects are more frequent in the gastrointestinal tract because that is the body system in which parasympathetic control predominates. The drugs are employed selectively because side effects occur consequent to blocking of both sympathetic and parasympathetic divisions of the autonomic nervous system (i.e., dryness of mouth, blurring of vision, diarrhea followed by constipation, urinary retention, anorexia, nausea, vomiting, fatigue,

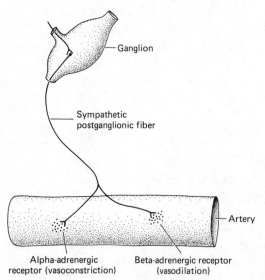

Ganglion

Sympathetic postganglionic fiber

Artery

Alpha-adrenergic receptor (vasoconstriction)

Beta-adrenergic receptor (vasodilation)

Fig. 6–4. Characteristics of the vascular receptors determine the response to sympathetic nerve stimulation.

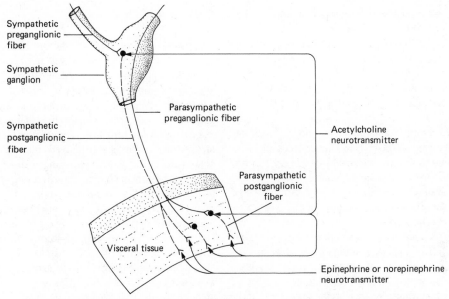

Fig. 6–5. Visceral innervation. Acetylcholine is the neurotransmitter at ganglionic sites in the sympathetic and parasympathetic nervous system and at tissue receptor sites affected by the parasympathetic nerves. Epinephrine or norepinephrine transmits impulses from the sympathetic nerves to the tissue receptors.

drowsiness, dizziness, and interference with sex functions).

ALLERGIC REACTIONS

Allergic responses are an important group of adverse drug reactions occurring during therapy. An allergic response is an abnormal manifestation of the immune response, and drugs may precipitate the reaction by acting as allergens. Drugs from protein sources (i.e., hormones) or small drug particles (haptens) that combine with body proteins are the allergens that interact with antibodies at tissue sites. The allergen-antibody interaction precipitates release of vasoactive intermediates (i.e., histamine, bradykinin) and causes fluid transudation into tissues and manifestations of the allergic response. The allergic reactions are comparable to those occurring with pollens and other antigenic substances and are classified either

as *immediate allergic reactions* or *delayed allergic reactions*.

Immediate Allergic Reactions

Immediate allergic responses occur when a drug allergen is administered to an individual having antibodies produced by prior use of the drug or a closely related pharmacologic agent. Immediate allergic reactions may occur with a single dose of the drug allergen in a sensitized individual. When the drug is being administered on a planned continuing schedule, administration is discontinued if an immediate allergic reaction occurs. *Anaphylaxis, urticaria,* and *angioedema* are immediate allergic responses, and the problems occurring with each type of reaction are a consequence of widely distributed allergen interacting with antibodies at tissue sites to cause fluid transudation.

Anaphylaxis. Dissemination of allergen to widely distributed internal tissue sites causes interaction with antibodies and rapid movement of fluid into tissues and depletion of plasma. Anaphylaxis is a life-threatening episode in which edema of the tracheobronchial structures narrows and finally obstructs the air passages. Concurrent dilation of capillaries rapidly moves fluid out of the vascular bed into tissues throughout the body. The sudden outflow of fluid depletes the circulating plasma volume and increases the viscosity of blood. The rapidly occurring sequence of physiologic changes can lead to cardiopulmonary failure within minutes unless therapy is instituted to halt fluid shifting and to open the airway. Anaphylaxis most frequently occurs when a drug is administered by a parenteral route because the drug immediately is distributed throughout the body by the circulating blood. Emergency treatment includes administration of epinephrine, which is a bronchodilator and a myocardial stimulant. Intensive use of supportive measures is planned until fluid gradually moves from peripheral capillaries and tissues into the circulation.

Urticaria. Generalized pruritic skin eruptions, or giant hives that itch intensely, are manifestations of urticaria. The problems occur when drug allergen and antibodies interact at superficial sites to release vasoactive substances and substances irritating to nerve endings in the skin (i.e., bradykinin). Therapy includes use of an antipruritic lotion to relieve the extreme discomfort of the patient and administration of an antihistamine to halt further activity of the vasoactive substance at tissue sites.

Angioedema. The allergic reaction described as angioedema is manifest as fluid accumulation in periorbital, oral, and respiratory tissues. As bronchial constriction gradually progresses, there is an obvious lengthening of the expiratory phase of respiration and wheezing as bronchial constriction increases. Angioedema may occur in concert with urticaria, or it may appear as a separate entity. Administration of an antihistaminic drug prevents progression of the problem, and natural appearance and function gradually return.

Delayed Allergic Reactions

In some individuals an allergic reaction to a particular drug may occur seven or more days after the drug initially is administered. Delayed allergic responses occur after the drug allergen has precipitated antibody formation. There is a gradual production of antibodies to the drug allergen and symptoms may emerge intermittently or gradually. When the delayed allergic response occurs in an individual requiring a drug for control of a health problem, the offending drug may be discontinued and an alternate drug may be prescribed for control of the patient's problem. In selected instances continued use of the drug may be planned when the drug is known to be highly selective for control of a devastating health problem. Concurrent plans for control of symptoms (i.e., antihistamines, skin lotions) may make therapy tolerable for the patient. The physiologic status of the patient is basic to decisions by the physician to discontinue or retain use of the drug when a delayed allergic reaction occurs. *Serum sickness, Arthus reaction,* and *rash and fever* are manifestations of delayed allergic responses.

Serum Sickness. Symptoms of serum sickness occur seven or more days after initial administration of a drug causing gradual low-level (titer) production of antibodies that interact with circulating drug. Serum sickness involves gradually emerging intermittent episodes of dyspnea, hypotension, generalized edema, joint pain, rash, and swollen lymph glands. Administration of an antihistaminic drug may prevent progression of the problems, but symptoms persist as long as the allergenic drug remains in the body. Antihistamines are usually given for the length of time known to be required for nearly complete elimination of the drug.

Arthus Reaction. Drug allergen interaction with antibodies at localized tissue sites may cause tissue necrosis by disruption of the blood supply. Spasticity, occlusion, and degeneration of blood vessels are precipitated by injection of the drug into a site having large quantities of bivalent antibodies.

Rash and Fever. The occurrence of the common problems of rash and fever in acutely ill patients makes it difficult to discriminate whether the problems are disease or drug related. Discontinuing drug use may alleviate the problems, and the assumption can be made that the drug was the precipitator of the problem. Continuing use of the drug is dependent on priority need for the particular drug for control of the patient's problem and the severity of the reaction.

Topical application of drugs may cause the production of antibodies in the cellular cytoplasm, which causes an allergic response at the site during subsequent drug application (fixed eruptions). Local applications of drugs may also sensitize the individual to subsequent systemic use of the same drug by releasing the drug into the deep tissues where it is absorbed. The production of antibodies that are available in the serum allows any of the foregoing types of allergic responses to occur with rechallenge by the drug or a close chemical relative of the drug originally employed.

DRUG INTERACTIONS

Drugs are agonists or antagonists that interact with receptors to elicit a response. Drugs have affinity for particular tissue sites, and a therapeutic concentration has efficacy in producing a response at selected receptor sites. Therapeutic effectiveness may be affected by the presence of other drugs or food, or differing factors in body systems that influence absorption, biotransformation, or excretion. Within the body drugs may interact to antagonize or enhance the action of other drugs. Although drug interactions are often viewed in terms of the adverse effects of the drugs, interacting drugs may be used concurrently for a desired increase in therapeutic response. The subject of drug interactions is the focus of intensive analysis and research at the present time.

Many drug interactions can be predicted on the basis of chemical or pharmacodynamic factors that influence the absorption, distribution, metabolism, or excretion of each of the drugs and changes that are probable when the drugs are administered concurrently. Drugs known to interact may be administered concurrently when precautions are taken to monitor drug effects or when dosage adjustment is planned to compensate for the altered response. Although the appearance of toxic effects is the most dramatic and most frequently described aspect of drug interactions, it is equally important that drug interactions may decrease the therapeutic benefit to the patient by decreasing the amount of drug available at receptor sites.

Drug Action Summation

The combined or concurrent action of drugs may intensify drug action or modify the incidence of adverse effects through *addition, synergism,* or *potentiation* of drug action. The terms are interpreted in a confusing variety of contexts in the literature; therefore, the definitions offered below are illustrated with examples of each mechanism to clarify the terms.

Addition describes the therapeutic effect of two drugs that is comparable to the effect attained when either drug is administered alone in an amount equivalent to the sum of the two drugs. Concurrent administration of the drugs allows lower dosage of either drug and consequently lessens the incidence of undesirable adverse effects commonly occurring when higher dosage is prescribed. For example, thiazide diuretics and antihypertensive drugs each can be used to control hypertension, but their use in combination controls hypertension and may allow reduction of the dosage of an antihypertensive agent that has disturbing side effects.

Addition of therapeutic effectiveness at lower dosage is an important factor in use of antineoplastic drugs to control cancer cell proliferation. Several combination dosages are employed to provide a multipronged attack on cancer cells. Lower dosage of each of the antineoplastic drugs allows longer periods of therapy with a lower incidence of adverse effects on normal body tissue during therapy.

Synergism describes the interaction of drugs at common receptor sites that intensifies the effect of drugs in disease control. The harmonious interaction of two drugs produces a response greater than that possible when either drug is used alone. For example, *ampicillin* has a bactericidal effect on gram-positive organisms, but the antibacterial effectiveness is broadened to control penicillinase-resistant bacteria when sodium *oxacillin* is administered concurrently.

Some combination drug products are designed to provide a synergistic action for control of persistent health problems. For example, *sulfamethoxazole-trimethoprim* (BACTRIM) is a combination drug available for control of urinary tract infections.

A common example of synergism is the use of diuretics in combination to improve or accelerate the removal of tissue fluid. *Hydrochlorothiazide* and *spironolactone* are frequently prescribed to be taken concurrently, and there is a combination tablet (ALDACTAZIDE) available. Each of the drugs acts at a different site in the renal tubule to prevent the reabsorption of sodium and water. As an added bonus, spironolactone lessens the losses of potassium ions occurring with use of the thiazides.

Additive or synergistic action of drugs may contribute to clinical problems. Concurrent administration of *atropine sulfate* and *meperidine hydrochloride* (DEMEROL), which has atropine-like (anticholinergic) side effects, causes dry mucous membranes, flushing, depressed respirations, and a decrease in intestinal motility. The problems are greater when the drugs are given concurrently than when either drug is used alone.

Knowledge of the possible intensification of drug action when more than one drug is used makes it possible to alert the patient to drug combinations to be avoided. For example, alcohol and other central nervous system depressants (i.e., sedatives, tranquilizers) may act synergistically to cause extreme drowsiness. The patient receiving any central nervous system depressant should know that ingestion of alcohol concurrently can cause drowsiness that endangers safety while doing tasks requiring alertness or while driving a motor vehicle.

Potentiation occurs primarily when drugs interact at common receptors to modify the metabolism or excretion of one of the drugs. Competition for protein-binding sites is an important interaction affecting responses to therapy. For example, *phenylbutazone* has a high affinity for albumin-binding sites, and displacement of oral anticoagulants may allow longer action time and bleeding can occur as the hypoprothrombinemia is potentiated.

Many of the drug interactions properly classified as antagonism result in potentiation of action of one of the drugs involved in the interaction. Some of the common problems will be presented with the discussion of drug antagonism.

Drug-Food Interactions

Drugs and foods may interact to adversely affect the therapeutic plan. For example, ingestion of large quantities of foods with high vitamin K content may inhibit the hypoprothrombinemic effect of oral anticoagulants; antacids may interfere with absorption of drugs (i.e., tetracycline) from the gastrointestinal tract. Some drug-food interactions are not clinically significant, but in some instances common foods (i.e., milk) may interfere with absorption of drugs from the gastrointestinal tract. The drug-food interactions having clinical significance are presented with discussion of drugs within the text.

Drug Antagonism

The opposing action of drugs in body tissues may be classified as *chemical antagonism, pharmacologic antagonism,* or *physiologic antagonism.*

Chemical antagonism is the combining or binding of two drugs that causes inactivation of the chemicals. For example, within the gastrointestinal tract both antacids and kaolin products bind a significant number of drugs and thereby limit the quantity available for absorption. Both groups of drugs have a large surface area, which favors adsorption. *Phenothiazine* tranquilizers and acidic drugs (i.e., phenylbutazone, nitrofurantoin, nalidixic acid, sulfonamides, dicumarol) are adsorbed by antacid and kaolin suspensions. *Kaolin* preparations also may impair absorption of the antibiotic *lincomycin* when the drugs are administered concurrently. Knowledge of chemical antagonism can be employed when planning administration to assure that the drug is given at least one hour before the product that may bind and inactivate it.

Pharmacologic antagonism is the competition of two drugs for a receptor that may allow the weaker drug to block access by the more potent drug. For example, narcotic action at the receptors in the medullary centers causes respiratory depression. Administration of narcotic antagonists for treatment of acute narcotic-induced respiratory depression blocks narcotic attachment to receptors at the center. The narcotic antagonists have a high affinity for the respiratory center receptors. Preferential attachment of the antagonists reestablishes the sensitivity of the centers, and the rate and depth of respirations improve.

Pharmacologic antagonism occurs when phenothiazine tranquilizers, tricyclic antidepressants, or amphetamines are used concurrently with the antihypertensive drug *guanethidine*. The drugs interfere with transport of guanethidine into the sympathetic nerve ending and negate its antihypertensive effect.

Physiologic antagonism is the opposing action of two drugs on body systems that allows cancellation of action by either drug. For example, the planned therapeutic effect of a vasoconstricting drug may be negated by concurrent administration of a pain-relieving drug with smooth muscle-relaxing properties. An alternate drug would be required if pain relief is needed by the patient receiving a vasopressor for maintenance of blood pressure levels.

The concept of physiologic antagonism can be used for the benefit of the patient without introducing changes in the natural physiologic status. For example, atropine sulfate can be administered to antagonize the smooth muscle spasms of the biliary tract often induced by morphine sulfate.

Enzyme Induction

Drugs may accelerate their own metabolism or increase the rate of metabolism of other drugs by inducing activity of the hepatic microsomal system. Rapid rates of biotransformation may decrease the intensity and duration of drug action, reduce drug toxicity, or contribute to the development of tolerance by increasing the rate at which drugs are converted to inactive metabolites.

The degree of enzyme induction and susceptibility to induction is genetically determined; therefore, problems with enzyme induction are not consistently evident in individuals receiving drugs described as causing interactions by enzyme induction. For example, inherited differences in genetic makeup are known to accelerate metabolism of the anticonvulsant drug *phenytoin* and the anti-inflammatory butaxones by the process of enzyme induction, but only those individuals susceptible to induction will require higher dosage to maintain therapeutic plasma levels of the drug.

Drugs can stimulate the activity of oxidizing enzymes and reduce the pharmacodynamic activity of another drug by accelerating its metabolic inactivation. Chronic use of drugs (i.e., alcohol, barbiturates, glutethimide, griseofulvin, phenytoin) maintains a consistently high level of enzyme activity and a predisposition to rapid metabolism of drugs requiring oxidizing enzymes for biotransformation. For example, alcohol is converted into *acetaldehyde* primarily by hepatic oxidizing enzymes; thus heavy drinkers have an increased level of oxidating enzymes. The continual demand for enzymatic metabolism of alcohol primes the enzymes, and during periods of sobriety drugs may be metabolized rapidly. Barbiturates and other sedatives may have less effect on the alcoholic when sober because oxidizing enzymes rapidly metabolize the drugs to inactive metabolites.

Dosage of drugs may be raised to compensate for the lower concentration occurring when the individual is predisposed to enzyme induction by prior use of inducing drugs, but problems arise when the inducing drug is discontinued. To avoid emergence of toxic effects of the second drug, the dosage is usually lowered when there is evidence that enzyme activity has returned to a normal level. For example, phenobarbital causes enzyme induction and with its administration the liver microsomes contain more oxidase and reductase. Normal sedative doses of *phenobarbital* reduce the concentration of coumarins in plasma and reduce their pharmacodynamic action. When phenobarbital is discontinued, the patient may hemorrhage if the oral anticoagulant is continued at previous levels because the enzyme system returns to a normal functional level. The anticoagulant is inactivated more slowly than when phenobarbital is inducing the enzymes required for coumarin metabolism.

Enzyme Inhibition

Drugs that inhibit enzyme activity prolong the time-action span of other drugs dependent on the enzymes for inactivation. Enzyme inhibition is seen more consistently in patients receiving drugs known to slow enzyme activity because the inhibition is drug induced rather than genetically determined. Enzyme inhibition may result from *competitive inhibition or noncompetitive inhibition* of drugs at hepatic enzyme sites.

Competitive Inhibition. A single very large dose of alcohol taken with another drug may inhibit the drug metabolism by competing with the drug for the enzymes of the oxidase system that metabolize alcohol. In addition to the depressant effect of alcohol on the central nervous system, the enzyme competition enhances the sensitivity to barbiturates and other sedatives when the individual is drinking heavily at the time of drug use. The synergistic action of alcohol and sedatives in the brain can cause death.

Noncompetitive Inhibition. Drugs can inhibit enzymes to the point where they are not available to act on a second drug that is dependent on the enzyme system for metabolism. The process is an example of noncompetitive inhibition. For example, *allopurinol* is a *xanthine oxidase inhibitor,* and the antineoplastic drugs *mercaptopurine* and

azathioprine are metabolized to uric acid analogs by *xanthine oxidase*. Absence of the enzyme activity because of allopurinol inhibition would cause toxicity of the antineoplastic drugs (i.e., fatal bone marrow aplasia) if the drugs were given concurrently at usual therapeutic dosage levels. Antineoplastics usually are prescribed at one fourth the usual dosage level when it is necessary to use allopurinol concurrently.

Excretion Inhibition

Interaction of drugs at active transport sites in the renal nephron may inhibit excretion of one of the drugs when drugs compete for a common transport site. For example, the blocking of tubular active carrier systems by *probenecid* has been used to therapeutic advantage. Probenecid lessens the secretion of aminosalicylic acid when the drugs are administered concurrently, and probenecid block of the carrier systems maintains circulating levels of *aminosalicylic acid* for a longer period of time.

The interaction of drugs at tubular sites can cause retention of drug and consequent toxic levels in the circulating fluids. For example, phenylbutazone may block secretion of the active metabolite (hydroxyhexamide) of the oral hypoglycemic drug *acetohexamide,* and a prolongation of hypoglycemic action occurs as the metabolite continues activity in circulating fluids:

Acetohexamide

> hydroxhexamide (active metabolite)

PHENYLBUTAZONE

Block

Renal tubule secretion

Urine

NURSING CARE

The foregoing discussion of mechanisms involved in adverse drug reactions allows analysis of problems and study of drugs within a pharmacodynamic frame of reference. Additional examples are presented in subsequent discussions throughout the text, and the presentations include nursing implications of drug action.

Preplanning for assessment of adverse drug reactions is an important aspect of the drug therapy regimen for each patient. Adverse reactions may simply constitute an annoyance for the patient, and simple nursing measures may alleviate the problem. For example, frequent mouth care or sucking on hard candy may lessen the discomfort of the dry mouth occurring when drugs with anticholinergic properties (i.e., belladonna alkaloids, phenothiazines) are given. When the therapeutic index of drugs is low (i.e., antineoplastics, oral hypoglycemics, insulin, antiarrhythmic drugs, digitalis) or the acutely ill patient has complex interrelated problems, it is essential to preplan for assessment of progress and emerging problems at closely scheduled intervals to identify early evidence of status changes indicating adverse reactions during drug therapy. For example, it is common practice to check the quality, regularity, and rate of the apical pulse before administration of *digitalis* as a precaution against giving the drug when bradycardia or arrhythmias have occurred as toxic manifestations of drug action.

Drugs may occasionally be used to control side effects that are unrelated to the primary action of the drug being employed for therapy. For example, administration of antacids is a routine part of the therapeutic plan for patients receiving glucocorticoids. The adrenal cortical hormone may be prescribed for a primary action in control of an inflammatory response, but the drugs also cause gastric hyperacidity. Concurrent administration of gastric antacids decreases the ulcerogenic potential of the glucocorticoids.

Additional Readings

Arndt, Kenneth A., and Jick, Hershel: Rates of cutaneous reactions to drugs. *J.A.M.A.*, **235**:918, March 1, 1976.

Bergman, H. David: Drug-induced diseases and disorders. *The Apothecary*, **89**:16, July–August, 1977.

Black, Curtis D.: Popovich, Nicholas G.; and Black, Marilyn C.: Drug interactions in the G I tract. *Am. J. Nurs.*, **77**:1426, September, 1977.

Deforges, Jane F.: Current concepts: genetic implications of G-6-PD deficiency. *N. Engl. J. Med.*, **294**:1438, June 24, 1976.

Evaluations of Drugs Interactions, 2nd ed. American Pharmaceutical Association, Washington, D.C., 1976.

Galton, Lawrence: Drugs and the elderly. *Nursing '76*, **6**:38, August, 1976.

Hartshorn, Edward A.: *Handbook of Drug Interactions*, 3rd ed. Drug Intelligence Publications, Hamilton, Ill., 1976.

Hussar, Daniel A.: Drug interactions: good and bad. *Nursing '76* **6**:61, September, 1976.

Isselbacher, Kurt J.: Metabolic and hepatic effects of alcohol. *N. Engl. J. Med.*, **296**:612, March 17, 1977.

Karch, Fred E., and Lasagna, Louis: Adverse drug reactions: a critical review. *J.A.M.A.*, **234**:1236, December 22, 1975.

Lenhart, Dorothy Garrahan: The use of medications in the elderly population. *Nurs. Clin. North Am.*, **11**:135, March, 1976.

Mattar, Mary E.; Markello, James; and Yaffee, Sumner J.: Pharmaceutical factors affecting pediatric compliance. *Pediatrics*, **55**:101, January, 1975.

Mouat, David: Evaluating dysfunction of the autonomic nervous system. *Geriatrics*, **33**:83, *April*, 1978.

Romankiewicz, John A.: Effects of antacids on gastrointestinal absorption of drugs. *Primary Care*, **3**:537, September, 1976.

Shimomura, Sam K., and Watanabe, Arthur S.: Adverse drug reactions. *Drug Intelligence Clin. Pharm.*, **9**:190, April, 1975.

Sibulkin, David: Drug eruptions. *Primary Care*, **5**:233, June, 1978.

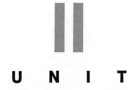

UNIT

Drugs Used to Maintain Hemodynamic Equilibrium

7

Cardiac Failure

Hemodynamic equilibrium is dependent on continual physiologic adjustments that maintain the cardiac output, vascular tone, and blood volume required to circulate blood in quantities sufficient to meet the continually changing metabolic activity. Tissue health is dependent on the adaptive responses that modify cardiac output, vascular tone, or blood volume to transport oxygen and nutrients and to remove metabolic wastes during varying activity periods.

Physiologic Correlations

CARDIAC OUTPUT

The heart is a high-energy physiologic pump that forcefully ejects blood at pressure adequate to perfuse the pulmonary and peripheral capillary beds. The rate of contraction and the stroke output volume affect the amount of blood pumped into the circulation. The average stroke output volume is approximately 70 ml/minute. At a contraction rate of 72 per minute, the total cardiac output per minute would be 5040 ml. The quantity of blood pumped into the aorta is directly related to the amount of blood in the ventricle at the end of the diastolic filling period (end-diastolic volume).

When the individual is at rest, approximately 5 liters of blood returns to the heart from the venous circulation each minute, and the heart pumps that volume of blood forward to the pulmonary and peripheral circulation. Blood distends the cardiac chambers and cardiac contraction is more forceful when activity increases the volume of blood entering the heart. In healthy young adults the heart can pump up to four times the normal amount of blood during periods of activity and the per minute volume entering the heart may rise 400 percent before the cardiac reserve, or pumping capacity, is exceeded. The increased rate and force of cardiac contraction are dependent on an increase in the coronary artery blood flow to the myocardium. In the presence of moderate coronary artery disease, the cardiac reserve may be only one and one-half times the resting capacity.

Cardiac Pressures

The venous blood pressure is approximately 5 mm Hg (mean value) at the junction of the superior and inferior vena cava and the right atrium (Fig. 7–1). The pressure is further reduced during filling of the atrial chamber. Contraction of the right atrium empties the blood through the tricuspid valve into the right ventricle. Closure of the tricuspid valve and right ventricular contraction elevate the chamber pressure. During systole the mean pressure of blood in the pulmonary artery is 15 mm Hg. When the ventricle relaxes, closure of the valve maintains the blood pressure high enough to move the blood through the pulmonary capillary bed and pulmonary veins and into the left atrium.

Contraction of the left atrium empties the blood through the bicuspid, or mitral, valve into the left ventricle. Closure of the bicuspid valve is followed by ventricular contraction, which elevates the blood pressure enough to propel it through the extensive arterial vascular system supplying capillary beds. Lower pressures at the capillary beds represent widespread distribution of the blood that is supplied by the arteries, but the pressure remains adequate to facilitate diffusion of electrolytes, oxygen, and nutrients at tissue sites.

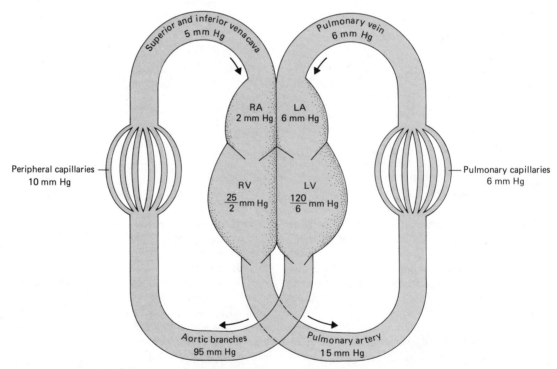

Fig. 7–1. Pressure in the right ventricle at systole propels blood through the pulmonary circulation. The higher pressure level in the left ventricle at systole provides the force required to propel blood through the extensive peripheral arterial circulation. Numerical values show ventricular systolic and diastolic levels and mean pressures for blood vessels.

Autoregulation of Cardiac Output

The inherent capacity of cardiac tissue to modify the contractile force in response to the changing quantities of blood in the heart chambers is described as *autoregulation*. When activity elevates the quantity of blood returning to the heart, the cardiac muscle fibers stretch to accommodate the greater volume of blood in the heart chambers. Within the limits of the cardiac reserve, the increased muscle stretching strengthens the force of contraction. The law of the heart as described by Frank-Starling points to the fact that an increased volume of blood stretching the cardiac muscle fibers during diastole will provide a stronger force of myocardial contraction during systole. The forceful contraction pumps a larger volume of blood into the aorta during systole.

Pacemaker Conduction Pathway

The pumping action of the heart occurs consequent to stimulation of the myocardium by impulses conducted from the sinoatrial (SA) node. The SA node is the "pacemaker," or initiator, of impulses in the coordinated heart. The impulse from the SA node initiates depolarization of the cardiac tissues and the tissue remains refractory until it can repolarize. A second stimulus arriving from the pacemaker during the refractory period cannot initiate depolarization.

An SA node–initiated impulse travels throughout the atria and provides the stimulus for atrial contraction. When the impulse reaches the atrioventricular (AV) node, there is a slight delay in transmission across the node before the impulse is conducted to the bundle of His and the Purkinje fibers to provide the stimulus for ventricular contraction.

Automaticity of Myocardial Cells

The SA and AV nodal cells have an intrinsic capacity for spontaneous depolarization, or *automaticity,* and the cells can achieve threshold potential without stimulation. Leakage of potassium ions from the cells allows attainment of threshold potential. The membrane becomes permeable to sodium ions when threshold is reached. Rapid entrance of the electrolyte into the cell causes the interior to become positively charged and the polar nature of the resting membrane is broken. Depolarization of the cell begins at one point and is conducted along the membrane as sodium permeability spreads sequentially. The syncytial arrangement of the myocardial cells allows rapid spread of electrical impulses unimpeded by membrane barriers.

Membrane Depolarization

Potassium, sodium, and calcium ions are involved in the electrical processes by which the action potential moves along the surface of the cell and into the cell to stimulate myocardial contraction. When the myocardial cell is stimulated, sodium ions cross to the intracellular surface of the membrane and a comparable amount of potassium ions cross to the extracellular surface (Fig. 7–2). Depolarization occurs as sodium ions increase the electropositive field along the inside of the membrane. Propagation of the action potential along the membrane and into the cell is accompanied by diffusion of calcium into the cell. In the presence of calcium ions (and magnesium ions), the muscle fibers contract.

Repolarization: The "Sodium Pump"

Electropositivity of the intracellular surface of the cell during early diastole is reversed by active extrusion of sodium ions concurrent with inward transport of potassium ions across the membrane (Fig. 7–2). The energy required for the active transport process is released by the hydrolysis of *adenosine triphosphate* (ATP) to *adenosine diphosphate* (ADP). The active transport mechanism is described as the "sodium pump," and the enzyme *sodium, potassium, adenosine triphosphatase* (Na+, K+, –ATPase) is the catalyst for the hydrolysis of ATP. Magnesium is a metallocoenzyme necessary for activation of ATPase activity. The "sodium pump" mechanism exchanges sodium and potassium ions across the membrane

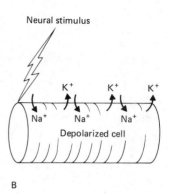

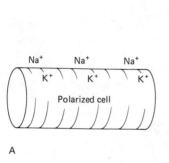

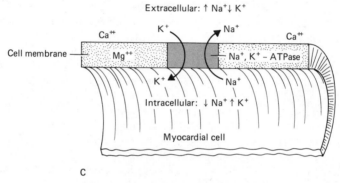

Fig 7–2. *A.* The ionic impermeability of the resting, or polarized, membrane is maintained by the net negative charge of the potassium ions on the inside and the net positive charge of the sodium ions on the outside of the membrane. *B.* Neural stimulation changes the membrane permeability, and the electrolytes are exchanged across the membrane. *C.* Repolarization occurs as the membrane enzyme (Na^+, K^+, -ATPase) initiates hydrolysis of ATP and the release of energy for transport of sodium and potassium ions across the membrane.

against a concentration gradient and the membrane returns to a resting state when the exchange is completed.

Autonomic Nervous System Controls

Cardiac responses to the changing demands of tissues for supplies of oxygen and nutrients are mediated primarily through autonomic nervous system control of pacemaker impulses. Balanced interaction between the parasympathetic and sympathetic divisions of the autonomic nervous system influences the number of conducted impulses that are required to increase or decrease cardiac output during periods of activity or rest.

Parasympathetic Nerve Control. Maintenance of cardiac output during rest periods represents the parasympathetic nerve control of cardiac tone mediated through the vagus nerve. Stimulation of the vagus nerve depresses cardiac activity by decreasing the number of impulses transmitted from the SA node and decreasing excitability of the AV node. The dual action decreases the number of impulses and slows the transmission of impulses to the ventricles (Fig. 7–3).

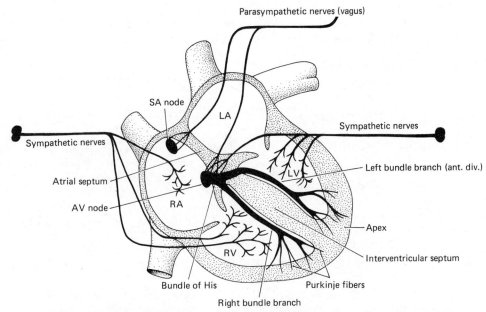

Fig. 7–3. The parasympathetic and sympathetic divisions of the autonomic nervous system mediate control of cardiac conduction and contraction through nerve endings distributed throughout the pacemaker and myocardial tissue.

The vagus nerve often is described as a wandering nerve because it provides approximately 75 percent of the parasympathetic nerve transmission pathway for control of widely distributed organ sites in the chest and abdomen. Stimulation of the afferent vagus nerve endings at any organ receptor mediates impulses to the medulla integrating center, and there is a consequent increase in vagal control mediated by the efferent nerve to the organ. For example, distention of the stomach or intestine can stimulate the vagus nerve endings and subsequent stimuli will increase motility of the gastrointestinal tract. Concurrent with the nerve transmission to the digestive tract, the vagus nerve branch to cardiac sites may decrease the number of impulses and slow the transmission of impulses through the SA and AV nodes. For example, a heavy meal distends the stomach, and the vagus nerve stimulation of motility and secretions facilitates digestion of the food. The concurrent vagus nerve effect on cardiac output is accompanied by a lower pulse rate and decreased cardiac output, which are clearly evident as the individual becomes lethargic and sleepy immediately following the ingestion of a heavy meal.

Sympathetic Nerve Control. Stimulation of cardiac activity to meet the requirements of increased physiologic work is mediated through the sympathetic division of the autonomic nervous system. Sympathetic, or adrenergic, receptors in cardiac tissue respond to the neurotransmitters: the norepinephrine released from nerve endings and epinephrine released into the bloodstream by the adrenal medulla.

Stimuli can originate as psychologic or physiologic factors that stimulate sympathetic nerve-mediated cardiac responses to meet body requirements during a short-term or a prolonged "alert" state. Sympathetic nerve stimulation accelerates the cardiac rate, conduction velocity, and contractile force to increase the cardiac output required for the circulation of blood providing the oxygen and nutrients for the higher metabolic work level.

Cardiac response occurs as the sympathetic neuro-transmitters stimulate receptors in the SA and AV nodal tissues and receptors scattered throughout myocardial tissue (Fig. 7–3). The increased pulse rate is an indicator of the cardiac response, and the individual shows alertness and physical readiness for the increased activity (i.e., increased depth and rate of respirations, increased muscle tension).

Pathophysiologic Correlations

CARDIAC FAILURE

Cardiac failure exists when, in the presence of adequate venous return to the heart, cardiac output is inadequate to meet the metabolic requirements for circulating blood. The severity of symptoms occurring consequent to cardiac failure is directly related to whether decompensation is acute or chronic, which, in turn, is related to the factor or factors leading to cardiac failure.

Compensatory Mechanisms

When cardiac output decreases, compensatory mechanisms are mobilized in a natural physiologic response to the decreased circulation to peripheral tissues. Sympathetic nerve activity accelerates the heart rate and redistributes blood by constriction of arterioles at renal, splanchnic, muscle, and cutaneous capillary beds. The process shunts blood to organs vitally involved in life-sustaining metabolic activities. In response to decreased renal blood flow, compensatory mechanisms acting directly through hormonal systems (i.e., antidiuretic hormone, the renin-angiotensin-aldosterone system) cause reabsorption of sodium and water at renal tubule sites and the process augments the intravascular blood volume. The resulting increased venous return to the heart lengthens myocardial fibers at the end of diastole and there is a transient increase in stroke volume output.

High-Output Failure

High-output failure may occur when the maximal cardiac output is insufficient to meet the high requirements for circulating blood in some extra-cardiac conditions (i.e., severe anemia, hyperthyroidism). Correction of the precipitating extracardiac problem reduces the metabolic requirements (i.e., transfusion of whole blood in anemia) and equalizes the relationship between cardiac output and tissue requirements for oxygen and nutrients.

Low-Output Failure

The most common type of cardiac failure is low-output failure. Impaired myocardial contraction force can occur consequent to decreased blood flow through the coronary arteries or resistance to emptying of the heart chambers. Either left heart failure or right heart failure interferes with forward movement of blood and precipitates symptoms related to deficiency of the blood supply required for physiologic function.

Left Heart Failure. Low cardiac output and incomplete emptying of the left ventricle increase the residual volume. The pressure of blood in the ventricle builds and the chamber becomes abnormally distended during diastole. When ventricular blood content stretches the muscle fibers beyond their ability to recoil forcefully, systolic contraction is diminished and cardiac output is reduced. Retention of blood in the ventricle at the end of diastole causes a progressive increase in the blood volume and an elevated pressure in the left atrium, pulmonary veins, and pulmonary capillary beds. The elevated blood pressure distends the capillaries and fluid transudates into the alveoli. The effect on respiration is directly related to the amount of fluid seeping into the alveoli and the ability of the lymphatics to remove the added fluid. The severity of symptoms is related to whether pulmonary fluid accumulation leads to interstitial edema (pulmonary congestion) or alveolar edema (pulmonary edema).

A commonly observed problem is the sequence of events occurring consequent to strenuous activity in individuals with a low cardiac reserve (i.e., elderly individuals). During activity, tissue requirements for oxygen and nutrients increase the heart rate. When the cardiac output is insufficient to meet tissue requirements, fatigue, weakness, or dizziness may alert the individual to the need to rest. The decreased cardiac output reflexly increases sympathetic nervous system stimuli and tachycardia, vasoconstriction, and sweating occur as physiologic compensatory responses. Continuing the activity beyond the point of decompensation gradually elevates the pulmonary venous pressure. Signs of pulmonary congestion (persistent cough, exertional or paroxysmal nocturnal dyspnea, orthopnea) may appear several hours later even though the individual rests after the period of activity.

Right Heart Failure.   Failure of the right ventricle increases the end-diastolic volume and lessens the contractile force of the right ventricle. Back pressure to the atria and the superior and inferior vena cava gradually distends systemic veins and the increased venous blood volume retards reabsorption of extracellular fluid at tissue sites. Hepatomegaly, splenomegaly, ascites, and engorgement of superficial veins (i.e., jugular) occur as the venous volume and pressure rise. Fluid transudates from the distended venules and capillaries into those sites providing the least resistance to fluid flow. The gradual outflow of fluid causes edema at dependent areas in peripheral tissues (i.e., ankles, gluteal areas).

Therapy

In an acute situation, use of drugs (cardiac glycoside, diuretic), restriction of sodium and fluid intake, and activity modification are required to improve the cardiac output and decrease fluid accumulation at pulmonary and peripheral sites. Elimination of the cause of congestive heart failure may be possible in some situations (i.e., surgical replacement of stenosed heart valves, treatment of hypertension), but many individuals with a low cardiac reserve will require continued treatment to maintain their cardiac output at a level sufficient for them to continue their normal activities of daily living. Diuretics play a vital role in acute or long-term control of circulating blood volume, and total body fluid volume. Diuretic therapy will be discussed in Chapter 14. The type and extent of underlying heart disease are important determinants of the individual's clinical response to treatment with digitalis glycosides.

Cardiac Glycosides

Digitalis glycosides were originally obtained from the foxglove plant and they have been employed for centuries for the control of cardiac problems. In 1785, William Withering first described the therapeutic action of digitalis, but only in the past 25 years have most of the pharmacologic mechanisms been clarified. Although the drug is frequently prescribed for control of cardiac failure, there is only limited knowledge of the specific changes effected at myocardial tissue sites. The complexity of hemodynamic factors involved in cardiac function (i.e., autonomic nervous system responses, conduction variables) complicates the process of delineating specific digitalis-induced responses.

The term *digitalis* is often employed to designate the entire class of cardiac glycosides that are obtained as active ingredients from various plants (i.e., digitalis, squill, strophanthus). Each of the glycosides consists of an aglycone, or genin (the core molecule), coupled with one to four sugar or saccharide molecules.

The aglycone is the source of the pharmacologic action of the glycoside. The aglycones in cardiac glycosides are steroids with similar structural features. The steroids are chemically similar to adrenocortical hormones, sex hormones, bile acids, and sterols. Although the sugar molecules attached to the aglycones differ, each sugar influences the solubility of the glycoside thereby affecting the absorption, distribution, cell permeability, and potency of the glycoside.

TERMINOLOGY

Chronotropic, dromotropic, and *inotropic* are the terms commonly employed to describe the effects of drugs on the heart. The terms are defined as follows:

Chronotropic: affecting the firing rate of the sinoatrial node (heart rate)

Dromotropic: affecting impulse conduction (conduction time)

Inotropic: affecting the strength of muscular contractility (force of contraction)

When the terms are utilized to describe drug effect, they are usually expressed as positive or negative outcomes. For example, digitalis has a *positive inotropic effect* (increased contraction force), *negative chronotropic effect* (decreased rate), and *negative dromotropic effect* (slowed conduction).

DRUG THERAPY

Cardiotonic is the term employed to describe the powerful stimulating action of drugs on the myocardium; the cardiotonic action is exemplified by digitalis and the cardiac glycosides. Because the drugs strengthen the force of systolic contraction and thereby improve cardiac output, they are employed primarily for control of acute heart failure and for long-term therapy to prevent recurrence of failure.

Digitalis glycosides also are used to protect the ventricular rate in the presence of atrial dysrhythmias (i.e., atrial fibrillation, atrial flutter). The glycosides slow transmission across the atrioventricular node and the number of impulses conducted from the atria to the ventricles is reduced.

Action Mode

The direct pharmacodynamic action of digitalis on cardiac tissue affects the excitation-conduction-contraction sequence. The glycosides inhibit the Na+, K+, −ATPase transport mechanism thereby lessening the exchange of sodium ions for potassium ions during repolarization. Intracellular accumulation of sodium ions activates the sodium-calcium ion-exchange mechanism. The removal of sodium ions from intracellular fluid is accompanied by an influx of calcium ions. The movement of calcium ions to the cellular reticulum favors the contraction of the myofibrils.

The digitalis glycosides have direct and indirect effects on the SA nodal tissue. The direct effects decrease the firing rate of the pacemaker and prolong transmission through the AV node. The indirect effects of the glycosides occur partially by their increasing the sensitivity of the carotid baroreceptors. A lower blood pressure stimulates the baroreceptors and there is an increase in vagal stimuli to pacemaker tissue. Concurrently there is a decreased responsiveness of the pacemaker tissue to sympathetic nervous system stimulation.

The effectiveness of digitalis in the control of ventricular response to atrial dysrhythmias also is represented by the direct and indirect effects of the glycosides. Digitalis directly decreases the AV node conduction velocity and prolongs the functional refractory period of the nodal tissue. The glycosides also reflexly increase vagal stimulation and reduce cardiac responses to sympathetic nerve stimuli. The dual action of digitalis delays conduction through the AV node and slows the ventricular contraction rate. When employed for treatment of atrial fibrillation, the ventricular response to atrial impulses can gradually be reduced from 200 beats/minute to 90 beats/minute by the glycoside.

Physiologic Outcomes

The positive effects of digitalis glycosides occur as a consequence of improved ventricular contractility and slowing of the heart rate. The increased contraction force of a dilated decompensated heart gradually returns it to near-normal size as its tension returns. Slowing of the heart rate is accomplished by a decrease in the sensitivity to sympathetic stimuli that induce tachycardia. The stroke volume increases as cardiac deceleration allows a more complete filling and the increased force of contraction assures a more complete emptying of the ventricles. A moderate fall in the diastolic blood pressure is a reflection of decreased vasoconstriction, and the widened pulse pressure indicates clearly the decrease in compensatory responses as cardiac output improves.

Venous pressure is reduced and circulation improves as blood returning to the heart enters the cardiac chambers without the resistance presented by ventricles incompletely emptied during systole. The improved pulmonary circulation facilitates gas exchange across the alveolar capillary membrane, slows the respiratory and pulse rates, and increases the vital capacity of the lungs. The return of normal circulation at the capillary beds also allows return of extracellular fluid to the venous circulation and tissue edema is reduced. As congestion in major organs is reduced, normal function returns. For example, decreased congestion in gastrointestinal tissues is accompanied by improved appetite and bowel elimination.

Improved blood circulation caused by digitalis also increases renal perfusion. As the circulating blood volume decreases, edematous fluid readily moves from tissue sites to the vasculature. The increased renal blood flow and mobilization of edematous fluid combine to accelerate urine formation, and copious amounts of urine with a low specific gravity often are eliminated by the patient about 24 hours after digitalis therapy is started.

Adverse Reactions

Digitalis glycosides have one of the lowest therapeutic indexes of all drugs. The therapeutic dose is approximately 35 percent of the toxic dose. About 20 percent of patients taking the glycosides exhibit some type of adverse reaction during the course of treatment.

The toxicity of the glycosides affects almost all body systems. Digitalis has a high toxic mortality rate in patients with cardiac failure. Measurements of serum digitalis concentrations aid in the recognition of digitalis toxicity when the data are interpreted in the context of the total clinical status of the individual. Patients who demonstrate serum glycoside concentrations about twice the mean therapeutic serum level are at a toxic level. Because the ratio between serum and myocardial glycoside concentration is relatively constant, serum glycoside concentration is a useful indicator of the drug concentration available for the myocardial receptors.

The *radioimmunoassay* technique employed in the laboratory has made it possible to measure serum levels of digoxin, digitoxin, and ouabain with great sensitivity and specificity. Antibodies, produced specifically in response to the stimulus of a drug given to a donor animal, provide an immune reaction with radioactively tagged drug plus the unknown amount of drug in the patient's serum to give a highly reliable measurement of a drug in the serum. To be effective, blood samples for the assay are drawn after sufficient time has elapsed for drug absorption and attainment of serum-tissue concentration equilibrium (i.e., six hours after oral administration of digoxin).

Digitalis Intoxication. The effects of elevated serum digitalis levels on brain tissues may precipitate gastrointestinal, neurologic, psychiatric, or visual problems. Although the effects, in general, are not serious problems, they may be harbingers of life-threatening cardiac toxicity. Manifestations of cardiac toxicity include a variety of atrial and ventricular arrhythmias and conduction disturbances caused by direct myocardial tissue effects or indirectly through the central nervous system cardiac control centers. When symptoms of toxicity appear, the drug should be discontinued. Therapy may be resumed when serum drug levels are within the normal range and symptoms subside.

Gastrointestinal Problems. Anorexia, nausea, and vomiting may be early manifestations of digitalis toxicity, and the problems occur in 20 to 30 percent of patients taking the glycosides. The problems occur secondary to the effects of high serum drug levels, which act on the chemoreceptor trigger zone in the medulla vomiting center. The symptoms can appear regardless of the route of administration of the drug. Anorexia often is the initial symptom described by the patient. It may be followed by nausea and excess salivation.

Gastrointestinal symptoms also may be caused by mechanisms other than central nervous system irritation. Orally administered digitalis may irritate the gastric mucosa and cause gastric distress or diarrhea. Elevated digitalis serum levels also cause slight vasoconstriction in some of the arterial beds, and the decreased blood supply may precipitate symptoms. For example, ischemia of the mesenteric tissue may cause abdominal pain or discomfort when serum levels are elevated.

Neurologic Problems. Easy fatigability, generalized muscle weakness, headache, drowsiness, vertigo, or confusion may occur early in digitalis intoxication as a consequence of the direct effect of elevated serum glycoside levels on brain cells. Additional evidence of the irritating effects on nerves appears as pain with paresthesias in the mandibular or lumbar area, or in the extremities. In addition to the neurologic problems, psychiatric manifestations may occur (i.e., apathy, depression, personality changes, irritability, insomnia) in individuals with a marginal blood supply to cerebral tissues (i.e., elderly patients with atherosclerosis).

Neurologic and psychiatric problems are prognostically important because they signal that digitalis toxicity is impending. Separating the problems and identifying them as related to digitalis toxicity may be a difficult task in situations where the clinical condition of the patient includes episodes of compromised circulation to cerebral tissues.

Visual Disturbances. Visual disturbances, as manifestations of toxicity, seldom occur with use of the modern purified glycosides. Because the problems can occur after gastrointestinal symptoms or cardiac arrhythmias, they may seem less important, from the patient's point of view, than other physiologic problems. It may be necessary to inquire about the presence of visual problems because patients seldom report them voluntarily. When queried, patients may describe difficulty in reading because of dimmed vision (amblyopia), blurred vision (diplopia), halos around dark objects, blind spots in the visual field (scotomata), or disturbances of yellow vision (xanthopsia) or of green and other color perception.

Cardiac Arrhythmias. Arrhythmias can occur when there are abnormal serum or tissue levels of the electrolytes affecting cardiac conduction and contraction (i.e., low potassium, high calcium, low or high magnesium ion levels). Hypokalemia is the electrolyte imbalance most commonly contributing to cardiac irritability. Toxic effects of digitalis may be diminished by administration of potassium chloride. When the serum potassium level is elevated to the normal range, potassium ions decrease binding of the glycoside to ATPase.

Cardiac arrhythmias occur in approximately 80 to 90 percent of patients with digitalis toxicity, and they arise as early manifestations of elevated drug levels in myocardial tissues. In toxicity most of the Na+, K+, −ATPase receptors may be blocked by digitalis and the inhibiting of repolarization increases myocardial irritability. Blocking of the receptors by the glycoside prevents the transfer of potassium ions into the cell and serum potassium levels are elevated.

When the individual is receiving a digitalis glycoside, any alteration in cardiac rhythm is suspected of being related to digitalis toxicity until proven otherwise. Arrhythmias of almost any known type may occur (i.e., atrial or ventricular tachycardia, ectopic beats in the atria or the ventricles, sinus bradycardia). In adults, premature ventricular contractions (PVCs) are the most common arrhythmia, occurring in approximately one third of patients with toxicity. Coupled beats (bigeminy) or multifocal PVCs are particularly characteristic manifestations of toxicity. Rhythm disturbances occur only at high serum levels in children and they are usually ectopic atrial or nodal beats. Ectopic beats occur as a consequence of increased automaticity of the myocardium secondary to excess tissue concentrations of digitalis.

Heart block, ventricular tachycardia, and ventricular fibrillation are life-threatening conduction disturbances. AV block occurs in 25 percent of the patients with drug-induced arrhythmias and the block to AV nodal impulse transmission may be partial or complete.

Hospitalized patients with digitalis-induced arrhythmias are placed on a cardiac monitor, and electrocardiographic (ECG) recordings are made when arrhythmias occur in any setting. Toxic levels of digitalis reduce the conduction velocity and increase the refractoriness of nodal tissue. The problem is evident as a prolonged PR interval on the cardiac monitor or on the ECG recordings. Shortening of the Q-T interval reflects excitability and reduced refractoriness of ventricular tissue. The direct effect of digitalis on repolarization is reflected by recordings that show deflection of the ST segment and the T wave in a direction opposite to that of the QRS complex.

Discontinuance of drug administration allows drug metabolism and elimination to lower the serum and tissue levels. After the drug is discontinued, the cardiac arrhythmia may subside in a period of time approximately equal to one half-life of the drug. Treatment of the arrhythmia depends on the hemodynamic consequences of the abnormal rhythm and the potential for emergence of serious arrhythmias. For example, antiarrhythmic drug therapy may be instituted when there are several PVCs per minute because the high level of myocardial irritability that they represent may lead to ventricular fibrillation and cardiac arrest. Further discussion of cardiac arrhythmias will be presented in Chapter 8.

Drug Interactions

The principal interactions of concern during digitalis therapy are those related to concurrent use of drugs that cause a decrease in serum potassium levels. Control of edema for the patient with congestive heart failure often requires the use of potent diuretics (i.e., ethacrynic acid, furosemide, thiazides) that accelerate urinary excretion of potassium. A similar loss of the vital electrolyte occurs during administration of the antifungal drug *amphotericin B* and during therapy with *glucocorticoids*. The hypokalemia resulting from use of the foregoing drugs predisposes myocardial tissue to toxic effects of digitalis glycosides.

Other drug interactions are less clearly or consistently problematic. There is some indication that the adsorbent action of *activated charcoal, cholestyramine,* or *kaolin-pectin* preparations may bind digitoxin and partially interfere with its absorption from the intestine. The coating action of gastric antacids containing *magnesium trisilicate* has been suggested as presenting a barrier to digitoxin absorption. Although the extent to which the drugs interfere with absorption may be variable, problems may be avoided by administration of oral digitoxin one and one-half to two hours before giving the interacting drugs.

Barbiturates may accelerate the rate of hydroxylation of digitoxin to digoxin at hepatic sites. Induction of the hepatic microsomal drug-metabolizing enzyme system is a common property of *phenobarbital, phenylbutazone,* and *phenytoin,* and their use concurrent with digitoxin may shorten the plasma half-life of the digitalis glycoside.

Normal serum and tissue calcium levels are crucial during digitalis therapy. Elevation of free calcium levels in the blood will enhance the effects of glycosides. Careful monitoring of serum calcium levels is indicated to avoid toxicity when the electrolyte is given parenterally to a patient who is also receiving digitalis.

Digitalization

In acute heart failure, a loading dose of a digitalis glycoside may be administered to promptly raise the drug level at myocardial tissue sites to the optimal level required to maintain compensation. The dosage selected for digitalization is directly related to the calculated maintenance dosage for the individual and to the elimination rate of the drug to be employed for therapy. For example, the patient who has not previously received a digitalis glycoside may receive a loading dose that is three times the maintenance dosage of digoxin in divided doses over a 24-hour period. One third of the digoxin loading dose is excreted in a 24-hour period; therefore, 66 percent of the dosage or two times the maintenance dosage remains in the body after the 24-hour period. To maintain the initial level, one maintenance dosage a day would be required to replace the amount of drug known to be excreted daily.

During digitalization, the patient's clinical status is monitored closely. The patient usually is on a cardiac monitor and periodic ECG recordings are taken. In those situations where the critical status of the patient requires titration of drug administration with the evidence of cardiac failure, a cumulative record of drug administration can be maintained as a safeguard against excess drug administration (Fig. 7–4).

In less acute situations the digitalis glycoside may be administered over a period of days on a schedule planned to gradually raise the serum drug level to a plateau within the therapeutic concentration. The half-life of the particular drug and the elimination rate are important considerations in predicting attainment of the plateau level. Ninety percent of the steady-state blood and body accumulation can be achieved after three half-lives if the drug is administered at intervals shorter than the half-life, and 99 percent of the plateau is reached by five half-lives of the glycoside. For example, the half-life range of digoxin is 32 to 48 hours and 99 percent of the plateau would be attained by daily administration of the drug for a period of six to ten days. These considerations also can be employed in monitoring the patient's status. Any significant changes in the variable parameters will become noticeable when four to five drug half-lives have elapsed.

Digitalis Preparations

The mechanism of action and therapeutic effects of all digitalis glycosides are essentially the same, but the drugs differ in routes of administration, absorption, metabolism, onset and duration of action, volume of distribution in the body, and rate of excretion. The particular dosage of the glycoside selected for control of heart failure or for slowing of the ventricular response to atrial dysrhythmias is based primarily on the lean body mass and renal function of the individual. After a therapeutic serum drug level has been attained, the maintenance dosage is planned to utilize the smallest quantity of drug required to replace that amount lost daily due to metabolic destruction or excretion.

Variations in the duration of action of the individual glycosides are determined mainly by the degree of plasma protein binding. Extensive pro-

Digitalization Schedule: Cumulative Record					
Time	Digoxin Dosage (mg)	Route	Cumulative Dosage (mg)	Heart Rate	Status
8:15 A.M.	0.5	IV	0.5	115	Mild failure
10:45 A.M.	0.125	IV	0.625	120	Mild failure
12 noon	0.125	IV	0.75	114	Tachycardia
5 P.M.	0.125	IV	0.875	108	Periodic failure
9 P.M.	0.25	PO	0.9	98	

Fig. 7–4. A graphic record of the digitalis dosage administered for control of acute cardiac failure provides a ready reference to the total amount of drug administered and status changes during intensive drug therapy.

tein binding of digitoxin (86 to 94 percent) provides a long duration of therapeutic action. Ouabain is not protein bound, and lanatoside C is only slightly bound to protein; their rapid excretion by glomerular filtration leads to a short duration of action.

The route of administration is based on the urgency of the clinical situation. Oral administration is the safest and most economical route, and the drugs are given orally whenever possible. The intravenous route is the preferred parenteral route because glycosides injected into the subcutaneous or intramuscular tissues are very irritating and absorption rates vary widely.

Digoxin and digitoxin are the most commonly prescribed digitalis glycosides. The FDA program for certification of dissolution rates before marketing oral formulations of digoxin (1974) and digitoxin (1977) has improved the reliability of absorption and consequently the bioavailability of the glycosides.

Digoxin (LANOXIN). Digoxin is the most frequently prescribed glycoside. The oral drug is readily absorbed from the gastrointestinal tract and the onset of therapeutic action occurs one hour after oral administration (Table 7–1). Low plasma protein binding (25 to 30 percent) allows rapid passage through the glomerular filtrate, and 80 percent of the drug is excreted unchanged in the urine. The remainder of the drug is excreted with bile or in the urine as inactive metabolites.

Renal function is a primary factor considered in the selection of digoxin for therapy because toxic levels can accumulate with compromised kidney function. Digoxin dosage usually is planned at the lower margin of the therapeutic range for elderly individuals because the renal clearance of drugs is less efficient in the older age group.

One of the major advantages of digoxin over digitoxin is the relatively short duration of action. In instances where toxicity occurs, only the time span of four to five half-lives (approximately seven days) is required, after discontinuing administration, for total elimination of the drug.

The range of the adult digitalizing dose with oral digoxin tablets is 0.5 to 1.25 mg administered in divided doses (i.e., every eight hours) over a 24-hour period. Intravenous digoxin may be administered for rapid digitalization, and the dosage range is 0.75 to 1.0 mg. The injectable form of digoxin contains 10 percent alcohol and must be diluted to lessen irritation of the vein. Slow intravenous injection of the drug (five to ten minutes) provides an initial effect within 15 to 30 minutes and a therapeutic peak drug level is present for one and one-half to five hours.

The average adult oral maintenance dosage of digoxin is 0.125 to 0.5 mg daily. The usual dosage for individuals with normal renal function is 0.25 mg administered once daily.

Radioimmunoassay may be done to monitor the serum levels of digoxin after digitalization. The therapeutic serum digoxin levels are 0.9 to 2.2 ng/ml. The low margin of safety of the glycoside can be seen by comparison of the therapeutic range with the toxic level, which includes all values above 3.0 ng/ml. In some patients, toxicity may occur with levels at 2.0 ng/ml.

Table 7–1.
Comparison of Orally Administered Digitoxin and Digoxin

Drug	Absorption (tablets)	Serum Half-Life ($t\frac{1}{2}$)	Plasma Protein Binding	24-hour Excretion Rate	Therapeutic Effect		
					Onset (hr)	Peak (hr)	Duration
Digitoxin	95 to 100%	6 to 9 days	86 to 94%	15 to 20%	2 to 4	8 to 12	14 to 21 days
Digoxin	< 80%	1.3 to 2 days	25 to 30%	33%	1 to 2	6 to 8	3 to 6 days

Digitoxin (CRYSTODIGIN, PURODIGIN). Digitoxin is the second most frequently prescribed digitalis glycoside. The drug is a relatively non-polar glycoside, and it is more lipid soluble and easily diffused across the lipid membrane of the intestinal mucosa (Table 7–1). Digitoxin is converted to water-soluble inactive metabolites (dihydrodigoxin) at hepatic sites. Metabolism involves excretion into the bile and reabsorption from the intestine (enterohepatic cycling), which contribute to the long duration of action. Most of the cardioinactive metabolites are excreted in the urine but some may be in the feces. These factors contraindicate the use of digitoxin in the presence of liver pathology but are the primary reason for utilizing the drug in the presence of kidney pathology. The blocking of the excretory pathway of digitoxin metabolites, although causing their retention, does not contribute to the hazard of toxicity because most of the metabolites are inactive.

The long serum half-life of digitoxin is a disadvantage when symptoms of digitalis intoxication occur. After the drug administration is discontinued, it takes four to five half-lives (30 to 45 days) for total elimination of the drug. Conversely, the long duration of action is a decided advantage in the ambulatory individual. The single daily dose is easy to remember, and if the dosage is omitted occasionally, there is no significant change in cardiac response.

For the individual who previously has not received a digitalis glycoside for three weeks, a loading dosage schedule is used for digitalization because daily administration of the digitoxin maintenance dose requires approximately 35 days to reach a steady-state plateau level. The adult digitalizing dose of oral digitoxin is 0.7 to 1.5 mg, given in divided doses over 48 hours. Intravenous administration of 0.7 to 1.2 mg will produce a therapeutic effect within 25 minutes after administration.

The average adult oral maintenance dosage is usually 0.05 to 0.30 mg/day. Monitoring of the effectiveness of digitoxin administration is based on therapeutic serum levels of 12 to 28 ng/ml, and the toxic serum levels are higher than 35 ng/ml.

Digitalis. Digitalis represents the dried leaves of *Digitalis purpurea*. It is the parent compound of the digitalis glycosides. Although it has been used for therapy for centuries, it is infrequently prescribed at the present time.

The standardized preparation of powdered digitalis is hydrolyzed in the stomach to digitoxin, gitoxin, and gitalin, and approximately 20 percent of the glycosides are absorbed from the gastrointestinal tract. Digitoxin is the principal glycoside liberated by the parent compound, and the time span of therapeutic effect closely resembles that of digitoxin (Table 7–1).

The adult digitalizing dosage is 1.55 gm, which is divided into three equal doses administered at six-hour intervals. The usual daily maintenance dosage for adults is 100 mg.

Acetyldigitoxin (ACYLANID). Acetyldigitoxin is slowly and incompletely absorbed from the gastrointestinal tract after oral administration. After administration therapeutic effects occur within two to six hours, and the peak action occurs in eight to ten hours. Approximately 10 percent of the drug is eliminated in the urine daily as metabolites, and the duration of action is 7 to 12 days.

The adult digitalizing dosage is 1.6 to 2.2 mg, which is divided into three or four equal doses administered over a 24-hour period. The maintenance dosage range for adults is 0.1 to 0.2 mg daily.

Lanatoside C (CEDILANID). Lanatoside C is a glycoside from *Digitalis lanata* in a form suitable for oral administration. Absorption from the gastrointestinal tract is lower and less consistent than that of other glycosides. Therapeutic effects are evident for a period of 16 to 72 hours after administration, and the urinary excretion rate is only 20 percent per day.

The digitalizing dosage range for adults is usually 8 to 10 mg, which may be given in divided doses daily for a 72-hour period. The adult maintenance dosage range is 0.5 to 1.5 mg daily.

Gitalin (GITALIGIN). Gitalin is a preparation for oral administration that is infrequently prescribed. Digitalization with gitalin is achieved usually by administration of 6 mg over a period of approximately 30 hours by giving an initial 40 percent of the total amount (2.5 mg) followed by increments of 0.75 mg at six-hour intervals. The adult dosage range is 0.25 to 1.25 mg daily.

Deslanoside (CEDILANID-D). Deslanoside is an injectable glycoside preparation made by hydrolysis of lanatoside C. Parenteral administration provides a therapeutic effect in 5 to 30 minutes, and a peak therapeutic level is attained in one to four hours. The duration of action is 16 to 36 hours, and 20 percent of the drug is eliminated daily.

The rapid onset of action provides glycoside at myocardial tissues for the emergency treatment of patients with acute heart failure. The adult digitalizing dose by intravenous or intramuscular injection is 1.6 mg. The drug injection may be given as a single dose intravenously, but the intramuscular dosage usually is divided, and half of the dosage (4 ml = 0.8 mg) is administered at two separate sites. The maintenance dosage is 0.4 mg daily, but the glycoside usually is converted to an oral formulation if it is feasible.

Ouabain Injection. Ouabain is a potent glycoside commonly prescribed for administration intravenously in emergency situations. After IV injection, a therapeutic effect is evident in three to ten minutes, and a peak therapeutic effect is attained in 30 to 60 minutes. Ouabain has a relatively short duration of action ($t\ 1/2 = 21$ hr). The dosage maximum for a 24-hour period is 1 mg. The drug initially may be administered intravenously at a dosage level of 0.25 to 0.50 mg followed by injections of 0.1 mg every 60 minutes to control cardiac failure. Oral digitalis glycoside usually is instituted as soon as the acute emergency has been alleviated.

NURSING INTERVENTION

Episodes of decompensation occurring consequent to cardiac failure exist on a continuum ranging from life-threatening events to transient episodes relieved by rest. Crisis intervention by members of the health team is indicated when acute heart failure precipitates fluid accumulation in the lungs and other vital organ tissues, but there are a higher proportion of less acute situations in which chronic cardiac failure periodically interrupts the normal health and living patterns of individuals. Nurses have opportunities, in a variety of health care settings, to evaluate the health maintenance plans of individuals with borderline compensation and to counsel them about their therapeutic regimen.

Initial Status Evaluation

While the patient with chronic cardiac failure is being interviewed, the data obtained should include specific statements about the tasks that the patient desires to accomplish but that seem unrealistic because decompensation occurs when the tasks are attempted. Data also should provide sample situations or factors that precipitate decompensation; specific indicators of decompensation that the patient describes as occurring during or following the precipitating events; and the measures generally employed to allow completion of the task without precipitating decompensation. The information should be explicit enough to allow interpretation, analysis, and planning for preventive measures with the patient after all data are gathered. For example, grocery shopping may be described by the elderly housewife as causing exhaustion. She may describe dyspnea, orthopnea, or swollen ankles as problems that occur later on each day that she goes shopping. Her remedy for the situation may be to take a nap before and after going shopping. These data provide a base line for discussion of activity modification as a factor in maximizing the effectiveness of digitalis therapy. Instruction or replanning with the patient will follow compilation of additional data related to her health status and activity tolerance.

The patient's motivation is a primary factor influencing the outcomes of the planned drug regimen. The data obtained by observation of the patient and by discussion of usual health care practices or management of previously prescribed therapies provide some indication of the patient's motivation level and of probable compliance with the drug therapy plan in the future.

Physical Examination.　A follow-up to the interview includes physical examination of the patient to obtain objective base-line data for assessing the effectiveness of the digitalis glycoside in maintaining cardiac compensation. The plan for conducting the examination is based on the search for the presence, or absence, of those problems predictably occurring when an individual has cardiac failure.

The primary problem is decreased cardiac output, and taking the apical pulse and blood pressure provides preliminary information about the adequacy of the heart as a pump. The extent to which cardiac output is meeting tissue requirements for blood can be evaluated by assessing the skin color and temperature, the quantity and specific gravity of the urine, and the behavioral responses of the patient (i.e., mental acuity, orientation, retention of information).

The physical examination also includes careful assessment for evidence of elevated venous pressure resulting from decompensation. The rate and depth of respirations provide preliminary information about the presence of fluid in the lung fields. Listening to the breath sounds with a stethoscope is required to define the extent of pulmonary fluid accumulation as defined by the presence of moist rales, rhonchi, or wheezes. Elevation of peripheral venous pressure can be assessed by observing the filling and distention of the jugular veins and the veins of the extremities. Digital compression of peripheral tissues allows definition of the amount of accumulated edematous fluid. Fluid accumulation in the abdominal cavity or organs (i.e., liver, bowels) can be defined by palpation and auscultation. Weighing the patient aids in assessing generalized tissue fluid accumulation.

Assessing Progress

Initial therapy for the individual without a history of heart failure, or for one who has not received digitalis for two to three weeks, may include a plan for digitalization. The administration of the glycoside at the high dosage required for prompt control of decompensation makes it necessary to monitor the patient for evidence of digitalis toxicity while assessing the effectiveness of therapy. The patient usually is on a cardiac monitor and periodic electrocardiographic recordings are taken during the period of digitalization. The clinical status of the patient is observed frequently to define physiologic or behavioral changes.

The pulse rate always is counted before digitalis is administered. It is preferable to count the apical pulse, but the most important factor is that the pulse be counted for a full minute. That practice provides an opportunity to assess the quality and regularity of the pulse while counting the rate. The primary reason for taking the pulse before administering digitalis is to assure that the drug-induced slowing of conduction across the AV node has not exceeded the planned therapeutic effect. The drug is withheld when the pulse rate is 60 beats/minute or lower in adults and 90 beats or lower in children, and the physician is informed of the heart rate. Because digitalis toxicity frequently includes myocardial irritability, the drug also is withheld when the pulse rate is markedly elevated over the previously recorded rate (i.e., pulse elevation from 72 to 100 beats/minute).

Acute decompensation requires the use of many therapies (i.e., oxygen administration, digitalis, sedatives, diuretics, fluid and sodium restriction), and nursing measures are utilized to decrease cardiac work (i.e., activity limitation, positioning for elevation of the upper trunk). Many procedures are required to monitor status changes (i.e, ECG, laboratory tests, chest x-ray). As the patient's condition improves, the procedures and therapies required for intensive therapy will gradually be employed more selectively.

The patient is the center of attention during an acute situation, and the individual may be content with a role of grateful, passive recipient while in distress. In the less intensive situation, health team planning can be more realistic when the patient participates as an informed consumer. As the patient's condition improves, the nurse can utilize the base-line data obtained during initial assessment of status to evaluate the individual's progress. A secondary gain from having the base-line data is the opportunity to share with the patient specific examples of improvement when positive outcomes occur during therapy.

Counseling

Setting guidelines with the patient for a balanced activity-rest schedule is an important aspect in maximizing digitalis effect and maintaining cardiac output. Realistic planning may allow the individual to accomplish tasks that are important to living patterns.

Many tasks can be accomplished if the pace is slowed and rest periods are planned during accomplishment of the overall task. In the supervised situation the patient's tolerance to increased activity can be monitored by taking the pulse and blood pressure before, during, and after the activity period. Compensatory responses precipitated by the activity are reflected by cardioacceleration, vasoconstriction, and sweating. When any activity causes the pulse rate to rise 20 beats/minute above the preactivity rate and to remain elevated for ten minutes while the patient is resting postactivity, the activity level probably has exceeded that desirable for the individual.

Specific information about the pharmacotherapeutic plan is presented as soon as the patient's condition permits involvement. Digitalis therapy usually is continued for long-term control of compensation and the person will be responsible for self-care after hospitalization. Each time the drug is administered, there is an opportunity to present a preplanned aspect of the total information to the individual, but in many instances discussion will occur naturally as evidence of the patient's curiosity about personal health care.

Instruction of the patient and a family member about the drug therapy regimen progresses more smoothly when the sessions are interactive and based on the individual's life situation. Scheduling of drug use and measures required to monitor drug effect (i.e, counting the pulse rate) are often easier for the patient to assimilate than the more complex descriptions related to drug effect, adverse effects, and problems that require that the physician be contacted (i.e., excess fatigue, nausea, vomiting, change in pulse rate or rhythm, visual changes).

Listing of the problems in a manner similar to the foregoing would be frightening to the individual, but the same information can be communicated in smaller segments while the patient is in the hospital. The most important factor in patient instruction is that the individual understand the planned effect of the drug. That information may be the basic reason therapy is continued when the individual is responsible for self-care without supervision in the day-to-day maintenance of the drug therapy plan.

Review Guides

1. Outline the assessment plan you would prepare for a patient who is being digitalized immediately after being admitted to the hospital with congestive heart failure.

2. Outline the physiologic problems that occur as a consequence of left heart failure and describe how the action of digitalis contributes to resolution of the problems.

3. Explain the reason for taking the apical pulse before administration of digitalis.
4. Describe the measures that would be employed to monitor drug effect when a child with heart failure is receiving digoxin.
5. List the problems that occur with digitalis toxicity in the order of their importance. Describe the terms that would be employed in instructing the individual how to identify those adverse effects when taking the drug at home.
6. Many patients who receive a digitalis glycoside also receive diuretics. Describe the plans that are appropriate for monitoring the patient's status when the drugs are employed concurrently.
7. Outline the physiologic factors that affect digitalis therapy in elderly individuals and the measures that would be employed to monitor the patient's status.
8. Explain the factors to be considered in counseling the patient who will be continuing digitalis therapy at home about progression of the activities of daily living.

Additional Readings

Braunwald, Eugene: Current concepts in cardiology: determinants and assessment of cardiac function. *N. Engl. J. Med.,* **296:**86, January 13, 1977.

Brown, Donald D., and Juhl, Randy P.: Decreased bioavailability of digoxin due to antacids and kaolin-pectin. *N. Engl. J. Med.,* **295:**1034, November 4, 1976.

Butler, Vincent P., Jr., and Lindenbaum, John: Serum digitalis measurements in the assessment of digitalis resistance and sensitivity. *Am. J. Med.,* **58:** 460, April, 1975.

Deberry, Pauline; Jefferies, Lenner P.; and Light, Margaret R.: Teaching cardiac patients to manage medications. *Am. J. Nurs.,* **75:**2191, December, 1975.

Dodge, Harold T., and Rubenstein, Simeon: Digitalis. *Am. Fam. Physician,* **9:**98, April, 1974.

Fozzard, Harry A., and Das Gupta, D. S.: Electrophysiology and the electrocardiogram. *Mod. Concepts Cardiovasc. Dis.,* **44:**29, June, 1975.

Goldfrank, Lewis, and Kirstein, Robert: The cardiotoxic emergency. *Hosp. Physician,* **13:**34, January, 1977.

Gorlin, Richard: Current concepts in cardiology: practical cardiac hemodynamics. *N. Engl. J. Med.,* **296:**203, January 27, 1977.

Gould, Lawrence: Guide to recognition of digitalis toxicity. *Hosp. Med.,* **13:**93, July, 1977.

Greenblatt, David J., and Smith, Thomas W.: Digitalis: clinical implications of new facts about an old drug. *Postgrad. Med.,* **59:**134, May, 1976.

Halkin, H.; Sheiner, L. B.; Peck, C. C.; and Melmon, K. L.: Determinants of the renal clearance of digoxin. *Clin. Pharmacol. Ther.,* **17:**385, April, 1975.

Hall, W.; Shappell, S.; and Doherty, J.: Effects of cholestyramine on digoxin absorption and excretion in man. *Am. J. Cardiol.,* **39:**213, February, 1977.

Hartel, G.; Kyllönen, K.; Merikallio, E.; Ojala, K.; Manninen, V.; and Reissel, P.: Human serum and myocardial digoxin. *Clin. Pharmacol. Ther.,* **19:** 153, February, 1976.

Huffman, David H.: Relationship between digoxin concentrations in serum and saliva. *Clin. Pharmacol. Ther.,* **17:**310, March, 1975.

Huffman, David H.; Crow, James W.; Pentikäinen, Pertti and Azarnoff, Daniel L.: Association between clinical cardiac status, laboratory parameters, and digoxin usage. *Am. Heart J.,* **91:**28, January, 1976.

Ingelfinger, Joseph A., and Goldman, Peter: The serum digitalis concentration—does it diagnose digitalis toxicity? *N. Engl. J. Med.,* **294:**867, April 15, 1976.

Katz, Arnold, M.: The ischemic myocardium: mechanism of early pump failure. *Hosp. Prac.,* **13:**83, June, 1978.

Kolata, Gina Bari: The aging heart: changes in function and response to drugs. *Science,* **195:**166, January 14, 1977.

Mechner, Francis: Patient assessment: examination of the heart and great vessels, part 1 (programmed instruction). *Am. J. Nurs.,* **76:**1, November, 1976.

Oparil, Suzanne: Digitalis assay and its clinical application. *Med. Clin. North Am.,* **60:**193, January, 1976.

Powell, Anne H.: Physical assessment of the patient with cardiac disease. *Nurs. Clin. North Am.,* **2:**251, June, 1976.

Rasmussen, Susan; Noble, R. Joe; and Fisch, Charles: The pharmacology and clinical use of digitalis. *Cardiovasc. Nurs.,* **11:**23, January–February, 1975.

Rosen, Michael R.; Wit, Andrew L.; and Hoffman, Brian F.: Electrophysiology and pharmacology of cardiac arrhythmias. 1. Cellular electrophysiology of the mammalian heart. *Am. Heart J.,* **88:**380, September, 1974.

———: Electrophysiology and pharmacology of cardiac arrhythmias. IV. Cardiac antiarrhythmic and toxic effects of digitalis. *Am. Heart J.,* **89:**391, March, 1975.

Schlant, Robert C., and Hurst, J. Willis: Assessment of cardiac function at the bedside. *Geriatrics,* **30:** 49, June, 1975.

Schwartz, Arnold; Lindenmayer, George E.; and Allen, Julius C.: The sodium-potassium adenosine triphosphatase: pharmacological, physiological and biochemical aspects. *Pharmacol. Rev.,* **27:**3, March, 1975.

Singh, R. B.; Dube, K. P.; and Srivastav, P. K.: Hypomagnesemia in relation to digoxin intoxication in children. *Am. Heart J.,* **92:**144, August, 1976.

Smith, Thomas W.: Digitalis toxicity: epidemioligy and clinical use of serum concentration measurements. *Am. J. Med.,* **58:**470, April, 1975.

Storstein, Liv: Studies of digitalis. III. Biliary excretion and enterohepatic circulation of digitoxin and its cardioactive metabolites. *Clin. Pharmacol. Ther.,* **17:**313, March, 1975.

———: Studies on digitalis. VIII. Digitoxin metabolism on a maintenance regimen and after a single dose. *Clin. Pharmacol. Ther.,* **21:**125, February, 1977.

Tanner, Gloria: Heart failure in the MI patient. *Am. J. Nurs.,* **77:**230, February, 1977.

Waxler, Rose: The patient with congestive heart failure: teaching implications. *Nurs. Clin. North Am.,* **2:**297, June, 1976.

Winslow, Elizabeth Hahn: Visual inspection of the patient with cardiopulmonary disease. *Heart Lung,* **4:**421, May–June, 1975.

8

Cardiac Arrhythmias

The patient population in most community hospitals includes an increasing number of people with cardiac rhythm disturbances. The upsurge is a reflection, at least in part, of improved diagnostic and treatment procedures. The survival of patients after heart attacks and the recovery of adults and children after intricate surgical procedures for correction of cardiac problems (i.e., congenital abnormalities, coronary artery occlusion) have increased the numbers of patients having arrhythmias during their hospitalization. Arrhythmias can occur as a consequence of cardiac tissue injury; thus acute myocardial infarction and cardiac surgery are associated with a high incidence of rhythm disturbances.

Almost all of the patients (90 percent) with an acute myocardial infarction in a coronary care unit have some form of arrhythmia in the early recovery period. At some time during the intensive care period, most of the patients (80 percent) have ventricular premature contractions that necessitate immediate administration of antiarrhythmic drugs. The decreasing incidence of fatalities in coronary care units reflects the expertise of personnel in recognizing and treating cardiac arrhythmias.

Physiologic Correlations

Cardiac arrhythmias are defined as *abnormalities in the rate, regularity, initiation site, or conduction pathway of a cardiac impulse that alters the sequence of myocardial tissue activation.* An understanding of cardiac arrhythmia pathogenesis necessitates consideration of the physiologic factors involved in the excitation-conduction-contraction sequence.

The normal cardiac cycle represents a stimulus-response continuum involving membrane polarity, electrical conduction, and mechanical contraction. A causal relationship exists between the events, which necessitates an orderly, stepwise progression for completion of the cardiac cycle. Membrane responses were discussed in Chapter 7, and they will be reviewed briefly to provide a frame of reference for the discussion of arrhythmias.

Membrane Polarity

The ionic impermeability of the resting myocardial cell membrane is such that a net negative charge occurs on the inside and a net positive charge occurs on the outside to produce a polarized membrane. The high intracellular concentration of potassium ions and the high extracellular concentration of sodium ions provide electrochemical gradients that act as the driving forces for movement of the electrolytes to the alternate sides of the membrane upon excitation. When the membrane permeability is changed as a result of stimulation, Na+-K+ exchange occurs due to the gradient. Because the rate of passage of positively charged sodium ions to the intracellular surface of the membrane is greater than the passage rate of potassium ions to the extracellular surface, the inner membrane becomes positive. The charge difference between the inner and the outer membrane surface is "lost" and the membrane becomes depolarized. The syncytial arrangement of cardiac cells allows each cell, during the depolarization process, to act as a stimulus to those fibers adjacent to it and the impulse is propagated in an orderly fashion throughout the myocardium.

During membrane repolarization sodium and potassium ions are reexchanged and polarity is restored. The membrane remains refractory until repolarization is complete. The end of the effective refractory period is related to the time when the membrane again can depolarize in response to an impulse.

The cells of the specialized conducting system are not dependent on external stimulation for initiation of depolarization. The cells have a property described as *automaticity* that allows spontaneous depolarization. The process involves the same exchange of sodium and potassium as described above for stimulus-initiated membrane responses. The primary difference lies in the spontaneous self-generation of impulses that causes depolarization of the specialized conducting tissues.

Spontaneous depolarization of the sinoatrial (SA), or sinus, node is more rapid than that of other specialized conduction tissues of the heart. The sinus node begins to repolarize during systole, and it produces an impulse immediately after other myocardial cells have ended their refractory period. The conduction cells discharge in response to the sinus node stimulus before attaining their spontaneous impulse threshold potential. The automaticity of the conduction cells is "overridden" by the SA impulse under normal conditions.

ELECTRICAL CONDUCTION VARIABLES

There are differences in the depolarization and conduction velocity of fibers in varying myocardial tissues. Fibers of the specialized conducting tissues of the atrial muscle, the Purkinje conducting system, which arborizes throughout the ventricles, and the muscle of the ventricles depolarize rapidly and they have a high conduction velocity.

Cells of the SA node and the atrioventricular (AV) node and the fibers of the atrioventricular ring and valve leaflets have a slower rate of depolarization, lower amplitude, slower conduction velocity, and a longer refractory period than the faster cardiac fibers described above. Changes in the electrical properties and in automaticity can occur in most cardiac fibers as a consequence of electrolyte imbalance, injury, drugs, or catecholamines that disrupt cellular function.

ELECTRICAL-MECHANICAL ACTIVITY

The rate of conduction through the specialized conduction system in the normal heart follows a progression that can be defined by analysis of the electrocardiogram (Fig. 8–1). The electrical events can be correlated with the mechanical events that follow conduction.

After initiation of conduction by the SA node, the ECG records a positive deflection, the P wave, which represents depolarization of the atria. The

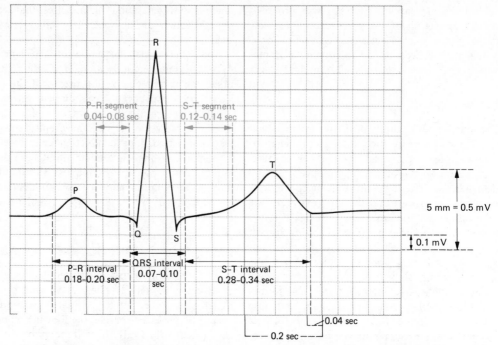

P–R segment
0.04–0.08 sec

S–T segment
0.12–0.14 sec

P

R

Q

S

T

5 mm = 0.5 mV

0.1 mV

P–R interval
0.18–0.20 sec

QRS interval
0.07–0.10
sec

S–T interval
0.28–0.34 sec

0.04 sec

0.2 sec

Fig. 8–1. Cardiac conduction time intervals related to the deflections of a typical electrocardiographic recording.

time span of atrial depolarization ranges from 0.08 to 0.12 second. As the impulse spreads, the atria contract to eject their residual blood content. Atrial systole is described as the "atrial kick," because the contraction contributes 15 to 20 percent of the stroke volume. The base line, or isoelectric span between the P wave and the slightly negative Q deflection, reflects impulse transmission through the AV node.

The QRS complex represents depolarization of the ventricles. Closing of the atrioventricular valves (bicuspid and tricuspid) correlates in time with the peak of the R deflection. Atrioventricular valve closure is followed by the first heart sound that can be heard when listening with a stethoscope at the apex of the heart. The QRS complex duration ranges from 0.04 to 0.1 second, which represents the time span required for depolarization of the ventricles before contraction is initiated.

Isometric contraction of the ventricles raises the chamber pressures sharply. When the pressures in the ventricles exceed those of the pulmonary artery and the aorta, the semilunar valves of those vessels open, and blood is ejected forward from the ventricles. Pressure in the ventricles continues to rise to the systolic contraction peak level. The semilunar valves close when the ventricular pressures decrease. Closure of those valves produces the second heart sound heard at the apex of the heart. Valve closure correlates with the time period on the ECG that indicates termination of the T wave. When ventricular pressures fall below those of the atria, the atrioventricular valves open, and rapid filling of the ventricles occurs during the diastolic period. Because the T wave represents repolarization of the ventricles, a stimulus can initiate conduction following the effective refractory period, which occurs shortly after the T wave deflection.

Electrical conduction is followed by mechanical contraction in each cardiac cycle. An electrical conduction problem can propagate a mechanical problem during the time period of the same cycle, or problems may continue into subsequent cardiac cycles. Disruption of the natural electrical-mechanical sequence may lengthen, shorten, or abort the series of events required for maintaining the normal cardiac cycle.

NEURAL STIMULATION

Parasympathetic Nerve Stimulation

The reciprocal interaction between the parasympathetic nerves and the sympathetic nerves allows prominence in control by that autonomic nervous system division which best meets the body requirements during varying period of activity. Parasympathetic nerve activity maintains the heart rate at the level required to meet body needs during moderate activity and resting periods. Deceleration of the heart rate is an outcome of release of the neurotransmitter *acetylcholine* at vagus nerve endings that act on inhibitory receptors of the SA node, atrial working muscle fibers, and the AV node to slow conduction.

Acetylcholine release increases the permeability of the myocardial cells to potassium ions and the cations rapidly leak out of the fiber to the external surface of the membrane. During each cardiac cycle, the exodus of the cation increases the negativity inside the cell to cause a transient period of hyperpolarization. Since fibers are not excitable, when membranes are hyperpolarized, there is a delay in the conduction time, slowing of SA node firing, and a lengthening of the refractory period of the AV node. When polarity is restored by return of the intracellular potassium ions, the affected cardiac fibers can respond again to stimulation.

Sympathetic Nerve Stimulation

Sympathetic nerve stimulation induces the release of neurotransmitter at the nerve endings and the transmitter hormone acts on the adrenergic receptors in the reactive tissue. The heart is richly innervated by postganglionic fibers of the sympathetic division of the autonomic nervous system. Sympathetic nerve endings are found in all types of cardiac fibers. The greatest density of nerve endings is found in atrial and nodal tissues.

Norepinephrine is the natural neurotransmitter at sympathetic nerve endings, but circulating *epinephrine* or *dopamine* also may elicit responses in tissues. Adrenergic receptors are classified as *alpha, beta,* or *dopaminergic receptors* on the basis of the different physiologic responses induced by a specific stimulating agent. The receptors are specific cellular structures with which neurotransmitter hormones interact in the responsive tissues. Each adrenergic receptor demonstrates a high affinity for a particular catecholamine agonist. The highly specific binding selectivity for a given agonist leads to a characteristic response.

Beta-adrenergic receptors further are designated as $beta_1$ or $beta_2$ receptors based on cardiac acceleration effects ($beta_1$) or smooth muscle relaxant effects ($beta_2$). Release of the neurotransmitter *norepinephrine* and its binding to the cardiac $beta_1$ receptors modify electrophysiologic properties of the working fibers of the atria and ventricles and of the specialized conducting system. The occupancy of the cardiac $beta_1$-adrenergic receptors by norepinephrine stimulates the activity of *adenylate cyclase*. The enzyme catalyzes the formation of *cyclic 3'–5' adenosine monophosphate* (cAMP) from *adenosine triphosphate* (ATP). The cAMP initiates the cellular events leading to an accelerated cardiac rate.

The most prominent effect of the beta-adrenergic receptor stimulation is an increase in the rate of sinus node firing. Also noted are an increase in the conduction velocity and shortening of the refractory period of the AV node. The increased rate of impulse passage through the AV node can be observed as a shortened P-R interval on the ECG. The rapid rate of sinus node initiation of conduction is accompanied by a faster rate of AV nodal transmission and impulses reach the ventricular conduction fibers at a rapid rate. Cardioacceleration occurs as a consequence of the increased sympathetic nerve stimulation.

Catecholamines raise the slope of depolarization of myocardial fibers. Release of norepinephrine during the time frame when cells are partially depolarized may raise the action potential amplitude and enhance automaticity of cardiac tissues. The catecholamine contributes to the irritability of working fibers and may cause ectopic foci to initiate abnormal impulses.

Pathophysiologic Correlations

Cardiac arrhythmias represent a wide variety of impulse initiation and conduction abnormalities. The seriousness of an arrhythmia is related to its effect on the hemodynamic equilibrium and to its potential for causing a life-threatening arrhythmia. Myocardial tissue hypoxia, ischemia, infarction, inflammation, and excess sympathetic nerve activity are the most common causes of arrhythmias. Treatment of the underlying disease process or correction of other causative factors may abolish or modify the abnormality.

ARRHYTHMIAS: ELECTROPHYSIOLOGIC PROBLEMS

Bradycardia

Bradycardia is considered to exist when the cardiac contraction rate is below 55 beats/minute. It can result from depressed conduction through any part of the myocardial conducting system. The low cardiac rate prolongs the ventricular diastolic filling time and there is a concurrent increase in stroke volume. The augmented stroke volume partially compensates for the reduced heart rate but there is a physiologic limit to the stroke volume adjustment. Bradycardia gradually decreases the cardiac output, and the patient may complain of dizziness or faintness, which results from the decreased blood supply to the cerebral tissues.

The low cardiac output also decreases perfusion of the coronary arteries. In persons with coronary artery disease the lower blood supply may precipitate anginal pain. When the patient has a very low cardiac rate (i.e., 40 beats/minute), cardiac failure can occur.

Digitalis toxicity may cause direct conduction bradycardia and vagus nerve–induced nodal (SA or AV) bradycardia. Discontinuing the drug may terminate the problems, but predominant vagus bradycardia may be controlled by the anticholinergic drug *atropine sulfate*. The drug can be employed to block the acetylcholine released by the vagus nerves. The interruption of parasympathetic vagal action leads to sympathetic nerve dominance, which may act to increase the heart rate.

Periodic, or episodic, sinus bradycardia occurs in elderly individuals with arteriosclerosis who have *carotid sinus syndrome*. The slow pulse rate results from excess sensitivity and stimulation of the baroreceptors in the carotid arteries. Excess sensitivity of the baroreceptors to external or internal pressure elicits parasympathetic nerve responses that slow the heart rate. Administration of *atropine sulfate* at the onset of bradycardia effectively may lessen the vagal stimulation of the heart, but patients with frequent or persistent bradycardia may require implantation of a pacemaker to consistently maintain their cardiac output.

Tachycardia

Tachycardia is considered to exist when the heart rate exceeds 100 contractions/minute. The rapid heart rate shortens the ventricular diastolic filling time and there is a decreased stroke volume output. The coronary arteries fill during diastole, and shortening of the diastolic period lessens the perfusion of the arteries.

Supraventricular tachycardias that occur as a consequence of AV node or atrial stimulation may be controlled by administration of digitalis glycosides, as was discussed in Chapter 7. Concurrent therapy with an antiarrhythmic drug (i.e., quinidine sulfate) may be planned when atrial flutter or atrial fibrillation is present. Rapid conduction occurring as an outcome of ventricular hyperactivity requires immediate therapy with antiarrhythmic drugs, because ventricular tachycardia can be a precursor for ventricular fibrillation and cardiac arrest.

Ectopic Beats

Ectopic foci may initiate extrasystoles by stimulation of fibers at any myocardial site that is irritated by local changes in tissues. The ectopic beats may appear as an expression of the natural automaticity of specialized conduction system tissue, or they may represent emergence of latent automaticity in working atrial or ventricular tissue. Ectopic beats, or extrasystoles, are abnormal or pathologic occurrences, but they represent an escape system of physiologic importance. Their occurrence represents a mobilization of the latent automaticity that provides protection against asystole when primary conduction fibers become abnormally depressed or dormant. For example, extreme sinus bradycardia results in a time lag between completion of repolarization and sinus node–initiated stimulation. The long period of time when fibers are excitable makes it possible for other fibers to initiate conduction. The new foci may provide a regular rhythm by setting the pace higher than the level previously conducted by the depressed sinus node.

The origin, frequency, and timing of the ectopic foci affect their importance to the conduction-contraction sequence of the cardiac cycle. The origin of an ectopic beat may be a myocardial site where there is a block to conduction in the fibers adjacent to an area of ischemia or infarction. Isolated fibers, which are not stimulated by normally conducted impulses, may initiate conduction by their inherent ability to fire spontaneously. The aberrant impulse provides the stimulus for an ectopic beat.

An extrasystole occurring immediately following the normally conducted, or generic, beat may eject so little blood that there is no evidence of the contraction at the level of the radial artery. When ectopic foci emit impulses during the time span when some of the myocardial fibers are refractory but other fibers have completed repolarization, stimulation of the excitable fibers can initiate an erratic, or fibrillatory, pattern (Fig. 8–2).

Premature contractions are named according to their myocardial site of origin. For example, an extrasystole originating in the atrial tissue is described as a premature atrial contraction (PAC) and that arising from a site in the ventricular tissue is referred to as a premature ventricular contraction (PVC). Premature impulses may arise from any myocardial site and periodically precipitate systolic contraction before normally conducted impulses stimulate contractions.

Premature Ventricular Contractions. Premature beats represent the most common form of rhythm disturbance, and the ventricular tissue is the most frequent site of premature contractions. The impulse follows a circuitous pathway in depolarizing fibers as they become excitable. The electrocardiographic pattern of a PVC usually shows an absence of the P wave and a wide, inverted QRS deflection (over 0.12 second) indicating an erratic conduction pathway. After a single PVC has occurred, there is usually a compensatory pause and the next sinus impulse arises at the time when it predictably would occur. The basic rhythmic conduction pattern is undisturbed by the premature ventricular contraction.

Ventricular hyperirritability is a major cause of concern because it progressively can decrease cardiac output and lead to cardiac arrest. Antiarrhythmic drugs (i.e., lidocaine hydrochloride intravenously) are usually started when the incidence of premature ventricular contractions is more than 5/minute. The incidence of multifocal PVCs or of PVCs that occur in a regular pattern related to the generic impulse (i.e., bigeminy, trigeminy, quadrigeminy) is an ominous indication of extensive ventricular hyperirritability. Cardiopulmonary resuscitative equipment is maintained in a state of readiness while antiarrhythmic drugs are administered to control the irritability of the ventricular tissues.

Reentry Pathways. In the rapid progression of impulses through the myocardial tissue, each cell stimulates an adjacent cell that has repolar-

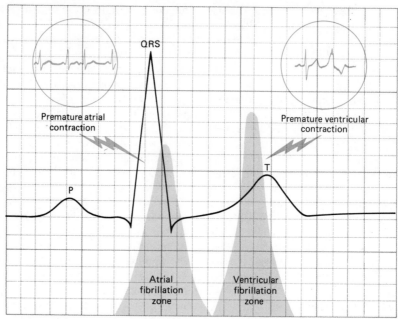

Fig. 8–2. Ectopic foci stimulating fibers of the atria or the ventricle at the time when some fibers are repolarized may precipitate a fibrillatory response in the myocardial tissue.

ized, and those cells, in turn, propagate the stimulus. The slowing of conduction in a myocardial cell, due to any local factor (i.e., injury), may allow the cell to remain refractory longer than adjacent cells. The refractory cell may block the passage of a stimulus reaching the area, and the impulse dies out. When the refractory period of a cell terminates, another impulse arriving at the fiber from an alternate route may stimulate its

depolarization. The process is called *reentry*. The new impulse may follow an aberrant conduction pathway in stimulating contraction. As long as the block remains, the cell is capable of conducting impulses that cause contractions by the reentry process. The specific therapeutic intervention depends on the extent to which the problem interferes with the patient's cardiac status.

Antiarrhythmic Drugs

Each of the drugs employed for control of arrhythmias is a potent agent with a low therapeutic index. The antiarrhythmic drugs in common use decrease automaticity of the myocardial tissue. The drugs also, by slightly different actions, prolong the effective refractory period.

DRUG THERAPY

Antiarrhythmic drugs can be divided into two basic types, or groups. The drugs in each group have similar effects on cardiac electrophysiology, electrocardiographic recordings, and hemodynamic parameters (Table 8–1). Group I drugs include *quinidine, procainamide,* and *propranolol.* Propranolol has properties generally similar to those of group I, but it also has effects that more closely resemble those of drugs in group II. Propranolol may be characterized as a subtype of the group I drugs. Group II drugs include *lidocaine* and *phenytoin.*

The status of the patient and the nature and extent of cardiac pathology influence the decision to utilize a particular antiarrhythmic drug. There is also a degree of predictability for clinical effectiveness that affects selection of a specific drug for control of a particular arrhythmia. *Quinidine* and *procainamide* are broad-spectrum antiarrhythmic drugs, and they have been found to produce good to excellent results in the control of supraventricular arrhythmias (i.e., premature atrial contractions, paroxysmal atrial tachycardia, atrial flutter and fibrillation, and junctional pre-

mature contractions or tachycardia). Both drugs have shown clinical effectiveness in control of premature ventricular contractions. Procainamide also provides excellent control of ventricular tachycardia.

Propranolol has been found to be effective in control of paroxysmal atrial tachycardia, ventricular contractions, and ventricular tachycardia and for the supraventricular and ventricular arrhythmias induced by digitalis toxicity. The group II drugs, *lidocaine* and *phenytoin,* show excellent clinical effectiveness in controlling ventricular arrhythmias (i.e., ventricular premature contractions, ventricular tachycardia, or the supraventricular and ventricular arrhythmias induced by digitalis toxicity).

Each of the antiarrhythmic drugs may be employed for therapy in acute care situations. With the exception of lidocaine, which is administered parenterally, each of the drugs may be employed

Table 8–1.

Effects of Antiarrhythmic Drugs on Cardiac Electrophysiology and Hemodynamics

Effects	Group I		Group II
	Procainamide Quinidine	Propranolol	Lidocaine Phenytoin
Electrophysiologic effects			
Automaticity	↓	↓	↓
Conduction velocity	↓	↓	→ or ↑
AV conduction time	→ ↑	→ ↑	→ or ↓
Excitability	↓	↓	→
Effective refractory period (ERP)	↑	↓	↓
Action potential duration (APD)	↑	↓	↓
ERP/APD	↑	↑	↑
ECG effects (duration)			
P-R interval	→ or ↑	→ or ↑	→ or ↓
QRS interval	↑	→	→
Q-T interval	↑	↓	→ or ↓
Hemodynamic effects			
Blood pressure	↓	→ or ↓	→ or ↓
Cardiac output	↓	↓	→ or ↓
LVEDP*	↑	↑	→ or ↑

Key: ↑ = increased; ↓ = decreased; → = no change.

* LVEDP = Left ventricular end-diastolic pressure.

for long-term therapy for ambulatory patients with arrhythmias.

Action Mode

Drugs in both groups I and II affect automaticity by decreasing spontaneous diastolic depolarization of the myocardial tissue. Slowing of the spontaneous depolarization rate reduces the firing frequency of the ectopic foci. The faster sinus impulses depolarize the myocardial cells so they are refractory to the impulse emitted from the ectopic foci. The drugs also increase the functional refractory period in relation to the duration of the action potential. *Group I* drugs also decrease automaticity by shifting the threshold potential voltage toward zero. Action of the drugs may slow conduction velocity of reentrant impulses by creating a bidirectional block to the passage of impulses. *Group II* drugs facilitate normal electrophysiologic activity by their effect on conduction velocity and refractory time. The drugs may decrease the activity of reentrant pathways by raising the membrane threshold to stimuli. The higher threshold may eliminate the unidirectional blocks that precipitate reentry.

The major actions of the drugs on myocardial electrophysiology can be monitored by ECG recordings. The action of *quinidine* and *procainamide* slows intraventricular conduction and prolongs repolarization, and the effect appears on the ECG as a prolonged QRS interval. When the administration of quinidine has produced a therapeutic serum drug level, the QRS interval becomes about 25 percent wider. *Propranolol, phenytoin*, and *lidocaine* accelerate repolarization. The effect of the drugs can be seen on the ECG as a slight decrease in the Q-T interval.

Each antiarrhythmic drug also shows some differing pharmacologic properties that affect its clinical usefulness. Some of the properties are related to effects on the autonomic nervous system. For example, each of the group I drugs, *quinidine, procainamide,* and *propranolol,* has an anticholinergic property. Because there is seldom a single target tissue specificity in the action of drugs, the properties of each drug may be mani-

fested in differing ways on the body systems. The following descriptions will focus on the differing characteristics of the drugs employed for control of arrhythmias.

Quinidine

Quinidine is the oldest of the antiarrhythmic drugs, having a long history of use for treatment of atrial arrhythmias. The drug frequently is employed to control atrial fibrillation, and it often spontaneously converts atrial fibrillation to normal sinus rhythm. Quinidine also may be employed to maintain the sinus rhythm after the fibrillatory pattern has been eliminated by cardioversion.

Action Mode. Quinidine has a direct action on myocardial fibers that increases the effective refractory period of atrial muscle fibers. The local anesthetic property of quinidine may contribute slightly to the depression of myocardial fiber responsiveness.

Quinidine also has an anticholinergic property that enhances the planned therapeutic effect of the drug on cardiac tissues. The anticholinergic action of the drug interferes with the vagus nerve activity that reduces the effective refractory period. By its direct and indirect action, quinidine provides the slower conduction rate required to control atrial fibrillation.

Quinidine has anti-alpha-adrenergic and anti-beta-adrenergic properties. Some of the effectiveness of quinidine in control of conduction may relate, in part, to the anti-beta-adrenergic action that decreases the myocardial response to sympathetic nerve stimulation. Quinidine action at alpha-adrenergic sites in the arteries contributes to the occurrence of hypotension during therapy.

Therapy Considerations. Quinidine is available for oral and parenteral use, but whenever possible the drug is given orally. The drug is a weak organic base and it is usually highly ionized in the pH of the stomach. A minimal amount of the drug is absorbed from the stomach, but absorption from the intestine is almost complete (approximately 95 percent). Peak plasma levels of the drug are attained in one to two hours (Table 8–2), and the myocardial activity peak is attained in four to six hours.

In acute situations, the patient may receive a loading dose of quinidine (i.e., 400 to 800 mg every two to three hours for five doses) in the first 24 hours, and the initial dosage is followed by a maintenance dosage (i.e., 200 mg four times per day). The drug has a relatively short half-life, which allows a steady-state plateau to be achieved in less than 24 hours, or 3.3 times the serum half-life of six to eight hours. Although the drug is highly bound to plasma proteins (80 percent), it is rapidly taken up by all tissues of the body with the exception of brain tissue.

Quinidine is a potent drug, and the patient's status is assessed regularly when therapy is initiated. Widening of the QRS interval more than 25 percent, hypotension, cardioacceleration, and allergic responses are the primary concerns when quinidine therapy is started. Assessment of the patient's status at the predictable time when serum levels are elevated (i.e., one hour after drug administration) and before administration of the next dose of the drug, when the serum drug level is lowest, provides a profile of the effectiveness of quinidine in controlling the cardiac problem.

Quinidine is metabolized in the liver by hydroxylation, and 20 to 50 percent of the unchanged drug is excreted in the urine. The pH of the urine is an important factor in elimination of the basic compound at renal tubule sites. When the pH of tubule urine is elevated, more of the drug diffuses back into the bloodstream and less is eliminated in the urine. In some instances, the presence of the metabolites in the urine gives it a brownish hue.

Preparations Available. Quinidine preparations include *quinidine sulfate* in the form of tablets and capsules and as extended-release tablets; *quinidine gluconate* (QUINAGLUTE) in extended-release tablets; *quinidine polygalacturonate* (CARDIOQUIN) in extended-release tablets; *quinidine gluconate injection* for intravenous infusion; and *quinidine hydrochloride* for injection.

Adverse Effects. Cardioacceleration may occur as a consequence of the anticholinergic property of quinidine. By antagonizing the vagus nerve–mediated slowing of conduction, quinidine increases the heart rate. Cardioacceleration also may reflect a reflex sympathetic nerve response to the reduction in cardiac output and the hypotension associated with quinidine administration.

Ventricular irritability can occur during therapeutic use of quinidine for control of atrial flutter or fibrillation. The anticholinergic action of quinidine interferes with the vagal influence that decreases conduction velocity and increases the effective refractory period of the AV node. As a consequence of the antivagal action of quinidine, there is increased conductivity at the AV node, and more flutter or fibrillatory impulses can traverse the node to be propagated to the ventricles. The ventricular tachycardia or ventricular fibrillation that can ensue is a serious complication of quinidine therapy. In clinical situations, the prob-

Table 8–2.
Oral Antiarrhythmic Drug-Dosage Response Factors

	Quinidine	Procainamide	Propranolol	Phenytoin
Adult dosage/day (gm)	0.8–2.4	2–4	0.04–0.24	0.3–0.4
Peak therapeutic effect (hr)	1–2	1–1.5	1–1.5	48–96
Therapeutic serum level (mcg/ml)	2.3–5	4–8	0.03–0.52	10–20
Serum half-life (hr)	6–8	2.2–3.5	2–3.5	13–24
Plasma protein binding (%)	60–80	15–20	90–95	50–85
Renal excretion (unmetabolized) (%)	20–50	50–60	<5	1–5

lem is modified by prior administration of digitalis glycosides, and the glycosides slow conduction through the nodal tissue.

Hypotension is a common problem during quinidine therapy. Because a sharp drop in blood pressure often occurs when the drug is administered intravenously, quinidine is given IV only to hospitalized patients who are under close supervision. Hypotension also occurs when patients receive quinidine intramuscularly or orally.

The problem most frequently occurring during oral quinidine therapy is diarrhea. Other symptoms of gastrointestinal irritation also occur frequently (i.e., nausea, loss of appetite, vomiting). Although the symptoms may be controlled by administration of the bitter-tasting drug with food, many individuals who are taking the drugs at home discontinue therapy because of the symptoms.

Quinidine is an alkaloid obtained from the bark of the cinchona tree, and it shares with quinine and similar alkaloids the propensity to produce toxic symptoms of *cinchonism*. The initial problems arise when serum levels of the drug are elevated. The early and most frequent symptoms are important because they are distressing to the patient (i.e., nausea, vomiting, anorexia, diaphoresis, abdominal pain). Symptoms can be severe when toxicity progresses. The major problems occur as a consequence of effects on the optic and auditory structures. The symptoms include marked tinnitus, vertigo, loss of hearing, blurring of vision, diplopia, photophobia, and altered color perception. The problems usually prompt the individual to seek medical attention, and discontinuing the drug gradually relieves the situation. Severe toxicity can cause headache, confusion, delirium, convulsions, or psychosis.

Allergic manifestations occur during quinidine therapy, and the drug allergen-antibody response can precipitate any of the problems of immediate allergic reactions (i.e., anaphylaxis, urticaria, angioedema) or those commonly occurring with delayed allergic reactions (i.e., serum sickness, rash, fever). A test dose of quinidine (i.e., 200 mg) may be administered to allow observation and assure that an allergic reaction does not occur before therapy is initiated.

Quinidine also causes thrombocytopenia, which is a manifestation of an indirect allergic response. Quinidine interacts with platelets and platelet antibodies, and the interaction causes lysis of the platelets. Petechial hemorrhages in the buccal mucosa may be an early clue to the problem, but bleeding episodes can be severe as the platelet count drops. After cessation of drug administration, platelet counts usually return to the normal range within seven to ten days.

The administration of quinidine to patients who have congestive heart failure or long-standing atrial fibrillation may be preceded by anticoagulation therapy. The plan is based on the possibility that the slow blood flow through the atria may have allowed formation of a thrombus. Quinidine-induced improvement in atrial contraction could precipitate a thromboembolic episode.

Interactions. The anticholinergic property of quinidine may be intensified to a level producing excess cholinergic blockade and consequent excess dryness of the mouth or constipation when anticholinergic drugs or drugs with anticholinergic properties are administered to an individual receiving quinidine. Belladonna alkaloids or phenothiazines, antihistamines, or tricyclic antidepressants, which have anticholinergic properties, enhance the anticholinergic properties of quinidine.

Quinidine interferes with acetylcholine action at the myoneural junction of skeletal muscles, and concurrent use of other drugs that affect the action of the neurotransmitter may cause neuromuscular blockade. When the patient is receiving quinidine, administration of the antibiotics kanamycin, neomycin, polymyxin B, or streptomycin, which have neuromuscular blocking properties, may cause muscle weakness. Prolonged apnea may occur during surgery when muscle relaxants (i.e., tubocurarine, succinylcholine) are administered to the patient who recently has received quinidine.

Concurrent administration of gastric antacids containing aluminum hydroxide may delay absorption of oral quinidine. Aluminum hydroxide slows gastric emptying and consequently delays transit of quinidine to the intestinal absorption sites.

Drugs that raise the pH of renal tubule urine (i.e., sodium bicarbonate, sodium lactate, thiazide diuretics, carbonic anhydrase inhibitors) may increase reabsorption of quinidine, a weak base, from the tubule urine. At the higher pH level, the amount of the free lipid-soluble form of the drug is increased, and it is more readily reabsorbed than the ionized form found at a lower pH level. The process raises the blood level of quinidine and prolonged Q-T intervals may be seen on the ECG.

During therapy with quinidine the synergistic action when other cardiac depressants (i.e., antiarrhythmic drugs) are administered may cause bradycardia or asystole. The myocardial depressant effect of rauwolfia alkaloids (i.e., reserpine) that occurs secondary to depletion of catecholamines may enhance the cardiac depressant action of quinidine. When the drugs are given concurrently, the patient should be monitored for adequacy of cardiac output. The vasodilating effects of all antihypertensive drugs may be potentiated when quinidine is used concurrently, and the patient should be monitored for evidence of hypotension.

Hypoprothrombinemia may occur in some patients receiving both quinidine and oral anticoagulants (i.e., warfarin). The problem occurs as a consequence of the action of each drug, which involves depression of the hepatic enzymes that synthesize the vitamin K–dependent factors required for the coagulation process.

Procainamide

Action Mode. Procainamide has pharmacologic properties similar to those of quinidine. Procainamide depresses the excitability of all cardiac tissue, and the conduction velocity is slowed in both the atrial and the ventricular specialized conducting system. The drug effectively suppresses automaticity in either atrial or ventricular tissue, and it is widely used for short-term and long-term treatment of arrhythmias.

Procainamide, like quinidine, has local anesthetic and anticholinergic properties. The local anesthetic property may contribute to the depression of membrane responsiveness to stimulation. The direct action of procainamide reduces conduction and the antivagal property maintains the prolonged effective refractory period by interfering with fiber responses to vagal stimulation.

Procainamide is widely employed for the control of atrial arrhythmias. It is employed also for emergency or long-term control of ventricular arrhythmias (i.e., ventricular tachycardia, premature ventricular contractions), and it has been found effective as a prophylactic antiarrhythmic agent for patients with acute myocardial infarction.

Therapy Considerations. Procainamide is available in forms for intravenous, intramuscular, or oral administration. The drug is prescribed for oral use in nonacute situations. The usual dosage is 250 to 500 mg administered at three-hour intervals. The oral drug is fairly well absorbed from the intestine (75 to 90 percent). Only 15 to 20 percent of the drug is bound to plasma proteins (Table 8–2), and the drug is readily distributed in highly vascular tissues (i.e., liver, spleen, kidneys, heart). Oral administration leads to a peak plasma concentration in one to one and one-half hours. The plasma drug level falls rapidly, and the drug has a relatively short half-life (2.2 to 3.5 hours). Without the use of a loading-dose regimen, a steady-state blood concentration is reached at about four times the half-life regardless of the size of the dose of procainamide. Maintenance of that level requires consistent administration of the drug exactly on the time schedule to avoid peaks and valleys in the drug concentration profile. The usual effective antiarrhythmic therapeutic serum level of procainamide is 4 to 8 mcg/ml. A serum drug level as high as 12 mcg may be required when the arrhythmia is unresponsive at lower levels. Serious toxicity is rare with serum drug concentrations below 12 mcg/ml.

The short time intervals between doses and the necessity for frequent monitoring of serum drug levels limit use of the drug to hospitalized patients. The hazards involved in poor patient compliance to the therapy plan outweigh the possible benefits of prophylactic use of procainamide for ambulatory patients.

In emergency situations involving ventricular arrhythmias (i.e., ventricular tachycardia) procainamide may be given parenterally as a loading dose to provide a prompt therapeutic serum drug level. The seriousness of the patient's cardiac status influences the route chosen. An intramuscular injection of procainamide provides a maximum effect in 15 to 60 minutes, but an intravenous bolus of drug provides an almost immediate effect.

An initial intravenous bolus of 100 mg of procainamide can be repeated every five minutes until the maximum cumulative dosage of 1 gm is reached. Intravenous bolus administration is usually discontinued when the arrhythmia is suppressed or adverse effects occur. Intravenous drug almost invariably causes a precipitous fall in blood pressure, and the injection is discontinued if the blood pressure falls more than 15 mm Hg, to prevent the cardiovascular collapse, convulsions, and coronary insufficiency that are known to be sequelae.

A constant-rate intravenous infusion of procainamide produces an effective serum drug concentration in six hours, and 90 percent of the steady-state concentration is reached in 12 hours. Whether the drug is given intramuscularly, by intravenous bolus, or by intravenous infusion in an emergency situation, the oral route is used for administration as soon as the arrhythmia is controlled.

The effectiveness of procainamide in control of an arrhythmia is monitored by following the P-R, QRS, and Q-T intervals on the cardiac monitor or ECG recording. Each of the intervals is prolonged at therapeutic drug levels. Slowing of the QRS time by more than 30 percent may indicate potential procainamide toxicity.

At termination of therapy with oral procainamide, which correlates with control of the arrhythmia, withdrawal is managed by using a gradually declining dosage scale. The procedure involves careful monitoring over a 72-hour period while drug levels are lowered. For example, when the drug is being administered at 375 mg every four hours, the dosage is changed, for a 24-hour period, to 250 mg every three hours, and during the final 24-hour period, the dosage is decreased to 250 mg every four hours. At the end of the time period, procainamide administration is discontinued.

Procainamide is hydrolyzed in the plasma to *p-aminobenzoic acid* and *diethylaminoethylamine,* and it is acetylated in the liver. There are differences in the rate of hepatic acetylation between individuals who are genetically fast acetylators and those who are slow acetylators. The fast acetylators have a significantly higher portion of a dose of procainamide in the circulation as the active metabolite, N-*acetylprocainamide* (NAPA), and the metabolite contributes to the antiarrhythmic activity of procainamide. Slow acetylators have a higher plasma content of procainamide than that of NAPA, and that difference is thought to contribute to the higher incidence of a lupus-like reaction during long-term use of procainamide in genetic slow acetylators.

Procainamide is eliminated by glomerular filtration and by renal tubule secretion. Between 50 and 60 percent of an oral dose of the drug is eliminated in the urine as unchanged drug. Approximately 15.6 percent is eliminated as the active metabolite NAPA, and 2 to 10 percent is eliminated as free and conjugated *p*-aminobenzoic acid.

The differences in metabolism rates between fast and slow acetylators are seen in urinary excretion of the drug. Fast acetylators eliminate a greater portion of drug as NAPA. The metabolite is more soluble than the unchanged parent drug. NAPA has a higher rate of passive reabsorption from the renal tubules, and that back diffusion adds to the content of the metabolite in the serum. Slow acetylators excrete a larger proportion of the drug unchanged.

Preparations Available. Procainamide is available as *procainamide hydrochloride* (PRONESTYL) in the form of tablets or capsules. *Procainamide hydrochloride injecton* is available for intramuscular or intravenous administration.

Adverse Effects. The most serious adverse effects occur with intravenous administration of procainamide. Marked hypotension occurs following bolus drug administration or during IV infusion. When the blood pressure falls more than 15 mm Hg, the drug is discontinued. Hypotension rarely occurs during use of oral forms of the drug.

The adverse cardiovascular effects during use of procainamide are toxic extensions of the planned therapeutic effects on conduction and contraction. Bradycardia, asystole, or heart block may occur during therapy, and the patients must be monitored closely to assure early recognition of the cardiac changes. Congestive heart failure is always a concern when drugs slow cardiac contraction in patients with a low cardiac reserve.

The anticholinergic properties of procainamide, like those of quinidine, can cause cardioacceleration by antagonizing the vagus nerve–mediated slowing of conduction. During intravenous administration, the decreased cardiac output and hypotension may precipitate sympathetic nerve stimulation, which increases the heart rate.

The anticholinergic property of procainamide also may interfere with vagal control that slows the conduction velocity and increases the refractory period of the AV node. Digitalis glycosides may be administered prior to procainamide to lessen the risk of ventricular arrhythmias when the drug is given to control atrial fibrillation or flutter.

The vagolytic effect of procainamide has an adverse effect on gastrointestinal motility. Interference with vagal tone can cause decreased peristalsis, abdominal distention, or paralytic ileus. The bitter taste of the drug and its irritation of the gastrointestinal tract are the cause of nausea, vomiting, or diarrhea that commonly occurs during therapy with the drug.

Procainamide has precipitated asthmatic attacks in individuals with bronchial asthma. Other allergic reactions include anaphylaxis, febrile reactions, serum sickness-like reaction, pruritus, and photosensitivity.

A systemic lupus-like syndrome, which is an autoimmune phenomenon, is associated with long-term use of procainamide. Previous to development of symptoms, tests for antinuclear antibodies (ANA) and lupus erythematosus (LE) preparations become positive. The syndrome is the most common side effect of long-term treatment with high dosage of procainamide, and it is estimated to occur in approximately 50 percent of the individuals taking the drug for more than six months. The incidence is high in those individuals who are slow acetylators of procainamide. Problems occurring with onset of the syndrome include afternoon fever, night sweats, polyarthritis, myalgia, pleuritic pain, pericarditis, and insomnia. The symptoms regress when the drug is withdrawn, and there is seldom any evidence of permanent vital organ damage. Tests for LE cells and ANA remain positive for some time after the symptoms have subsided.

Some of the problems that can occur with use of procainamide are infrequently observed, and discontinuing use of the drug reverses the symptoms. Problems related to the central nervous system (i.e., psychosis, hallucinations, giddiness, confusion, malaise, mental depression) or blood dyscrasias (i.e., agranulocytosis, leukopenia, bone marrow plasmacytosis, thrombocytopenia) are reported as occurring infrequently during therapy.

Interactions. Most of the interactions described as occurring during administration of quinidine could occur with use of procainamide, but there are few reports of interactions between procainamide and other drugs. The anticholinergic property of procainamide suggests the need to observe the patient for evidence of drug interactions when anticholinergic agents (i.e., belladonna alkaloids) or drugs with anticholinergic properties (i.e., phenothiazines, antihistamines, tricyclic antidepressants) are administered concurrently. The patient should be observed for adequacy of salivation and peristaltic activity when the drugs are given.

Procainamide has a neuromuscular blocking property, and there may be diminished acetylcholine activity at the motor system myoneural junction when drugs with a neuromuscular blocking property are administered concurrently. When procainamide is used with drugs affecting acetylcholine activity at the motor end plate (i.e., kanamycin, neomycin, polymyxin B, streptomycin), the patient should be observed for evidence of muscle weakness or fatigue.

Procainamide excretion is less affected by the pH of tubule urine than is quinidine, but tubule reabsorption of procainamide can occur when the pH of tubule urine is elevated. When drugs that raise the pH of urine are given concurrently (i.e., thiazide diuretics, carbonic anhydrase inhibitors, sodium bicarbonate, sodium lactate), more procainamide is reabsorbed from the tubule urine. Conversely, drugs that acidify the urine (i.e., ascorbic acid) may somewhat increase its elimination and lower the half-life. Any major changes in the patient's urinary pH indicate the need for assessing the patient for evidence of toxicity or for ineffectiveness of procainamide therapy.

Combinations of antiarrhythmic drugs are sometimes employed for control of rhythm disturbances. When drugs with cardiac depressant effects are used during the time the patient is receiving procainamide, cardiac conduction and contraction patterns should be monitored regularly.

Propranolol

Action Mode. Propranolol is a beta-adrenergic blocking agent used to control the cardiac arrhythmias and cardioacceleration caused by sympathetic nerve stimulation. Propranolol combines reversibly with the receptors and blocks the access of the norepinephrine to them. Release of norepinephrine at beta-adrenergic receptors of the SA node and other conduction tissue normally increases automaticity, decreases the effective refractory period, and increases contractility. Those effects are muted when propranolol is administered. The drug prolongs the refractory period of the SA node and the AV node and it decreases ventricular automaticity.

Propranolol also exerts a direct membrane effect independent of the beta-adrenergic blocking action. The drug has a local anesthetic property that may have some slight effect on the stabilization of myocardial cell membranes effected by propranolol in the control of automaticity.

The drug is used for control of many of the arrhythmias occurring as toxic manifestations of digitalis therapy, (i.e., supraventricular tachyarrhythmias). Because it increases the refractory period of the AV node it also is useful for the control of ventricular response to atrial fibrillation or flutter.

Many cardiac arrhythmias occur secondary to beta-adrenergic stimulation, and propranolol provides effective control of the excess stimulation. The drug also is considered to be the mainstay of therapy for control of the anginal pain occurring in patients with coronary arteriosclerosis or atherosclerosis. Propranolol blocking of sympathetic nerve stimulation reduces oxygen consumption by reducing the strength of contraction and decreasing the heart rate. The reduction in cardiac work reduces the metabolic rate of the myocardium, and there is a more even ratio between the supply and demand for blood flow through the coronary arteries.

Therapy Considerations. Propranolol is available in forms allowing administration orally or intravenously, but the oral drug is employed more frequently. Because absorption from the intestinal tract may be delayed when the drug is ingested with foods, the drug is administered before meals and at bedtime. Intestinal absorption is nearly complete (90 percent), and the drug is widely distributed in body tissues. Propranolol readily crosses the blood-brain barrier and the placenta barrier.

Propranolol is metabolized in the liver, lungs, and kidneys, and the processes include many complex steps involving several active metabolites. Considerable variation is found in the rate of metabolism of propranolol, and some of the differences are related to the rate of passage through the liver. The drug that is absorbed from the intestinal tract enters the portal circulation and travels to hepatic sites. Propranolol is avidly extracted from the blood entering the sinusoids, and liver tissue may sequester up to 30 mg of the drug before hepatic sites are saturated. One of the considerations of therapy plans is to provide adequate drug (> 10 mg every six hours) to provide the amount known to remain at liver-binding sites and allow additional drug for therapeutic effect at cardiac sites.

Propranolol has a relatively short serum half-life (Table 8–2), and a steady-state concentration can be attained in approximately 12 hours by periodic administration of the drug. A peak effect on cardiac tissue is attained one to one and one-half hours after oral administration of the drug.

Propranolol is 90 to 95 percent bound to plasma protein. Most of the drug is metabolized before excretion. Less than 5 percent of the unchanged drug appears in the urine. Propranolol and its metabolites also are excreted in breast milk.

The dosage of propranolol is adjusted to achieve a resting pulse of 60 to 65 beats per minute, and the dosage range for reaching that level varies widely (i.e., 40 mg to 600 mg/24 hours). The initial dose usually is small because there is an unknown amount of beta-adrenergic blockade being introduced into an unknown environment of adrenergic activity. Dosage is gradually increased, but a drop in blood pressure to under 100 mm Hg systolic may preclude or postpone dosage increments. Dosage is considered adequate when there is at least a 10 percent fall in the resting heart rate. When the drug is administered to control angina pectoris, dosage increments may be planned at three- to seven-day intervals. An optimum response often occurs when the dosage reaches 160 to 240 mg/day given in four divided doses. The dosage level for control of arrhythmias may be considerably lower (i.e., 10 to 30 mg three to four times/day). At the termination of long periods of drug therapy, the dosage is gradually decreased over a two-week period. Sudden withdrawal of the large dosage employed for control of anginal pain may cause myocardial infarction or arrhythmogenic sudden death.

Preparations Available. Propranolol is available for oral use as *propranolol hydrochloride* (INDERAL) tablets. It also is available as *propranolol hydrochloride* in ampules for intravenous use.

Adverse Effects. Propranolol action causes a marked decrease in cardiac output and a consequent decrease in systolic blood pressure. During therapy, individuals may have a reduction in activity tolerance because the usual sympathetic nerve compensatory mechanisms are lessened by the blocking action of the drug. When strenuous activity is attempted, the individual may experience light-headedness, vertigo, syncope, weakness, and fatigue.

Administration of propranolol to individuals with a low cardiac mechanical reserve may precipitate symptoms of heart failure. The cardiac depressant effects of the drug contribute to increased diastolic blood volume and the increased cardiac work may cause heart failure. The drug also may suppress cardiac conduction at a level causing sinus arrest, bradycardia, or AV nodal block.

Blocking of adrenergic responses may cause the individual who takes insulin for control of diabetes to have unheralded hypoglycemic episodes. The problems arise because there is no protective catecholamine-induced glycogenolysis to provide glucose, and the warning symptoms also are absent when sympathetic nerve responses are impaired (i.e., increased pulse, diaphoresis, blood pressure changes).

Propranolol may cause diverse gastrointestinal symptoms including transient episodes of nausea, vomiting, epigastric distress or abdominal cramps, constipation, or flatulence. The problems usually are relieved by decreasing the dose of the drug.

The serious problems occurring during therapy are visual disturbances, hallucinations, paresthesias of the hands, fever with myalgia, or sore throat. Beta-adrenergic blockade at bronchial sites can precipitate episodes of asthma in persons with a history of bronchial asthma or chronic obstructive lung disease.

Propranolol administration at high dosage or for long periods of time may cause symptoms of depression (i.e., malaise, insomnia, weakness, lassitude, fatigue) or overt psychosis. Tinnitus, alopecia, and peripheral artery insufficiency are problems that are disturbing to patients during long-term therapy. In most instances, the problems are reversed when drug therapy is discontinued.

Interactions. Propranolol antagonizes both the hypotensive and positive inotropic effects of levodopa by antagonizing the beta-adrenergic properties of the dopamine that is formed during levodopa administration. Propranolol also antagonizes the beta-stimulation action of isoproterenol at cardiac and bronchial sites, and it also blocks the stimulation action of epinephrine at cardiac sites.

Propranolol and phenothiazines, when used concurrently, can produce an additive hypotensive effect. The beta-blocking action in combination with the alpha-blocking property of phenothiazines decreases vascular responses to sympathetic nerve stimulation. Propranolol also enhances the hypotensive action of antihypertensive agents. The catecholamine-depleting action of reserpine also could add to the beta-adrenergic blocking action of propranolol.

Propranolol has an anticholinergic property that has minimal effect on its action during therapy. Anticholinergic drugs (i.e., atropine sulfate, tricyclic antidepressants) may counteract the beta-blocking action of propranolol that causes bradycardia by reestablishing the parasympathetic-sympathetic nerve balance.

Propranolol intereferes with carbohydrate metabolism, and the drug may increase or decrease blood glucose levels. The effect on glucose levels occurs independent of the beta-blocking action of propranolol. The variation in blood glucose levels when propranolol is administered makes it necessary to monitor individuals receiving insulin or oral hypoglycemics carefully during therapy. Propranolol also prolongs the hypoglycemic effect of insulin by interfering with catecholamine-induced glycogenolysis.

Propranolol affects acetylcholine activity at the motor nerve terminal. Concurrent administration of depolarizing muscle relaxants (i.e., decamethonium, succinylcholine) or nondepolarizing muscle relaxants (i.e., gallamine triethiodide, pancuronium) or drugs with muscle-relaxant properties can cause muscle weakness and fatigue.

The blocking of the beta-adrenergic vasodilating effect by propranolol can synergize the potent vasoconstrictor effects of ergot alkaloids (i.e., CAFERGOT) that are employed to relieve migraine headaches. Propranolol also competes with aspirin for the anti-inflammatory receptor sites.

Lidocaine

Action Mode. Lidocaine is a local anesthetic that is frequently prescribed for short-term arrhythmia control. The drug is used primarily in emergency situations where ventricular arrhythmias pose a threat to life. Lidocaine is effective in the control of ventricular tachycardia, premature ventricular contractions, and digitalis-induced ventricular arrhythmias.

Lidocaine is chemically similar to procainamide, and procainamide often is used to maintain control of a ventricular arrhythmia after an initial period of therapy with lidocaine. The primary effects of lidocaine administration are a decrease in the automaticity in the Purkinje fibers and an elevation of the ventricular fibrillatory threshold.

Therapy Considerations. Lidocaine is administered as an intravenous bolus, intravenous infusion, or intramuscular injection. When the drug is administered by intramuscular injection into the deltoid area, effective blood levels are attained in five to ten minutes. The peak effect occurs in 15 minutes and a therapeutic effect is maintained for 90 to 120 minutes. Injection of lidocaine into the gluteal muscle produces a slower and less reliable therapeutic effect than deltoid muscle injection.

The rapid onset of action when the drug is administered as an intravenous injection (45 to 90 seconds) and the short duration of action (20 minutes) allow control of life-threatening arrhythmias by readministration of the drug at short time intervals. When given intravenously, the plasma half-life of lidocaine is 10 to 15 minutes, and repeated bolus injections calculated on the basis of 1 mg/kg of body weight may be given until the cumulative maximum of 5 mg/kg is reached.

The initial bolus, or loading dose, of lidocaine is followed by intravenous infusion if the arrhythmia persists. Intravenous infusion at 2 to 4 mg/minute provides a therapeutic blood level and attainment of a steady-state concentration in 8 to 24 hours. The range of steady-state therapeutic serum levels of lidocaine is 2 to 5 mcg/ml, and levels above that range rapidly lead to toxic effects of the drug.

Lidocaine is almost exclusively metabolized by the microsomal enzymes in the liver. Since approximately 90 percent of the drug is rapidly metabolized, the rate of hepatic blood flow becomes an important factor in the blood concentration of the drug. The active metabolite, *monoethylglycinexylidide* (MEGX), has a serum half-life similar to that of lidocaine, and it contributes to the therapeutic action of the drug. MEGX is metabolized in the liver, and it is excreted in the urine as the active metabolite *glycinexylidide* (GX). The importance of the active metabolites relates to their contributions to the therapeutic effect of lidocaine and to the central nervous system toxicity that can occur during administration of the drug.

Lidocaine, like other local anesthetics, has a high affinity for adipose tissues, and it also is widely distributed in highly perfused body tissues (i.e., kidney, lungs, liver, heart). The wide distribution in tissues results in a short half-life for therapeutic effectiveness of the drug. The distribution characteristics also affect dosage calculations, because serum levels may be somewhat higher in lean individuals than in those who are obese.

During the time of intravenous infusion, the patient is monitored regularly for status changes. To avoid inadvertent rapid infusion, the intravenous usually has a double clamp setup, or the drip rate may be controlled by an automatic pump. Lidocaine (2 percent) is diluted in a sterile intravenous solution (i.e., dextrose in water) and a minidrip setup may be used to allow delicate titration of the flow rate with the frequency of ectopic beats.

A graphic record is maintained while the lidocaine infusion is running. A clear profile of the incidence and characteristics of the arrhythmia, the amount of drug being infused per minute, and other relevant factors (i.e., concurrent drug administration, changes in the patient's status) is recorded in a correlated time sequence to allow rapid analysis of the cardiac response to therapy during any time period.

Preparations Available.   Lidocaine is available as *lidocaine hydrochloride injection* (XYLOCAINE). The preparation may be in the form of a prefilled syringe for bolus injection, or it may be in a vial requiring dilution before administration as an intramuscular injection or intravenous infusion.

Adverse Effects.   Stimulation and depression of the central nervous system are the most common adverse effects of lidocaine therapy. The incidence of the adverse effects is highest in the first 48 hours of therapy, but symptoms may appear at any time the patient is receiving the drug. Somnolence, tremulousness, drowsiness, disorientation, slight deafness, or paresthesias provide early clues to the toxic effects of lidocaine. Higher levels of lidocaine at brain sites can cause depression of inhibitory influences on motor pathways, and convulsions, coma, or respiratory arrest may occur. Modifying the dosage or discontinuing the drug usually relieves the symptoms.

Hypotension, conduction disturbances, bradycardia, tachyarrhythmias, and heart block are cardiovascular problems that may occur during therapy with lidocaine. The cardiac status of the patient influences the decision to discontinue lidocaine therapy, employ alternate drug therapy, or continue lidocaine infusion and implement supportive measures for control of the adverse effects.

Interactions. Lidocaine usually is employed for emergency or short-term therapy, and other drugs may be administered during the emergency situation. When antiarrhythmic drugs are given concurrently, there may be an intensification of the cardiac-depressant effects of lidocaine. Drugs that have a potential for slowing hepatic blood flow may prolong the half-life of lidocaine.

Phenytoin

Action Mode. Phenytoin has been used for many years as an anticonvulsant, and currently is employed selectively for control of cardiac arrhythmias. Phenytoin is thought to reduce ectopic pacemaker automaticity by increasing potassium conductance during diastole thus preventing spontaneous diastolic depolarization. The drug enhances AV conduction and decreases ventricular automaticity.

Phenytoin is one of the primary drugs employed for control of supraventricular tachycardia or ventricular premature systoles that occur as cardiotoxic effects of digitalis. Phenytoin is particularly useful because it shortens the refractory period of the AV node and improves conduction in the digitalis toxic cardiac tissue.

Therapy Considerations. Phenytoin may be administered orally or intravenously for arrhythmia control. The high pH of phenytoin solution (pH 11 to 12) precludes intramuscular administration, and the high alkalinity also makes it advisable for the solution to be injected into the largest available vein to avoid phlebitis.

Approximately 90 to 100 percent of the oral drug is absorbed from the small intestine within six hours after ingestion. Phenytoin is distributed in adipose tissue and in highly vascular organs (i.e., heart, liver, brain, kidney). Fifty percent of the drug in the plasma is bound to proteins (Table 8–2). Because phenytoin becomes sequestered in body tissues and is highly bound to plasma proteins, 48 to 96 hours are required to attain the plasma level required for peak therapeutic effect.

Daily administration of the oral drug for from 5 to 15 days is required before the plasma drug level reaches a steady-state therapeutic concentration. The prolonged time period reflects the slow rate of metabolism and the long half-life for elimination of phenytoin.

Phenytoin is metabolized in the liver by deethylation and hydroxylation. The principal metabolite is *5-phenyl-5-parahydroxyphenylhydantoin* (HPPH), and the glucuronic conjugate of HPPH is excreted in the urine. The urine content of HPPH can be measured to identify the source of problems when plasma levels show variation. An increase in urine HPPH content occurs when metabolism is accelerated, and the urine HPPH content is lower when metabolism of phenytoin is decelerated by interacting drugs.

Immediate control of arrhythmias with phenytoin requires intravenous administration to attain the therapeutic serum level of 10 to 20 mcg/ml (Table 8–2). The drug is given as a slowly administered intravenous bolus (maximum = 50 mg/min). Because plasma levels cannot be monitored effectively during intravenous infusion and prolonged infusion irritates the veins, an IV bolus dosage of 100 mg every five minutes may be given. The dosage may be repeated until the arrhythmia is abolished, an estimated plasma level of 18 mcg/ml is reached, or toxicity appears. The onset of hypotension is an indication for discontinuing administration of the drug. Usually a cumulative total of 1000 mg is given over the first 24 hours and 500 mg may be given on the following day.

Intravenous administration of phenytoin is hazardous even with the precautionary use of electrocardiographic monitoring. Fatalities from respiratory arrest, arrhythmias, and hypotension have occurred. The life-threatening problems occur more frequently in patients with low serum albumin concentrations or patients who have been hospitalized for long periods of time. The toxicity may be partly attributable to the propylene glycol solvent vehicle in the intravenous preparations.

The initial loading dose of the drug is followed by administration of the oral drug on a daily basis to maintain suppression of the arrhythmia. The effectiveness of phenytoin in reducing the refractory period of the AV node can be observed by noting the shortened Q-T interval on the cardiac monitor or ECG recordings.

Preparations Available.   Phenytoin is available as *phenytoin* oral formulations prepared by many manufacturers as tablets, chewable tablets, extended release tablets, and oral suspensions. *Phenytoin sodium* (DILANTIN) is available as capsules, tablets, and extended-release tablets, and in ampules or prefilled syringes containing solutions for parenteral use.

Adverse Effects.   Phenytoin causes few adverse effects when administered orally in dosages recommended for arrhythmia control, but problems can occur with high serum drug levels (> 20 mcg/ml). The most common adverse effects are nystagmus and diplopia. High serum drug levels (i.e., > 30 mcg/ml) can precipitate problems with coordination and balance (i.e., tremor, unsteady gait, ataxia). Most of the problems are reversible when the drug is discontinued, but ataxia may be a chronic problem.

Phenytoin is irritating to the gastric mucosa, and nausea frequently is a problem during oral drug therapy. Taking the drug with a snack or with a large glass of water helps to alleviate the discomfort.

Mild megaloblastic anemia may occur during long-term therapy. Phenytoin inhibits activity of the intestinal conjugate enzymes involved in conversion of *polyglutamates* to the readily absorbed *monoglutamates,* and the enzyme inhibition reduces absorption of folic acid from the intestine. The resultant megaloblastic anemia that occurs in some patients is modified by concurrent adminis-tration of folic acid during therapy with phenytoin.

Interactions.   Several drugs can alter phenytoin biotransformation by inhibiting or inducing the hepatic microsomal enzymes involved in metabolism. Inhibition of phenytoin metabolism allows cumulation and serum drug levels may be elevated to the toxic range. There may be as much as a 50 percent increase in the serum half-life when metabolism is retarded and the individual continues to take the drug on a regular schedule. Oral anticoagulants, phenylbutazone, methylphenidate, chlordiazepoxide, diazepam, chloramphenicol, disulfiram, and some of the sulfonamides can inhibit phenytoin metabolism at hepatic sites. In genetically slow acetylators, isoniazid inhibits parahydroxylation of phenytoin in the liver.

Phenytoin metabolism may be accelerated by drugs that induce hepatic microsomal enzymes, and rapid metabolism decreases the therapeutic serum levels of phenytoin. Alcohol ingestion (in alcoholics), carbamazepine, or folic acid may increase the rate of phenytoin metabolism when the drugs are used concurrently.

Phenobarbital has a variable effect on phenytoin biotransformation when the drugs are administered concurrently. In some individuals, the enzyme induction caused by phenobarbital accelerates phenytoin metabolism, but in other individuals the serum phenytoin level may be elevated as a consequence of phenobarbital inhibition of the microsomal enzymes. The variability may be related to the total amount of the drug used in a given time period.

Concurrent administration of phenytoin with other drugs may accelerate metabolism of those drugs and decrease their therapeutic effect. For example, phenytoin may decrease the serum levels and the half-life of dicumarol and may accelerate the metabolism of vitamin D, doxycycline, and some glucocorticoids (i.e., dexamethasone).

Phenytoin administration concurrent with insulin or sulfonylurea hypoglycemics can cause hyperglycemia. The blood glucose level is elevated by phenytoin inhibition of insulin secretion. Phenytoin stimulates the ATP "sodium pump" at pancreatic beta cells, and the decreased intracellular sodium reduces the excitability necessary to allow insulin production by the pancreatic cells.

Bretylium Tosylate

Bretylium tosylate (BRETYLOL INJECTION) is an adrenergic neuron blocking agent that is employed when other antiarrhythmic drugs fail to control ventricular arrhythmias. The drug has positive inotropic, chronotropic, and dromotropic effects that differ from other antiarrhythmic drugs. It blocks neurotransmitter release from the postganglionic adrenergic neuron and that action decreases automaticity and raises the threshold to ventricular fibrillation. The refractoriness of cardiac fibers also may be useful in abolishing reentrant arrhythmias.

The drug dosage is calculated on the basis of 5 to 10 mg/kg of body weight and that dose is given intravenously or intramuscularly. Immediately after administration of the drug there is a rapid release of catecholamine from the adrenergic neurons that causes a temporary increase in the automaticity of cardiac fibers, a transient increase in conduction velocity, and a sudden, sharp elevation of the systolic and diastolic blood pressure. Postural hypotension, which is a common adverse effect, occurs as a consequence of the drug-induced decrease in sympathetic nerve control of cardiac output. Nausea, vomiting, nasal congestion, muscle weakness, and mental confusion also occur during therapy. High concentrations of the drug can cause a curarelike paralysis with muscle weakness and fatigue.

Verapamil

Verapamil (ISOPTIN) is a relatively new antiarrhythmic drug that acts selectively to inhibit the depolarizing calcium current. The drug directly blocks the slow inward channel for calcium movement and alters the electrophysiologic properties of automatic myocardial fibers.

Verapamil has been particularly effective in control of supraventricular arrhythmias that result from reentrant impulses. The drug depresses conduction through the AV node and that action interrupts the reentrant circuits. The prolongation of nodal conduction time can be seen as a lengthened P-R interval on the ECG.

The drug is administered in oral or intravenous doses of 80 mg two to three times a day. Maximum plasma drug levels are attained two hours after oral administration, and the drug is rapidly distributed in body tissues.

The drug is metabolized by demethylation at hepatic sites and most of the metabolites are excreted in the bile (80 percent). The remaining metabolites are excreted in the urine and drug elimination usually is complete at the end of 48 hours. The elimination half-life of the major metabolites is ten hours. Transient mild hypotension is the most common adverse effect and bradycardia also may occur during therapy.

Disopyramine

Disopyramine phosphate (NORPACE) is a relatively new oral antiarrhythmic drug that acts like the group I drugs, quinidine and procainamide. Disopyramine decreases the conduction velocity and prolongs the action potential duration of myocardial fibers.

The drug effectively suppresses all types of ectopic impulses and is particularly useful in control of ventricular extrasystoles. Administration of the drug to patients with chronic ischemic heart disease may reduce the frequency of episodic ventricular tachycardia.

Adults may initially be given a loading dose of 300 mg followed by 150 mg at six-hour intervals. The usual daily dosage is 400 to 800 mg. When the drug therapy is being changed to disopyramine, the initial dose is given six to twelve hours after the last dose of quinidine sulfate and three to six hours after that of procainamide.

Disopyramine is metabolized in the liver. More than half of the unchanged drug is excreted in the urine. The most distressing adverse effect from the patient's point of view is the dryness of the mouth that occurs as a consequence of the anticholinergic properties of the drug. The major adverse effect is severe hypotension.

NURSING INTERVENTION

Identification and control of arrhythmias are recurrent concerns in intensive care units where patients are monitored closely for status changes following major surgery or acute medical crises (i.e., myocardial infarction). The availability of sophisticated monitoring devices provides objective data that facilitate definition of the progression and hemodynamic consequences of disturbances in cardiac rhythm. Electronic monitoring of cardiac conduction patterns, cardiopulmonary and intra-arterial pressures, and cardiac output supplies data that allow continual adjustments in the dosage of antiarrhythmic drugs as changes occur in cardiac conduction and hemodynamic parameters.

There are numerous situations in which arrhythmias occur within the framework of intermediate, chronic, or ambulatory care of patients with diverse health problems. Chronic heart disease, coronary artery stenosis, debilitation, and acute physiologic stress are some of the risk factors that increase the potential for emergence of cardiac rhythm disturbances. Identification of arrhythmias and assessing the effectiveness of drugs in control of rhythm disturbances can be a vital aspect of nursing care in any health care setting.

The seriousness of an arrhythmia is related to its effect on cardiac output and the possibility of its progression to a life-threatening disruption of ventricular conduction. For example, the heartbeat may be irregular when atrial fibrillation is controlled by digitalis, but sufficient blood is ejected with each ventricular contraction to meet physiologic needs. Although an antiarrhythmic drug (i.e., quinidine) may be prescribed for control of the fibrillation pattern, the adequacy of cardiac output lessens the concern about the arrhythmia. Frequent premature ventricular contrac-

tions also may have minimal effect on cardiac output, but the ventricular irritability they represent portends the possibility of ventricular fibrillation and cardiac arrest. Intensive therapy is indicated for control of ventricular ectopic beats occurring more frequently than six times per minute.

Initial Status Evaluation

In the acute situation, control of the arrhythmia is the focus of health team activities. It also is important to obtain information about the previous health status and functional level of the patient as base-line data for analysis of physiologic and behavioral changes during therapy. The cardiac status and the initial anxiety of the patient may preclude obtaining information for assessing the cardiac and extracardiac responses to therapy. Family members, relatives, or close friends may be able to provide relevant information, and it usually is comforting to them to feel they are contributing to the patient's care. Provocative questioning is useful in directing the interview of individuals whose anxiety about a loved one's progress makes it difficult to volunteer information. For example, direct questioning may be required to ascertain whether the patient's confusion and sluggish verbal responses are related to the present crisis or to a previous health problem (i.e., stroke) that affected cerebral tissue perfusion.

When the interview is conducted, psychologic support of the family or friends is a meaningful outcome of the interaction. The data obtained during the interview must be carefully analyzed to delete irrelevant information volunteered by the distraught interviewees and to determine the information that is pertinent to the patient's immediate care and the data that will provide a base line for ongoing assessment of progress. It is possible that the input may contain clues to factors that contributed to the onset of the acute cardiac incident. For example, the patient's wife may have responded in the affirmative to the initial inquiry by the physician about whether her husband had been taking the prescribed anti-arrhythmic drug. If, during the interview, she indicates that he has been treating an annoying cold for two days, it is important to ascertain the measures he employed to treat the cold. If it is found that the patient's self-medication plan included drugs with a potential for causing extracardiac symptoms or interacting with the antiarrhythmic drug (i.e., nasal decongestant, antihistamines), the information should be communicated promptly to the physician.

Physical Examination. The physical examination provides objective data for evaluating the effectiveness of the antiarrhythmic drug regimen. The examination includes evaluation of the cardiac rhythm pattern and the effects of the arrhythmia on cardiovascular dynamics.

Listening to the cardiac sounds with a stethoscope at the apex of the heart is an essential part of the examination. Specific details of the sounds that characterize the arrhythmia are useful in later definition of changes. When the patient is on a cardiac monitor, it is a useful practice to draw a sample of the basic pattern on a piece of adhesive tape and attach it to the top of the monitor for future reference. Taking an ECG rhythm strip (leads II and V_1) provides a base line for definition of the basic rhythm and the arrhythmia pattern. Measurement of the key intervals on the rhythm strip allows specific comparison during antiarrhythmic drug therapy.

The effect of the arrhythmia on cardiac output can be analyzed by comparing the heart rate, rhythm, and strength of contraction with the pulse rate, rhythm, and strength. The blood pressure and the apical-radial pulse (taken during the same minute by two people) provide information about the adequacy of each cardiac contraction in filling the peripheral arteries. The characteristics of distal pulses (i.e., pedal pulse) also provide information about the adequacy of arterial filling.

Capillary filling can be defined by pressing on the fingernail and checking the time required for color to return when the pressure is released. The adequacy of tissue perfusion can be monitored by observing the color of superficial tissues (i.e., skin, nailbeds, lips, buccal mucosa), measuring the urine output, and evaluating mental acuity.

Assessing Progress

A primary concern during therapy is the assessment of the effectiveness of drug therapy in control of the arrhythmia. The practice of frequent-interval monitoring allows early identification of changes in cardiac function. When the apical pulse is taken as part of the planned objective assessment of the patient's status, it is possible to identify bradycardia, tachycardia, irregular conduction patterns of atrial fibrillation, or the interruption of the normal heartbeat by premature ventricular contractions. The assessment can be validated by viewing the pattern on the cardiac monitoring or by running a short ECG rhythm strip. ECG validation of monitor patterns is essential for definition of fine changes in intervals or complexes. The rhythm strips taken by the nurse and the 12 lead recordings taken periodically by the laboratory technician provide comparative data about changes in the conduction pattern and the effect of the antiarrhythmic drugs on the cardiac rhythm.

When there is evidence of a decrease in cardiac output, the patient's care includes measures to conserve energy and to support physiologic efforts toward compensation. Administration of oxygen to the patient may decrease the myocardial hypoxia that contributes to the arrhythmia potential of irritable heart tissue.

Each of the antiarrhythmic drugs decreases automaticity and also decreases myocardial contractility. Excess prolongation of the P-R interval or widening of the QRS complex ($>$ 25 to 30 percent) provides the "alert" that conduction has slowed. Analysis of the heart sounds heard with a stethoscope at the apex of the heart also provides a valuable guide for early definition of cardiac decompensation. For example, when the patient is receiving a lidocaine intravenous infusion for control of premature ventricular contractions, the first and second heart sounds representing sinus node–initiated beats may be normal at the apex and the premature ventricular contractions are clearly identifiable interruptions in the sinus rhythm. Suppression of the ectopic beats by the lidocaine may return the rhythm to a regular and uninterrupted beat with normal heart sounds. Continued infusion of the lidocaine can cause cardiac decompensation and early signs of heart failure that are evident when listening to the heart sounds. An additional filling sound that occurs when the atrium empties into the ventricle forewarns of decompensation. The sound, called a *ventricular diastolic gallop,* is the earliest sign of a decrease in ventricular contractility. The ventricular diastolic gallop usually is associated with a succession of alternating strong and weak beats, which are described as *pulsus alternans.* Slowing of the lidocaine infusion rate usually leads to disappearance of the ventricular diastolic gallop and pulsus alternans, and myocardial contractility improves. The foregoing example provides a frame or reference for assessment of myocardial contractility during therapy with each of the antiarrhythmic drugs.

Counseling

Antiarrhythmic drugs are most frequently employed for short-term control of rhythm disturbances associated with myocardial infarction or cardiac surgery, but individuals may receive the drugs for long-term control of arrhythmias associated with chronic cardiac problems. The drugs do not correct the underlying problem but they are effective in decreasing rhythm disturbances.

Knowledge that there is a basic heart problem usually motivates the ambulatory patient to maintain the antiarrhythmic drug therapy regimen. When the patient is being prepared to maintain the antiarrhythmic drug therapy plan at home, the details of instructions are influenced by the particular plan for therapy.

It is helpful to the patient if all the essential information, about cardiac and extracardiac problems related to the particular antiarrhythmic drug, is communicated in a relaxed interactive session allowing the patient to clarify personal concerns about the drug and heart function (Fig. 8–3). The interactive pattern also allows presentation of suggestions for alleviating some of the problems related to the side effects of the drug (i.e., taking a large glass full of water with phenytoin to decrease gastric irritation). Explicit statements about the problems that must be reported to the physician can be made less threatening to the patient if the rationale for informing the physician is presented as allowing for the physician to make changes in drug dosage or to use measures that can alleviate untoward symptoms.

Discussions of activity modification are highly individualized and the measures adopted are dependent on the cardiac status of the individual. It is predictable that the ambulatory patient who is receiving an antiarrhythmic drug for suppression of automaticity also will have some loss of myocardial contractility. It is important to prepare the individual to monitor the effects of daily activities on the maintenance therapy. The individual must be prepared to recognize early signs of cardiac failure (i.e., fatigue, ankle edema, shortness of breath, paroxysmal nocturnal dyspnea) and understand the importance of prompt contact with the physician when problems arise.

Ambulatory patients who are taking antiarrhythmic drugs are periodically and regularly examined to ascertain the effectiveness of the drug regimen. The patient who fully understands the importance of this contact in attaining the desired therapeutic objectives can become motivated to comply with the scheduled appointments for evaluation of progress.

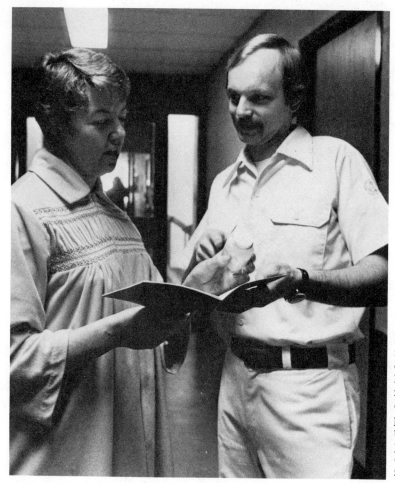

Fig. 8–3. The nurse's counseling of the patient who is to continue drug therapy after hospitalization should allow frequent informal interactive discussion of the drug therapy plan and the implications of the plan to the person's living patterns. (Courtesy, Northeastern University College of Nursing, Boston.)

Review Guides

1. Describe the electrophysiologic events occurring with premature ventricular contractions and the changes on the ECG that indicate effectiveness of lidocaine in controlling the arrhythmia.
2. Outline a plan for monitoring the status of a patient who is receiving lidocaine hydrochloride by intravenous infusion at 3 mg/minute for control of premature ventricular contractions.
3. Explain the rationale for the transition and the plan for assessment when a patient's drug therapy is changed from lidocaine to procainamide.
4. Explain the factors that influence plans for dosage scheduling when the patient is receiving procainamide.
5. List two primary concerns and the plans that would be employed for monitoring the patient's status when bretylium is being administered.
6. Outline the factors that would be considered when counseling a construction worker who is being discharged from the hospital with a prescription for propranolol about his drug therapy plan.
7. Outline a plan for assessing (interviewing and examining) the effects of drug therapy, during a clinic visit, when an individual is taking quinidine.

8. Formulate a list of questions that could be used during a clinic visit to obtain information about adverse effects and drug interactions when an individual is taking phenytoin.

Additional Readings

Adler, Jack: Patient assessment: abnormalities of the heartbeat (programmed instruction). *Am. J. Nurs.,* **77**:1, April, 1977.

Ahlquist, Raymond P.: Present state of alpha and beta adrenergic drugs. II. The adrenergic blocking agents. *Am. Heart J.,* **92**:804, December, 1976.

——: Present state of alpha and beta adrenergic drugs. III. Beta blocking agents. *Am. Heart J.,* **93**:117, January, 1977.

Alexander, Sidney: Ventricular premature beats: when is drug treatment justified? *Postgrad. Med.,* **60**:68, September, 1976.

Anderson, Gary A.: Use of lidocaine in ventricular arrhythmias. *Am. Fam. Physician,* **13**:118, June, 1976.

Aranda, Juan M.; Befeler, Benjamin; Castellanos, Agustin, Jr.; and Sherif, Nabil El: His bundle recordings: their contribution to the understanding of human electrophysiology. *Heart Lung,* **5**:907, November–December, 1976.

Arnsdorf, Morton F.: Electrophysiologic properties of antidysrhythmic drugs as a rational basis for therapy. *Med. Clin. North Am.,* **60**:213, March, 1976.

Aviado, Domingo M., and Salem, Harry: Drug action, reaction and interaction. 1. Quinidine for cardiac arrhythmias. *J. Clin. Pharmacol.,* **15**:477, July, 1975.

Coodley, Eugene L., and Snyder, Stuart: Propranolol and management of arrhythmias. *Am. Fam. Physician,* **14**:146, November, 1976.

Crouthamel, William G.: The effects of congestive heart failure on quinidine pharmacokinetics. *Am. Heart J.,* **90**:335, September, 1975.

Data, Joann L.; Wilkinson, Grant R.; and Nies, Alan S.: Interaction of quinidine with anticonvulsant drugs. *N. Engl. J. Med.,* **294**:699, March 25, 1976.

Devitt, Denis G., and Shand, David G.: Plasma concentrations and the time course of beta-blockade due to propranolol. *Clin. Pharmacol. Ther.,* **18**:708, December, 1975.

Ferrer, M. Irené: Axioms on heart block. *Hosp. Med.,* **13**:25, July, 1977.

Gelband, Henry, and Rosen, Michael R.: Pharmacologic basis for the treatment of cardiac arrhythmias. *Pediatrics,* **55**:59, January, 1975.

Ghose, Manash Kumar: Pericardial tamponade. A presenting manifestation of procainamide-induced lupus erythematosus. *Am. J. Med.,* **58**:581, April, 1975.

Giardina, Elsa-Grace V.; Dreyfuss, Jacques; Bigger, J. Thomas, Jr.; Shaw, James M.; and Schreiber, Eric C.: Metabolism of procainamide in normal and cardiac subjects. *Clin. Pharmacol. Ther.,* **19**:339, March, 1976.

Greenblatt, David J.; Bolognini, Victoria; Koch-Weser, Jan; and Harmatz, Jerold S.: Pharmacokinetic approach to the clinical use of lidocaine intravenously. *J.A.M.A.,* **236**:273, July 19, 1976.

Han, Jack: Management of cardiac arrhythmias. *Am. Fam. Physician,* **13**:128, January, 1976.

Hoffman, Brian F.; Rosen, Michael R.; and Wit, Andrew L.: Electrophysiology and pharmacology of cardiac arrhythmias. III. The causes and treatment of cardiac arrhythmias. A. *Am. Heart J.,* **85**:115, January, 1975.

——: The causes and treatment of cardiac arrhythmias. B. *Am. Heart J.,* **85**:235, February, 1975.

——: VII. Cardiac effects of quinidine and procaine amide. A. *Am. Heart J.,* **89**:804, June, 1975.

——: Cardiac effects of quinidine and procaine amide. B. *Am. Heart J.,* **90**:117, July, 1975.

Hutcheon, Duncan E.: Cardiovascular drug interactions. *J. Clin. Pharmacol.,* **15**:129, February–March, 1975.

Krone, Ronald J., and Kleiger, Robert E.: Prevention and treatment of supraventricular arrhythmias. *Heart Lung,* **6**:79, January–February, 1977.

Lefkowitz, Robert J.: B-adrenergic receptors: recognition and regulation. *N. Engl. J. Med.,* **295**:323, August 5, 1976.

Luchi, Robert J.; Entman, Mark L.; Harrison, Donald C.; and Eknoyan, Garabed: Use of cardioactive drugs in acute myocardial infarction. *Heart Lung,* **5**:44, January–February, 1976.

Marriott, Henry J. L.: Bedside recognition of cardiac arrhythmias. *Geriatrics,* **30**:55, June, 1975.

Mattea, Judith, and Mattea, Edward: Lidocaine and

procainamide toxicity during treatment of ventricular arrhythmias. *Am. J. Nurs.,* **76:**1429, September, 1976.

Neasman, Annie R.; Schobel, Ruth C.; and Lemberg, Louis: Arrhythmias in the coronary care unit. VI. Physiologic basis for the use of antiarrhythmic drugs. *Heart Lung,* **5:**496, May–June, 1976.

Pfeifer, Henry J.; Greenblatt, David J.; and Koch-Weser, Jan: Clinical use and toxicity of intravenous lidocaine. *Am. Heart J.,* **92:**168, August, 1976.

Roos, Julius C., and Dunning, Arend J.: Effects of lidocaine on impulse formation and conduction defects in man. *Am. Heart J.,* **89:**686, June, 1975.

Rosen, Michael R.; Hoffman, Brian F.; and Wit, Andrew L.: Electrophysiology and pharmacology of cardiac arrhythmias. V. Cardiac antiarrhythmic effects of lidocaine. *Am. Heart J.,* **89:**526, April, 1975.

Rosen, Michael R.; Wit, Andrew L.; and Hoffman, Brian F.: Electrophysiology and pharmacology of cardiac arrhythmias. VI. Cardiac effects of verapamil. *Am. Heart J.,* **89:**665, May, 1975.

Sinno, M. Ziad, and Gunnar, Rolf M.: Hemodynamic consequences of cardiac dysrhythmias. *Med. Clin. North Am.,* **60:**69, January, 1976.

Surawicz, Borys: Arrhythmias and antiarrhythmic therapy in context. *Hosp. Pract.,* **11:**59, June, 1976.

Ten Eick, Robert E.; Singer, Donald H.; and Solberg, Lloyd E.: Coronary occlusion: effects on cellular electrical activity of the heart. *Med. Clin. North Am.,* **60:**49, January, 1976.

Vyden, John K.; Mandel, William J.; Hayakawa, Hirokazu; Nagasawa, Koichi,; and Groseth-Dittrich, Marsha: The effect of lidocaine on peripheral hemodynamics. *J. Clin. Pharmacol.,* **15:**506, July, 1975.

Walinsky, Paul: Acute hemodynamic monitoring. *Heart Lung,* **6:**838, September–October, 1977.

Westfall, Una Elizabeth: Electrical and mechanical events in the cardiac cycle. *Am. J. Nurs.,* **76:**231, February, 1976.

Winkle, Roger A., and Harrison, Donald C.: Beta blockers in the treatment of acute arrhythmias. *Heart Lung,* **6:**62, January–February, 1977.

Wit, Andrew L.; Hoffman, Brian F.; and Rosen, Michael R.: Electrophysiology and pharmacology of cardiac arrhythmias. IX. Cardiac electrophysiologic effects of beta adrenergic receptor stimulation and blockade. A. *Am. Heart J.,* **90:**521, October, 1975.

———: Cardiac electrophysiologic effects of beta adrenergic receptor stimulation and blockade. B. *Am. Heart J.,* **90:**665, November, 1975.

———: Cardiac electrophysiologic effects of beta adrenergic receptor stimulation and blockade. C. *Am. Heart J.,* **90:**795, December, 1975.

Wit, Andrew L.; Rosen, Michael R.; and Hoffman, Brian F.: Electrophysiology of cardiac arrhythmias. VIII. Cardiac effects of diphenylhydantoin. A. *Am. Heart J.,* **90:**265, August, 1975.

———: Cardiac effects of diphenylhydantoin. B. *Am. Heart J.,* **90:**397, September, 1975.

9

Peripheral Artery Constriction

Hypertension is a major public health problem. It is estimated that 24 million Americans have hypertension, but only three million of those individuals are receiving adequate therapy for blood pressure control. Hypertension is the leading preventable cause of sickness, premature disability, and death in the United States. In individuals with untreated hypertension, the heart must pump blood against sustained peripheral arterial resistance. That increased workload is associated with a high incidence of cardiac enlargement and failure. Sustained blood pressure elevation also accelerates atherosclerotic changes. The disruption of vessel integrity is associated with a high incidence of arterial thrombosis, embolization, aneurysm, or hemorrhage at vital organ sites (i.e., renal, cerebral, retinal tissues).

Physiologic Correlations

Activation of interrelated physiologic reflex control mechanisms maintain the systemic blood pressure in response to changes in circulating blood volume. The primary physiologic control mechanisms are the sympathetic nervous system reflexes, the renin-angiotensin-aldosterone (RAA) system, and the vascular pressure receptor feedback systems. The mechanisms act at cardiac, renal, arterial, and venous sites to maintain the systemic blood pressure.

Vascular Resistance

The primary factors that determine the level of arterial blood pressure are the cardiac output and the peripheral vascular resistance: $BP = CO \times PVR$. The key factor in vascular resistance is the radius of the blood vessel. Larger vessels have a lower resistance and smaller vessels have a higher resistance. Because of their number and their radius, the arterioles account for most of the resistance in the arterial circulation.

The degree of smooth muscle contraction within arteriole walls controls their radius, and sympathetic nerve activity controls the vascular muscle contraction. Increased sympathetic tone constricts the arteries and arterioles, or *resistance vessels,* and the action is reflected in elevation of the diastolic blood pressure. Concurrent sympathetic nerve stimulation constricts the veins, or *capacitance vessels.* That action decreases their capacity and the rate of venous return to the heart is increased. The higher volume of blood in the left ventricle at the end of diastole increases the stroke volume, and the change is reflected in an elevated systolic blood pressure. Constriction of arterioles or tension, causes an increased force of blood flow in the intervening systemic arteries. The elevated arterial tension and arteriolar constriction may balance and peripheral perfusion may remain unchanged. At renal sites, glomerular blood flow often is diminished because both afferent and efferent arterioles constrict. The increased resistance in afferent and efferent glomerular arterioles is associated with an elevation in the intraglomerular pressure.

Sympathetic Neurotransmission

In the sympathetic nerve pathways, afferent fibers transmit impulses to the central nervous system, and efferent fibers transmit impulses from central control centers to the arterioles, venules, heart, and other body tissues. The efferent pathways of the sympathetic nerve tracts have preganglionic and postganglionic fibers (Fig. 9–1). The neurotransmitter at the ganglionic junction is acetylcholine. Norepinephrine is the mediating hormone between the postganglionic fiber and the arteriolar smooth muscle. Norepinephrine action at the alpha-adrenergic receptors of either arteries or veins causes constriction.

The biosynthesis of norepinephrine occurs in the terminal varicosities of the postganglionic neuron (Fig. 9–1). Norepinephrine is synthesized from tyrosine by a series of enzymatic reactions. In response to a sympathetic nerve impulse, norepinephrine is released from the storage vesicle of the neuron varicosity, and the impulse is transmitted to the adrenergic receptors at tissue sites.

Some of the norepinephrine escapes into the circulation where it is readily deactivated, or metabolized, by the enzyme catochol-O-methyl-transferase (COMT). The uptake of norepinephrine into the neuron varicosity is facilitated by an energy-dependent "amine pump" mechanism. Most of the neurotransmitter returns to the storage vesicle where it remains available for release to transmit subsequent impulses. Some of the norepinephrine in the neuron varicosity is metabolized in the mitochondria by the enzyme *monoamine oxidase* (MAO). The inactive metabolites *normetanephrine* (NMN) and *vanillylmandelic acid* (VMA) are released in to the plasma and they are excreted in the urine.

Renin-Angiotensin-Aldosterone System

The close physiologic link between the renin-angiotensin hormonal pressor system and aldosterone secretion provides a vital mechanism for regulation of the plasma volume and vasoconstriction. Reduced glomerular filtration, low sodium content in the fluid of the distal tubules, or sympathetic nerve stimulation that occurs in response to decreased circulating blood volume, each can activate the renin-angiotensin-aldosterone (RAA) system.

The initiating factor in the reflex control mechanism is the release of the proteolytic enzyme *renin* from the juxtaglomerular cells of the nephron arterioles. At renal sites and in the circulation, renin cleaves the substrate *angiotensinogen* to form *angiotensin I*. The action of enzymes in the plasma and pulmonary tissues converts angiotensin I to the potent vasoconstrictor substance *angiotensin II*. Circulation of the potent pressor hormone to vascular tissues causes constriction of arterioles and venules (Fig. 9–2). The initial action of angiotensin II at widespread vascular beds of the skin and splanchnic and renal tissues increases the circulating plasma volume. Continued renin release and concurrent sympathetic nerve stimulation increase the cardiac output and sustain the constriction of the arterioles and veins. Sympathetic nerve stimulation at beta-adrenergic receptors of renal tissues maintains the release of renin from the nephron juxtaglomerular cells.

Angiotensin II also accelerates the adrenal cortical biosynthesis of *aldosterone,* and the potent sodium-retaining hormone acts at sites in the distal tubule to increase the reabsorption of so-

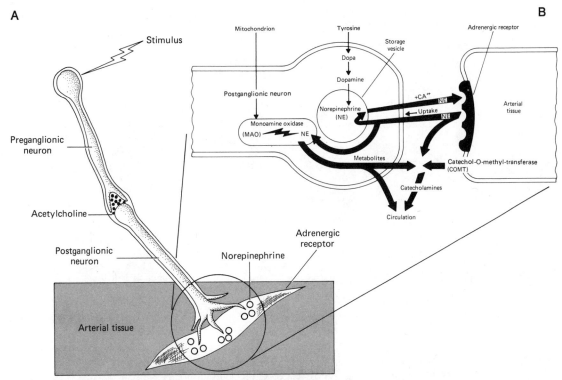

Fig. 9–1. *A.* Schematic diagram of a sympathetic nerve fiber. Acetylcholine transmits impulses at the sympathetic nerve ganglion, and norepinephrine transmits the impulses from the nerve ending to the tissue adrenergic receptor. *B.* The biosynthesis, release, and metabolism of norepinephrine occur at the neuron-tissue junction.

dium ions and water and the excretion of potassium ions. The activity of aldosterone increases the extracellular fluid volume and elevates the arterial blood pressure. Although the renin-generated release of aldosterone often is related to the osmolality, or sodium concentration, of tubule fluid, renin release can occur in response to other stimuli at the renal tissues (i.e., sympathetic nerve stimulation). Aldosterone activity under those circumstances can cause an inappropriate reabsorption of sodium that leads to hypervolemia.

Pressure and Volume Receptor Responses

There are clusters of nerve endings, at clearly delineated sites in the major blood vessels, that are sensitive to the stretching and the velocity of stretch in the vascular wall. (Fig. 9–2). The receptors in the arteries (i.e., carotid, aorta) are called *baroreceptors,* and the receptors in the veins (i.e., vena cava) and atrium are called *volume receptors.* The baroreceptors respond more readily than the volume receptors to changes in the circulating plasma volume.

The receptors send afferent impulses to the vasomotor control centers in the medulla, and efferent impulses modify the factors affecting stretch of the blood vessel. For example, a decrease in circulating blood volume reduces the afferent impulses from the carotid and aortic baroreceptors. The physiologic response is a decrease in parasympathetic nerve activity and an

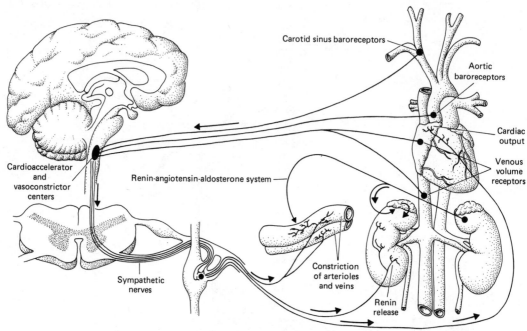

Carotid sinus baroreceptors

Aortic baroreceptors

Cardiac output

Venous volume receptors

Cardioaccelerator and vasoconstrictor centers

Renin-angiotensin-aldosterone system

Sympathetic nerves

Constriction of arterioles and veins

Renin release

Fig. 9–2. Schematic illustration of reflex control mechanism responses to decreased circulating blood volume and the associated effects on cardiac, renal, and vascular tissues.

associated increase in the heart rate. Simultaneously there is an increase in sympathetic nerve stimulation that increases ventricular contractility.

The combined neural changes increase the cardiac output and increase the driving pressure of blood flow to peripheral tissues.

Pathophysiologic Correlations

Hypertension, the term employed to describe persistent diastolic blood pressure elevation, encompasses both the secondary and essential types. Secondary hypertension is associated with controllable problems or curable diseases (i.e., unilateral renal parenchymal disease or renovascular disease, coarctation of the aorta, pheochromocytoma, primary aldosteronism, Cushing's disease, eclampsia, use of oral contraceptives). Treatment of the basic causative factor usually leads to alleviation of the hypertension.

Ninety percent of individuals with hypertension have essential, or primary, hypertension. The

basic cause of essential hypertension remains elusive despite intensive search for the cause. The consistently elevated diastolic blood pressure readings reflect the increased peripheral resistance associated with sustained constriction of arteries and arterioles. Although the vascular status of the individual mimics a sustained level of sympathetic nerve activity, circulating catecholamine levels are not consistently elevated. It has been postulated that the vascular constriction may be attributed to heightened receptor sensitivity to norepinephrine without an increase in the biosynthesis of the neurotransmitter hormone. Once the disease becomes established, sensitized hypertensive patients overact physiologically to psychologic or physiologic stresses.

Prolonged arterial constriction progressively causes anatomic changes that maintain the arterial resistance. Hypertension accelerates and aggravates arteriosclerosis and atherosclerosis, and there may be an increase in atherosclerotic placque formation. When the individual has mild or moderate untreated hypertension, the media of the small arteries and arterioles becomes thickened, or hypertrophied, by hyperplasia of the smooth muscle. An associated increase in the hyaline content leads to progressive narrowing of the arterial lumen. The process contributes to the incidence of sclerosis, obstruction, or aneurysm at vital arterial sites. For example, benign nephrosclerosis may reduce the large volume of blood flow required by the natural filtration processes of the kidney. There may be a gradual and progressive loss of functioning nephrons secondary to ischemia of the renal tissue. The cerebral arteries have a segmental distribution of the smooth muscles, and some areas are devoid of a muscular coat. When pressure is increased, the nonmuscular portions of the arteries dilate. Excess pressure can lead to tissue ischemia, cerebral edema, or petechial hemorrhages into the brain tissues. Changes also may occur in the aorta, and the vessel loses the compliance required to accommodate changes in blood flow. Problems are particularly evident in the proximal aorta where the arterial

wall contains more elastic than smooth muscle fibers. The aorta becomes a distended, stiff-walled, noncompliant vessel. Excessive distention of the aorta impinges on the lumen of afferent vessels and reduces the blood flow through the arterial branches.

Continued pumping of the blood against excess resistance leads to enlargement of the heart, or *cardiomegaly*. Fifty to eighty percent of individuals with untreated mild hypertension develop cardiomegaly. The size and number of coronary arteries remain unchanged, and the tissues in the enlarged heart may become hypoxic. Untreated individuals have five to six times the risk, as compared with treated on normotensive persons, of developing major cardiac events (i.e., angina pectoris, infarction, cardiac failure).

There are some subclassifications of individuals with essential hypertension. For example, individuals may be classified as having increased renin activity, suppressed renin production, expanded plasma and extracellular volume, or augmented cardiac output. The subclassifications are of interest in the search for the "ideal" antihypertensive drug therapy.

Hypertensive Levels

Hypertension is a problem in all age groups. In recent years there has been considerable effort expended in case finding. The objective of the search is to increase the number of individuals

Table 9-1.
Levels of Blood Pressure Indicating Hypertension

Age	Systolic Pressure (mm Hg)	Diastolic Pressure (mm Hg)
1 month to 3 years	110 (or above)	65 (or above)
3 years to 6 years	120	70
6 years to 8 years	125	80
8 years to 11 years	130	80
11 years to 13 years	140	80
13 years to 15 years	140	85
15 years to 55 years	140	90
55 years or above	140	100

Table 9–2.

Relationship of Diastolic Pressure to Hypertensive Status

Hypertension Level	Diastolic Pressure Range
Borderline	90–100 mm Hg
Mild	90–104 mm Hg
Moderate	105–114 mm Hg
Moderately severe	115–129 mm Hg
Severe	>130 mm Hg

who are receiving treatment for their hypertension. The overall goal is prevention of the devastating cardiovascular consequences of untreated hypertension. Although the original concern was that adults have their blood pressure taken for diagnostic purposes, the programs have expanded to include young children and adolescents. The change occurred when epidemiologic studies indicated that hereditary and environmental factors are associated with hypertension. Blood pressure readings can be affected by emotional state, exercise, and other factors, but there are general age-related guidelines that can be employed in screening programs for hypertension (Table 9–1).

The diagnosis of hypertension is made only after the blood pressure level has been determined on at least three separate occasions. The process is referred to as *casual blood pressure determinations* because they are taken without special preparation of the patient and without regard to time or environmental factors. The range of diastolic readings provides a general guide for description of the hypertensive level of the individual. Most individuals fall into the "borderline" and "mild" hypertension groupings (Table 9–2).

Malignant Hypertension

Malignant hypertension is a life-threatening clinical syndrome characterized by severe diastolic blood pressure elevation (> 130 mm Hg) and varying degrees of renal, retinal, and cerebral tissue involvement. The initial pathophysiologic mechanisms of the blood pressure elevation may be diverse, but the onset of malignant hypertension is a medical emergency. The earliest symptom in 85 percent of individuals with malignant

hypertension is severe generalized headache. The malignant nature of the syndrome is indicated by the presence of arteriolitis and arteriolar fibroid necrosis that impairs the function of vital organs. The syndrome threatens the integrity of the cardiovascular system, and it may be associated with progressive target-organ deterioration (i.e., retinopathy, renal failure, encephalopathy, heart failure).

Partial destruction of the renal arterioles activates the RAA system, and there is a self-sustaining production of renin. The persistent blood pressure elevation causes further renal damage and intense activation of the RAA system. The extent of nephron destruction is a prognostic factor in malignant hypertension. The rapid, progressive deterioration in nephron function is associated with an elevation in the blood urea nitrogen (BUN) and serum creatinine levels and the appearance of protein and red blood cells in the urine samples.

Changes in the retina provide some clues to the extent of the cerebral tissue damage. When the examination of the retina shows hemorrhages and exudates, the syndrome may be classified as *accelerated hypertension*. Papilledema indicates the presence of cerebral edema with encephalopathy and finalizes the diagnosis of malignant hypertension. In addition to the problems related to retinal changes, the effects of cerebral ischemia and edema impair consciousness, and the individual may be drowsy, confused, or comatose. Many patients are agitated and unable to sleep as hypertensive encephalopathy progresses.

Emergency care of the patient includes use of rapid-acting diuretics and parenteral administration of potent antihypertensive drugs. Lowering of the blood pressure is planned on a graded scale because the diminished compliance of the arterioles in the hypertensive patient does not allow adjustment to rapid changes in blood flow. For example, when the desired blood pressure level for the individual is 150/90 mm Hg, the reduction may be planned to lower the blood pressure from the initial level to one half the desired level during the first hour of therapy. During the following 24-hour period, drug dosage is planned to gradually lower the pressure to the desired level. The bed may be tilted into a head-up position to take advantage of the orthostatic hypotension that occurs earlier than the decrease in supine blood pressure.

Reduction of the blood pressure causes the glomerular filtration rate to fall slightly when therapy is initiated. Usually there is an increase in the serum creatinine level and the BUN may rise to 20 percent over the pretreatment level. The lower pressure promotes healing of vascular lesions and there is a subsequent improvement in renal function. Following the acute episode, therapy is planned to maintain the diastolic blood pressure between 80 to 100 mm Hg with adequate renal function.

Antihypertensive Drugs

Drug therapy that is tailored to the needs and tolerance of the individual can reduce blood pressure effectively in almost all situations. Therapy is directed at control of blood pressure with consequent relief of symptoms and reduction of long-term cardiovascular complications of the disease.

DRUG THERAPY

Elevated blood pressure must be lowered, and therapy consists of selecting the drugs that will be most effective and least deleterious to the individual. Dosage of antihypertensive drugs is gradually increased until the desired effect is attained, maximum therapeutic dosage level is reached, response reaches a plateau, or unacceptable side effects supervene. The antihypertensive drugs decrease vasomotor tone by diverse complex mechanisms. It is important to recognize that the drugs provide control of hypertension, but they are not curative. When the drugs are discontinued by the patient with essential hypertension, the blood pressure will gradually return to pretreatment levels.

The therapeutic regimen for an individual is based on the course, stability, duration, and level of hypertension. In general, the therapeutic aim is to maintain the blood pressure at approximately 130/85 mm Hg when measured in the supine and standing position. The vascular compliance is an important factor in determining the blood pressure level that will maintain tissue perfusion in each individual situation.

The antihypertensive drugs have varied effects on the blood pressure. During therapy the hypotensive effects of the drugs may be greater when the person is in the erect than in the supine position. The drugs compromise the normal mechanisms that provide the rapid adjustments in blood pressure that are required at the time of positional changes. The hypotensive effects of the drugs may be more evident when the person quickly changes body position. For example, dizziness may occur when the person assumes an erect position after squatting or sitting, and the change in blood pressure is described as *orthostatic hypotension*. The change in pressure that occurs when the person has been standing still for a short period of time, or when the person quickly rises from a recumbent position to a standing position, is described as *postural hypotension*.

Antihypertensive drug therapy follows a clearly defined approach, generally described as empiric but effective. The guidelines are based on current knowledge of the mechanisms of essential hypertension and the actions of antihypertensive drugs. The *stepped-care plan* involves the gradual addi-

---

Step 1: Long-acting diuretic (i.e., chlorthalidone, thiazide)
   –Add–
Step 2: Methyldopa, or propranolol, or reserpine, or clonidine, or guanethidine, or prazosin
   –Change to– (if above drugs are inadequate or produce undesirable adverse effects)
Step 3: Long-acting diuretic (i.e., chlorthalidone, thiazide)
   Propranolol
   Hydralazine
   –Add– (if inadequate)
Step 4: Guanethidine

---

tion of drugs when blood pressure control indicates the need for more intensive therapy.

The stepped-care plan provides direction for treatment of mild to moderate hypertension by using a diuretic for a two-to-four-week trial period. The addition of an adrenergic-blocking agent for reduction of peripheral vascular resistance is indicated when the blood pressure persists to be in the range of 140 to 199 mm Hg systolic and 90 to 114 mm Hg diastolic. The therapeutic plan is revised if the patient does not respond to the drug therapy indicated in step 1 and step 2. The individual with moderately severe or severe hypertension (systolic range = 200 to 240 mm Hg+; diastolic range = 115 to 130 mm Hg+) requires the more intensive therapy indicated by the combination of two or three of the antihypertensive agents with a diuretic drug.

Diuretic Therapy

Elevated serum sodium concentrations are known to play a role in the production and control of hypertension. Restriction of dietary sodium intake may lower pressure to normal levels in some individuals with mild hypertension, but the thiazide diuretics are the mainstay of antihypertensive drug therapy. The thiazides and the other diuretics with a similar action (i.e., chlorthalidone, quinethazone) are frequently employed as initial therapy for blood pressure control. Fifty to seventy percent of individuals with mild hypertension will respond to therapy with diuretics without the occurrence of significant adverse effects.

The initial effect of diuretic therapy is a reduction in circulating blood volume with a consequent lowering of cardiac output. At the distal tubule, thiazides block the active reabsorption of sodium, and the process raises the amount of sodium, chloride, and water remaining in the tubule urine. Because active reabsorption of sodium is inhibited, there is an increased rate of potassium secretion in exchange for sodium at the tubule membrane. Acceleration of potassium secretion lowers serum levels of the electrolyte. To prevent the occurrence of hypokalemia, potassium chloride supplements often are prescribed, and the individual is encouraged to increase the daily intake of foods with a high potassium content.

The thiazides are employed as initial therapy for individuals with mild or moderate hypertension, and they may be used with other antihypertensive drugs (i.e., guanethidine) for initial therapy of severe hypertension. Their use with other antihypertensive drugs is in example of a therapeutic drug interaction. The thiazides have some direct vascular relaxing effects, and thiazide-induced lowering of circulating blood volume also potentiates the action of the antihypertensive drugs. When thiazides are used, dosage of the other antihypertensive drugs often may be lowered to levels causing fewer adverse effects without lessening effective control of blood pressure levels. Each of the antihypertensive drugs causes retention of sodium and water, and the concurrent use of the thiazides controls the secondary volume expansion. A small amount of plasma volume depletion appears to be necessary to reduce drug resistance and to obtain maximum effect of the antihypertensive drugs. The thiazides maintain that therapeutic margin. A detailed discussion of diuretics is presented in Chapter 14.

DIRECT ARTERIOLE DILATORS

The drugs that act primarily on smooth muscle of the arterioles to decrease peripheral vascular resistance include *hydralazine, diazoxide, prazosin,* and *nitroprusside.* The drugs reduce peripheral resistance by a selective dilation of precapillary arterioles. The direct arteriole dilators lower the blood pressure in both the supine and upright positions. The drugs lower peripheral arteriole resistance more than other drugs, and there is a greater percentile fall in diastolic blood pressure than in systolic blood pressure.

Hydralazine

Hydralazine is the best known of the drugs providing a direct relaxant effect on arteriole smooth muscles. Until recently, it was the only direct vasodilator approved for use in hypertension control. Hydralazine usually is employed with a diuretic and another antihypertensive drug for control of moderately severe or severe hypertension.

Action Mode. Hydralazine action is associated with widespread dilation of precapillary arterioles. The drug interferes with calcium ion transport across the smooth muscle membrane, and the reduced calcium level diminishes the active state of contraction in the arteriole muscle fibers.

The hypotensive effect of hydralazine activates the baroreceptor reflexes, and there is a subsequent increase in sympathetic nerve discharge. The accelerated sympathetic nerve stimuli increase cardiac output by increasing the rate and force of myocardial contraction. Concurrent sympathetic nerve stimulation at nephron sites increases the rate of renin secretion from the juxtaglomerular cells. The sympathetic nerve-induced cardiac effects are unopposed by the drug, but the vascular constriction effects of sympathetic stimuli and of angiotensin II are modified by the action of hydralazine. When hydralazine is used without other drugs, the patient may complain of the discomfort caused by palpitations and dyspnea on slight exertion. In individuals with coronary artery insufficiency, the increased myocardial oxygen consumption may cause sufficient myocardial ischemia to precipitate angina pectoris.

Hydralazine often is employed in conjunction with drugs that block adrenergic stimulation. The combination decreases the effect of the vasodilator on cardiac output and renin release. The antihypertensive drugs that interfere with both alpha- and beta-adrenergic receptor stimulation (i.e., methyldopa, guanethidine) may be used with hydralazine, but propranolol is more often employed because of its selective beta-adrenergic-blocking action. Propranolol offers the advantage of interrupting sympathetic nerve stimulation of the heart without suppressing the effect of sympathetic nerve stimulation on venous alpha-adrenergic receptors. Retention of the venous responses maintains the vasoconstriction required to prevent postural hypotension.

The decreased arteriolar pressure effected by hydralazine causes sodium and water retention by alteration of intrarenal hemodynamics. The secondary aldosteronism that is precipitated by the activity of the renin-angiotensin-aldosterone system also is associated with retention of sodium and water. Diuretics are used with hydralazine to counteract the volume expansion that is a predictable problem during therapy.

Therapy Considerations. Hydralazine is available in forms for parenteral or oral administration, but it is most commonly used by the oral route. The initial oral dosage range is 30 to 80 mg/day. The short serum half-life of three to six hours necessitates administration of hydralazine three to four times per day. The lower dosage is planned to avoid adverse effects of the drug, and the dosage may be gradually increased at weekly intervals to the daily maintenance dosage of 100 to 200 mg. The dosage maximum is 300 to 400 mg/day during short-term therapy, and the maximum level is lower (200 mg/day) during long-term therapy. The maximum dosage is considered to reduce the incidence of a lupus erythrematosus-like syndrome that occurs more frequently during long-term therapy at higher dosage.

The oral drug is well absorbed from the intestine. A large portion of the drug is eliminated by metabolism in the intestinal wall and liver prior to traveling to the systemic circulation. Distribution in the body tissues is somewhat uneven. The increase in blood flow that occurs in cerebral, coronary, renal, and splanchnic arterioles indicates a higher drug concentration in the arteriole muscle tissues at those sites.

The onset of action after initial oral drug administration is 30 to 60 minutes, and a peak effect occurs in three to four hours. Hydralazine is metabolized in the liver by hydroxylation and acetylation. Differences occur in the rate of hydralazine acetylation between those individuals who are genetically fast acetylators and those who are slow acetylators. Although the serum half-life of hydralazine is a relatively short period of three to six hours, individuals who are slow acetylators can have elevated plasma drug levels for a much longer period of time. Those individuals may require only a twice-a-day dosage regimen to maintain therapeutic plasma drug concentrations.

Hydralazine may be administered parenterally in hypertensive emergencies when the patient is unable to take the drug orally. Administration of a bolus of drug (i.e., 20 to 40 mg at 0.5 to 1 mg/minute) usually produces evidence of the hypotensive effect in five to ten minutes. Hydralazine also may be administered by a continuous intravenous infusion (i.e., 50 to 100 mg/liter), and the flow rate is titrated to the changes in blood pressure. Intramuscular injections usually are administered initially at the level of 10 mg, and the onset of action occurs in five to ten minutes.

Preparations Available. Hydralazine hydrochloride (APRESOLINE) is available for oral use in tablet forms. *Hydralazine hydrochloride* (APRESOLINE) also is available in ampules of solution for intramuscular or intravenous administration.

Adverse Effects. Generalized severe headache, which is caused by cerebral arteriole dilation, is common during the first few days of therapy. As therapy continues, the headache usually abates. Patients should be warned that they may experience headache, palpitations, and mild postural hypotension two to four hours after taking the first dose of hydralazine. The patients also can be told that the effects will lessen gradually and that they will not be a problem after the drug has been taken for about a week.

Other common problems include nausea, dizziness, and sweating. Less common adverse effects include flushing, nasal congestion, lacrimation, conjunctivitis, localized edema (i.e., periorbital, genital, ankle), muscle cramps, and numbness and tingling of the extremities.

During the early weeks of therapy, some patients have an influenza-like syndrome with fever, muscle and joint aching, and edema. Ten percent of individuals who take hydralazine for more than two months have an acute rheumatoid episode. Both the influenza-like syndrome and the rheu-

matoid state subside when drug therapy is discontinued.

The 10 to 20 percent of patients on prolonged therapy who have a lupus erythmatosus-like syndrome probably represent slow acetylators of hydralazine. Previous to the onset of symptoms of the autoimmune phenomena, patients have positive tests for antinuclear antibodies (ANA) and positive lupus erythematosus (LE) preparations. Problems occurring with the onset of the syndrome include afternoon fever, night sweats, polyarthritis, myalgia, pleuritic pain, pericarditis, and insomnia. The symptoms regress when the drug is withdrawn, and there is seldom any residual organ damage. Tests for LE cells and ANA remain positive for some time after the symptoms subside.

Diazoxide

Diazoxide is a nondiuretic thiazide that is administered intravenously for control of hypertension. The drug has a rapid action that lowers blood pressure within minutes in crisis situations.

Action Mode. The action of diazoxide on the muscle fibers of the precapillary arterioles is similar to that of hydralazine. Diazoxide interferes with calcium ion transport across the smooth muscle membrane, and the diminished level of calcium interferes with the contraction of the smooth muscle fibers.

The hypotensive effect of diazoxide also is similar to that of hydralazine. The decreased pressure caused by diazoxide induces a reflex sympathetic nerve response that is mediated through the arterial baroreceptors. There is an increase in cardiac output and increased production of renin during diazoxide administration. The drug also causes excess sodium and water retention. Concurrent administration of an adrenergic-blocking agent and a diuretic modifies the problems with cardioacceleration and fluid retention.

Diazoxide is the drug most commonly employed for control of blood pressure in hypertensive emergencies or for control of severe hypertension. The drug is used for short-term therapy, and an oral antihypertensive agent may be given concurrently to assure continuation of blood pressure control when parenteral administration of diazoxide is terminated.

Diazoxide administration is associated with an initial drop in renal blood flow and glomerular filtration. Although the effect on renal function is related to the initial fall in blood pressure, the renal flow rate improves even though the pressure remains low.

Therapy Considerations. The serum albumin binding of diazoxide is high (90 percent), and intravenous administration is planned to provide the drug for therapeutic effect while considering the high affinity for serum albumin binding. The drug may be injected rapidly (within 30 seconds) as a bolus of 300 mg. The same dosage may be repeated in 30 minutes if the pressure response is less than that desired for the patient. Additional drug may be given intravenously at four-hour intervals using the rapid administration method for injection.

An alternate method for intravenous administration of diazoxide is to give 75 mg of the drug and to inject 150 mg every five minutes until the desired hypotensive effect is obtained. Usually a therapeutic response occurs when 300 to 600 mg of the drug has been administered, but more than that amount may be given.

The onset of action when the drug is administered intravenously is from three to five minutes. The patient is monitored closely during the period when the drug is being administered. There is an initial sharp drop in pressure, and the blood pressure is taken every minute until the maximum hypotensive level stabilizes. Monitoring is essential to ascertain the lowest hypotensive level attained and to assess the effect of that blood pressure level on the patient's status. After the low pressure level has stabilized, the pressure is taken every five minutes until it begins to rise. Hourly pressures usually are taken until the drug is re-administered.

The blood pressure level usually rises gradually over a period of 10 to 30 minutes, and it slowly returns to pretreatment levels over a 2-to-12-hour period if additional drug is not given. Ambulatory patients are asked to remain in the supine position for 30 minutes after the drug is given, and the patient's standing blood pressure is taken before surveillance is terminated.

Diazoxide usually is administered into the largest available vein to minimize the irritating effects of the strongly alkaline solution (pH 11.6). Extravasation of the drug into the tissues causes pain and a burning sensation that persist for one to two hours.

Ease of administration, rapidity of onset, and a high degree of effectiveness make diazoxide an ideal agent for rapid lowering of the blood pressure in a hypertensive emergency. In situations where a precipitous drop in blood pressure would be hazardous for the patient (i.e., cerebral or coronary insufficiency), the dosage and the intervals between drug administration may be modified to avoid a sudden drop in pressure.

Preparations Available. Diazoxide (HYPERSTAT) is available only in solutions for intravenous injection. The solutions contain sodium hydroxide for pH adjustment to assure solubility.

Adverse Effects. Diazoxide decreases gastric motility by a mechanism similar to its action on arteriolar muscle tissue, and constipation, flatulence, or abdominal distention may be problematic. The effects of diazoxide on uterine muscle may decrease contractions when the drug is employed to control the hypertension associated with toxemia of pregnancy. Administration of oxytocic drugs usually overcomes the uterine inertia and reinstitutes labor. The safety of diazoxide for use during human pregnancy has not been established.

Diazoxide inhibits the release of insulin from the pancreas, and a transitory hyperglycemia, lasting up to 12 hours, may occur with intravenous administration of the drug. The patient's blood and urine sugar levels usually are monitored when the drug is administered for more than 48 hours.

Extrapyramidal symptoms can occur with high dosage of diazoxide. The problems vary from restlessness to fully developed parkinsonian symptoms (i.e., oculogyrus, trismus, rigidity, tremor). The symptoms abate when the drug is discontinued. Other neurologic problems include anxiety, insomnia, polyneuritis, paresthesias, and pruritus.

The tachycardia, palpitations, moderate postural hypotension, or anginal pain that may occur during therapy are related to the effect of the drug on cardiovascular dynamics. Diazoxide is considered to be relatively nontoxic, and the usual short-term therapy limits the incidence of adverse effects that would be natural to a drug with similar properties.

Prazosin

Prazosin is an oral drug that has recently been released for control of hypertension. The drug is useful for control of mild, moderate, and moderately severe hypertension.

Action Mode. The drug is thought to inhibit activity of the enzyme *phosphodiesterase* that is required for hydrolysis of *cyclic adenosine phosphate* (cAMP) and *cyclic guanosine monophosphate* (cGMP). The increased levels of cAMP and cGMP in the smooth muscle cells of precapillary arterioles interfere with contraction. Prazosin is thought to have a sympatholytic effect, because there is less reflex sympathetic nerve activity than that occurring with hydralazine or diazoxide.

Prazosin may be employed alone or with a diuretic for blood pressure control. During therapy there is a greater hypotensive effect when the person is in the upright position than in the supine position.

Therapy Considerations. Prazosin is absorbed well from the intestine when administered orally. The drug is highly bound to serum proteins (97 percent), and it is widely distributed in body tissues.

The initial dose of prazosin may cause syncope and sudden collapse within 30 to 90 minutes after taking the drug; therefore, a small initial dosage

usually is given (i.e., 1 mg). The dosage may be increased at two-week intervals until the daily maintenance dosage level is reached (i.e., 20 mg ÷ 2 to 3 doses). The hypotensive effect of the drug is evident within two hours of ingestion, and there is a maximum decrease in the blood pressure in two to four hours.

Prazosin is metabolized in the liver by demethylation. The conjugates reenter the intestine with the bile, and 90 percent of the drug metabolites are excreted in the feces. Prazosin has a short half-life (two to four hours), and it is probable that the attainment of therapeutic hypotensive levels with a three-times-a-day schedule is partially related to the hypotensive effect of active metabolites.

Preparations Available. Prazosin (MINIPRESS) is available in capsules for oral administration. The capsules contain 1 mg, 2 mg, or 5 mg of the drug.

Adverse Effects. The most prominent adverse effects of prazosin are dizziness, headache, weakness, nasal congestion, and palpitations. Postural hypotension, which is preceded by tachycardia, is relatively common.

Patients should be forewarned that the first dose of the drug may lead to dizziness, weakness, or fainting. The problems are related to the drop in blood pressure that may occur 30 to 90 minutes after the drug is taken. The problems may last up to an hour, and any activities that could jeopardize safety should be avoided (i.e., driving an automobile).

Nitroprusside

The drug is employed for control of hypertension in a variety of emergency situations. Nitroprusside predictably provides an effective antihypertensive action.

Action Mode. The direct vasodilator action of nitroprusside relaxes the smooth muscles of the precapillary arterioles and the postcapillary venules. The venodilation decreases the quantity of blood returning to the heart. Dilation of the capacitance vessels also allows peripheral venous pooling of blood, and tilting of the bed into a head-up position maximizes the hypotensive effect of nitroprusside. The modification of position commonly is employed in an acute emergency situation where immediate control of blood pressure is essential to the life of the patient.

Venodilation decreases the stroke volume and cardiac output. In the supine position, the decreased cardiac output may contribute appreciably to the hypotensive effect of the drug. The cardiac output is reduced more in the upright position and that effect may contribute as much as the decreased peripheral vascular resistance to the lowering of blood pressure.

Therapy Considerations. Nitroprusside is administered by intravenous infusion with the drip rate titrated to the level of blood pressure. The average flow rate of the drug solution (50 to 150 mg/liter) is initially adjusted to 10 mcg/minute. The flow rate is increased by 10 mcg every five minutes until the desired hypotensive level is attained. The infusion rate is controlled by using an infusion pump or a microdrip regulator.

The onset of drug effect is instantaneous, and monitoring of the blood pressure is continuous during the period of infusion. The potency of the drug is an indication for mobilization of precautionary measures against inadvertent administration of excess amounts of the drug. The effects of the drug are dissipated within a few minutes (one to three minutes) when the infusion is stopped, and the blood pressure returns to the pretreatment level in 5 to 15 minutes. In the event of an inadvertent overshoot of the hypotensive effect, stopping the drug infusion and elevating the patient's legs may raise the pressure quickly.

Precautions are taken to protect the solution from deterioration during administration. Covering the bottle and tubing with aluminum foil or other opaque material protects it against the destructive effects of room light. Solutions are used only for 4 to 12 hours because they are unstable and deteriorate rapidly.

Nitroprusside is metabolized to *cyanogen* by enzymes in the red blood cells and other tissues. The cyanogen is rapidly metabolized, by the enzyme *rhodenase* at hepatic sites, to the inactive metabolite *thiocyanate*. The metabolite has a serum half-life of four to seven days, and it is slowly eliminated by the kidneys. Blood thiocyanate levels are monitored when the drug is administered for more than 48 hours. Drug administration usually is discontinued when the thiocyanate level is elevated (> 10 mg/100 ml) because toxic symptoms can occur as the level rises (i.e., nausea, fatigue, weakness, stupor, slurred speech, tinnitus, muscle spasms, disorientation, psychosis). Administration of nitroprusside at high doses (> 3 mg/kg BW) can increase the blood cyanogen content to levels that cause tissue anoxia and the release of acid metabolites.

Preparations Available. Sodium *nitroprusside* (NIPRIDE) recently became available as a commercial preparation. It is supplied in a vial of drug that is diluted for intravenous administration.

Adverse Effects. Rapid reduction of blood pressure during administration may cause confusion and somnolence, and the problems are prominent in individuals with hypertensive encephalopathy. Rapid infusion of the drug may cause nausea, retching, abdominal pain, palpitations, tachycardia, headache, dizziness, restlessness, anxiety with sweating, or muscle twitching. The symptoms abate when the drug infusion rate is slowed or when the drug infusion is halted temporarily. The rapid hypotension can be hazardous for patients with severe atherosclerosis.

SYMPATHETIC NERVE INHIBITORS

Clonidine, methyldopa, guanethidine, and *reserpine* act by varying mechanisms to inhibit impulse transmission through sympathetic nerve pathways. The antihypertensive effect of the drugs is an expression of their interference with norepinephrine neurotransmission.

Clonidine

Clonidine acts at medullary and peripheral adrenergic sites to control hypertension. It is useful for control of mild, moderately severe, and severe hypertension. The drug usually is employed with a diuretic or other antihypertensive agents.

Action Mode. Clonidine acts by stimulating the alpha-adrenergic receptors in the medullary cardiac and vasomotor control centers. The drug reduces the number of cardioaccelerator and vasoconstrictor impulses that are transmitted. Clonidine reduces blood pressure in both the standing and supine positions, and there is an associated bradycardia. During therapy with clonidine, there is a diminution, but not complete blockade, of sympathetic nerve impulse output from the medulla. Cardiovascular reflexes remain functional, and physiologic stimuli (i.e., position changes, exercise) can reflexly elevate the blood pressure.

Therapy Considerations. Clonidine is absorbed rapidly from the intestine after oral administration. The drug is a basic lipid-soluble drug and it has a high volume of distribution in body tissues. The initial daily dosage is small (0.1 to 0.2 mg) and the dosage is gradually increased to the maintenance level of 0.2 to 0.8 mg/day. The moderately long serum half-life (12 to 20 hours) makes it possible to administer the drug on a twice-a-day schedule.

The onset of hypotension occurs within 30 to 60 minutes after oral administration, and the peak hypotensive effect is evident for from two to four hours. The drug effect is more prominent when the patient is in the upright position, and the hypotension represents the decreased resistance of arterioles and venules. The decrease in blood pressure is associated with a decreased heart rate.

Clonidine is metabolized in the liver and four inactive metabolites have been identified. Twenty percent of the metabolites are eliminated by the bile into the feces after enterohepatic circulation. Approximately 48 percent of the unchanged drug and 32 percent of the metabolites are excreted in the urine.

Preparations Available. Clonidine (CATAPRES) is available for oral use in tablet form. The tablets are scored to allow their use with varying dosage prescriptions.

Adverse Effects. The most prominent adverse effects during therapy with clonidine are dry mouth and sedation. The sedative effect may subside as therapy continues, but drowsiness is a persistent problem for the patient. Some patients refuse to take the drug because drowsiness interferes with activities of daily living. Patients should be informed that alcohol and other sedatives can potentiate the central nervous system depressant effects of the drug. Patients also should be cautious about performing tasks that could jeopardize safety while mental acuity is reduced.

During therapy, parotid gland pain, sleep reversal, constipation, and impotence in male patients can be problems. Some male patients find the disruption of sexual activity intolerable and they discontinue taking the drug.

One of the major problems with the use of clonidine is the hazard of a withdrawal syndrome with rebound hypertension that occurs 12 to 48 hours after the drug is discontinued abruptly. The syndrome is associated with the sudden increase in the levels of circulating catecholamines following cessation of the inhibitory action of clonidine. Gradual reduction of the dosage over a two-to-three-day period allows a slower physiologic readjustment to the catecholamine levels. It is important to instruct patients to take the drug regularly and not to omit the dosage at any time during therapy. A reminder to get the prescription refilled in time to maintain a supply of drug on hand may help them to avoid the withdrawal syndrome. The drug generally is not prescribed for individuals known to be unreliable or noncompliant with prescribed therapies.

Interactions. The tricyclic drugs act as competitive inhibitors of clonidine. Concurrent use of tricyclic antidepressants may antagonize the hypotensive effect of clonidine.

Methyldopa

Methyldopa usually is employed with a thiazide diuretic for control of mild hypertension. It also is used with a diuretic and another antihypertensive drug for control of moderately severe, severe, and malignant hypertension.

Action Mode. Methyldopa is metabolized to *alpha-methyldopamine* and then to *alpha-methyl-norepinephrine* (a-mNE). The active metabolite a-mNE stimulates central inhibitory alpha-adrenergic receptors in the medulla. The interference with norepinephrine activity at the receptors is similar to that of clonidine. Methyldopa is a potent inhibitor of sympathetic outflow from the medullary centers. It also reduces plasma renin activity by competing with norepinephrine at renal tissues.

The sympathetic reflexes are reasonably well maintained, and physiologic activity can stimulate reflex responses in the cardiovascular system. Methyldopa lowers the systolic and diastolic blood pressure in both the supine and standing positions.

Therapy Considerations. Methyldopa is available in forms for intravenous and oral administration, but it is infrequently used intravenously. Dosage of the oral tablets is planned with consideration of the variation in intestinal absorption of the oral drug. The average amount of drug absorbed is 50 percent of the oral dosage, and the remainder is excreted in the feces.

Administration of the oral drug (0.75 to 2 gm) requires a three-to-four-times-a-day schedule because of variability in responses. The serum half-life of the drug is short (two hours) and serum levels show little correlation with drug action. The hypotensive activity is partially attributable to the effect of active metabolites. The hypotensive effect of the drug is evident 6 to 12 hours after oral administration. The peak effect occurs in three to six hours and the hypotensive effect lasts for 8 to 12 hours. It may take from one to four days for the full effect of the drug to be established. When drug administration is discontinued, the blood pressure returns to the pretreatment level in 48 hours.

Methyldopa is metabolized in the liver and kidneys. Most of the drug is excreted unchanged in the urine, but there are some conjugates eliminated. Metabolites in the urine may cause a red color in the toilet bowl when the commonly used oxidizing cleansers are in the water.

Preparations Available. Methyldopa (ALDO-MET) is available in tablet form for oral administration. *Methyldopate hydrochloride* (ALDOMET) is available in ampules for intravenous administration.

Adverse Effects. The most prominent adverse effects are dry mouth and sedation. The sedative effect occurs within the first 48 to 72 hours of therapy, but it gradually abates. Methyldopa also causes disturbances in mental acuity manifest as greatly impaired ability to concentrate, problems with reading, difficulty with simple calculations, and lapses of memory.

Postural hypotension, constipation, and abdominal cramps also are common problems. Both male and female patients have problems with decreased libido, and male patients sometimes have problems with impotence.

Fever, which is a manifestation of an immunologic response, occurs in the early days of therapy. The patient may have influenza-like symptoms with general malaise, shaking chills, and a markedly elevated temperature. The episode continues until the drug is discontinued.

Fever associated with hepatic dysfunction is a serious toxic effect that occurs in a small number of patients (1 percent). The problems arise within 12 to 20 days after therapy is initiated, and the symptoms are undistinguishable from those of viral hepatitis. The syndrome is rarely severe and usually is reversible with cessation of drug therapy. The incidence of the toxic effect has decreased since newer drug preparations have been formulated.

A relatively large number of patients on methyldopa therapy (25 percent) have an elevated Coombs' test when therapy is continued for four or more months. There may be no clinical abnormalities, but the blood cannot be cross-matched. A small number of patients (5 percent) develop hemolytic anemia that is slowly reversible when the drug therapy is discontinued.

Interactions. Methyldopa may potentiate the sedative effects of haloperidol when the drugs are used concurrently. Both drugs prevent dopamine from reaching its central neurotransmitter receptor, and patients may have varying mental problems when haloperidol is added to methyldopa therapy.

Concurrent use of monoamine oxidase inhibitors (i.e., pargyline, furazolidine) may cause hypertension and excitement because there is excess norepinephrine in the adrenergic neuron as a consequence of the action of each drug.

Concurrent therapy with levodopa and methyldopa may increase the incidence of vomiting and grogginess caused by each of the drugs when it is used alone. The patients should be closely monitored and a reduction in drug dosage may be required to alleviate the problems.

Guanethidine

Guanethidine is a potent inhibitor of sympathetic nerve transmission. It is employed with a diuretic in the control of moderate and severe hypotension.

Action Mode. Guanethidine utilizes the norepinephrine reuptake mechanism, or "amine pump," for transportation into the adrenergic neuron (Fig. 9–3). Norepinephrine that remains free in the myoneural junction is rapidly deactivated by action of the enzyme *catechol-O-methyltransferase* (COMT). Within the varicosity of the adrenergic neuron, guanethidine binds to the norepinephrine storage vesicles. The drug depletes

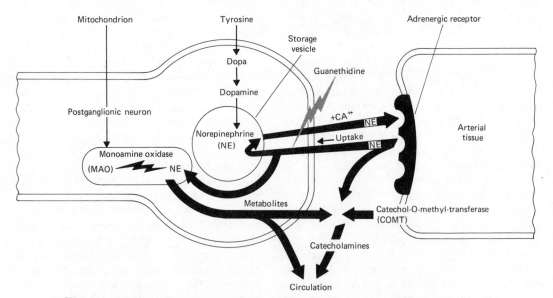

Fig. 9–3. Guanethidine prevents norepinephrine release and reuptake at the myoneural junction. Norepinephrine is deactivated by enzyme activity and released into the circulation.

norepinephrine stores and diminishes the quantity of norepinephrine available for release in response to sympathetic nerve stimulation.

The action of guanethidine provides a sympathetic nerve block that suppresses the reflexes that control resistance and capacitance vessels. The decrease in total peripheral vascular resistance diminishes the responses to upright posture and exercise. Guanethidine action causes a moderate fall in diastolic pressure in the supine position and a reduction in the systolic and diastolic pressures in the standing position.

Therapy Considerations. Guanethidine has a very long serum half-life (five to ten days) that allows the daily drug dosage (10 to 300 mg) to be given as a single dose. Absorption of the drug from the intestine is variable (5 to 60 percent), and the onset of hypotensive effect is slow (48 to 72 hours). The daily dosage schedule allows a steady-state serum drug concentration to be attained in about 15 days, and dosage changes may be made at five-to-seven-day intervals. Dosage adjustments are based on periodic recordings of the blood pressure taken in both the recumbent and erect positions and after controlled exercise.

A loading dose may be administered to the hospitalized patient with severe hypertension. The larger dosage results in control of hypertension within three days. A diuretic is administered concurrent with the loading dosage to decrease the sodium and water retention that can counteract the hypotensive effect of guanethidine.

The unabsorbed drug is excreted in the feces. Up to 30 percent of the unchanged drug may be excreted by the kidneys.

Preparations Available. Guanethidine sulfate (ISMELIN) is available in tablet form. *Guanethidine monosulfate* is available as a tablet containing hydrochlorothiazide.

Adverse Effects. The most frustrating problem for the patient is the urgency that accompanies bowel movements three to five times each day. The hypermotility of the intestinal tract is associated with eating, and it can lead to fecal incontinence. An anticholinergic drug (i.e., atropine sulfate) may be required to alleviate the problem.

Postural, orthostatic, and exercise hypotension is a frequent problem. The hypotension is particularly evident during dosage adjustment, and the patient should be instructed to change positions slowly to avoid falling. Bradycardia is also frequently present and it can potentiate the dizziness that occurs with position changes.

Generalized muscle weakness often occurs and is most evident upon arising in the morning. Male patients may have retrograde ejaculation, and they often refuse to take the drug.

Interactions. The hypotensive effect of guanethidine can be reversed by the tricyclic antidepressants and by amphetamine, chlorpromazine, and methylphenidate. The drugs displace guanethidine from the peripheral neuron sites or inhibit uptake of guanethidine into the nerve endings.

Rauwolfia Alkaloids

The rauwolfia alkaloids include *alseroxylon, deserpidine, rauwolfia serpentina, rescinnamine, reserpine,* and *syrosingopine.* Reserpine is the most commonly used of the group of drugs, and the discussion will focus on the therapeutic use of reserpine as a prototype for each of the drugs in the grouping. The drugs were the mainstay of antihypertensive drug therapy until drugs with fewer adverse effects were introduced.

Action Mode. Reserpine depletes stores of norepinephrine by slowly releasing the neurotransmitter from storage vesicles into neuronal tissue where it is inactivated by monoamine oxidase (Fig. 9–4). The drug acts at hypothalamic, medullary, and peripheral postganglionic sites by a similar mechanism. By depletion of depots of norepinephrine, reserpine action lessens the amount of norepinephrine available for impulse transmission when the sympathetic nerve is stimulated. The hypotensive effect of reserpine is due more to its peripheral than central actions. The

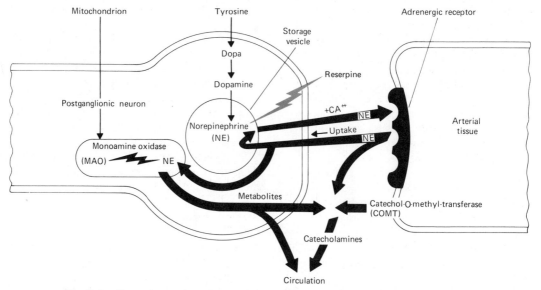

Fig. 9–4. Reserpine depletes the norepinephrine stores in the vesicles of the sympathetic neuron varicosities at peripheral sites.

drug produces sedation and tranquility by depleting serotonin at hypothalamic and medullary sites. Those effects are useful adjuncts to therapy. Reserpine is employed with an oral diuretic for control of mild or moderate hypertension.

Therapy Considerations. Reserpine is available for oral or intramuscular administration, but the drug is more commonly administered orally. Several weeks are required for maximum hypotensive effect when the drug is given orally, and the residual effects require several weeks to dissipate after drug therapy is discontinued. The initial dosage range usually is 0.5 to 1 mg daily, and doses are given two to three times a day. The dosage usually is adjusted downward at weekly intervals. The daily maintenance dosage is 0.25 mg, given in two to three divided doses. The long duration of action makes it possible for the drug to be given in a single oral dose.

Initial administration of reserpine causes a rapid outpouring of norepinephrine and the neuron is depleted of the neurotransmitter. When

reserpine is administered intramuscularly, the sudden release of norepinephrine may cause a sharp, though brief, rise in blood pressure and cardiac arrhythmias may be precipitated. After the initial effect, moderate hypotension and bradycardia occur.

Preparations Available. Reserpine (LEMI-SERP, RAU-SED, RESERPOID, SANDRIL, SERPASIL) is available in tablets or elixir for oral use and as a solution for intramuscular injection. *Rauwolfia serpentina* (RAUDIXIN), *alseroxylon* (RAUWILOID), *deserpidine* (HARMONYL), and *rescinnamine* (MODERIL) are available as tablets for oral administration.

Adverse Effects. Mental depression is a major concern during therapy. Patients and their family members should be aware of the signs of depression (i.e., early-morning awakening, with fatigue and inability to return to sleep, disinterest in food, depressed physiologic function). Drug therapy is discontinued at the first evidence of depression.

The drug seldom is employed for therapy when the person has a history of mental depression.

There is a high incidence of nasal congestion, bradycardia, and diarrhea during therapy with reserpine. Parenteral administration is associated with an increased secretion of gastric acid, and gastrointestinal hemorrhage may occur.

Patients complain about headaches, bizarre dreams, and drowsiness that interfere with their ability to continue life activities during therapy.

Interactions. The initial release of norepinephrine may potentiate the antivagal action of quinidine and cause cardioacceleration and arrhythmias if the initial dosages of the two drugs are given concurrently. The vasodilating effect of quinidine (and other vasodilators) may potentiate the hypotensive effects of reserpine. Concurrent administration of either digitalis or quinidine to the patient who is receiving reserpine may cause excess bradycardia.

The sedative effect of reserpine potentiates the central nervous system depressant effects of barbiturates, alcohol, or narcotics. Central nervous system excitability can occur with concurrent use of tricyclic antidepressants or monoamine oxidase inhibitors.

Monoamine Oxidase Inhibitor

Pargyline hydrochloride (EUTONYL) is employed principally for the control of severe hypertension when patients are refractory to other drugs. The drug has limited use because adverse effects are severe and common during therapy.

Pargyline is a monoamine oxidase inhibitor that acts at central and peripheral sites. The mechanism of action involves inhibition of the enzyme monoamine oxidase (MAO), which metabolizes norepinephrine, and there is an elevated level of NE in the neuron. The effect of pargyline action is a slowdown of norepinephrine synthesis. The more recently synthesized NE is preferentially released when the neuron is stimulated, and pargyline action decreases the supply of recently synthesized norepinephrine available for impulse transmission.

Pargyline hydrochloride is available as oral tablets. Administration of the daily dose (50 to 75 mg) is required for 4 to 21 days before the therapeutic orthostatic hypotension is achieved. Tolerance to the drug occurs readily. When the drug is discontinued, there are residual effects for a period of three weeks.

Pargyline causes the same adverse effects shared by other adrenergic inhibitors. The major adverse effect during therapy with pargyline is a hypertensive crisis that can occur when the patient ingests foods or drinks with a high tyramine content (i.e., aged cheese, wine). Pargyline inhibition of MAO decreases the enzyme activity required to prevent the release of large amounts of NE when the additional tyramine accelerates its biosynthesis.

Pargyline potentiates the effects of many drugs. Adverse effects can occur with the concurrent use of hypoglycemic agents, narcotics, sedatives, antihistamines, tricyclic antidepressants, or alcohol. Pargyline also may unmask schizophrenia.

Ganglionic Blocking Agents

Mecamylamine hydrochloride (INVERSINE) and *trimethaphan camsylate* (ARFONAD) act by stabilizing the postsynaptic membrane at the sympathetic nerve ganglion to raise the threshold against acetylcholine that is released by the preganglionic neuron. Drug action blocks impulse transmission to the postganglionic neuron fibers.

Many of the adverse effects of the drugs are directly related to nonselective ganglionic blocking of transmission in the autonomic nervous system. Acetylcholine is the transmitter at the ganglion of the sympathetic nerves and also the transmitter at both the ganglion and tissue receptors of the parasympathetic nerves. Blocking of acetylcholine-mediated transmission in the adrenergic fibers produces a rapid hypotensive effect, but concurrent blocking of transmission in cholinergic fibers produces many adverse effects.

Dryness of the mouth, nose, and throat is bothersome to the patient, but persistent vomiting, urine retention, adynamic ileus, cycloplegia, tachycardia, and severe orthostatic hypotension are serious problems. The nonselectivity of action lessens the usefulness of the drugs for control of blood pressure, and they are employed principally for treatment of hypertensive crises (i.e., dissecting aneurysm).

Baroreceptor Sensitizers

Alkavervir (VERILOID) and *cryptenamine* (UNITENSEN) are veratrum alkaloids that stimulate the baroreceptors in the carotid and aortic sinuses. Drug action at the arterial receptors improves their responsiveness to fullness or stretch. When pressure in the arterial sinuses is elevated, impulses travel to the cardioinhibitory centers in the medulla. The centers then emit efferent impulses that lower the systolic and diastolic blood pressures and slow cardiac contraction by decreasing the sympathetic tone and increasing the vagal tone.

The drugs are potent antihypertensive drugs, but they are infrequently employed for control of hypertension because patients find the adverse effects intolerable (i.e., persistent nausea, vomiting, epigastric distress, hiccups, salivation, hyperhidrosis, blurred vision, paresthesias). When the veratrum alkaloids are given to patients taking digitalis or quinidine concurrently, arrhythmias and excess bradycardia may occur.

Alpha-Adrenergic Blockers

Phenoxybenzamine hydrochloride (DIBENSYLINE) and *phentolamine mesylate* (REGITINE) occupy alpha-adrenergic receptors and their action prevents activation by norepinephrine. The drugs act primarily at receptors of the arterioles of the skin, mucosa, intestine, and kidney to prevent constriction of the resistance vessels. The drugs are utilized only when hypertension is secondary to an excess release of catecholamines (i.e., with pheochromocytoma or with clonidine withdrawal crisis).

Phentolamine is short acting (15 minutes) and usually is administered by constant intravenous infusion. Phenoxybenzamine binds tenaciously

with the receptors, and an intravenous bolus of drug produces a prolonged period of effectiveness. Orthostatic hypotension and reflex tachycardia can occur during therapy with either drug. Short-term use usually does not cause the hypermotility of the intestines, nasal congestion, and miosis that are known to be adverse effects of the drugs.

Beta-Adrenergic Blockers

Propranolol hydrochloride and *metoprolol tartrate* are the beta-adrenergic blocking agents currently employed for treatment of persons with hypertension. The therapeutic effects of the drugs are related to the decrease in the cardiac response to sympathetic nervous system stimulation and to the suppression of renal secretion of renin. The drugs cross the blood-brain barrier, and a central action may contribute to the therapeutic effect.

Propranolol Hydrochloride (INDERAL). The drug usually is used with a thiazide diuretic or other antihypertensive drugs. The initial daily oral dosage is 80 mg and that dosage is gradually increased until the desired response is attained. The usual daily maintenance dosage is 160 to 180 mg. The beta-adrenergic blocking action of propranolol is nonselective, and its action at pulmonary beta$_2$ receptors can produce bronchoconstriction in susceptible persons. Propranolol is commonly used for control of cardiac arrhythmias. A detailed discussion of the drug is presented in Chapter 8.

Metoprolol Tartrate (LOPRESSOR). The drug has a more potent action at cardiac beta$_1$ receptors and less activity at pulmonary beta$_2$ receptors than propranolol. Because it is more cardioselective, it is used in preference to propranolol for treatment of persons susceptible to bronchospasm associated with beta$_2$ blockade. The drug action is not entirely cardioselective, and persons with chronic respiratory problems (i.e., bronchial asthma) may require a beta$_2$ agonist to provide bronchodilation during therapy. Metoprolol is initially administered orally at a daily dosage of 100 mg. The usual daily maintenance dosage is 200 to 400 mg, divided for administration two to three times per day.

REGIONAL ARTERIAL DILATION

Cyclandelate, dihydrogenated ergot alkaloids, isoxsuprine, niacin, nicotinyl alcohol, nylidrin, *papaverine* (and its congeners), and *tolazoline* (Table 9–4) are employed for dilation in particular regions of the arterial circulation. The drugs generally are used for dilation of arterioles in the cerebral tissues or in extremities.

The drugs have been employed, with varying degrees of success, in attempts to improve the behavior and cognitive function of elderly indi-

Table 9–4.
Regional Vasodilator Drugs: Selected Dosage-Response Factors

Drug	Adult Daily Dosage	Action Mode	Adverse Effects
Cyclandelate (CYCLOSPASMOL)	400 to 800 mg ÷ 2 to 4 (capsules)	Nonspecific relaxation of peripheral arterial smooth muscle	Gastric pain and eructation, flushing, tingling, headache, dizziness, sweating, weakness, tachycardia
Dihydrogenated ergot alkaloids (HYGERGINE)	3 mg ÷ 3 (sublingual tablets)	Arterial alpha-adrenergic-receptor blocking	Nausea, vomiting, sublingual irritation, sinus bradycardia
Isoxsuprine hydrochloride (VASODILAN)	30 to 80 mg ÷ 3 to 4 (tablets)	Nonspecific relaxation of arterial smooth muscle	Dizziness, hypotension, tachycardia, abdominal distress, occ. rash
Niacin (NIAC, NICOCAP)	300 to 400 mg ÷ 2 (tablets, extended-release capsules)	Nonspecific relaxation of dermal vessel musculature in blush area and extremities	Flushing of face and neck, tingling, gastric upset, rash, urticaria
Nicotinyl alcohol (RONITACOL)	150 to 300 mg ÷ 3 (elixir)		
Nylidrin hydrochloride (ARLIDIN)	9 to 48 mg ÷ 3 to 4 (tablets)	Arteriole beta-adrenergic-receptor stimulation in skeletal muscles	Nausea, vomiting, palpitations, tachycardia, hypotension, dizziness, trembling, nervousness
Papaverine (CERESPAN, KAVRIN, PAVABID, PAVACAP, PAVERINE, VASAL, VASOSPAN)	300 to 450 mg ÷ 2 to 3 (tablets, elixir, extended-release capsules)	Direct relaxation of arterial smooth muscle	Nausea, drowsiness, rash, headache, vertigo, lethargy, malaise, increased heart and respiratory rate, constipation, diarrhea
Congeners: ethaverine hydrochloride (ETHATAB); dioxyline phosphate PAVERIL)	300 to 600 mg ÷ 3 ⁣ 600 to 2000 mg ÷ 3 to 4		
Tolazoline hydrochloride (PRISCOLINE, TOLPAL)	100 to 300 mg ÷ 4 to 6 (tablets, extended-release tablets)	Direct relaxation of arterial smooth muscle, sympathetic blocking	Chilliness, headache, paresthesias of scalp, nausea, vomiting, diarrhea, cardiac arrhythmias

viduals with advanced arteriosclerosis or atherosclerosis of cerebral vessels. The results of studies make it difficult to evaluate whether the moderate improvements in patients' functional status are related to the drugs or to other variables (i.e., increased personal attention, concerted efforts to involve the patients in environmental activities).

The drugs also have been employed for treatment of varying arterial problems that cause symptoms associated with localized tissue ischemia (i.e., Buerger's disease, arteriosclerosis, intermittent claudication, nighttime muscle cramps). Controlled studies are needed to more clearly define the effectiveness of the drugs in treatment of transitory or nonacute circulatory problems. The recent advances in surgical arterial bypass procedures have minimized use of the drugs for control of highly disruptive circulatory problems.

NURSING INTERVENTION

Many individuals have their first inkling that there is a health problem when they are told about a blood pressure elevation at the time of a routine physical examination or while participating in a hypertension screening program. The diagnosis is made by the physician after periodic blood pressure evaluation following the initial discovery of an elevation. Many of the individuals are asymptomatic when they are informed that they have essential, or primary, hypertension. The diagnosis and the plan for therapy communicate clearly to a "healthy" individual that there is a chronic health problem that must be dealt with in everyday living.

The problem of deepest concern to health professionals is the high rate of noncompliance with therapy after the disease has been identified. From the patients' point of view, it is difficult to maintain a plan of therapy that requires the long-term use of drugs when there are no symptoms, and the drugs make them feel worse rather than better. Concurrent modifications in favored living patterns that are imposed by prescribed changes in dietary, smoking, and activity patterns can make the individuals resentful and resistive to therapy. It is little wonder that the noncompliance rate is often as high as 50 percent of the individuals with essential hypertension.

Studies of the hypertensive patient population have indicated that more than two thirds of the individuals partially or completely default in taking the prescribed drugs because of misinformation, misunderstanding, or lack of knowledge. In a few clinic situations, the noncompliance rate was reduced to a minimum by careful planning of measures to help the patients follow the prescribed regimen.

In health care settings the efforts of each professional complement those of others who are assisting the person to maintain the blood pressure control plan. The challenge to each professional is to improve patients' compliance to antihypertensive drug therapy plans.

Initial Status Evaluation

The initial contact with the person who has essential hypertension affords an opportunity to determine those factors that will influence implementation of the therapeutic plan. An open interactive discussion with the individual allows an opportunity to ascertain the person's knowledge of the disease and the rationale for the therapeutic plan. An important element in the interchange is definition of the person's perceptions or misconceptions about folk remedies, drug action, dietary restrictions, or activity limitations. There is a rich opportunity, during the discussion, to reinforce the individual's knowledge about the disease and the effectiveness of drug therapy in decreasing the cardiovascular complications of hypertension.

Some individuals are visiting more than one physician for control of concurrent health problems, and it is necessary to ascertain the various therapies being employed for health maintenance. Information about use of prescription drugs (i.e., oral contraceptives) and the independent use of over-the-counter drugs (i.e., nose drops, cough syrups) is important in considering drug interactions or factors contributing to the hypertensive level.

When hypertension is diagnosed while the patient is being treated for an intercurrent medical problem, it is important to determine whether the person previously has been treated for hypertension. It also is important to ascertain whether a previously diagnosed patient has followed the prescribed antihypertensive drug regimen. When an individual indicates that there has been a partial or complete omission of the drug therapy plan, it is essential that specific details of the reasons for noncompliance be elicited.

It may assist patients to express particular problems if inquiry is directed at specific variables that can be predicted on the basis of their life circumstances. Common problems are inability to find a babysitter for young children, timing of appointments that interferes with scheduled employment hours, transportation costs, or the cost of medication. Individuals living on a marginal income may find the cost of clinic or office visits, transportation, or drugs prohibitive. For example, the daily use of hydrochlorothiazide and the use of methyldopa three times a day costs approximately $150 per year.

An indication that the person is unconvinced that the benefits of treatment justify the side effects, expense, and inconvenience of drug therapy should be explored carefully to ascertain the particular factors that are frustrating the patient. It may be possible to mobilize available services to modify the time burden or the cost of therapy to the individual.

Blood Pressure Assessment. An early definition of basal, or resting, blood pressure levels provides guidelines for antihypertensive drug therapy. The basal blood pressure is determined by analysis of *serial pressures*. For example, the hospitalized patient may have the blood pressure taken four times a day for four days. The sporadic or exceptionally high readings are deleted, and the remaining pressure levels are averaged to define the basal blood pressure level. In the home situation, the patient or a family member may take the blood pressure twice a day for two weeks. It is usual to have the person come to the clinic or office at the end of the first week to evaluate the reliability of home recordings. The readings during the second week are averaged, after deletion of the sporadic high readings, to determine the basal blood pressure.

Assessing Progress

Blood pressure readings during therapy are compared with those obtained previous to therapy. An ongoing graphic record of pressure levels allows health team members and the patient to evaluate progress. The blood pressure and pulse are taken before each administration of the drug in the initial phase of dosage-response assessment. It is important to briefly note on the graphic chart any variables that relate to changes in pulse or blood pressure levels (i.e., restless, drowsy, confused, elevated temperature). In addition to providing relevant factors about the cardiovascular status, the annotated graphic record provides an indication of tissue perfusion and the cause of variant readings.

Blood pressure monitoring procedures are directed at identifying the effectiveness of antihypertensive drug therapy and the hypotensive level that occurs with activity or position changes. The antihypertensive drugs have a varying intensity of effect on standing and supine pressures, and the monitoring plan includes taking pressures in each position. For example, the blood pressure is taken when the individual is supine for five minutes, immediately after moving to a standing position, and two minutes after standing. Initial evaluation may include taking the blood pressure in each arm to assure that the use of a different limb will not influence readings.

Each of the antihypertensive drugs causes some degree of postural hypotension because the arterioles are less responsive to the reflex sympathetic nerve stimulation associated with position changes. Precautions should be taken when the hospitalized patient is assisted from a supine to a standing position during the initial days of drug dosage adjustment. The patient should rise (or be assisted to rise) slowly to a sitting position on the edge of the bed with feet dangling for a short period. If no dizziness occurs, it is possible for the patient to stand safely. Standing near the bed for ten minutes allows an adequate time period for assessment of readiness to move forward without symptomatic hypotension. The onset of dizziness necessitates lying down with the head elevated on pillows. Flexing and exercising the legs moves venous blood toward the heart, and a subsequent attempt to rise may be uneventful.

The predictability that potent antihypertensive drugs will cause postural hypotension often is capitalized on during intensive therapy for severe or malignant hypertension. The head of the bed may be tilted to a 45-degree angle by placing blocks under the legs of the bed, and the position intensifies the hypotension level attained.

Assessment of exercise hypotension levels may be planned for ambulatory patients. For example, the pressure is taken in a supine position, two minutes after standing, and immediately after controlled exercise (i.e., running or hopping in place until slightly winded). The blood pressure then is taken while the person remains standing erect following the exercise.

Counseling

The data obtained in base-line assessment provide a valuable guide for instruction of the patient about the particular antihypertensive drug therapy plan. Each aspect of the therapeutic plan should be discussed with the person, and the goal of therapy should be expressed as frequently as possible: *to decrease the blood pressure level.* The patient may be more actively involved in the discussion when helped to view therapy as making the difference between a productive life and future disabling illness. Discussion of the planned regimen will be more palatable for the patient when it is clearly stated that many problems will subside after the initial days of therapy, and that measures can be taken, or dosage can be modified, to reduce some of the problems that arise.

Specific measures to avert the hazard of fainting and injury when postural or orthostatic hypotension occurs should be discussed with the patient. It is helpful if the specific procedures employed during the initial days of therapy, to protect the individual from falling when dizziness occurs, are reiterated. The necessity of sitting or squatting at the first sign of dizziness also should be discussed.

The varying activities of everyday living may increase the incidence of orthostatic hypotension, and the patient should be advised to exercise the feet and lower legs when standing for long periods of time. It also is useful to describe positions or activities that should be avoided because there is compression of the veins (i.e., squatting to do chores, sitting with legs tightly crossed). When pooling of blood in the extremities persistently causes orthostatic hypotension, the individual may find toe-to-thigh ace bandages or support hose helpful. Excessively high environmental temperatures or hot showers can exaggerate vasodilation and intensify hypotension.

It is very important that the patient understand the need for periodic evaluation of the effectiveness of the therapeutic regimen. The initial "checkup" periods may be planned at two-week intervals, but the intervals between examinations by the physician usually are lengthened as therapy stabilizes. Throughout the discussion, the focus is on how the person will manage the regimen, because the drugs are effective only if the drug therapy plan is implemented by the individual.

Review Guides

1. Formulate a plan for instruction of the ambulatory patient about guanethidine therapy. Include the rationale for use of the drug, adverse effects, and drug interactions in the plan.
2. Outline the factors that must be considered when preparing the patient, who is leaving the hospital, to maintain an antihypertensive drug therapy plan that includes chlorthalidone, hydralazine, and guanethidine.
3. Describe how you would explain to the patient who is receiving reserpine that she also must take the prescribed diuretic when she argues that tissue fluid has lessened and urine volume is normal.
4. Outline the measures that can be taken to decrease orthostatic hypotension during antihypertensive drug therapy.
5. Plan a scheduled sequence for taking the patient's blood pressure when assessing the effectiveness of the antihypertensive drug on blood pressure levels.
6. Outline a plan for administration of the drugs when there is a new prescription for the patient to receive reserpine and quinidine. Explain the rationale for the administration plan.
7. List the measures that would be implemented when monitoring the status of a patient receiving diazoxide intravenously.
8. Describe the observations that would be appropriate when assessing the progress and problems when the patient is receiving the following drugs for long-term therapy: clonidine, hydralazine, methyldopa.

Additional Readings

Barnes, Robert W.: Evaluating peripheral arterial occlusive disease. *Postgrad. Med.,* **59:**98, February, 1976.

Botwin, Elaine Dobbins: Should children be screened for hypertension? *Am. J. Maternal Child Nurs.,* **1:**152, May/June, 1976.

Caldwell, John R.: Drug regimens for long-term therapy of hypertension. *Geriatrics,* **31:**115, January, 1976.

Corea, Anna L.: Current trends in diet and drug therapy for the dialysis patient. *Nurs. Clin. North Am.,* **10:**469, September, 1975.

Dhar, Sisir K., and Freedman, Philip: Clinical management of hypertensive emergencies. *Heart Lung,* **5:**571, July–August, 1976.

Dollery, C. T.; Davies, D. S.; Draffan, G. H.; Dargie, H. J.; Dean, C. R.; Reid, J. L.; Clare, R. A.; and Murray, S.: Clinical pharmacology and pharmacokinetics of clonidine. *Clin. Pharmacol. Ther.,* **19:**11, January, 1976.

Dormois, John C.; Young, James L.; and Nies, Alan S.: Minoxidil in severe hypertension: value when conventional drugs have failed. *Am. Heart J.,* **90:**360, September, 1975.

Fisch, Irwin R., and Frank, Jess: Oral contraceptives and blood pressure. *J.A.M.A.,* **237:**2499, June 6, 1977.

Freis, Edward D.: Reserpine in hypertension: present status. *Am. Fam. Physician,* **11:**120, June, 1975.

Frohlich, Edward D.: Hypertensive crisis. *Hosp. Med.,* **13:**32, January, 1977.

Garrison, Glen E.: Peripheral artery insufficiency. *Hosp. Med.,* **11:**64, March, 1975.

Gottlieb, Thomas B., and Chidsey, Charles A.: The clinician's guide to pharmacology of antihypertensive agents. *Geriatrics,* **31:**99, January, 1976.

Gould, Lawrence, and Reddy, C. V. Ramana: Phentolamine. *Am. Heart J.,* **92:**397, September, 1976.

Grim, Clarence E.: Office management of hypertension. *Am. Fam. Physician,* **14:**90, July, 1976.

Harris, Raymond: Treatment of hypertension in geriatric patients. *Clin. Med.,* **83:**9, July, 1976.

Hayes, Arthur H., Jr., and Schneck, Dennis W.: Antihypertensive pharmacotherapy. *Postgrad. Med.,* **59:**155, May, 1976.

Henrich, William L.; Cronin, Robert; Miller, Paul D.; and Anderson, Robert J.: Hypotensive sequelae of diazoxide and hydralazine therapy. *J.A.M.A.,* **237:** 264, January 17, 1977.

Jones, Linda Newell: Hypertension: medical and nursing implications. *Nurs. Clin. North Am.,* **11:** 283, June, 1976.

Keith, Thomas A., III: Hypertension crisis. *J.A.M.A.,* **237:**1570, April 11, 1977.

Koch-Weser, Jan: Drug therapy: diazoxide. *N. Engl. J. Med.,* **294:**1271, June 3, 1976.

———: Drug therapy: hydralazine. *N. Engl. J. Med.,* **295:**320, August 5, 1976.

Kohli, Romesh K., and Elwood, Charles M.: Treating acute hypertensive crisis with sodium nitroprusside. *Am. Fam. Physician,* **15:**141, January, 1977.

Kumar, G. Krishna; Dastoor, Firdaus C.: Robayo, Juan Rodriquez; and Razzaque, Mohammed A.: Side effects of diazoxide. *J.A.M.A.,* **235:**275, January 19, 1975.

Lieberman, Ellin: Children with hypertension. *Am. Fam. Physician,* **12:**99, October, 1975.

Long, Madeleine L.; Winslow, Elizabeth H.; Scheuhing, Mary Ann; and Callahan, Jule A.: Hypertension: what patients need to know. *Am. J. Nurs.,* **76:**765, May, 1976.

McLain, Larry G.: Drugs in the management of hypertensive emergencies in children. *Clin. Pediatr.,* **15:**85, January, 1976.

Mehta, Pradeep K.; Mamdani, Bashir; Shansky, Ronald M.; Mahurkar, Sakharam; and Dunea, George: Severe hypertension. *J.A.M.A.,* **233:**249, July 21, 1975.

Mitchell, Ellen Sullivan: Protocol for teaching hypertensive patients. *Am. J. Nurs.,* **77:**808, May, 1977.

Myers, Martin G.: New drugs in hypertension. *Can. Med. Assoc. J.,* **116:**173, January 22, 1977.

Nies, Alan S.: Clinical pharmacology of antihypertensive drugs. *Med. Clin. North Am.,* **61:**675, May, 1977.

Nukherjee, Dipak; Feldman, Michael S.; and Helfant, Richard H.: Nitroprusside therapy. *J.A.M.A.,* **235:**2406, May 31, 1976.

O'Malley, K.; Segal, J. L.; Israili, Z. H.; Boles, M.; McNay, J. L.; and Dayton, P. G.: Duration of hydralazine action in hypertension. *Clin. Pharmacol. Ther.,* **18:**581, November, 1975.

Page, Lot B.; Yager, Henry M.; and Sidd, James J.: Drugs in the management of hypertension. *Am. Heart J.,* part I, **91:**810, June, 1976; part II, **92:**752, July, 1976; part III, **92:**252, August, 1976.

Peart, W. Stanley: Renin-angiotensin system. *N. Engl. J. Med.,* **292:**302, February 6, 1975.

Pettinger, William A.: Drug therapy: clonidine, a new antihypertensive drug. *N. Engl. J. Med.,* **293:**1179, December 4, 1975.

Ram, Chitta Venkata S.: Newer antihypertensive drugs. *Heart Lung,* **6:**679, July–August, 1977.

———: Report of the task force on blood pressure control in children. *Pediatrics,* **59:**(suppl., pp. 797–820), May, 1977.

Recommendations for a National High Blood Pressure Program Data Base for Effective Antihypertensive Therapy. Department of Health, Education, and Welfare Publication No. 74–593 (National Institutes of Health). U.S. Government Printing Office, Washington, D.C., 1973.

Rodman, John S.: Methyldopa hepatitis. A report of six cases and review of the literature. *Am. J. Med.,* **60:**941, June, 1976.

Rossi, G. Victor: Hypertension development, classification and treatment: antihypertensive drugs. *Am. J. Pharm.,* **147:**65, May–June, 1975.

Shank, Linda F., and Ludewig, J.: Hypertension. *Nurs. Clin. North Am.,* **9:**677, December, 1974.

Ward, Graham W.; Bandy, Patricia; and Fink, Janis W.: Treating and counseling the hypertensive patient. *Am. J. Nurs.,* **78:**824, May, 1978.

Weidmann, Peter; Hirsch, David; Beretta-Piccoli, Carlo; Reubi, Francois C.; and Ziegler, Walter H.: Interrelations among blood pressure, blood volume, plasma renin activity and urinary catecholamines in benign essential hypertension. *Am. J. Med.,* **62:**209, February, 1977.

Woosley, Raymond L., and Nies, Alan S.: Drug therapy: guanethidine. *N. Engl. J. Med.,* **295:**1053, November 4, 1976.

Ziesche, Susan, and Franciosa, Joseph A.: Clinical application of sodium nitroprusside. *Heart Lung,* **6:**99, January–February, 1977.

Zweifter, Andrew J., and Ester, Murray D.: Factors influencing the choice of antihypertensive agents. *Postgrad. Med.,* **60:**81, July, 1976.

10

Coronary Artery Constriction

Myocardial ischemia and infarction are the primary causes of deaths due to heart failure. Coronary artery disease is the factor most commonly interfering with the delivery of oxygen to the myocardial tissue. Angina pectoris may be the earliest sign of an arterial disease that is disrupting the distribution of the blood that is required for myocardial tissue perfusion.

Physiologic Correlations

Cardiac activity is a physiologic example of perpetual motion. The coronary arteries and arterioles that arborize through the myocardium maintain a continual state of hyperemia to meet the nutritive and oxygen requirements of the active cardiac muscle. The large arteries determine the transmural blood flow distribution in endocardial and epicardial tissues, and the arterioles provide the resistance that determines the rate of blood flow. Blood perfusion is comparable in the epicardium and the endocardium, but the endocardium consumes a greater amount of oxygen.

Blood is supplied to the myocardium by the right and left coronary arteries that branch off the aorta immediately distal to the aortic valve (Fig. 10–1). The *left anterior descending branch of the left coronary artery* is located in the grooves between the ventricles on the anterior surface of the heart. The artery provides blood for perfusion of the anterior left ventricle and a major portion of the interventricular septum. The *circumflex branch of the left coronary artery* is located in the groove between the left atrium and the left ventricle, and smaller branches travel anteriorly and posteriorly. The circumflex artery perfuses the left atrium and the lateral wall of the left ventricle. The *right coronary artery* is located in the grooves between the right atrium and the right ventricle. It also travels to the posterior aspect of the interventricular septum. The artery supplies blood to the right atrium, the major portion of the right ventricle, and the inferior segment of the interventricular septum.

The coronary arteries fill during the diastolic

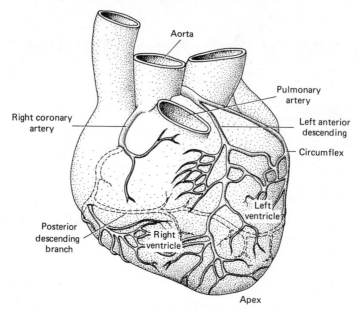

Fig. 10–1. The right and left coronary arteries branch off the aorta and travel throughout the myocardium to supply blood to the epicardial and endocardial tissues.

phase of the cardiac cycle, and the pressure in the aorta is directly proportional to the filling of the arteries. The heart rate also influences the adequacy of arterial filling. Tachycardia shortens the diastolic period and decreases the arterial filling time. Bradycardia may diminish coronary artery filling when there is a decreased cardiac output.

Myocardial oxygen utilization is directly related to the *coronary blood flow,* the *oxygen content of arterial blood,* and the *amount of oxygen extracted from the arterial blood.* Cardiac tissues extract the maximal amount of oxygen (65 to 70 percent) from arterial blood that passes through the myocardium, and that level cannot be increased appreciably during stress. The oxygen-carrying capacity of blood also is maximal in healthy individuals with a normal hemoglobin level. The only remaining parameter that can be modified, to increase the availability of oxygen for increased cardiac work, is the coronary blood flow.

The resistance of the coronary arterioles is high under basal conditions, and there is a remarkable capacity for dilation in response to stress. The hypoxia of myocardial tissue that occurs as a consequence of additional cardiac work is associated with dilation of the coronary arterioles. The hypoxic stimulus to vasodilation is so strong that it overrides the sympathetic stimulus for vasoconstriction during stress. The wider radius of the arterioles increases the blood flow and the oxygen supply available for the increased metabolic work of the heart. Dilation of the arterioles in response to requirements for additional oxygen constitutes a *cardiac blood flow reserve.*

Myocardial oxygen consumption and cardiac work are related. The primary determinants of oxygen consumption are the *systolic wall tension, heart rate,* and *velocity of myocardial contraction.* Systolic wall tension during the cardiac cycle is determined by the systolic pressure, the ventricular diameter, and the thickness of the ventricular muscle. The time interval of systolic wall tension is governed by the velocity of contraction and the heart rate. The myocardial oxygen consumption is directly proportional to those factors.

Pathophysiologic Correlations

Dilation of the arterioles can increase the blood supply to the myocardium of the normal heart up to five times prestress level. When the arteries and arterioles are incapable of dilating in response to stress, there is a decrease in the reserve blood supply to those segments of myocardium serviced by the constricted vessels.

The heart is an aerobic tissue, but it can employ anaerobic glycolysis during short periods of ischemia. The lactic acid products of anaerobic metabolism and the chemical irritants (i.e., bradykinin, histamine) released by the ischemic tissue stimulate cardiac nerve receptors. Impulses that are transmitted to the central nervous system provide the stimuli for the typical pain radiation patterns of angina pectoris. The radiation, or distribution, of the pain follows a pattern that represents the common origins of the involved tissues. The heart, neck, jaw, and arms originate in the same embryonic tissues and receive pain nerve

fibers from the same segments of the spinal cord. The characteristics of the pain and the patient's history of precipitating factors are the primary basis for the diagnosis of angina pectoris because the only other fairly consistent finding is a depression of the S-T segment on the electrocardiogram.

Ninety percent of the persons with angina pectoris have significant atherosclerosis involving one or more of the coronary arteries. Cardiac involvement is a manifestation of the generalized atherosclerotic process in arteries throughout the body (Fig. 10–2).

The atherosclerotic processes reduce the distensibility of the coronary vessels, and the blood flow reserve varies widely between segments of the myocardial tissues. As the intraluminal disease progresses, the route for blood flow gradually becomes limited. The development of collateral channels between smaller arteries provides alternate routes for blood flow when arterial narrow-

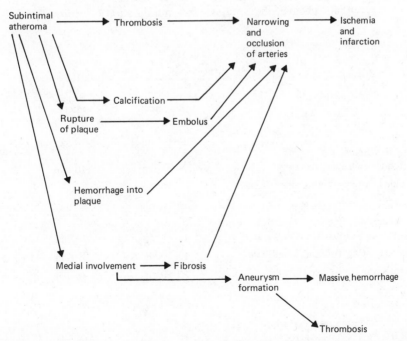

Fig. 10–2. Subintimal atheroma causes progressive intraluminal changes in arteries throughout the body.

ing diminishes the blood supply. The collateral vessels modify the incidence of infarction by partially supplying the blood required for increased cardiac work.

Antianginal Drugs

The myocardial hypoxia that is associated with angina pectoris represents a disproportion between the supply of available oxygen and the oxygen requirements of myocardial tissues during periods of stress. The use of antianginal drugs is an integral part of an overall plan for the control of factors contributing to the incidence of myocardial ischemia (i.e., obesity, stress, smoking, atherosclerosis).

DRUG THERAPY

Nitrates, beta-adrenergic blockers, and *antilipemics* are the agents selectively employed to reduce myocardial hypoxia. Although each of the agents can effectively modify some of the factors contributing to myocardial ischemia, the nitrates are the mainstay of therapy. The nitrates and the beta-adrenergic-blocking drugs have a positive effect on myocardial oxygen consumption, but they do not change the functional capacity of the stenosed coronary arteries. The antilipemic drugs are employed selectively to control progression of the atherosclerotic process.

NITRATES

The primary aim of therapy with the nitrates is to decrease the metabolic demands on the heart during stress and to improve perfusion of ischemic areas of the myocardium. The major differences between the varying formulations of nitrates relate to the route of administration and to the onset and duration of action (Table 10–1).

Table 10–1.
Nitrates: Selected Dosage-Response Factors

Drug	Dosage	Therapeutic Effect	
		Onset	Duration
Inhalant			
Amyl nitrate	0.18–0.3 ml	30 sec	3–5 min
Sublingual Nitrates			
Erythrityl tetranitrate (CARDILATE)	5–15 mg	5–10 min	2–3 hr
Isosorbide dinitrate (ISORDIL, SORBITRATE)	2.5–10 mg	2–5 min	1–2 hr
Nitroglycerin (NITROGLYN, NITROSTAT)	0.15–0.6 mg	1–3 min	9–11 min
*Oral Nitrates**			
Erythrityl tetranitrate (CARDILATE)	15–60 mg	30 min	3–4 hr
Isosorbide dinitrate (ISORDIL, SORBITRATE)	10–60 mg	15–30 min	4–6 hr
Mannitol hexanitrate (NITRANITOL)	30–60 mg	15–30 min	4–6 hr
Nitroglycerin, extended release (NITRO-BID, NITRONG)	1.6–6.5 mg	60–80 min	8–12 hr
Pentaerythritol tetranitrate extended-release (PERITRATE, PENTAFIN, PENTRITOL)	10–40 mg	30–60 min	12 hr

* Liver inactivation causes variable onset and duration of action.

Sublingual Nitrates

Erythrityl tetranitrate, isosorbide dinitrate, and *nitroglycerin* are available in forms for sublingual use. When the tablet is placed under the tongue, the lipid-soluble drug is rapidly absorbed. The drug is taken up by the lymphatics and within minutes the nitrate is circulating to systemic sites of action. Nitroglycerin is the drug most frequently employed for prevention or relief of the anginal pain associated with myocardial ischemia. Nitroglycerin will be discussed as the example of the actions, adverse effects, and interactions of the nitrates.

Nitroglycerin

Action Mode. The direct action of nitroglycerin on smooth muscles of the vasculature causes dilation of the systemic veins, dilation of the systemic arterioles, and dilation of nonsclerotic arteries and collateral channels at cardiac sites. Dilation of the systemic veins decreases venous return to the heart, and more blood remains in the peripheral venous circulation. The decrease in cardiac blood volume reduces the radius and the pressure of the left ventricle and the systolic ejection time is shortened. Dilation of the systemic arterioles reduces the peripheral vascular resistance and lowers the pressure in the arterial circulation. The left ventricle ejects blood against less pressure and the ventricular wall tension is lower during systole. The combined effects of the systemic arterial and venous dilation may decrease the left ventricular work index as much as 22 percent, and there is a marked decrease in myocardial oxygen consumption.

Recent studies indicate that the nitrates also selectively dilate the large nonsclerotic epicardial arteries and the drugs decrease resistance in the small arterioles and collateral coronary vessels. The action on the coronary arterial circulation leads to intramyocardial regional redistribution of blood to ischemic areas.

Therapy Considerations. The sublingual tablet is the most frequently prescribed form of nitroglycerin, but the drug is also available as an extended-release tablet and as an ointment for topical application. Nitroglycerin dosage regulation differs from that of most of the other drugs used for therapy because the patient is actively involved in determination of the smallest dosage that will provide relief of anginal pain. The patient needs explicit instructions about the use and storage of nitroglycerin at the initial time that the drug is prescribed.

The prevention of myocardial ischemia is a major objective for use of the nitrates, and patients are instructed about prophylactic use of the drug. Allowing the intact sublingual tablet to dissolve under the tongue immediately before a situation known to precipitate anginal pain (i.e., strenuous physical activity, exposure to the cold wind, sexual intercourse) usually allows the person to be pain free during a half-hour period of activity.

Nitroglycerin is the cornerstone for control of pain in angina pectoris. The sublingual drug is most effective when it is used at the onset of chest discomfort or pain, and it usually provides complete relief of the anginal pain. Patients are instructed to repeat the initial dose at five-minute intervals if pain is unrelieved. The recommended maximum of tablets for each pain episode is three doses because the vasodilation that is caused by that total dosage is associated with headache and hypotension. The short duration of drug action (30 minutes) makes it possible to repeat the dosage sequence at the onset of subsequent pain episodes. The patient is advised to cease activity and to take the drug while sitting. Although standing motionless would be the best position for increasing peripheral venous blood pooling, the orthostatic hypotension induced by the drug makes it advisable to take measures to avoid falling if dizziness occurs.

Patients are instructed to carry a supply of the tablets with them at all times. The tablets are unstable at temperature extremes and exposure to light, and precautions must be taken to protect them against deterioration. The patient is instructed to carry a small daily supply in an amber bottle with a tightly fitting metal screw cap. The synthetic filler can be left in the bottle, but the person is cautioned against replacing it with cotton, which absorbs nitroglycerin. The person can remove a small supply for use and store the remainder in a cool room where the temperature range is between 15° and 30° C (59° to 86° F). The nitrates cause vasodilation in the buccal membranes, and the slight burning, stinging, or tingling provides an indication of the freshness of the tablets. The absence of pain relief and of the buccal sensation can be used as an indication that the tablets have deteriorated. Patients should be made aware of the fact that the amount of drug that is effective for any given amount of pain should still be effective days later for the same amount of pain if the tablet potency is unchanged and the coronary arteries are not further stenosed. When precautions are taken to protect the tablets from heat, light, and moisture, they should retain their potency for up to six months.

Nitroglycerin ointment 2 percent (NITRO-BID, NITROL) is applied to a 15-cm-by-15-cm (6-by 6-in.) area on the chest, abdomen, back, arm, or thigh for slow cutaneous absorption of the drug. Nitroglycerin is taken up by the cutaneous lipids, which become the sustained-release media for the drug. A 2.5-cm (1-in.) ribbon of the drug provides 12.5 mg of nitroglycerin. The effect on systemic vascular dilation is evident in 15 minutes and the antianginal effects last for three hours. The ointment is applied prophylactically previous to activity or before retiring to prevent nocturnal angina. Administration sites are rotated to avoid skin irritation, and friction is avoided when applying or removing the ointment to avoid acceleration of drug absorption. Dosage regulation is based on the thickness of the layer of ointment that is required to reduce the blood pressure by 10 mm Hg and raise the pulse by 10 beats per minute. The vital sign assessment is made while the individual is in a sitting position to maximize peripheral venous pooling. The pulse and blood pressure are taken one hour after application of the ointment, and those levels are compared with the vital signs taken in the same position immediately before application of the ointment.

Tolerance is known to occur with use of the nitrates. The loss of therapeutic effect is associated with a decrease in the venodilating action of the drugs. To regain the therapeutic effect of the nitrates, the person may be advised by the physician to discontinue use of the nitrate for two to five days when physical activity and other angina-precipitating events can be avoided. The omission period usually restores vascular nitrate sensitivity. Reuse of the drug may be accompanied by the headache, dizziness, and flushing of the face that commonly occur with initial use of the nitrates. The incidence of tolerance is negligible when nitrates are used intermittently, but both tolerance and cross-tolerance may occur with regularly scheduled use of oral formulations.

Adverse Effects. A pounding headache, dizziness, and flushing of the face often occur during the initial days of therapy with nitrates. Headache and flushing of the face occur as direct consequences of arterial dilation. Dizziness or syncope occurs as a consequence of the hypotension caused by generalized vasodilation. The problems are somewhat modified by initiation of therapy with small dosage of the drugs.

Therapy with the nitrates also occasionally causes tacyhcardia. The heart rate is accelerated when hypotension stimulates the baroreceptor reflex mechanisms and efferent sympathetic nerve impulses stimulate the heart.

Interactions. Alcohol potentiates the vasodilating effects of the nitrates. Individuals who are taking the drugs should be advised that ingestion of alcohol close to the time of nitrate use may cause dizziness or syncope.

Oral Nitrates

Erythrityl tetranitrate, isosorbide dinitrate, mannitol hexanitrate, nitroglycerin, and *pentaerythritol tetranitrate* are available as oral tablets and as extended-release capsules or tablets (Table 10–1). The drug enters the portal circulation after being absorbed from the intestine. Much of the nitrate is degraded by hepatic enzymes before it reaches the systemic circulation. The higher dosage of the oral formulations, overcomes some of the loss due to hepatic metabolism, and a therapeutic level of the drug is available for systemic action.

The oral drugs may be prescribed when sublingual tablets are required frequently during a 24-hour period for control of anginal pain. Although the oral tablets decrease the number of sublingual tablets required, patients usually are advised to carry a small supply of sublingual drug for use during breakthrough pain episodes. The oral drugs usually are taken on a regularly scheduled basis, and additional dosage of the oral form may be taken previous to stressful pain-precipitating events that cannot be avoided.

Adverse effects common to the nitrates may be less severe with use of the oral forms than those occurring with use of the sublingual forms of nitrates. The slower absorption and release of nitrates at systemic sites produce a less acute vasodilation effect. The oral forms cause gastric irritation, and nausea or vomiting may occur during therapy.

BETA-ADRENERGIC-BLOCKING DRUGS

Propranolol

Propranolol (INDERAL) is the only beta-adrenergic-blocking agent currently available in the United States for control of angina pectoris. It is employed primarily when patients have incapacitating anginal pain despite the use of sublingual or oral nitrates. The drug is effective in blocking the sympathetic nerve stimuli that increase cardiac work during exercise or emotional stress. When used in conjunction with the nitrates, propranolol has a positive effect on the primary determinants of myocardial oxygen consumption (Table 10–2), and there is a subsequent reduction in the incidence of anginal pain.

Action Mode. Propranolol decreases sympathetic nerve stimulation by combining reversibly with the cardiac beta-adrenergic receptors. By blocking access to the receptors by the sympathetic nerve neurotransmitters *norepinephrine* and *epinephrine*, the drug blocks the cardioacceleration natural to increased activity. Propranolol action prolongs the refractory period of the sino-atrial and atrioventricular node and that effect on conduction slows the heart rate.

The decreased rate of cardiac contraction is accompanied by an increase in the ventricular volume, but the effect may be minimized by the concurrent use of the nitrates, which reduce the ventricular volume. The action of propranolol also blocks the reflex sympathetic responses that occur when the vasodilating effect of the nitrates lowers the blood pressure.

The net effect of the combined actions of propranolol and the nitrates is a reduction in the ventricular volume, ventricular contractility, systolic blood pressure, and heart rate (Table 10–2). The drugs act synergistically to markedly decrease myocardial oxygen consumption and reduce the frequency and severity of anginal episodes.

Therapy Considerations. Patients are able to do more pain-free physical work when taking propranolol because the drug effect delays the appearance of the imbalance between myocardial oxygen supply and demand. Sustained work (i.e., 15 minutes) raises the heart rate–pressure ratio

Table 10–2.

Comparison of the Cardiac Effects of Nerve Stimulation, Nitrates, and Propranolol

	Sympathetic Nerve Stimulation	Nitroglycerin	Propranolol
Left ventricular volume	↑	↓	↑
Systolic blood pressure	↑	↓	↓
Left ventricular contraction	↑	↑ (reflex)	↓
Heart rate	↑	↑ (reflex)	↓

to a level that may cause anginal pain, but the pain would appear up to five minutes earlier without the beta-adrenergic-blocking action of propranolol.

The initial daily dosage of propranolol is low (i.e., 30 to 80 mg ÷ 3 or 4), and the drug is usually administered before meals and at bedtime. Dosage increments of from 10 to 40 mg/dose may be made at three-to-seven-day intervals. Regulation of the dosage is based on the amount of drug required to inhibit the heart rate elevation in response to stress (i.e., mental problem solving). The general guideline is a decrease in the resting pulse rate of 20 beats per minute. The minimum heart rate that is considered acceptable is approximately 50 beats per minute. The usual dosage of propranolol is between 120 mg and 240 mg daily. The end point of dosage adjustment is the relief of anginal pain, a pulse rate of 50 beats per minute, or the onset of significant adverse effects of the drug.

At termination of therapy with propranolol, the drug is withdrawn gradually over a period of three days to avoid exacerbation of angina pectoris. Acute myocardial infarction also has occurred several days after abrupt withdrawal of the drug. To avoid the problems associated with abrupt withdrawal of propranolol, the patient should be advised to maintain the drug administration plan without interruption at any time.

Adverse Effects. Propranolol is used only when moderate or severe anginal pain interferes with the person's life-style because there are significant adverse effects associated with the use of the drug. Sinus bradycardia, heart block, gastrointestinal symptoms (i.e., nausea, abdominal cramping, diarrhea), postural hypotension, and bronchospasm may occur during therapy. The gastrointestinal disturbances may subside with reduction of the drug dosage. The occurrence of bronchospasm is highest in individuals with a history of asthma and the problem can precipitate acute symptoms in individuals with chronic obstructive lung disease.

The beta-adrenergic-blocking effects of propranolol suppress the normal sympathetic reflex

response to hypoglycemia in individuals with diabetes. Masking of the symptoms (i.e., sweating, increased heart rate, anxiety) that usually provide the "alert" that moves the person to ingest a carbohydrate may necessitate modification of the propranolol dosage. A detailed discussion of the actions, adverse effects, and interactions of propranolol is presented in Chapter 8.

ANTILIPEMIC DRUGS

The metabolic pathways of the major lipoproteins are closely interrelated. The types of lipid disorders are classified by the characteristic elevations in plasma levels of chylomicrons, very-low-density lipoproteins, intermediate-low-density lipoproteins, low-density lipoproteins, and high-density lipoproteins (Table 10–3).

At the present time, dietary regulation is the cornerstone of therapy. Dietary restrictions can reduce the plasma levels in almost all persons with hyperlipoproteinemia. The long-term effects on prevention or recession of atherosclerosis are currently under intensive study.

Dietary management is initiated and continued for two to six weeks when lipid levels are elevated. When plasma levels of lipids remain high in individuals known to have extensive coronary artery atherosclerosis, drug therapy may be added to the therapeutic regimen. The combined diet and drug therapy is aimed at reducing the lipid levels by approximately 15 percent in the first four to six weeks of therapy without the onset of side effects.

The primary concern in the treatment of individuals with extensive coronary artery disease is the protection of coronary blood flow reserve by preventing progression of the atherosclerotic process. The drugs employed for therapy *increase lipoprotein catabolism* or *decrease lipoprotein production.*

Cholestyramine resin, colestipol hydrochloride, dextrothyroxine, sitosterols, and *probucol* are the drugs employed to increase lipoprotein catabolism, or clearance, from the plasma. Each of the drugs has been employed for control of the elevated beta- and prebeta-lipoprotein levels that

Table 10–3.
Drug and Diet Therapy for Lipid Disorders

Type	Plasma Lipoprotein Values	Diet	Drugs
I	Elevated chylomicron level	Low-fat, high-carbohydrate diet	none
II	Elevated beta-lipoprotein, low-density lipoprotein, and cholesterol levels	Low-cholesterol, low-saturated-fat, high-polyunsaturated-fat diet	Cholestyramine, colestipol, dextrothyroxine, niacin, sitosterols, probucil
III	Elevated abnormal form beta-lipoprotein, triglyceride, and cholesterol levels	Low-calorie, low-cholesterol, high-polyunsaturated-fat diet	Clofibrate, niacin
IV	Elevated prebeta-lipoprotein, very-low-density protein, and triglyceride levels	Low-calorie, low-cholesterol, high-polyunsaturated-fat diet	Clofibrate, niacin
V	Elevated chylomicron, triglyceride, and cholesterol levels	Low-calorie, low-fat, low-carbohydrate, high-protein diet	Niacin

are known to increase the risk of coronary artery disease in type II hyperlipoproteinemia.

Clofibrate and *niacin* (nicotinic acid) are the drugs employed to decrease lipoprotein production. The drugs are used for control of type III and IV hyperlipoproteinemia. Niacin also is used for treatment of persons with a type V lipid disorder. Both drugs are employed as an adjunct to dietary restrictions (Table 10–3).

Cholestyramine Resin

Action Mode. *Cholestyramine resin* (CUEMID, QUESTRAN) is an oral anion-exchange resin. The drug remains in the intestinal lumen and the resin complexes with bile acids. Cholestyramine resin releases chloride ions in exchange for the bile acids, and that binding increases the clearance of the low-density lipoproteins present in the bile. The new resin complex is excreted with the feces.

Therapy Considerations. Cholestyramine resin is employed with a low-cholesterol, low-saturated-fat, high-polyunsaturated-fat diet for treatment of type II hyperlipoproteinemia. The drug initially is given at low dosage (i.e., 16 gm/day ÷ 2 to 4 doses) and the dosage is increased at two-to-three-week intervals by 4 to 8 gm until the maximum dosage of 32 gm/day is reached.

The drug is supplied in a powdered form that has an unpleasant taste and odor. The drug can be made somewhat more palatable by mixing it in lemonade, fruit juice, or a pulpy fruit (i.e., applesauce). The drug can be mixed with carbonated beverages, but it will foam excessively unless the powder is sprinkled carefully on the top of the liquid and stirred gently.

Therapy with cholestyramine resin is one of the most expensive of the antilipemic drug therapy plans. The usual dosage schedule costs the person approximately $30 to $40 per month.

Adverse Effects. Constipation is one of the most common adverse effects, and it can be particularly distressing when the drug is used by elderly patients. Stool softeners or laxatives may decrease the undesirable problems of impaction, straining at stool, and enlargement of hemorrhoids in elderly persons.

Most of the gastrointestinal problems (i.e., nausea, vomiting, abdominal cramping, and distention) can be controlled by decreasing the dosage frequency. There have been reports of the rare occurrence of serious steatorrhea, intestinal obstruction, and hyperchloremic acidosis.

Interactions. The resin may bind other drugs administered orally. Iron, acids, or neutral drugs (i.e., digoxin, levothyroxine, sodium warfarin, phenylbutazone, tetracycline, thiazide diuretics) may be absorbed by the resin. Administration of drugs can be planned one hour before or four to six hours after administration of the resin to assure adequate drug absorption. Long-term therapy with the drug also interferes with the absorption of fat-soluble vitamins that are dependent on the presence of bile in the intestine (i.e., vitamins A, D, K).

Colestipol Hydrochloride

Colestipol hydrochloride (COLESTID) is a bile sequestrant with actions, adverse effects, and interactions similar to those of cholestyramine resin. The drug is supplied in water-soluble beads and usually is administered initially at a dosage level of 5 gm two to four times a day. The dosage may gradually be increased to 10 gm three to four times per day.

Dextrothyroxine

Dextrothyroxine sodium (CHOLOXIN) is a derivative of thyroxine. Administration of the drug at a low dosage level provides control of type II hyperlipoproteinemia without causing the accelerated metabolic effects common to the thyroxine group. The Coronary Drug Project of the National Heart and Lung Institute has advised against use of the drug for patients with coronary artery disease. In their studies there was a high cardiovascular mortality rate when the drug was taken by patients with a history of myocardial infarction. The drug is useful for selected individuals with elevated lipid levels in the absence of coronary artery disease.

Action Mode. The drug decreases plasma cholesterol levels, increases the metabolism and clearance of hepatic cholesterol, and increases the removal rate of low-density lipoproteins.

Therapy Considerations. At initiation of therapy there is a time lag of approximately two to four weeks before evidence is seen of the effect of dextrothyroxine on plasma lipid levels. The initial oral drug dosage is low (1 to 2 mg/day) and the dosage is increased monthly by 1-to-2-mg increments to the usual maintenance level of 4 to 8 mg/day. The maximum effect on plasma cholesterol levels occurs in two to three months. The cost of the drug is relatively low ($12 to $14/month) at the usual maintenance dosage level.

Adverse Effects. Acceleration of angina pectoris and arrhythmias have occurred in persons with a history of heart disease. Dextrothyroxine has also caused glucose intolerance, abnormal liver function tests, glycosuria, and neutropenia.

Interactions. Dextrothyroxine enhances the effect of oral anticoagulants. The process may include an increase in the affinity of the anticoagulant receptor sites on plasma albumin, and the longer period of albumin binding maintains drug in the serum for prolonged action. It is estimated that the dosage of oral anticoagulants can be reduced by one third to avoid elevation of the prothrombin levels when the drugs are used concurrently.

Sitosterols

Sitosterols (CYTELLIN) is a plant sterol similar in structure to cholesterol. When employed in therapy of type II hyperlipoproteinemia, the maximum effect on plasma cholesterol levels occurs in two months. Sitosterols inhibits the absorption of cholesterol from food sources in the intestine. It is thought to act by competing for cholesterol absorption sites. The drug action in the intestine also interferes with the reabsorption of biliary cholesterol.

The oral liquid form of the drug is administered at a dosage of 6 gm one-half hour before meals and at bedtime. The palatability of sitosterols may be increased by mixing the drug with milk, coffee, tea, or fruit juice when there are no contraindications to the use of those liquids. Adverse effects of the drug are limited to a mild laxative effect of the methylcellulose used as the dispensing agent in the preparation. The stools are bulky and light tan.

Clofibrate

Clofibrate (ATROMID-S) is an oral drug employed for reducing the plasma lipid levels of individuals with hypertriglyceridemia. The Coronary Drug Project of the National Heart and Lung Institute has advised against the use of the drug for individuals with atherosclerotic coronary artery disease because a high incidence of serious adverse effects occurred in the study population.

Action Mode. The specific mode of action of the drug is unclear. It inhibits the biosynthesis of cholesterol, accelerates the catabolism of low-density lipoproteins, and decreases the hepatic production of very-low-density lipoproteins. The inhibition of cholesterol synthesis enhances the mobilization of cholesterol and increases its flow out of tissue deposits. The exodus of cholesterol from tissue stores decreases the size of superficial tuberous xanthomata. The usual dosage of the drug is 1.5 to 2 gm/day divided into two doses.

Adverse Effects. Serious adverse effects have occurred during therapy with clofibrate. Cholelithiasis occurred in a significant number of persons during the Coronary Drug Project study. There also was a small, but significant incidence of arrhythmias, new angina pectoris, intermittent claudication, peripheral vascular disease, thromboembolic events, and leukopenia during the course of the study.

Approximately 10 percent of the patients taking the drug have nausea or dyspepsia, and diarrhea also occurs. More than half of the patients have a gain in weight as a consequence of an increased deposition of subcutaneous fat. Dermatitis, dry skin, brittle hair, alopecia, sore muscles, fatigue, influenza-like symptoms, and decreased libido also are problems during therapy with clofibrate.

Interactions. The use of clofibrate with oral anticoagulants may enhance the hypoprothrombinemic effects of the anticoagulant by displacing the drug from albumin-binding sites. The dosage of the anticoagulant may require reduction by one third to prevent bleeding when the drugs are used together. Clofibrate also displaces other drugs (i.e., phenytoin) from albumin-binding sites.

Nicotinic Acid (Niacin)

Nicotinic acid (NICOLAR) has a broad spectrum of effectiveness in control of lipid disorders, and it has been employed for treatment of individuals with types II, III, IV, or V hyperlipoproteinemia. Some limitation in use has occurred because there is a high incidence of adverse effects during therapy with niacin.

Action Mode. The antilipemic dosage exceeds that required for vitamin supplementation with nicotinic acid. Within four to six hours after therapy with niacin is initiated, there is a decrease in the plasma triglyceride concentration and a decrease in the synthesis of very-low-density lipoproteins.

Niacin has an indirect lowering effect on intermediate-low-density lipoproteins and low-density lipoproteins. The therapeutic effect is evident in the changes in plasma levels several days after therapy is initiated.

Therapy Considerations. Dosage usually is initiated with 100 mg of nicotinic acid given three times a day with meals or with cold liquids. Dosage increments of 300 mg are made at four-to-seven-day intervals. The maintenance dosage of the drug is 3 to 6 gm/day, which usually is divided into three doses. The cost of maintenance therapy is usually as low as $7 per month, which is considerably lower than the cost of the other antilipemic drugs.

Adverse Effects. Intense cutaneous flushing and pruritus often occur one to two hours after the tablet is ingested. The problems gradually regress as tolerance to the superficial vasodilating effects of the drug develops. Although gastrointestinal symptoms do occur, they usually are transient problems and can be decreased by taking the drug with meals or chewing the tablets and taking a full glass of water.

During the Coronary Drug Project a significant incidence of arrhythmias occurred in the patient population, which was comprised of individuals with coronary artery disease. Serious problems also include hyperuricemia, glycosuria, activation of gastric ulcers, and an increase in skin pigmentation.

Probucol (LORELCO)

The drug is employed primarily for the control of hypercholesterolemia and elevated levels of low-density lipoproteins. It is a relatively new drug that is useful for the treatment of patients with combined hypercholesterolemia and hypertriglyceridemia.

Action Mode. The exact mechanism of action of the drug is unclear but it is thought to act by increasing the cholesterol and bile acid excretion in the feces. It may inhibit the transport of cholesterol from the intestine as well as inhibiting the early stages of its synthesis.

Therapy Considerations. The drug is intended for long-term use. The daily dosage of 1 gm is divided for administration two times a day with meals. Plasma drug levels are less variable, and they are higher when the drug is taken with food. The plasma drug concentrations stabilize within three to four months when the dosage is taken regularly for that period of time. Base-line cholesterol and triglyceride levels usually are evalu-

ated prior to the start of therapy to provide base lines for assessing the effectiveness of the drug. The daily cost of therapy for the person taking the drug is about twice that of clofibrate.

Adverse Effects. The most common adverse effects are transient gastrointestinal disturbances (i.e., flatulence, nausea, vomiting, abdominal pain, diarrhea). Clinical studies show that approximately 2 percent of the patients discontinue taking the drug because of the gastrointestinal problems.

NURSING INTERVENTION

Assessment and Counseling

Sublingual nitrates (i.e., nitroglycerin) are widely used for control of the sporadic pain episodes associated with coronary artery disease. Each individual should be carefully instructed at the time therapy is initiated about the disease, personal risk factors requiring control (i.e., smoking, obesity), precipitating events that can be modified, and the effects of the drug. It is usual to plan recontact with the person to assure understanding of the extensive amount of information and to assess individual progress. The overall objective is to provide a basis for the individual to make sound judgments in implementing the plan for use of drugs prescribed for control of the cardiac problem. Adequate knowledge is essential for the person's maintenance of the plan for prophylaxis and relief of pain.

Angina pectoris may have a different meaning to the nurse than it does to many of the persons with the problem. The physiologic reality impels the nurse to view the problem in terms of myocardial hypoxia. Many patients view angina pectoris as a sensation that is precipitated by particular life events, builds to a peak, and sometimes gradually subsides with cessation of the activity and a period of rest. Persons with that perception of the problem do not have sufficient understanding of their coronary artery disease and of the action of nitroglycerin to comply with the therapeutic plan.

Periodic assessment of the effectiveness of therapy with the patient allows an opportunity to provide information and to correct misconceptions about the use of nitroglycerin. Although there are predictable precipitating factors (i.e., physical exertion, emotional excitement, eating a heavy meal, sexual intercourse, mental stress, nightmares), the discussion will be more productive if the patient is encouraged to identify those personal life situations that most frequently cause anginal pain.

Most persons describe discomfort or distress rather than pain in discussing their experience with angina pectoris. When encouraged to be explicit, the descriptions indicate that the "discomfort" is felt in the neck or jaw and radiates to the shoulder and the upper arm. The sensation in the arm and hand often is described as an ache, numbness, or tingling sensation. The retrosternal sensations are described by patients as constricting, tight, or heavy, and there is often some description of feeling unable to breathe. Although the patterns of pain differ between individuals, the radiation pattern is relatively consistent in each individual.

The importance of the explicit discussion of the personal precipitating events and pain patterns is that it assures the person's awareness of the problems associated with insufficient coronary artery blood flow. The person's input also provides a base line for discussing the need to contact the physician when the pain patterns change or when an episode is unrelieved by nitroglycerin. Both progression of the coronary artery occlusion and the occurrence of myocardial infarction are possible reasons for pain to persist unrelieved by nitroglycerin.

The effectiveness of the drug is dependent on its being fresh, and it is important to discuss with the person the measures that can be taken to assure the viability of the nitroglycerin content of the drug when it is required. It is useful to have the person describe explicitly the manner in which the drug is carried for emergency use. Some patients have been found to store the tablets in a facial tissue or in a flat metal container with other drugs (i.e., aspirin), in attempts to make retrieval of the drug convenient or to avoid showing that medication is being carried. A detailed description of the factors that cause deterioration of nitroglycerin is an essential part of the discussion of drug use and storage. The person should be informed of the effectiveness of an amber bottle with a tightly fitted screw cap in retaining drug potency.

The control of personal risk factors is often a problem for the individual. A simple directive to lose weight and to stop smoking leaves the person with two major long-term habits that should be changed. Individuals usually move forward in thinking about change when they perceive that the professional knows the difficulty entailed in changing the lifelong patterns. It also is helpful if the nurse assists the person in identifying specific measures that can be taken as initial steps in modification of those habit patterns. Some individuals also may benefit from a referral to a community clinic when they have difficulty with dieting or cessation of smoking.

Many persons have difficulty accepting the prophylactic use of sublingual nitroglycerin tablets preactivity. It may facilitate the discussion if the person is asked to identify life situations that could be avoided to decrease the incidence of anginal attacks. Further discussion can focus on the prophylactic use of nitroglycerin as allowing continuance of those activities that cannot be avoided. Prophylactic use of the drug can contribute to improving the quality of life for the individual with angina pectoris.

The length of the combined assessment and counseling session described above will vary as the person's learning needs differ. The important component is the individual's readiness for unsupervised use of the drugs in a safe and effective manner.

An important consideration when examining the individual with atherosclerosis of the coronary arteries is that the cardiac problems are early signs of a generalized atherosclerotic process. Physical examination should include evaluation of perfusion in all body tissues. Auscultation of the major arteries can provide valuable information about blood flow. The

turbulence caused by atherosclerotic involvement is evident in rushing sounds, or bruit, in contrast to the absence of sounds when laminar flow is present in uninvolved arteries.

Review Guides

1. Describe how nitroglycerin action relieves pain using terms that could be understood by most patients.
2. Outline the specific factors about the use and storage of nitroglycerin that must be discussed with the patient.
3. Explain how the person can be helped to understand how a tablet placed under the tongue can relieve pain or prevent exercise-induced pain.

4. Formulate a plan for instructing a patient about the use of an oral nitrate, a sublingual nitrate, and propranolol for control of the individual's problem with cardiac ischemia.
5. Explain the specific factors about the rationale for use of an oral nitrate, dietary restriction, and cholestyramine resin that should be described to the patient with type II hyperlipoproteinemia.

Additional Readings

Allendorf, Elaine Erickson, and Keegan, M. Honor: Teaching patients about nitroglycerin. *Am. J. Nurs.,* **75**:1168, July, 1975.

Aronow, Wilbert S.: Treatment of angina pectoris: pharmacologic approaches. *Postgrad. Med.,* **60**:100, November, 1976.

Battock, Dennis J.: Levitt, Peter W.; and Steele, Peter P.: Effects of isosorbide dinitrate and nitroglycerin on cerebral circulatory dynamics in coronary artery disease. *Am. Heart J.,* **92**:455, October, 1976.

Benditt, Earl P.: The origin of atherosclerosis. *Sci. Am.,* **236**:74, February, 1977.

Brown, Michael S., and Goldstein, Joseph L.: Receptor-mediated control of cholesterol metabolism. *Science,* **191**:150, January, 1976.

Cairns, John A.; Fantus, Ivan George; and Klassen, Gerald A.: Unstable angina pectoris. *Am. Heart J.,* **92**:373, September, 1976.

Clark, Marie Castellan: Chest pain. *Heart Lung,* **4**:956, November–December, 1975.

Conti, Charles R.: Medical management of angina. *Resident Staff Physician,* **21**:57, October, 1975.

Epstein, Stephen E.; Kent, Kenneth M.; Goldstein, Robert E.; Borer, Jeffrey S.; and Redwood, David R.: Reduction of ischemic injury by nitroglycerin during acute myocardial infarction. *N. Engl. J. Med.,* **293**:29, January 2, 1975.

Fleischmajer, Raul: Hypolipidemic drugs. *Am. Fam. Physician,* **17**:188, February, 1978.

Gelfand, Maxwell L.; Kloth, Howard; and Goodkin, Louis: The medical treatment of angina pectoris. *Am. Fam. Physician,* **13**:84, April, 1976.

Gray, Richard; Chatterjee, Kanu; Vyden, John K.; Ganz, William; Forrester, James S.; and Swan, H. J. C.: Hemodynamic and metabolic effects of isosorbide dinitrate in chronic congestive heart failure. *Am. Heart J.,* **90**:346, September, 1975.

Harvengt, C., and Desager, J.-P.: Colestipol in familial type II hyperlipoproteinemia: a three-year trial. *Clin. Pharmacol. Ther.,* **20**:310, September, 1976.

Hazzard, William R.: A pathophysiologic approach to managing hyperlipemia. *Am. Fam. Physician,* **14**:78, August, 1976.

Houser, Doris: What to do first when a patient complains of chest pains. *Nursing '76,* **6**:54, November, 1976.

Kise, Monica Swartz: Drug therapy in the treatment of angina pectoris. *Nurs. Clin. North Am.,* **11**:309, June, 1976.

Lees, Robert S., and Lees, Ann M.: Therapy of hyperlipidemias. *Postgrad. Med.,* **60**:99, September, 1976.

Levy, Robert I.: The meaning of lipid profiles. *Postgrad. Med.,* **57**:34, April, 1975.

McDonald, Charles D., Jr.: Current management of angina pectoris. *Clin. Med.,* **83:**9, April, 1976.

Pennock, Ronald S.: Optimum therapy for angina pectoris. *Am. Fam. Physician,* **14:**102, August, 1976.

Reddy, Sudhakar; Curtis, Edward I.; O'Toole, James D.; Matthews, Robert G.; Salerni, Rosemarie; Leon, Donald F.; and Shaver, James A.: Reversibility of left ventricular asynergy by nitroglycerin in coronary artery disease. *Am. Heart J.,* **90:**479, October, 1975.

Reichek, Nathaniel: Long-acting nitrates in the treatment of angina pectoris. *J.A.M.A.,* **236:**1399, September 20, 1976.

Ross, Russell, and Laurence, Harker: Hyperlipidemia and atherosclerosis. *Science,* **193:**1094, September 17, 1976.

Shakir, K. M. Mohamed, and Margolis, Simeon: Hyperlipoproteinemia. *Primary Care,* **3:**277, June, 1976.

Taggart, Eleanor: The physical assessment of the patient with arterial disease. *Nurs. Clin. North Am.,* **12:**109, March, 1977.

Walton, Christine, and Hammond, Betsy: Angina: teaching your patient how to prevent recurrent attacks. *Nursing '78,* **8:**32, February, 1978.

Warren, Venkat, and Goldberg, Emanuel: Intractable angina pectoris. *J.A.M.A.,* **235:**841, February 23, 1976.

Winsor, Travis, and Berger, Harvey J.: Oral nitroglycerin as a prophylactic antianginal drug: clinical, physiologic, and statistical evidence of efficacy based on a three-phase experimental design. *Am. Heart J.,* **90:**611, November, 1975.

Yeshurun, D., and Gotto, A. M., Jr.: Drug treatment of hyperlipidemia. *Am. J. Med.,* **60:**379, March, 1976.

Zelis, Robert; Liedtke, James A.; Leaman, David M.; Babb, Joseph D.; and Roberts, Barbara H.: Angina pectoris: diagnosis and treatment. *Postgrad. Med.,* **59:**179, May, 1976.

11

Red Blood Cell Deficiency

A relatively well-balanced diet supplies the basic materials (i.e., amino acids, minerals, vitamins) that are required for red blood cell building or *erythropoiesis*. Nutritional anemia is a common health problem associated with a disproportion between the supply of nutrients and the additional requirements for nutrients during normal periods of accelerated erythropoiesis in the human life-cycle. Hereditary factors, disease processes, or drugs that cause bleeding or affect the bioavailability of nutrients also can cause a deficiency in the quantity of circulating red blood cells.

Physiologic Correlations

Erythropoiesis

Red blood cell development takes place primarily in the red bone marrow. Rapid cell division and synthesis of hemoglobin characterize the development of *erythroblasts* from *hemocytoblasts* during the earliest phases of red blood cell development (Fig. 11–1). The gradual maturation of the cells leads to development of anucleate *reticulocytes* or *normoblasts* that rapidly synthesize hemoglobin. In the natural replacement continuum, the red blood cell maturation may circumvent reticulocyte production and proceed by developing normoblasts from the erythroblasts. Reticulocyte production is higher when renal release of *erythropoietin* stimulates development of red blood cells in the bone marrow. At the time of their release in the vasculature, the *mature erythrocytes* are hemoglobin-laden biconcave discs capable of transporting oxygen to body tissues.

Nutrient Requirements

Building of a red blood cell framework, or stroma, capable of surviving 120 days of inching through minute capillaries is dependent on the availability of amino acids, minerals (i.e., copper), and vitamins. The principal vitamins involved in construction of the stroma are folic acid and vitamin B$_{12}$.

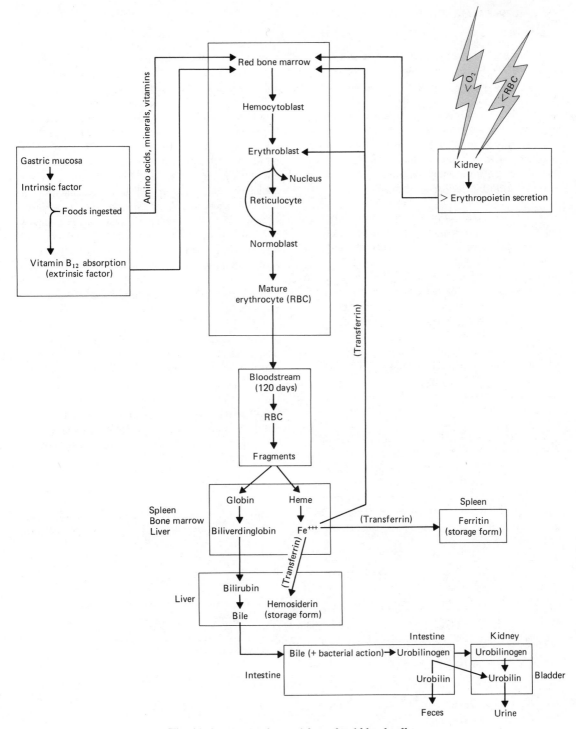

Fig. 11–1. Production and fate of red blood cells.

Folic Acid Utilization. Folic acid is available in many foods (i.e., liver, kidneys, yeast, leafy green vegetables). The folate *polyglutamates* from food sources are enzymatically hydrolyzed in the intestinal tract to *monoglutamates,* which are readily absorbed from the intestine. The folates are methylated in the liver, and the transport and storage form (5-methyl-tetrahydrofolic acid) travels to the bone marrow to supply the necessary building blocks for erythropoiesis.

Vitamin B_{12} Utilization. Food sources provide vitamin B_{12} in a coenzyme, protein-bound form. The action of gastric acid and proteolytic enzymes frees the vitamin from the protein bond. The vitamin attaches to the glycoprotein known as *intrinsic factor* that is secreted by the gastric mucosa. The glycoprotein–vitamin B_{12} complex travels readily through the intestine to receptors in the wall of the lower ileum. During a short period of receptor attachment, the vitamin is absorbed. Vitamin B_{12} travels to the body tissues (i.e., nerves) and to the bone marrow where it functions with other components to build the red blood cell stroma.

Iron Utilization. Dietary iron is taken up by the body in direct proportion to the need for replenishment of stored iron or for the production of red blood cells. Ten percent of the daily dietary intake of iron is absorbed in healthy adults, and that amount may be doubled in growing children. Plasma iron is firmly bound to the *transferrin* that carries it to the bone marrow for synthesis of hemoglobin or to the storage sites in the liver and spleen (Fig. 11–1).

The total body iron content of the adult is 3 to 5 gm, and one half of that amount is in the circulating hemoglobin. Approximately 27 percent of the total body iron content is in the bone marrow or in the storage forms *hemosiderin* in the liver and *ferritin* in the spleen. The remainder of the iron is in the functional units of skeletal muscle (16 percent) or in the myohemoglobin of striated muscles (5 to 7 percent). Because of the quantity of stored iron in the body, as little as 1 mg of dietary iron each day can maintain balance in healthy persons.

Iron Recycling. The anucleate erythrocytes are incapable of repair or reproduction. After about 120 days of travel in the circulation, the plasma membrane of the cell ruptures and the fragments spill into the bloodstream. The body is frugal with iron supplies, and the iron content of disintegrated red blood cells is recycled (Fig. 11–1). Although some iron travels with bile into the intestine, most of the mineral is returned to the liver during enterohepatic recycling of the bile. Only minute amounts of iron are lost in the feces or urine.

Hematologic Status Evaluation

Analysis of the structure of the erythrocytes and their number in relation to the quantity of

Table 11–1.

Normal Erythrocytes and Iron Values in Adults

	Males	Females
Blood		
Erythrocyte count	4.6–6.2 million/cu mm	4.2–5.4 million/cu mm
Hemoglobin (Hb)	14–18 gm/100 ml	12–16 gm/100 ml
Hematocrit (Hct)	40–54 ml/100 ml	35–47 ml/100 ml
Plasma		
Iron	50–140 mg/ml	Same
Total iron-binding capacity	250–380 mg/ml	Same
Transferrin saturation	35–40%	Same

circulating plasma provides a base line for determining the hematologic status of the individual. The term *normocytic* is employed to describe the normal size of the mature red blood cell in the circulation at the end of the maturation process. The number of red blood cells in the circulation is reflected by the erythrocyte count. The normal number of erythrocytes in the blood differs slightly between adult males and females (Table 11–1).

The color that is provided by the normal inclusion of hemoglobin (Hb) in erythrocytes is described as *normochromic* and the hemoglobin level can be colorimetrically measured to determine the quantity present in the red blood cells. The normal level of hemoglobin content of the erythrocytes is slightly lower in adult females than in adult males. The hematocrit (Hct) level reflects the ratio of the volume of packed red blood cells in a volume of plasma, and it allows definition of the adequacy of the circulating blood volume.

Pathophysiologic Correlations

A deficiency of erythrocytes can result from any factor that causes losses of large quantities of blood from the circulation. Transfusions of whole blood may be required when bleeding or disintegration of erythrocytes occurs as a consequence of accidental injury, disease processes (i.e., cancer, hemophilia), drug-induced hemolysis, or genetic abnormalities in cell structure (i.e., sickle cells).

Chronic health problems (i.e., bleeding hemorrhoids, gastritis, gingivitis) may cause asymptomatic or "silent" losses of small quantities of erythrocytes and reduce the number of circulating red blood cells. The health status of the individual is dependent on the ability of the hematopoietic system to compensate for the blood losses.

There is a growing concern among health professionals about the persistence of the widespread problem of iron-deficiency anemia associated with inadequate intake of iron-containing foods. It has been estimated that 95 percent of all preschool children and women of childbearing age have iron intakes below the standards set by the Food and Nutrition Board of the National Academy of Sciences. Blacks rated markedly lower than whites on tests of hemoglobin and hematocrit levels.

Iron-Deficiency Anemia

Low energy level and episodes of dizziness or fainting may be the first evidence of the person's anemic status. The decreased quantity and the smaller size of erythrocytes reduce the supply of oxygen-carrying hemoglobin, and body tissues gradually are deprived of the vital oxygen supply for their metabolic processes. The decrease in blood volume may cause symptomatic orthostatic hypotension.

Laboratory examination of the blood of the person with iron-deficiency anemia characteristically shows hypochromic, microcytic red blood cells. The deficiency in quantity and size of the red blood cells is reflected in a low erythrocyte count, low hematocrit level, and low hemoglobin content of the red blood cells. A biochemical analysis of plasma samples is required to confirm iron deficiency as the causative factor. In iron-deficiency anemia, the plasma iron concentration is below the normal range (Table 11–1), and the level may be as low as 5 to 40 mg/ml. The saturated and unsaturated portions of transferrin comprise the total iron-binding capacity (TIBC), and elevation of the level (i.e., 350 to 500 mg/ml) is an indication that insufficient iron is available to combine with transferrin. The amount of transferrin saturation may be considerably below the normal range (i.e., 4 to 15 percent).

Adults may seek medical attention when fatigue and decreased work performance interfere with their life-style. The effects of iron-deficiency anemia in infants or children initially may be viewed by their parents as willful behavior problems and insufficient concentration on activities to allow quiet play. Boys between four and six years old are slow in starting tasks and they are repetitive in their play. Girls at the same age level are slow in organizing their play and they have a short attention span during complex activities. The inability to concentrate in both sexes can have an adverse effect on learning ability at a time in the normal developmental pattern when acquisition of new knowledge is relatively high. Young schoolchildren who are anemic often are irritable and apathetic underachievers in school.

Chronic iron-deficiency anemia is associated with changes in varying body tissues. Soreness of the tongue, abnormal redness of the lips with cracking at the outer corners of the mouth (cheilosis), dysphagia, and dystrophy of the nails and skin are relatively common problems in the presence of long-standing anemia.

Megaloblastic Anemia

Deficiency of the vitamins required for initial red blood cell building may cause the release of large, nucleated, irregularly shaped red blood cells into the circulation. The macrocytic cells can be formed when there is a deficiency of either folic acid or vitamin B_{12}.

Deficiency of folic acid represents an insufficient intake of the vitamin in the diet. The appearance of the megaloblastic red blood cells and a serum assay that shows a low folate content are the primary factors in the diagnosis of the folic acid deficiency as the cause of the anemia.

The absence of the intrinsic factor required for vitamin B_{12} absorption from the intestine is the cause of the megaloblastic anemia associated with vitamin B_{12} deficiency. The absence of the vitamin in the serum suggests the presence of the specific hematologic problem called *pernicious anemia*. The diagnosis is made after a specific test of vitamin B_{12} absorption from the intestinal tract. The absence of radioactive vitamin B_{12} in the 24-hour specimen of urine after the person has taken the radiotagged vitamin orally indicates that none of the drug was absorbed. A subsequent test that includes administration of the vitamin with intrinsic factor leads to a normal content of the vitamin in the 24-hour specimen when the individual has pernicious anemia (Schilling test). A final test of the fasting gastric content of hydrochloric acid may be performed because there is an absence of hydrochloric acid (achlorhydria) in persons with pernicious anemia.

Specificity in diagnosis is important because folic acid administration will lead to normal red blood cell maturation, but it will not reverse the neurologic changes associated with vitamin B_{12} deficiency. Pernicious anemia is a chronic health problem requiring lifelong treatment.

The problems that occur with pernicious anemia include weakness, pallor, and lethargy. The neurologic damage that occurs in the absence of vitamin B_{12} represents a gradual progression from an inability to produce myelin to a gradual destruction of the nerve axon and the nerve head. The neurologic problems can range from uncomfortable paresthesias or incontinence to disabling unsteadiness of gait and paralysis. The prognosis is dependent on the extent of nerve damage before drug therapy is instituted.

Antianemic Drugs

ORAL IRON THERAPY

Ferrous sulfate, ferrous fumarate, ferrous gluconate, and *ferrocholinate* are the oral drugs employed for replacement of iron when the person has microcytic hypochromic red blood cells associated with a deficiency of the iron needed for hemoglobin synthesis. The drugs also are employed prophylactically during periods when deficient intake of nutrients or acceleration of growth indicates the need for supplemental iron supplies.

Therapy Considerations. The uptake of iron from the intestinal tract increases when the body content of iron is low. When the stores of iron are lowest, up to 70 percent of the drug may be absorbed. The presence of food in the gastrointestinal tract may slow absorption, so the drugs are usually administered before meals. Infants or young children initially may receive the drug with formula or food in an attempt to gradually build the tolerance of the intestinal mucosa to the drug. After the first few days of therapy, the drug gradually is given on a between-meal or formula-feeding schedule. The plan seems to decrease the incidence of gastrointestinal disturbances. Ascorbic acid can influence the absorption or utilization of iron, and it tends to reduce the gastrointestinal effects that commonly appear during iron therapy.

The primary sites of absorption of iron preparations are the stomach, duodenum, jejunum, and proximal ileum. The iron is absorbed directly into the circulating blood where it is oxidized to the ferric state. The ferric iron travels in plasma in combination with the beta-globulin *transferrin*, which carries it to the bone marrow or to storage sites in the liver and spleen.

The iron that is taken up by the bone marrow of the person with iron-deficiency anemia is rapidly utilized in hemoglobin synthesis. The iron may appear in the hemoglobin of circulating reticulocytes within four to eight hours after oral administration of the drug. The rapid inclusion of iron in hemoglobin gradually becomes slower as the hemoglobin level rises toward the normal level.

Approximately 25 mg of elemental iron content of the drug must be utilized daily to raise the hemoglobin to the desired therapeutic response of a 1 percent increase in the hemoglobin level each day. The drug dosage is planned at a level high enough to provide the 25 mg for absorption while allowing for irregularities in drug absorption.

The maximum erythropoietic response to oral iron administration is attained during the second and fourth weeks of therapy. The replenishment of body stores of iron in the liver and spleen may take 12 to 18 months beyond the time that the anemia is completely corrected. The initial dosage may be reduced to a maintenance dosage that is one third to two thirds of the original dosage level after the hemoglobin concentration returns to the normal level for the individual. The maintenance dosage usually is taken for a period of 12 months.

The patient should be informed that the iron that is not absorbed from the gastrointestinal tract will be excreted. The feces are a dark green color, which at a casual glance resembles the dark tarry feces that occur when there is a high content of digested blood. The iron content of the feces will not produce a guaiac test reaction because that test is an assay of the peroxidase activity of the hemoglobin from disintegrated red blood cells.

Solutions of iron preparations stain the teeth unless they are well diluted. Water or fruit juice can be used as a diluent, and the solution can be taken through a straw to diminish its contact with the tooth enamel. Iron elixirs are usually given from a dropper that is supplied with the bottle. When it is necessary to dilute the elixir, water is the only diluent used.

Preparations Available. The content of elemental iron in each of the products employed for therapy varies according to the type of preparation and the manufacturer of the drug (Table 11–2). The ferrous preparations are considered to be more effective and less astringent and irritating to the gastrointestinal mucosa than the ferric salts.

Ferrous sulfate (FER-IN-SOL, FEOSOL) is the least expensive of the iron preparations. It is available as capsules, sugar-coated tablets, extended-release capsules, enteric-coated tablets, elixir, and syrup. Extended-release and enteric-coated forms are used selectively because the drug may remain intact until it passes the primary sites of absorption. The drug absorption rate beyond the proximal ileum is very slow. Administration of the drug with meals or after meals may be preferable to the use of the slow-release forms for individuals having problems with nausea. Sixty milligrams (20 percent) of a 300-mg tablet of ferrous sulfate is in the form of elemental iron. The oral solutions of ferrous sulfate facilitate the administration of the drug to children and to adults who are unable to swallow tablets.

Ferrous sulfate dosage may initially be low, and dosage increments may be made gradually after

Table 11–2.
Daily Dosage of Oral Iron Preparations

	Ferrocholinate	Ferrous Fumarate	Ferrous Gluconate	Ferrous Sulfate
Adults	990 mg	600–800 mg	600–1800 mg	300–1500 mg
Children 6 to 12 years old	990 mg	100–300 mg	300–900 mg	120–600 mg
Children under 6 years old	104 mg	100–300 mg	100–300 mg	120–300 mg
Ferrous iron content	12%	33%	11.5%	20%

four to five days in an attempt to avoid the adverse effects of the drug. The dosage of ferrous sulfate for premature infants and poorly developed infants is calculated on the basis of 3 to 6 mg/day when the drug is used prophylactically. Children under six years old usually receive 300 mg of ferrous sulfate daily. The dosage for children 6 to 12 years old and pregnant women is twice that amount (600 mg/day). Adults usually receive the daily dosage (Table 11–2) in three divided doses.

Ferrous fumarate (IRCON, TOLERON) contains 33 percent ferrous iron. The drug sometimes is better tolerated than other ferrous salts. Ferrous fumarate is available in tablets, chewable tablets, and extended-release tablets. The daily oral dose (Table 11–2) is divided into three or four doses taken before meals.

Ferrous gluconate (FERGON) contains 11.5 percent ferrous iron. It often is employed for persons having gastrointestinal symptoms when taking ferrous sulfate. It is available as capsules, tablets, or liquid. Infants and children under six years old usually receive 100 to 300 mg of ferrous gluconate daily. Children between the ages of 6 and 12 and pregnant women receive 300 to 900 mg daily. The daily oral dosage (Table 11–2) usually is divided into one to four doses.

Ferrocholinate (CHEL-IRON, FERROLIP) contains 12 percent ferrous iron. The drug often is better tolerated than either ferrous gluconate or ferrous sulfate. Ferrocholinate is available as a liquid, syrup, or tablets. Infants or children under six years old usually receive 104 mg of ferrocholinate daily. Adults and children over six years old receive 990 mg of ferrocholinate daily, and the drug is given three times a day before meals.

Adverse Effects. Gastric irritation is the most frequent problem occurring with the use of the oral iron preparations. Mild nausea, diarrhea, or constipation frequently occurs at initiation of therapy, but the problems sometimes subside as therapy continues. Patients occasionally complain of abdominal cramps and the discomfort may be persistent enough to require changing to a different, better-tolerated product.

Interactions. Concurrent administration of gastric antacids to the individual receiving an iron preparation may raise the pH of the stomach and duodenal contents. The decrease in acidity can interfere with absorption of the iron at those sites.

Concurrent administration of tetracycline with iron preparations interferes with absorption of either drug. Separation of the times for drug administration, to allow use of tetracycline two to three hours before the iron preparation is given, protects against the drug interaction.

PARENTERAL IRON THERAPY

Iron dextran injection and *iron sorbitex* are the two forms of iron available for parenteral administration. Use of the injectable forms is planned only when the individual is unable to take drugs orally or when gastrointestinal pathology precludes oral drug administration. Either iron dextran or iron sorbitex may be administered intramuscularly but only iron dextran can be administered intravenously.

The total parenteral dosage of elemental iron is calculated on the basis of the person's iron-deficiency level and the body weight. The calculated total dosage is given over a carefully scheduled time period. The cautious dosage calculation is essential because there is no normal physiologic mechanism for elimination of the excess systemic iron content. The iron exceeding the amount required for hemoglobin synthesis or storage will be deposited in body tissues for long periods of time.

Intramuscular injection of the iron preparations causes staining of the tissues unless precautions are taken to avoid the leakage of the iron back through the injection tract. A preliminary step is to place a new 19- or 20-gauge needle on the syringe after the drug is withdrawn from the ampule. At the time of injection the "Z tract" technique is employed. The subcutaneous tissues are firmly pushed aside before the needle is inserted. The drug is injected deeply into the gluteal muscle at the upper outer quadrant. When the needle is removed and the pressure on the tissues is released, the return of the tissues to their natural position occludes the injection tract. A scheme for alternating the sites for each injection also can prevent tissue staining.

Iron Dextran. Iron dextran (IMFERON) is a ferric hydroxide–dextran complex that contains 50 mg of elemental iron per milliliter. Although the drug can be given by the intramuscular or the intravenous route, it rarely is administered intravenously.

The drug is absorbed from the intramuscular injection site over a period of approximately three weeks. Absorption takes place in two fairly distinct phases, which involve absorption into the lymphatic system. Sixty percent of the drug is absorbed during the first three days when the local tissue inflammation accelerates lymphatic removal of the drug from the injection site. Most of the remaining drug is more slowly absorbed by phagocytosis over the following one to three weeks. The process moves the drug to the lymphatic system and gradually it enters the bloodstream to be delivered to hematopoietic tissues. The iron is incorporated into hemoglobin or stored in the liver and spleen to replace iron reserves.

Intravenous administration of iron dextran leads to the incorporation of the iron into the

hemoglobin of reticulocytes at approximately the fourth day after administration. The maximum effect on hemoglobin synthesis is evident by the tenth day. The hemoglobin level may rise 1.5 to 2.2 gm/ml during this time period. The rate of rise in the hemoglobin level then slows to about half that initially present until it reaches the normal level for the individual.

Adverse effects are infrequent, but some of the problems are persistent and severe. Intramuscular injection can cause pain and severe inflammation at the injection site. Staining of the skin can persist for years after the injection. Intravenous administration can cause phlebitis, venospasm, and pain along the course of the vein.

Hypotension, arthralgias, lymphadenitis, and allergic reactions (i.e., fever, urticaria, anaphylaxis) have occurred after injection of iron dextran. The occurrence of allergic reactions has led to the use of an initial test dose while the person is under close supervision. The dosage of 25 mg is given by the route being employed for administration of the drug (IM, IV), and the individual is observed for evidence of an allergic response. Therapy is started if there is no reaction to the test dose of iron dextran.

The intramuscular injections for adults usually are from 1 to 4 ml of iron dextran daily. The usual dose of 2 ml provides 100 mg of elemental iron, and the injections are continued daily until the calculated total dosage of elemental iron has been given.

Iron Sorbitex. Iron sorbitex (JECTOFER) provides 50 mg of elemental iron in each milliliter of drug. The intramuscular dosage of the drug is rapidly absorbed from the injection site, and approximately 95 percent of the drug is absorbed at the end of a 24-hour period. The absorbed drug enters the bloodstream and the lymphatic system. Peak serum levels are attained within two hours after the injection, and bone marrow uptake of the drug occurs within 24 to 48 hours. The quantity of iron that is utilized varies with the level of iron deficiency, and there can be as high as a 66 percent utilization of the iron for hemoglobin synthesis when there is a severe iron deficiency.

The iron is stored primarily in the liver and spleen, but some of the iron also is stored in the intestinal, pulmonary, and renal tissues.

Thirty percent of the injected drug is excreted in the urine within 24 hours after the injection. The presence of the drug in the urine may turn the urine black when it is allowed to stand exposed to air and light.

Adverse effects include nausea, vomiting, flushing of the face, headache, diarrhea, and a transient alteration in taste perception. The drug solution has a pH 7.2 to 7.9 and it may cause pain at the site of injection. Large dosages of the drug (i.e., 200 mg) seldom are administered because the high dosage can cause malaise, muscle cramps, temperature elevation, sweating, palpitations, precordial pressure sensations, and hypotension. The problems usually occur one-half to two hours after the drug is administered but they generally subside in a few hours.

Iron sorbitex usually is administered intramuscularly once each day until the maximum calculated dosage has been given. Single-incident administration may be planned on the basis of 1.5 mg/kg of body weight.

FOLIC ACID THERAPY

Action Mode. *Folic acid* is a B complex vitamin that is employed for therapy of megaloblastic anemia occurring as a consequence of deficiency of the vitamin. Folic acid is essential for the biosynthesis of nucleic acids during the early phases of erythrocyte maturation.

Therapy Considerations. The oral drug is enzymatically hydrolyzed to folate monoglutamate, which is absorbed rapidly from the proximal portion of the small intestine. Liver methylation changes the drug to the active tetrahydrofolic acid, which is the transport and storage form of the vitamin. Tetrahydrofolic acid is widely distributed in all body tissues and approximately 50 percent of it is stored in the liver tissues.

Excess drug is excreted in the urine unchanged, and up to 50 percent of an oral dose exceeding 2.5 mg may be lost in the urine. The drug also is found in the milk of lactating mothers.

Within the first 24 hours after administration of the drug, the person experiences a feeling of well-being. The bone marrow maturation of normal red blood cells is apparent within 48 hours after initiation of drug therapy. Production of reticulocytes is rapid after two to five days of therapy. The serum folate levels gradually rise from the low level commonly associated with megaloblastic anemia (<0.002 mcg/ml) to the normal serum folate level (0.005 to 0.015 mcg/ml).

The initial oral dose for adults and children is 0.25 to 1 mg daily. The dosage for pregnant women and lactating mothers may be at the higher level of the dosage range to prevent megaloblastic anemia and the associated damage to the fetus during the last trimester of pregnancy. Infants may receive 100 mcg daily and children under four years old may receive 300 mcg/day. Adults and children over four years old usually receive 400 mcg of folic acid daily.

Preparations Available. *Folic acid* (FOLVITE) is available as tablets for oral administration or as sodium folate in solution for intramuscular or intravenous use. The high pH (8 to 10) makes it necessary to inject the drug deeply into the tissues when the solution is administered intramuscularly. Folic acid is administered orally unless there is pathology of the gastrointestinal tract that could interfere with absorption.

Adverse Effects. Folic acid is relatively nontoxic. There have been allergic reactions during therapy (i.e., skin rash, itching, general malaise, bronchospasm) but the incidence of the side effects has been rare.

Interactions. Administration of folic acid to patients who concurrently are receiving phenytoin may accelerate the metabolism of the anticonvulsant. The low phenytoin levels can interefere with seizure control.

Leucovorin is the *formyl* derivative and the active form of folic acid. Any of the drugs that are folic acid antagonists (i.e., methotrexate, pyrimethamine, trimethoprim) can cause toxic effects that affect red blood cell maturation, and leucovorin could be used to diminish or counteract the toxic effects of those drugs. Leucovorin is employed primarily to maintain the natural erythropoietic maturation process during therapy with antineoplastic drugs (i.e., methotrexate).

The term *leucovorin rescue* has been popularized to describe the use of the drug in cancer therapy. The drug enters normal cells and "rescues" them from the toxic effects of the folic acid antagonist that is concurrently being employed for cancer therapy. The preferential inclusion in normal cells rather than into tumor cells occurs because there is a difference in membrane transport mechanisms between the two types of cells.

The drug is administered intramuscularly 6 to 36 hours after the infusion of the antineoplastic drug. The dosage administered is based on the protocol established for treatment of the particular patient with cancer.

Leucovorin also is employed when an inadvertent large dosage of a folic acid antagonist (i.e., methotrexate) has caused toxic blood levels. The antidote dosage of leucovorin is based on the calculation of an equal weight to that of the toxic dose of the drug. The best "rescue" occurs when the leucovorin is given within one hour of the overdose. The measure usually is ineffective when it is delayed for more than four hours.

VITAMIN B₁₂ THERAPY

Vitamin B₁₂ with intrinsic factor, cyanocobalamin, and *hydroxocobalamin* are the drugs primarily employed for reversal of the megaloblastic red blood cell formation characteristic of pernicious anemia. Vitamin B₁₂ also is a constituent of many vitamin formulations used for prophylaxis or treatment of nutritional deficiencies.

Crude liver extract, which contains 2 mcg of cyanocobalamin activity in each milliliter, and liver extract, which contains 20 mcg/ml, were administered parenterally for many years for the treatment of patients with pernicious anemia. In recent years, use of the liver products has become obsolete because the synthetic vitamin preparations provide a more controllable quantity of the vitamin. The incidence of hypersensitivity reactions also was relatively high when the liver extracts were employed for therapy.

Vitamin B₁₂ with Intrinsic Factor

The addition of intrinsic factor to vitamin B₁₂ or cobalamin provides the glycoprotein required for absorption of the vitamin from the intestinal tract. Without the addition of intrinsic factor, patients with pernicious anemia could not respond to oral vitamin therapy.

One oral unit of the drug combination provides 15 mcg of cyanocobalamin activity with 300 mg of intrinsic factor concentrate. The drug travels to the receptors in the wall of the lower ileum where the vitamin is absorbed into the blood. Vitamin B₁₂ is rapidly bound to the beta-globulin *transcobalamin I* in the plasma. Although the oral drug could be ideal in treatment of pernicious anemia, 50 percent of the patients develop intestinal antibodies to the intrinsic factor and become refractory to the oral therapy. Parenteral therapy with vitamin B₁₂ avoids that problem.

Vitamin B₁₂

Cyanocobalamin and *hydroxocobalamin* are synthetic injectable forms of vitamin B₁₂, commonly employed for treatment of pernicious anemia. Hydroxocobalamin may be employed for initial therapy because it produces a sustained serum cobalamin level. Cyanocobalamin is the drug form that usually is used for long-term therapy.

Action Mode. The drugs provide the vitamin B₁₂ required as a coenzyme in the production of nucleic acids for the maturation of red blood cells. The coenzyme also is required for the regeneration of tetrahydrofolate from its inactive storage form. In the presence of vitamin B₁₂, nucleic acids and tetrahydrofolate are available for maturation of normal red blood cells.

Therapy Considerations. The administration of vitamin B_{12} gradually raises the serum level of cobalamin from the low level that is associated with megaloblastic anemia and neural damage (100 pg/ml) to the normal serum range for the vitamin (200 to 900 pg/ml). Improvement in the hematologic status of the person is evident in the feeling of wellness that is present within 24 hours after the initiation of therapy. The bone marrow begins to produce normocytic cells within 48 hours. There is an increase in the production of reticulocytes within two to five days after therapy is initiated. Drug therapy also arrests the progress of nerve deterioration. The extent of neurologic improvement depends on the amount of nerve damage present at initiation of therapy, but there usually is a decrease in paresthesias and tingling sensations in the periphery.

Most of the injected drug travels to the liver where it is converted to the coenzyme, and most of the drug (50 to 90 percent) is stored in the liver. Small amounts are distributed in varying body tissues. Approximately 95 percent of an injected dose of the vitamin is retained in the body. When the drug is administered in amounts exceeding the binding capacity of the plasma, liver, and other body tissues, the excess free vitamin B_{12} is excreted in the urine.

Preparations Available. *Cyanocobalamin* (BE-TALIN 12 CRYSTALLINE, REDISOL, RUBRAMIN PC, RUVITE, SYTOBEX) and *hydroxocobalamin* (AL-PHAREDISOL, NEO-BETALIN 12, SYTOBEX-H) are available in forms for subcutaneous or intramuscular injection. The drugs have a similar vitamin B_{12} activity and the dosage is similar for both drugs. The quantity and frequency of drug administration is planned to raise and maintain the erythrocyte count above 4.5 million/mm³. The dosage for adults is 30 mcg for five to ten days, and the injection may be given subcutaneously or intramuscularly. A maintenance dosage of 100 to 200 mcg usually is administered intramuscularly at monthly intervals. Lifelong therapy is required to prevent neurologic damage, and persons with pernicious anemia may need help to see the need for treatment as their general health improves.

Adverse Effects. The vitamin preparations are considered nontoxic even when administered in large doses. Mild transient diarrhea may occur. There have been some instances of peripheral vascular thrombosis, itching, transitory exanthema, urticaria, and anaphylaxis. An intradermal sensitivity test may be done before initiation of therapy if the person has a history of allergy. In severe megaloblastic anemia, intensive therapy with the vitamin may cause hypokalemia, and potassium replacement may be required.

NURSING INTERVENTION

Assessment and Counseling

Iron-deficiency anemia is a persistent public health problem that is present in individuals from all socioeconomic groups. Nurses can be instrumental in alleviating the problem by counseling individuals about the periods in their normal life-cycle when there is an elevation in the requirements for iron intake. Individuals may respond more readily when they are given specific information about the reality of the problem and its relevance to their health maintenance. In many instances the intake of iron-rich foods or use of an easily absorbed iron preparation may prevent iron-deficiency anemia. The counseling by the nurse can be based on the predictable requirements for iron at varying stages of the normal growth and development continuum.

Comparison of the changing iron requirements with the iron needs of the normal nonanemic adult can facilitate communication of information about iron requirements. As little as 1 mg of iron may be absorbed from the nutrients available in the gastrointestinal tract during a 24-hour period. The iron replacement is directly related to the total body iron content. Iron losses through excretion are minimal and only the amount that is lost each day is absorbed for replacement. The ordinary diet readily provides a sufficient amount of iron (1 to 16 mg daily) to allow absorption of the amount that is required each day by the healthy adult.

Cyclic Changes in Iron Requirements. Numerous pregnant women of all socioeconomic and ethnic groups have an insufficient dietary intake to meet the normal nutrient demands of pregnancy and the nutrient requirements of the unborn child. Dietary improvement and supplements of folate and iron in expectant mothers may decrease the incidence of pregnancy anemia. Improving the mother's nutritional status also can reduce the high incidence of low-birth-weight babies. During pregnancy the body requirements for iron increase to approximately 17 to 37.5 mg/day. The blood profiles of mothers immediately predelivery often show lower iron values than is usual for adult women. The lower values reflect the depletion of iron stores by the demands of a normal pregnancy.

Most iron reserves are obtained by the fetus during the last two months of gestation. Before birth the fetus takes what it needs from the nutrient stores of the mother. The fetus is quite efficient in acquiring an adequate supply of iron even if the mother's blood is iron deficient.

Premature infants may be iron deficient because of an insufficient iron reserve gathered from the mother before their early birth. The premature infant has a more rapid growth rate than an infant born at term. The fragile hematologic status of the premature infant makes it necessary to supply elemental iron regularly. The premature infant's blood is so precious and well guarded that an exact record of the amount of blood that is lost with the removal of samples for laboratory tests is recorded on the infant's clinical record.

The full-term infant's hemoglobin level ranges from 14 to 22 gm/100 ml at the time of birth. The mechanism for regulating erythropoiesis does not function fully for some time after birth and the number of circulating red blood cells gradually declines. More red blood cells die than can be replaced. The striking increase of plasma ferritin levels that begins immediately after birth reflects the recycling of iron from the catabolism of erythrocytes. The infant is considered anemic when the hemoglobin concentration falls below 11 gm/100 ml and the hematocrit is less than 33 percent.

Production of new red blood cells by the bone marrow is insignificant until about two months of age when growth becomes rapid. As the vascular volume increases, the hemoglobin mass is diluted. The growth of muscle requires an increased quantity of iron for myoglobin formation. The need for iron is great when the infant is two months old, and the requirements remain high throughout the first year of the infant's life. The rapid growth raises the iron requirements of the infant to 1.5 mg/kg/day.

There are limited natural sources of iron for the infant under one year of age. The addition of ferrous sulfate to cereals during their manufacture would provide an ideal method of supplying infants with iron, but ferrous sulfate is a pro-oxidant that readily converts fatty acids in the cereals to organic acids. The cereal becomes rancid within a short period of time. Commercially available cereals are fortified with organic iron salts and they contain iron (0.6 to 22 mg iron per dry ounce), but the bioavailability of the organic iron is low. Less than 1 percent of the iron from the fortified cereals is absorbed.

Cow's milk supplies only 0.5 mg of iron per liter and that is insufficient to supply the iron requirements of the growing infant. The best source of the mineral is the iron-containing commercial formulas that offer easily absorbed ferrous sulfate. The formulas can supply the vital mineral to infants under 12 months old. Nursing infants require supplemental iron.

Preschool children consume limited quantities of iron-containing foods (i.e., meat, eggs). Iron-deficiency anemia is still rampant in children one to three years of age. Supplemental iron may be required during the entire period of childhood growth. The continual expansion of the blood volume requires a proportionate increase in iron for hemoglobin synthesis.

The normally menstruating woman loses from 10 to 60 ml of blood every month. The monthly physiologic loss of iron is about 20 mg. The loss of iron may require absorption of approximately one additional milligram of iron daily.

The rapid growth and muscular development of the adolescent male may periodically raise the daily iron requirements to a high level (1.5 to 23 mg/day). Ingestion of foods seldom is a problem in teen-age males, but it is necessary to direct their attention to the advisability of increasing the intake of iron-rich foods as substitutes for some of their carbohydrate favorites.

The elderly present more complex problems in analyzing iron requirements. Individuals who are living on a marginal income may have a poor nutritional intake. Perhaps the most meaningful approach to assisting the elderly to maintain their hematologic status is to advise them to have a regular annual physical examination. Asymptomatic blood loss is one of the major contributors to the anemic status of the older age group.

The predictable cyclic changes that occur in the growth and development patterns can be employed as a base line for discussion of individual nutritive needs. It is particularly important to counsel parents about the inclusion of iron-rich foods or the use of iron supplements during the early childhood period when iron requirements are high. Correction of deficiencies at that time may change the statistical incidence of iron-deficiency anemia.

Review Guides

1. Outline the factors that would be considered when assessing the iron requirements of members of a three-generation household.
2. Outline the factors that would be included in a response to the inquiry about the use of an oral concentrated vitamin preparation from a person with pernicious anemia.
3. Formulate a plan for instructing the mother of a young child about the administration of an oral iron preparation and the effects of the therapy.
4. Describe the method, employed for intramuscular administration of parenteral iron preparations and the rationale for use of the procedure.
5. Describe the predictable effects of administration of iron, folic acid, and vitamin B_{12} preparations on the maturation of erythrocytes. Include the specific changes in the hematologic status in the description.

Additional Readings

Beutler, Ernest: Genetic disorders of human red blood cells. *J.A.M.A.*, **233:**1184, September 15, 1975.

Brophy, Michael, H., and Süteri, Pentti K.: Pyridoxal phosphate and hypertensive disorders of pregnancy. *Am. J. Obstet. Gynecol.*, **121:**1075, April 15, 1975.

Cerami, Anthony, and Peterson, Charles M.: Cyanate and sickle-cell disease. *Sci. Am.*, **232:**45, April, 1975.

Crosby, William H.: Pica. *J.A.M.A.*, **235:**2765, June 21, 1976.

Erbe, Robert W.: Inborn errors of folate metabolism. *N. Engl. J. Med.*, **293:**part I, p. 753, October 9, 1975; part II, p. 807, October 16, 1975.

Garratty, George, and Petz, Lawrence D.: Drug-induced immune hemolytic anemia. *Am. J. Med.*, **58:**398, March, 1975.

Haut, Arthur: Iron deficiency anemia. *Am. Fam. Physician*, **11:**136, April, 1975.

Herbert, Victor; Colman, Neville; Spivack, Morton; Ocasio, Edgar; Ghanta, Vijava; Kimmel, Kenneth; Brenner, Lois; Freundlich, Joanne; and Scott, John:

Folic acid deficiency in the United States: folate assays in a prenatal clinic. *Am. J. Obstet. Gynecol.,* **123:**175, September 15, 1975.

Iyengar, Leela, and Rajalakshmi, K.: Effect of folic acid supplement on birth weights of infants. *Am. J. Obstet. Gynecol.,* **122:**332, June 1, 1975.

Jacobs, A.; Path, F. R. C.; and Worwood, M.: Medical progress: ferritin in serum: clinical and biochemical implications. *N. Engl. J. Med.,* **292:**951, May 1, 1975.

McFarlane, Judith M.: Everyday care of the child with sickle cell anemia. *Pediatr. Nurs.,* **2:**9, January–February, 1976.

Muss, Hyman B., and White, Douglas R.: Iron deficiency anemia in adults. *Am. Fam. Physician,* **17:** 174, February, 1978.

Orkin, Stuart H., and Nathan, David G.: Current concepts: the thalassemias. *N. Engl. J. Med.,* **295:**710, September 23, 1976.

Oski, Frank A.: Anemia in children. *Hosp. Pract.,* **11:**63, December, 1976.

Provisor, Arthur J.: Childhood anemia. *Am. Fam. Physician,* **14:**124, October, 1976.

Rios, Ernesto; Lipschitz, David A.; Cook, James D.; and Smith, Nathan J.: Relationship of maternal and infant iron stores as assessed by determination of plasma ferritin. *Pediatrics,* **55:**694, May, 1975.

Scrimshaw, Nevin S., and Young, Vernon R.: The requirements of human nutrition. *Sci. Am.,* **235:**50, September, 1976.

Sesso, Anna M., and Silverio, John: Facts and opinion: iron deficiency anemia: how long must it be with us? *J. Gynecol. Nurs.,* **4:**37, January–February, 1975.

Shaninpour, Nayereh: The adult patient with bleeding esophageal varices. *Nurs. Clin. North Am.,* **12:**331, June, 1977.

Smith, David W. E.: Reticulocyte transfer RNA and hemoglobin synthesis. *Science,* **190:**529, November 7, 1975.

12

Vascular Thrombosis and Clotting Problems

The deep veins of the legs and pelvis are common sites of venous thrombosis in hospitalized patients. Early ambulation of patients after surgical procedures and passive or active leg exercises for those patients who are confined to bed have somewhat decreased the incidence of venous thrombosis.

Eighty-five percent of the emboli in the pul-monary circulation arise from thrombosis in one of the veins in the lower extremities. It is estimated that peripheral venous thrombosis that causes acute pulmonary embolism occurs in 500,000 hospitalized patients each year in the United States. Approximately 10 to 20 percent of those episodes are terminal events.

Physiologic Correlations

Clotting of blood at the site of injury to a blood vessel (i.e., intravenous needle injection site) is a physiologic protective mechanism that maintains the integrity of the vasculature. The coagulation process involves a series of complex interactions between the clotting factors that precipitate fibrin clot formation. Specific numerical designations for the clotting factors have been recommended by the International Committee on Nomenclature of Blood Clotting Factors in an attempt to estab-lish a common language in discussions of the coagulation process (Table 12–1).

Tissue injury initiates the coagulation processes through an *extrinsic pathway* and an *intrinsic pathway* that lead to clot formation (Fig. 12–1). Tissue injury initially mobilizes the clotting factors of the extrinsic pathway and a blood clot may be formed within 15 seconds. Although all the factors required for blood coagulation are present in the blood, the secondary response, which is

Table 12–1.

Blood Clotting Nomenclature

Factor*	Common Synonyms
I	Fibrinogen
II	Prothrombin
III	Thromboplastin
IV	Calcium
V	Plasma prothrombin converting factor, proaccelerin
VII	Proconvertin
VIII	Antihemophilic factor A, platelet cofactor I
IX	Plasma thromboplastin component, Christmas factor, antihemophilic factor B
X	Stuart factor
XI	Plasma thromboplastin antecedent, antihemophilic factor C
XII	Hageman factor
XIII	Fibrin-stabilizing factor, fibrinase
Platelets	Thrombocytes
Profibrinolysin	Plasminogen
Fibrinolysin	Plasmin

* Roman numeral designation recommended by the International Committee on Nomenclature of Blood Clotting Factors.

mediated through the intrinsic pathway, requires from one to three minutes to produce clotting.

Extrinsic Coagulation Pathway

Thromboplastin (factor III), which is released from the tissues at the site of vascular injury, initiates the coagulation process of the extrinsic pathway by activating *Stuart factor* (factor X). The process requires the presence of *calcium ions* (factor IV) and *proconvertin* (factor VII). The activated Stuart factor, calcium ions, and *plasma prothrombin converting factor* (factor V) are involved in the formation of the protective enzyme *thrombin*. The formation of thrombin is a key factor in the coagulation process. Thrombin converts *fibrinogen* (factor I) to the *fibrin* that forms the matrix of the clot. The presence of *fibrin-stabilizing factor* (factor XIII) causes the serum to exude from the fibrin clot and it becomes firm and insoluble.

Intrinsic Coagulation Pathway

Tissue injury activates *Hageman factor* (factor XII), which is the initial clotting factor of the intrinsic coagulation pathway. Hageman factor activates *plasma thromboplastin antecedent* (factor XI) to convert *plasma thromboplastin component* (factor IX) to an active form. The activated plasma thromboplastin component, *antihemophilic factor A* (factor VIII), phospholipid, and *calcium ion*s (factor IV) activate *Stuart factor* (factor X). The steps in the coagulation process that follow the activation of Stuart factor are similar to the processes of the extrinsic coagulation pathway (Fig. 12–1). The strong impetus to thrombin formation accelerates conversion of *fibrinogen* to *fibrin* and assures sufficient clotting to protect the integrity of the vasculature.

Clot Dissolution

Clots are temporary "plugs" at the site of tissue injury. The clot remains for a short period of time and gradually it is fragmented by the biochemical action of substances that are liberated from the tissues in a process described as *fibrinolysis*. *Profibrinolysin*, which is liberated from the tissues, activates the *fibrinolysin* that enzymatically lyses the clot (Fig. 12–1).

Vitamin K Synthesis

Vitamin K_1 is a precursor that is required for hepatic synthesis of several clotting factors (factors II, VII, IX, X). The primary source of the vitamin is the residue of vitamin K-rich foods in the intestinal tract (i.e., cabbage, cauliflower, spinach, kale, cheese, tomatoes, egg yolk, fish, liver). The foods provide the materials from which enteric bacteria synthesize the vitamin K_1 that is required for the hepatic generation of the clotting factors. An intact intestine and the presence of the bacteria are required for vitamin K_1 synthesis. The latter condition is not met by the sterile intestine of the newborn and vitamin K_1 is administered after birth to correct the deficit.

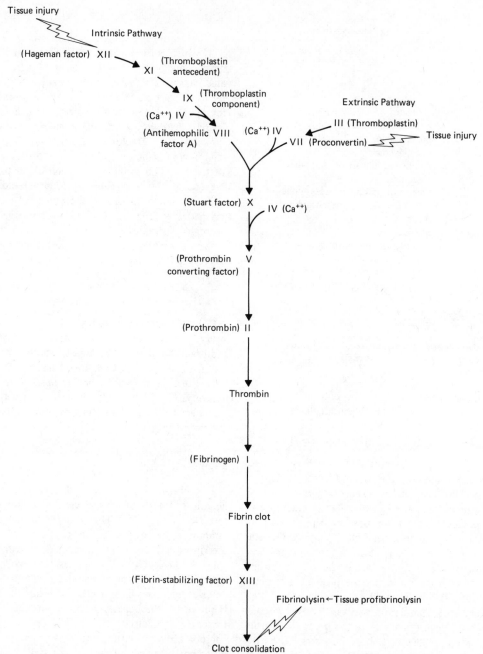

Fig. 12–1. The coagulation events lead to the generation of thrombin and fibrin formation. Release of enzymes gradually causes dissolution of the insoluble fibrin clot.

Pathophysiologic Correlations

Clotting Factor Deficits

The repetitive pattern of the extrinsic and intrinsic coagulation pathways allows clotting when some of the factors are missing. Genetic factors can cause serious defects in the intrinsic pathway in some persons. The occurrence of consequent coagulation problems depends on the clotting factor that is absent. For example, some males have a deficit of *antihemophilic factor A* (factor VIII) or *antihemophilic factor B* (factor IX). The sex-linked genetic defects of the intrinsic coagulation pathway are expressed in males. When either of the vital clotting factors is missing, spontaneous bleeding can occur with minor tissue trauma. In contrast, the absence of *antihemophilic factor C* (factor XI) or *Hageman factor* (factor XII), which are recessive traits in both males and females, causes no bleeding problems.

Vascular Thrombosis

Thrombosis can occur in either the venous or arterial circulation. The implications to the health status of the person depend on the size and location of the thrombus and its effect on blood flow to the tissues. The primary difference between venous and arterial thrombosis is related to the velocity of blood flow, which affects thrombus development and the liberation of emboli.

The endothelium of the blood vessels has a protein layer of cells that carry a negative charge. That charge tends to repel the clotting factors and the platelets. The negative charge of the endothelium is a natural antithrombolic protective property of the vasculature. A roughened area or injury to the intima of the blood vessel results in a break in the protective layer of cells. The loss of the normal negative electrical charge of the endothelium allows platelets to adhere to the cell wall.

Platelets have a stickiness that causes them to adhere to each other, and the platelets aggregate to form a localized intravascular mass. Adenosine diphosphate (ADP) that is released from the platelets is thought to be the basic factor causing the aggregation and the formation of a white permeable mass of platelets. A second phase occurs as larger amounts of ADP are released. There is a massive irreversible aggregation of platelets and an impermeable clump is formed. The platelet mass formation is independent of the coagulation process.

The release of thrombin from the platelets initiates the coagulation process. The clot that forms on the surface of the platelet clump consists of erythrocytes and leukocytes entrapped in the fibrin strands formed by the action of thrombin. The leukocytes phagocytize or ingest the platelets and within 24 hours the mass may be comprised of fibrin and platelet debris. The end result of the process is the formation of a mixed thrombus that has a white head, a red body, and a red flowing tail. The characteristics of the thrombus may vary according to the quantity of platelets, red blood cells, leukocytes, and fibrin that are present.

Venous Thrombosis. The primary cause of venous thrombosis is the stasis of blood at sites of increased pressure (i.e., the pressure on the calf veins when the patient lies supine during a long surgical procedure). A typical venous thrombus has a small white head representing the clumping of platelets at the wall site, a red body, and a long, free-flowing tail. The red thrombus has blood cells distributed at random throughout the fibrin meshwork.

The blood in the venous circulation moves at a low flow velocity. The slow blood flow allows the thrombus to increase in size by forward propagation and retrograde extension. Segments of the loosely structured red thrombus easily break off and travel through the venous circulation to the smallest vessel that resists their passage (i.e., pulmonary arterioles). The clinical implications of the embolus may be mild to severe depending on the location and the effect on hemodynamics at the tissue site.

The life-span of a venous thrombus depends on the processes of phagocytosis and fibrinolysis, which slowly dissolve the clot. During the period of clot dissolution, segments of the thrombus may break off and travel as emboli in the venous circulation.

Arterial Thrombosis. The high velocity of blood flow in the arterial circulation interferes with the building of a fibrin clot atop the clump of platelets, and the thrombus consists primarily of aggregated platelets and fibrin strands. There may be a small red body representing accumulation of a few tenacious fibrin strands and blood

cells, but the rapid blood flow sweeps away most of the activated plasma coagulation factors.

Arterial thrombi form at sites where the intimal surface is rough or where the endothelium has been denuded by surgical procedures (i.e., removal of endothelium for prosthetic heart valve insertion). The primary cause of irregularities or roughness of the endothelium is atherosclerosis. Thrombosis may occur distal to atherosclerotic elevations into the intima of the artery. The mural thrombi contribute further to intimal thickening and the decreased elasticity of the artery. An arterial thrombus may fragment and shower the circulation with platelet-fibrin emboli, but the incidence is lower than embolization from venous thrombi.

Anticoagulants

The purpose of anticoagulant therapy, when there is clinical evidence of a thrombus or embolus, is to suppress the activity of the blood coagulation sequence that propagates and extends existing clots. The anticoagulant drugs also are employed as prophylaxis when patients are at high risk of having a thromboembolic incident (i.e., prolonged immobility, previous vascular thrombosis, major orthopedic, gastrointestinal, or cardiac surgery). The drugs act at differing sites in the coagulation process to interfere with new clot formation. They do not affect the formation of the platelet clump that is the primary base of thrombi formed at the site of endothelial injury.

DRUG THERAPY

The anticoagulant drugs include *heparin*, which is administered parenterally, and a group of drugs commonly referred to as the *oral anticoagulants*. The oral drug group includes both *coumarin* and *indandione* derivatives, which have similar pharmacologic properties and clinical applications.

The anticoagulant effect of heparin is immediate; therefore, it usually is employed as initial therapy when a thrombus or embolus is present. The oral anticoagulants have a slower onset of

action, and they are commonly used as therapy subsequent to a short period of heparin therapy.

Heparin

Heparin sodium is the purified extract of the physiologic substance from *porcine intestinal mucosa* or *bovine lung tissue*. The livestock source is a primary factor in the rapidly rising cost of therapy with the drug. The source becomes important also when there is excess prolongation of the coagulation process during therapy because it requires more of the antidote (protamine sulfate) to neutralize heparin that is obtained from bovine lung tissue than that obtained from porcine intestinal mucosa.

Action Mode. Heparin has the highest negative electrostatic charge of any substance that can be safely injected into the body. Heparin binding inactivates the positively charged protein *thrombin* (Fig. 12–2). In combination with antithrombin (factor III), heparin inhibits activation of Stuart factor (factor X) and the conversion of prothrombin (factor II) to thrombin. The action of heparin on thrombin indirectly interferes with the reaction between activated plasma thromboplastin

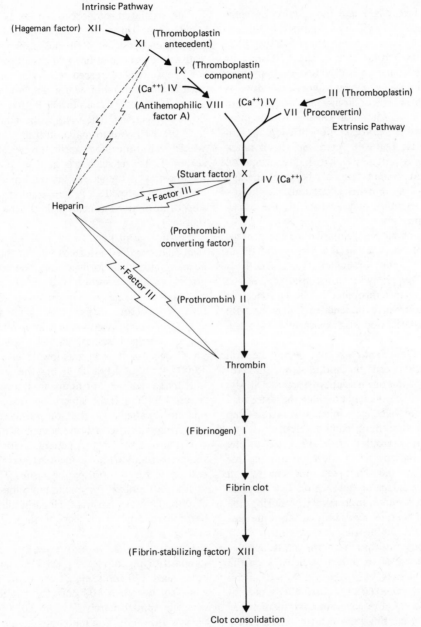

Fig. 12–2. Heparin interferes with the action of factor X, and it independently, or in union with antithrombin III, interrupts the formation of thrombin.

antecedent (factor XI) and thromboplastin component (factor IX), which is catalyzed by thrombin.

Heparin has a diuretic property that may be related to its depression of aldosterone production. The diuresis is evident when the drug is administered in large dosage to patients with edema and sodium retention. During therapy there is an increased urinary excretion of sodium chloride and water. Diuresis begins 36 to 48 hours after therapy is initiated and it may continue 48 hours beyond termination of heparin therapy when the patient remains edematous. Slight potassium ion retention may accompany the excretion of sodium ions.

Heparin is employed primarily for the prevention of clot formation distal or proximal to an established thrombus or embolus. It currently is being used frequently at low dosage levels as prophylaxis against thromboembolic episodes for selected postoperative patients and persons with evidence of arterial stenosis (i.e., carotid stenosis).

Therapy Considerations. Aqueous heparin sodium solution can be administered intravenously by injection or infusion, or subcutaneously. A repository form, which provides the drug in a gelatin-dextrose vehicle, is injected into the deep subcutaneous or intramuscular tissues.

Blood-clotting profiles are done prior to the initiation of therapy to provide a base line for therapy and to rule out preexisting coagulation problems. The effect of heparin on the coagulation process is monitored regularly during the initial days of therapy regardless of the route employed for drug administration.

The *clotting time* has been the most popular method for assay of the effect of heparin on the coagulation process, but the *activated partial thromboplastin time* (PTT) currently is considered to provide a more accurate analysis of heparin effect. The clotting-time determination represents the time required for the person's blood to form a clot in a test tube. The normal clotting time is from three to six minutes, and the aim of therapy is to prolong the clotting time from two to two and one-half times the normal range.

The partial thromboplastin time is an assessment of the thrombin generation pathway or fibrin formation. The PTT measures the intrinsic pathway of coagulation, and prolongation of the PTT represents decreased activity of those clotting factors that are required for activation of Stuart factor (factor X). The normal PTT range is from 30 to 40 seconds. The therapeutic aim is to prolong the PTT and to maintain it at a level that is within two times the normal range (60 to 80 seconds). The exact levels may vary in different laboratories as the assay methods change, but the above levels provide a general guide for comparisons of normal levels against those attained during therapy.

The dosage of heparin for prophylaxis is lower than that required after coagulation factors have been mobilized to form a clot. The prophylactic dose (i.e., after insertion of a prosthetic valve or great-vessel surgery) may be continued for the time period (four to five days) when the hazard of thromboembolic episodes is known to be greatest. The dosage is sometimes described as a "minidose" because it is at the low level of 5000 to 15,000 units of heparin. It may be administered initially as soon as four hours after surgery. There is less bleeding from superficial tissues in postoperative patients at the low dosage than that occurring with use of oral anticoagulants.

Heparin therapy for patients with a known venous thromboembolic incident may be continued up to ten days after the insult. That period of time is required for maximum adhesion of the clot to the vascular wall. Heparin therapy may be prolonged when the person must remain bedridden.

Heparin dosage is expressed in units. The standard of potency set by the USP is that there be at least 120 units/mg of the drug. A general guide for dosage is 100 units/kg of body weight, which is approximately 7500 to 10,000 units for the average adult. The initial dosage may be based on the calculation of individual requirements by weight, but subsequent dosage is based on the adequacy of anticoagulation.

Prior to initiation of therapy it is important to plan with the laboratory for obtaining the patient's blood for white blood cell count when one is prescribed. The blood sample should be taken within two hours after heparin administration because the leukocytes tend to disappear in heparinized blood.

The intravenous route is most commonly employed for administration of heparin to hospitalized patients. When the drug is administered intravenously, there is an immediate effect on coagulation. The quantitative effect on coagulation is proportional to the heparin dosage. The serum half-life of the drug is dose dependent. For example, when the drug is administered intravenously at a dosage of 100 units/kg of body weight, the serum half-life of the drug is one hour. At an intravenous dosage level of 400 units/kg the serum half-life is two and one-half hours. The difference in serum half-life provides the basic guideline for intermittent drug administration. A relatively large dosage is required to maintain suppression of coagulation factors when the drug is administered at four-to-six-hour intervals. The PTT returns to the normal range within three to four hours after the last dose of the drug is administered intravenously.

An indwelling catheter or a pediatric scalp vein needle is usually inserted and taped in place when intermittent intravenous administration of heparin is planned. The tubing has a "Y" shunt, or "heparin lock," with a rubberized cap that allows penetration by a needle at the time of drug administration. A small syringe is employed for dosage measurement to assure preparation of the exact amount of heparin. The drug (i.e., 5000 to 15,000 units every four to six hours) is injected slowly at a rate of 1 to 2 ml/minute to minimize the pain associated with venous irritation by the drug. Intermittent intravenous administration causes peaks and valleys in plasma drug levels. The PTT taken one hour after administration may be high (i.e., five times normal) while the test done one hour before the next dose may be within the therapeutic range. The blood samples for the PTT assay are taken at a precise time prior to each dose that is administered during the first few days of dosage regulation.

Heparin may be diluted for infusion with dextrose, sodium chloride, Ringer's solution, or 1/6 molar sodium lactate, but it is incompatible with most other intravenous solutions. The initial drug solution (i.e., 10,000 to 20,000 units of heparin in 1 liter of solution) is run slowly at 1 ml/minute. The anticoagulant effect of the drug is evident in two to three hours. The PTT level, which is obtained four hours after the infusion is started, provides the guide for regulation of the infusion rate to adjust the amount of drug administered. A microinfusion pump (i.e., Holter pump) is often employed to maintain the intravenous flow of heparin solution at a steady rate and to protect against inadvertent infusion of a high dose of heparin.

Intravenous infusion is more confining for the patient than intermittent injection, but it provides a more even anticoagulant drug level. The incidence of bleeding episodes is lower with the steady suppression of coagulation than it is with the less even pattern found with the intermittent intravenous injection of heparin.

Subcutaneous injection of heparin delivers the drug into the adipose tissue. There is a time lag before the drug is absorbed and the effect on coagulation becomes measurable. The initial dosage usually ranges from 10,000 to 20,000 units of heparin. One half of that amount of drug may be administered in subsequent injections that are given at eight-hour intervals. Precautions are taken to inject the drug into the adipose tissues and to avoid the local irritation, hematoma formation, and tissue slough that can occur when the drug is injected into superficial tissue layers. With the exception of a 5-cm (2-in.) circumference around the umbilicus, the abdomen provides an abundance of subcutaneous fat for the injection. The administration sites are carefully alternated to decrease the formation of tissue depots of heparin.

Most nurses employ a "bunch-the-skin" technique for administration of the drug subcutaneously. A 1.25-cm-long (0.5-in.) 26-gauge needle, which is inserted perpendicularly into a 1.25-cm (0.5-in.) roll of tissue, delivers the drug to the target tissue layer. The drug is injected without aspirating and the tip of the needle is held steady

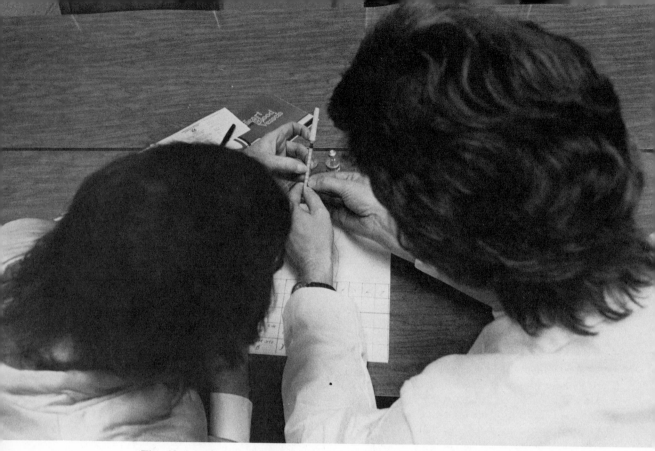

Fig. 12–3. The nurse's counseling of the patient who is to continue the use of subcutaneous heparin after the period of hospitalization should include information about the drug, safety measures that are to be used during the injection, and methods for alternating the injection sites. (Courtesy, Northeastern University College of Nursing, Boston.)

to prevent tissue trauma during the injection. After administering the drug, the needle is withdrawn while simultaneously releasing the skin fold. Light pressure for three to five minutes, without massage, after withdrawal of the needle allows observation for bleeding from the injection site. The use of ice in a plastic glove for a five-minute period both before and after the injection frequently is employed to decrease bleeding from the injection site. When subcutaneous administration of heparin is discontinued, the PTT level returns to the normal range within 12 to 24 hours after the last injection of the drug. When patients are to self-administer heparin subcutaneously at home, their instruction should include guided practice to assure their familiarity with safe procedures (Fig. 12–3).

A "Z" tract technique can also be utilized for administration of heparin into the abdominal subcutaneous tissues. The procedure involves the use of the same precautions described for the "bunch-the-skin" technique, but a larger fold of skin is grasped and lifted upward. The five-eighth-inch, 26-gauge needle is inserted at a 45-degree angle to the skin surface.

The repository form of heparin is administered deeply into the subcutaneous tissues. The drug seldom is administered intramuscularly because that highly vascular tissue bleeds easily. The initial dosage usually ranges from 30,000 to 40,000 units and subsequent doses often are 20,000 units given at 12- or 24-hour intervals. The onset of anticoagulant action occurs within two to four hours after the initial injection.

Most of the heparin in the circulation is bound to plasma proteins. A large amount of the drug is taken up by the mast cells, which serve as storage depots for the drug. The rapid movement to storage sites is the reason that a higher initial dosage of the drug is required for a prompt anticoagulant effect.

Heparin is metabolized by hepatic enzymes (i.e., heparinase) to *uroheparin,* which has approximately one half the anticoagulant activity of heparin. Twenty percent of the drug and its metabolites is excreted in the urine.

An abnormally shortened clotting or activated partial thromboplastin time can occur when therapy with heparin is terminated abruptly. Gradual reduction of dosage usually is planned to avert the hazard of a thromboembolic incident associated with the transient increase in coagulation activity.

Intramuscular injections of other drugs are avoided whenever possible during therapy with heparin. When they are unavoidable, use of the deltoid muscle makes detection of bleeding easier than when the injection is made into the gluteal or thigh muscle. Administration of a drug intramuscularly, to a patient receiving intermittent intravenous or subcutaneous doses of heparin, can be planned to precede the heparin dosage by one hour. That practice allows the drug to be administered when the anticoagulant effect of heparin is at the lowest level.

Preparations Available. Heparin sodium (HEPATHROM, HEPRINAR, LIPO-HEPIN, PANHEPRIN) is available as an aqueous solution in ampules, vials, and in disposable units for injection. The repository form of heparin (LIQUAEMIN SODIUM) provides heparin in a gelatin-dextrose vehicle.

Adverse Effects. The most dangerous adverse effects that occur during heparin therapy are related to the action of the drug on the coagulation process. The evidence of bleeding may be minor ecchymosis or there may be major hemorrhagic complications. The incidence of bleeding episodes is highest in persons with blood dyscrasias or occult lesions. History taking and blood-clotting pro-files are done prior to the administration of the initial dose of the drug whenever possible in an attempt to identify potential bleeding problems. During therapy incisions, injection sites, urine, stools, and menstrual flow should be monitored to identify excess bleeding as a consequence of the decreased coagulation of blood.

Transient alopecia has occurred in the third to fourth month of therapy with heparin. Long-term therapy (i.e., over six months) at high dosage levels has caused osteoporosis and spontaneous fractures of the ribs and vertebrae.

Allergic reactions, which were fairly common with older preparations of heparin (i.e., urticaria, rhinitis, lacrimation, arthralgia, bronchospasm, chest pain, hypotension, anaphylaxis), rarely occur with the newer refined preparations. A trial dose of 1000 units of heparin may be given to the patient when there is a question about the possibility of an allergic reaction. Intravenous administration of heparin has occasionally caused thrombocytopenia. There have been isolated incidents of an unusual hypersensitivity reaction that occurred from seven to ten days after the initial dose of heparin. Sudden pain and cyanosis occurred on the same side as the thrombosis within 15 to 30 minutes after the drug was injected.

Heparin Antidote. The best protection against hemorrhagic incidents is careful monitoring of the effect of the drug on the coagulation process in conjunction with frequent examination of the patient for evidence of bleeding (i.e., ecchymosis, bleeding gums, occult blood in the feces). Bleeding can occur when the clotting time or PTT is within the therapeutic range, and it is always a potential problem when the suppression of coagulation processes is excessive.

Drug administration is discontinued when there is evidence of bleeding or the PTT is unduly prolonged. Cessation of drug administration allows return of the coagulation activity within a few hours.

Protamine sulfate is a strongly basic drug that is a specific antidote for heparin. The drug combines tenaciously with heparin to form salts devoid of anticoagulant activity. Inactivation of circulating heparin occurs within five minutes of protamine sulfate injection.

Protamine sulfate diluted in normal saline may be administered intravenously when major bleeding exists or threatens. The usual dosage is 1 mg of protamine sulfate for each 100 units of heparin. The dosage is calculated on the basis of the last dose of heparin administered.

The maximum dosage of protamine sulfate is 100 mg because it can produce an anticoagulant effect beyond that dosage level. Protamine sulfate can inhibit activation of factor V by activated factor X when it is present in the circulation in excess of heparin for its binding. Adverse effects of protamine sulfate are hypotension, vasodilation, bradycardia, and dyspnea.

Interactions. Aspirin decreases the adhesiveness of platelets. Administration of the drug during heparin therapy can contribute to the incidence of bleeding. The anticoagulant activity of heparin can be decreased by concurrent administration of digitalis, quinine, penicillins, tetracyclines, antihistamines, or nicotine.

Oral Anticoagulants

Two groups of anticoagulants are generally administered orally for control of coagulation. The *coumarin derivatives* (acenocoumarol, dicumarol, phenprocoumon, warfarin sodium, warfarin potassium) and the *indandione derivatives* (anisindione, diphenadione, phenindione) have similar pharmacologic characteristics and comparable therapeutic clinical applications.

Action Mode. The oral anticoagulants indirectly affect the generation of the clotting factors by competing with vitamin K_1 utilization that is required for their synthesis in the liver (Fig. 12–4). By inhibiting their production, the oral anticoagulants interfere with the activation of *prothrombin* (factor II), *proconvertin* (factor VII), *plasma thromboplastin component* (factor IX), and *Stuart factor* (factor X). The antithrombosis effect of the oral anticoagulants is related primarily to the low concentration of factor X that is crucial for progression of the coagulation mechanisms. Because the drugs affect factors in the intrinsic and extrinsic pathways of the coagulation process, they prolong both the *activated partial thromboplastin time* and the *prothrombin time*.

The prothrombin time (PT) assays the extrinsic pathway that activates most of the clotting factors inhibited by the oral anticoagulants. The normal PT level is related to the assay of a control or standardized sample of blood. The control value ranges from 11 to 14 seconds. The therapeutic aim is to maintain the PT level within one and one-half to two and one-half times the control. The anticoagulant therapy produces a prolongation of the prothrombin time that is described as *hypoprothrombinemia*.

The indications for use of the oral anticoagulants are the same as those for heparin therapy. They are employed for the prevention of clot formation distal or proximal to an established thrombus or embolus. The drugs are also used in prophylaxis of venous thrombosis and as protection against arterial or cardiac thrombi in situations where the endothelium has been removed by surgical procedures. Therapy with the oral anticoagulants often follows a short period of treatment with heparin.

Therapy Considerations. The dosage of the oral anticoagulants varies with the particular drug employed for therapy (Table 12–2). It is usual for the initial dosage to be twice the maintenance dosage level, and the higher dosage is given for the first two days of therapy. At the end of that time period, a blood sample is taken to determine the prothrombin time. Approximately six to seven days are required to attain smooth control of the prothrombin level. Throughout the period of therapy with oral anticoagulants in the hospital setting, there is a regularly scheduled plan for monitoring the patient's status and the effectiveness of the drugs in controlling clot formation. The patient's tissues and body cavities are ex-

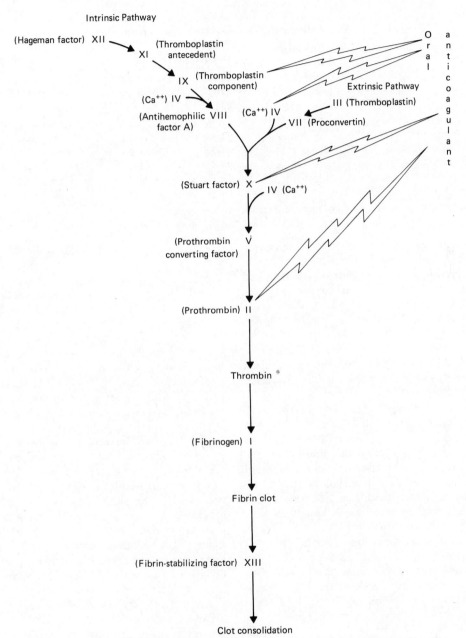

Fig. 12–4. Oral anticoagulants interfere with the activity of factors **II, VII, IX,** and **X** in the coagulation pathways.

Table 12–2.

Oral Anticoagulant Drug-Dosage Response Factors

Drug	Maintenance Dosage (Adults) (mg)	Hypoprothrombinemia		Serum Half-Life
		Peak (Hr)	Duration after Therapy (Days)	
Acenocoumarol	2–10	36–48	2–4	24 hr
Anisindione	25–250	48–72	1.5–3	3–5 days
Dicumarol	25–200	24–96*	2–10	1–2 days
Diphenadione	2.5–5	48–72	15–20	20 days
Phenindione	50–100	36–72	2–4	5–10 hr
Phenprocoumon	0.75–6	48–72	4–7	6.5
Warfarin	2–10	24–36	4–5	36–44 hr

* Highly variable due to dose-dependent kinetics.

amined regularly for evidence of bleeding and all stools are tested for the presence of occult blood.

The prothrombin time initially is monitored daily and the hematocrit value is assessed three times each week. The drug usually is administered in the evening (i.e., at 8 P.M.) to allow time for the return of the prothrombin level report before the next daily dosage of the drug is prescribed. The drug dosage gradually becomes standardized as the prothrombin maintains a steady level each day.

There is predictability in the progression of clotting factor suppression. The clotting factors must be inhibited to within 4 to 9 percent of normal before there is adequate control of coagulation. The initial peak effect on the prothrombin level primarily reflects suppression of factor VII, which has a plasma half-life of from one to five hours. Suppression of factors IX and X requires from five to seven days because their half-life is 20 to 40 hours. Factor II has a long half-life (60 hours), and it is suppressed to 9 percent of the normal level before the drugs have a full anticoagulant effect. Larger doses of the drug prolong the duration of action but have no added effect on the onset of clotting-factor suppression.

The serum half-life of the drug and that of the clotting factors affect the duration of the latent period after therapy is terminated. It takes from six to seven days for the clotting factors to return to their normal levels. Each of the drugs has a different half-life and that affects the duration of action.

Most of the oral anticoagulants are well absorbed. *Dicumarol* is an exception because it is slowly and incompletely absorbed. The anticoagulants in the circulation are almost completely bound to plasma albumin. In addition to being distributed in the liver, lungs, spleen, and kidneys, the drugs cross the placenta and are found in the milk of nursing mothers. Heparin is the preferred drug for pregnant women or nursing mothers because it does not cross the placenta nor does it appear in breast milk.

The drugs are metabolized by hepatic microsomal enzymes, and the drug or the metabolites are excreted in the urine. The metabolites of *anisindione* and *phenindione* may impart a red-orange color to alkaline urine. Increasing the oral intake of water or fruit juice lessens the problem. The patient should be told about the possibility of urine discoloration because the red tinge appears somewhat like diluted blood. Handling of the tablets also colors the palms of the hands an orange-yellow hue.

Resistance to the effects of the anticoagulants occurs in some patients. A higher dosage of the drug is required to attain the therapeutic prothrombin level. The resistance may be associated with genetic abnormalities in the anticoagulant–vitamin K_1 receptor site or with increased drug metabolism and excretion rates.

Preparations Available. The coumarin derivatives *acenocoumarol* (SINTROM), *dicumarol, phenprocoumon* (LIQUAMAR), *warfarin sodium* (COUMADIN, PANWARFIN), and *warfarin potassium* (ATHROMBIN-K) are available as tablets for oral administration. Warfarin sodium also is available in a powdered form for reconstitution and injection. The indandione derivatives *anisindione* (MIRADON), *diphenadione* (DIPAXIN), and *phenindione* (HEDULIN) are available as oral tablets.

Adverse Effects. Bleeding problems are the most common adverse effects of the oral anticoagulants. The problems represent extension of the pharmacologic properties of the drugs. Bleeding usually occurs when the prothrombin level is excessively prolonged but it can occur when the prothrombin time is within the therapeutic range in patients with occult lesions (i.e., chronic gastritis). The bleeding can range from minor ecchymotic sites to major hemorrhagic episodes.

Adverse effects of the coumarin derivatives occur infrequently. Diarrhea is the most common problem. Gastrointestinal disturbances (i.e., nausea, vomiting, anorexia, abdominal cramping, ulcerations of the mouth), alopecia, dermatitis, urticaria, or fever may occur during therapy with the coumarins. Leukopenia occasionally has occurred with each of the coumarin derivatives except *warfarin*.

The coumarin derivatives are more commonly employed for therapy because use of the indandione *phenindione* has been associated with a relatively high incidence of serious adverse effects. The chemical similarity between the varying indandione derivatives makes it necessary to monitor patients for signs of adverse effects during therapy with each of the drugs. The indandiones may be used for treatment of patients receiving tolbutamide or phenytoin because the coumarins cause those drugs to accumulate in the body.

The indandione derivatives can cause serious dermatologic reactions (i.e., rash, severe exfoliative dermatitis), hematologic reactions (i.e., leukopenia, leukocytosis, agranulocytosis), nephropathy (i.e., acute tubular necrosis), and hepatotoxicity (hepatitis, jaundice). The drug is discontinued immediately if there is evidence of fever, skin rash, leukopenia, eosinophilia, or agranulocytosis. Persons receiving the drug are instructed to notify their physician when there is marked fatigue, fever, chills, or sore throat. The diversity of adverse effects that have been reported as being related to the indandiones makes the drug suspect when new symptoms occur during therapy.

Oral Anticoagulant Antidote. Bleeding that occurs during therapy with the anticoagulants is carefully evaluated. The treatment of bleeding depends on the urgency of the situation. The appearance of any uncontrollable bleeding necessitates discontinuing the use of the drug. Excessive blood loss may require whole-blood transfusions, but fresh frozen plasma supplies the clotting factors that have been suppressed during anticoagulant therapy. *Vitamin K₁* administration may accompany infusion of the plasma in an attempt to reestablish synthesis of the clotting factors. Some of the anticoagulants have a long duration of action and the continued administration of vitamin K_1 may be required to reverse the drug action (Table 12–2). The clinical status of the patient is evaluated carefully before administration of vitamin K_1 because the reactivation of clotting factor synthesis that it produces is followed by a period of refractoriness to the anticoagulants due to the competitive nature of vitamin K_1 and the anticoagulants. Reinstitution of therapy will be followed by the same time lag in anticoagulant effect as that occurring when therapy previously was initiated.

Vitamin K_1 is available in forms for parenteral or oral administration. The oral forms of the vitamin may be employed when the prothrombin level indicates excess hypoprothrombinemia, but parenteral administration usually is planned when there is a bleeding episode. *Phytonadione* (AQUA-MEPHYTON, KONAKION, MEPHYTON) may be given intramuscularly (i.e., 5 to 50 mg) or administered intravenously (i.e., 5 to 25 mg) in emergency situations. The drug effect on clotting factor synthesis requires four to five hours when the drug is administered by the parenteral or oral route. *Menadiol sodium diphosphate*, K_4, (KAPPADIONE, SYNKAYVITE) and *menadione*, K_3 (KAPPAXIN, KAYQUINONE, KOLKLOT) also may be employed for vitamin K_1 replacement but their rapid rate of hepatic metabolism makes them less effective than phytonadione.

Interactions. The availability of vitamin K from the intestine is necessary for the smooth control of clotting factor synthesis by the oral anticoagulants. Therapeutic hypoprothrombinemia is dependent on the maintenance of a controlled suppression of key clotting factors. The absorption of vitamin K from the intestine can be inhibited by disease states that decrease the availability of bile salts required for the absorption of the vitamin. Vitamin K–rich foods can provide an excess of the vitamin and antagonize the effects of the oral anticoagulants. Most of those foods (fish, fish oils, tomatoes, cheese, kale, cauliflower, cabbage, spinach, egg yolk, liver) are not ingested in excess quantities by most individuals.

Bleeding during therapy with the oral anticoagulants can be potentiated by the concurrent use of drugs that have a high ulcerogenic potential. The salicylates, indomethacin, and the pyrazolones (i.e., sulfinpyrazone, oxyphenbutazone, phenylbutazone) may contribute to the incidence of bleeding from new or occult gastric irritation sites when they are used with the oral anticoagulants.

Hypoprothrombinemia and bleeding during therapy with the oral anticoagulants may be potentiated by concurrent use of drugs that *displace them from plasma protein-binding sites* (salicylates, sulfonamides, chloral hydrate, indomethacin, mefenamic acid, clofibrate, or dextrothyroxine); drugs that *displace them from their binding sites and decrease platelet aggregation* (sulfinpyrazone, oxyphenbutazone, or phenylbutazone); or drugs that *inhibit their metabolism by hepatic microsomal enzymes* (tricyclic antidepressants, chloramphenicol, allopurinol, disulfiram, or metronidazole).

The effect of the oral anticoagulants can be inhibited by drugs that *decrease their absorption* from the gastrointestinal tract (cholestyramine); drugs that *accelerate their metabolism by inducing hepatic microsomal enzymes* (barbiturates, glutethimide, carbamazepine, rifampin, or griseofulvin); or drugs that *increase plasma levels of vitamin K_1* (estrogens or oral contraceptives). Diuretics reduce the response to the anticoagulants by reducing the excess plasma fluid and concentrating the clotting factors.

Platelet Aggregation Inhibitors

Dextran 75 (GENTRAN 75), *dextran 70* (MACRODEX), and *dextran 40* (RHEOMACRODEX) are glucose polymers that are employed to prevent the formation of thrombi. The drug adheres to the vascular endothelium and to the surface of platelets. The presence of the dextran on the platelet membranes decreases their mobility and their adhesiveness. Dextran may also alter the structure of fibrin formed during its administration. The fibrin clots have a coarser fibrin network and the clots are dissolved at a more rapid rate than those that are formed prior to the infusion of dextran.

Dextran 75, dextran 70, and dextran 40 have differing molecular weights as indicated by their number designation. Dextran 40, which has the lower molecular weight (40,000), is the more commonly used dextran formulation. Although dextran 40 initially is rapidly excreted (60 percent in six hours), 20 percent of the drug molecules are larger than the maximum weight of molecules that can pass through the glomerulus of the nephron ($> 50,000$ molecular weight). Unexcreted molecules remain in the circulation and subsequent administration of dextran 40 leads to accumulation of the drug to an effective level. Administration of dextran at a dosage level of 500 ml/day (10 percent solution) intravenously for eight days provides a serum concentration of 8 mg/ml.

The drug frequently is given to surgical patients in an intravenous infusion that may be started preoperatively, continued during surgery, and repeated daily for up to five days postoperatively. The termination of therapy is correlated with the time the patient is fully ambulatory. When the patient is to be on a longer period of bed rest, the drug may be infused intravenously every two to three days until the patient is ambulatory.

Dextran increases the blood volume and decreases the viscosity of blood. Hemodilution has a positive effect on venous stasis and perfusion of the microcirculation, but it may increase the cardiac work load. During therapy with dextran, the intake and output of fluid are monitored daily and the hemoglobin and hematocrit levels are evaluated at least three times each week. The patient's incision is regularly observed for evidence of bleeding.

Fluid overload can cause hemodilution on about the fourth or fifth day of therapy. The blood values may show a decreased hemoglobin value (i.e., 10 gm/100 ml) and a low hematocrit value ($<$ 35 percent of normal). The increased fluid volume may precipitate pulmonary edema when the patient has a low cardiac reserve.

Mild allergic reactions (skin eruptions, asthma-like symptoms) may occur during therapy with dextran. The incidence of anaphylactic reactions is negligible. A small number of patients have hematoma formation or generalized edema around the incision site.

Investigational Drugs. Clinical trials indicating the thrombosis retardant effect of *dipyridamole* and *hydroxychloroquine* and the nonsteroidal anti-inflammatory drugs *aspirin, sulfinpyrazone,* and *phenylbutazone* have generated a high level of interest in further investigation. The results of the early trials suggest that the drugs may be used to prevent the development of arterial and venous thrombosis.

The drugs prevent the second phase of platelet aggregation, which is associated with accelerated adenosine diphosphate (ADP) activity. The ADP that is released in that phase causes massive platelet aggregation and they produce platelet plugs by adhering to the platelets previously clumped on the vessel wall. The drugs also are thought to inhibit prostaglandin activity. The prostaglandins are intermediates for the release of ADP.

Aspirin has been found equally effective in dosage ranges of 600 to 2400 mg and 300 and 3600 mg. The effect is evident from four to seven days after a single oral dose of the drug. Aspirin produces an irreversible defect in the platelets. It also appears to inhibit the platelet surface enzyme (glucosyl transferase) that is required for platelet adhesion to surfaces. At high dosage levels, aspirin is thought to inhibit glucose utilization in the platelets.

Dipyridamole (PERSANTIN) action is different from that of the other drugs. Dipyridamol inhibits glucose utilization or metabolism by the platelets and increases their level of *cyclic adenosine monophosphate* (cAMP). The effect on glucose utilization and cAMP is thought to be the basis for dipyridamole interference with platelet adhesiveness.

Clinical trials are being planned to study the effectiveness of the drugs and the dosage levels required for their therapeutic effect. Some of the known adverse effects of the drugs may preclude their use for the prevention of thrombosis.

Thrombolytic Enzymes

Fibrinolysin (THROMBOLYSIN). The drug, which is prepared by activating the human blood plasma factor, has both profibrinolysin-activator and fibrinolytic, or plasmin, properties. It is employed for its action of converting proteins of the clot to peptides and amino acids. The effects on clot disintegration make it a useful drug for the treatment of thrombophlebitis, phlebothrombosis, pulmonary embolism, and thrombosis of the arteries. The drug is effective when it is used within five days of the thrombotic incident. Older clots are resistant to the drug action.

The usual intravenous dosage of the drug is 50,000 to 100,000 units/hour, and that dosage is continued for a period of one to six hours per day. The usual course of therapy is three to four consecutive days. After that time, antistreptokinase titers begin to rise in response to the streptokinase that is employed in activating the plasma factor in preparation of the drug.

The clotting time and PTT time are evaluated daily when dosages exceeding 200,000 units/day are employed for therapy. The most common adverse effect during therapy is a febrile reaction that occurs within three to eight hours after the start of the intravenous infusion.

Streptokinase-Streptodornase (VARIDASE). The drug is designed for topical and localized application to remove clotted blood or fibrinous tissue accumulations that are associated with trauma or inflammation. The drug is available as a solution for intramuscular injection and as a solution or jelly for buccal or topical application. The periodic flushing of surface cavities may be planned to remove nonadherent necrotic tissue and increase the drug contact with the underlying surfaces.

Urokinase (ABBOKINASE) and *Streptokinase* (STREPTASE). The drugs are enzymes that have been employed in selected clinical situations to dissolve or remove clots. They have been used for the dissolution of acute massive pulmonary emboli and thrombi in the deep leg veins. The treatment is dependent on early identification of the thrombosis because thrombi that are over four days old have started organizing and cannot be lysed completely.

Urokinase has been the more useful of the enzymes. The drug is a direct plasminogen activator. It is extracted from human urine, and the extraction is time consuming and expensive. The drug is particularly useful in acutely ill patients in whom the natural lytic processes, which usually occur in weeks, may be delayed for months. A 12-hour intravenous infusion can lyse pulmonary emboli, increase pulmonary capillary perfusion, and decrease the hemodynamic abnormalities associated with the pulmonary embolus.

Streptokinase acts indirectly on plasminogen. It is administered by continuous intravenous infusion. A large unit dose (250,000 to 600,000 units) may be infused over a period of 10 to 30 minutes, and the infusion rate then is decreased (100,000 units/hour) during the subsequent 24-hour infusion period. Streptokinase is a secretory protein of hemolytic streptococci and it is antigenic in most patients. The frequency of exposure to streptococcal antigens provides most individuals with circulating antibodies that react with the drug. The high dosage of the drug is employed to provide enough streptokinase to neutralize the antibodies and also allow an excess to act on the thrombus or embolus. Therapy with the drug is followed by a marked increase in streptokinase antibodies and that precludes subsequent therapy with the drug for at least three to six months.

Streptokinase has been administered by intra-arterial infusion close to the site of a vascular thrombus in an attempt to avoid some of the problems with generalized systemic infusion. The dosage of the drug is 1/100 of the dosage required for intravenous infusion, and the low drug level has been found to effectively lyse fresh occlusions.

Fibrinolysis Inhibitor

Aminocaproic acid (AMICAR) is employed to decrease excess fibrinolysis caused by accelerated profibrinolysin activity. The drug competes with activators of profibrinolysin to inhibit excessive formation of fibrinolysin.

The drug is useful for maintaining the integrity of clots that have formed in the central nervous system after the rupture of an aneurysm. Retention of the clot prevents rebleeding during the time interval when plans for control measures are being formulated (i.e., surgery, hypertension control). The drug has also been employed to maintain the normal plasma level of fibrinogen (130 mcg/ml) when the coagulation factor is lowered by major obstetrical complications or surgery.

Aminocaproic acid (5 to 30 gm/day) is administered orally or by slow intravenous infusion. The oral drug is well absorbed, and a peak plasma level is attained in two hours. The drug is excreted unchanged in the urine. The high urine concentration provides a therapeutic advantage in the control of bleeding from the genitourinary tract. Aminocaproic acid inhibits the profibrinolysin activator (urokinase) in the tract and thereby can enhance clot formation at the highly vascular sites after genitourinary surgery.

The major adverse effect of aminocaproic acid is generalized thrombosis, which is an extension of its pharmacologic effect. Hypotension, conjunctivitis, nasal congestion, diarrhea, erythema, pruritus, and rash may occur during therapy.

Procoagulants

The absence or depressed production of one or more clotting factors can cause uncontrollable bleeding. For example, congenital deficit of the clotting factors causes persons with hemophilia to hemorrhage into the joints, muscle or soft tissues, gastrointestinal tract, and other body tissues in response to minimal injury. The frequency of the intermittent life-threatening problems interrupts their life patterns. In the last few years there has been a trend toward self-therapy for persons with hemophilia. Intravenous injection of the missing clotting factor at home promptly at the earliest sign of bleeding has decreased the expense, dependence, and joint deformities that previously were associated with inpatient hospital treatment for bleeding episodes.

The particular product required for the replacement of the missing clotting factor is defined before replacement, and the clotting factor assay after treatment allows an evaluation of the coagulation status. The goal is to maintain the factors within 10 to 20 percent of normal in persons with congenital or acquired clotting-factor deficiencies.

Clotting-Factor Replacement

Factor IX complex (KONYNE, PROPLEX) contains the clotting factors II, VII, IX, and X in concentrations 24 times those of normal human plasma. The clotting factors are absent or minimally active in individuals with hemophilia B, or Christmas disease.

Factor IX complex is administered intravenously and the dosage is 30 to 60 units/kg of body weight. The maintenance dosage ranges from 5 to 10 units/kg of body weight injected intravenously twice a day.

Administration of factor IX is associated with a high risk of hepatitis (50 percent) and thromboembolic incidents. Slow administration of the intravenous dosage can decrease the problems of fever, chills, rash, flushing, or tingling that occur when the drug is injected rapidly. Anaphylactic reactions have been reported with the administration of the drug.

Antihemophilic factor (FACTORATE, HEMOFIL, HUMAFAC, PROFILATE) is employed primarily to provide factor VIII to individuals with hemophilia A. Replacement of the factor is required when bleeding into the tissues around the joints occurs or when there are other manifestations of severe bleeding. The dosage of antihemophilic factor is 4 to 5 units/kg of body weight, which can raise the plasma level of factor VIII to within 10 percent of normal. A level that is at least 40 percent of normal is required to provide hemostasis in the presence of hemorrhage. The drug may also be administered to individuals with acquired factor VIII–inhibiting factors. Adverse effects are rare but chills and fever may occur during therapy.

NURSING INTERVENTION

Thrombosis may occur in any situation where the patient is immobilized, but the intraoperative period frequently is the time when venous thrombosis occurs. Attempts have been made to decrease the prolonged venous stasis that is natural to lying supine on the operating table during a protracted surgical procedure. In some instances electrical stimulation of the calf muscles has been employed during surgery in an attempt to maintain the muscle contraction that moves venous blood from the small veins of the lower legs to the central veins. There is general agreement that placing a blanket roll under the patient's feet can effectively decrease compression on the lower leg veins while the patient is on the operating table. In the immediate postoperative period, frequent position changes and exercising of the extremities can maintain the venous blood flow at a velocity discouraging thrombus formation.

Initial Status Evaluation

The assessment of the patient's vascular and pulmonary status is an essential aspect of the nursing care of persons at high risk of thromboembolic episodes. The same assessment also provides a base line for evaluating the effectiveness of anticoagulant therapy. It is essential to define whether prophylactic anticoagulant therapy is protecting against thrombosis or whether treatment is controlling the extension of an existing thrombus and protecting against embolization.

Specific attention to the integrity of the venous circulation is necessary for identifying changes that occur. Measuring the circumference of the calf and thigh of both legs allows comparisons that can provide clues to covert changes not otherwise discernible. Marking the skin with a ballpoint pen at the level where each limb is measured allows a reliable comparison with subsequent measurements of the limbs.

An increase in calf size of 12 to 15 cm is suggestive of a problem with venous flow. Further assessment can be done by flexing the patient's knee slightly and forcefully dorsiflexing the foot. The maneuver causes calf muscle compression on the veins and the patient may express discomfort or pain (Homan's sign). The test is useful but not completely reliable. It can be negative in the presence of deep-vein thrombosis.

Occlusion of the soleal, posterior tibial, or peroneal veins may be accompanied by edema distal to the thrombus, and there may be pain on muscle movement. Thrombosis of the larger vessels of the leg may be almost silent and the limb may be edema free. When measurements and observations indicate the presence of tissue

fluid, elevation of the limb to a 45-degree angle for ten minutes will speed drainage when the fluid accumulation is due to problems other than thrombosis (i.e., varicose veins). The obstruction of blood flow will cause the measurement to remain unchanged after elevation when deep venous thrombosis is causing the problem. When the foregoing assessment shows positive indicators of venous occlusion, the findings should be discussed promptly with the physician.

The regularly scheduled leg exercises and quadriceps contraction exercises of patients who are confined to bed afford an opportunity to ask the patient whether there is any discomfort in the extremities during the activities. It is estimated that 50 percent of the patients who have discomfort in the legs do not volunteer information about it. Many patients will self-diagnose the problem as related to previous leg exercises or other activities. The patient's statement of discomfort on muscle movement is particularly important because it may provide the only clue to deep vein thrombosis prior to embolization.

The initial assessment of the patient's respiratory status provides a base line for evaluating changes. A pulmonary embolus will cause disruption of the hemodynamics involved in gas exchange. The patient's complaints will vary according to the size of the pulmonary artery that is occluded. The physical findings at the time of embolization may be subtle and nonspecific (i.e., tachypnea, rales, tachycardia, fever). The patient's symptoms may provide a clearer guide to the problem (i.e., dyspnea, cough, pleural pain, hemoptysis). The suggestion of a problem as determined by careful assessment should promptly be discussed with the physician because the earliest signs are evidence of a life-threatening clinical entity.

Counseling

Each contact with the hospitalized patient provides an opportunity to prepare the individual for continuing therapy with an anticoagulant at home. On a day-to-day basis, the necessary information can be provided in an unhurried and nonthreatening manner.

It is important that the person understand the rationale for the anticoagulant therapy. The patient who understands the action of the drug as related to the prevention of clot formation can participate in discussion of measures that can be implemented to enhance that action, for example, planning to interrupt long periods of automobile travel at half-hour intervals to allow ten-minute periods of walking, or flexing and extending the legs when prolonged periods of standing are unavoidable.

Discussion of usual living patterns allows analysis of practices that promote venous stasis and counteract the effectiveness of the drug (i.e., crossing the legs, wearing knee-high-stockings, sitting for protracted periods of time). Alternative practices can be discussed when the individual has difficulty with a complete change in habit patterns. For example, crossing the ankles provides a reasonable substitute for leg crossing and there is minimal venous compression.

There are numerous drugs that can interact with the oral anticoagulants. The patient need not learn the entire list of those drugs, but the person should be aware that the possibility of drug interactions makes it necessary to avoid the use of over-the-counter drugs while taking an oral anticoagulant. Because there are over 400 salicylate-containing over-the-counter drugs, the inadvisability of taking any nonprescribed drug must be stressed. The person who customarily takes aspirin for relief of pain or control of fever can take the nonsalicylate *acetoaminophen* as a substitute.

The patient should be told to inform any dentist or new physician that an anticoagulant is being taken. The hazard of obtaining a prescription for an interacting drug is lessened when those professionals are aware of the drug therapy. They will also take precautions against bleeding when necessary procedures are performed (i.e., tooth extraction).

Discussions with the patient provide an opportunity for identifying personal life situations that may present the hazard of a bleeding episode while the anticoagulant is being taken (i.e., falling, use of saws, scissors, razors). The focus on the person's real-life situation can provide guidelines that are relevant and useful to the individual. The discussion should include measures for the control of minor bleeding when it occurs (i.e., applying ice or pressure). The person should be told that the physician is to be contacted when there are frequent episodes of minor bleeding or when bleeding is not controlled with the usual simple measures.

Many patients are well informed about measures they should use to monitor external and internal bleeding, but they are unaware that the physician is to be contacted for less than gross hemorrhage. They must be told that unusual or uncontrolled bleeding is an indication to stop taking the drug and to notify the physician promptly. Examples of bleeding should be explicit (i.e., bleeding from the nose, skin, rectum, vagina, blood in the urine or vomitus, black and tarry stools, extensive bruising of the skin, excessive and unusual menstrual flow). Obscure back pain also can be a sign of retroperitoneal hemorrhage; therefore, the person is advised to report any new symptom to the physician. The information can be shared straightforwardly when the person is made aware of the relationship between the oral anticoagulant therapy and the nurses' frequent inspection of the incision or intravenous injection sites, guaiac testing of stools, inspection of the urine, and observation of the skin for ecchymotic areas.

The importance of uninterrupted use of the prescribed anticoagulant and the regularly scheduled tests of the coagulation status (PT, PTT) must be emphasized. Equally important is the periodic examination and evaluation of the therapeutic plan during attendance at the clinic or the physician's office. Individuals who travel frequently should be reminded to take an adequate supply of the drug with them and to arrange for laboratory tests if they are due to be taken during the travel period. Carrying an American Heart Association anticoagulant alert card or wearing a Medic-Alert tag allows treatment based on the particular drug being employed for coagulation control when emergency situations arise.

Review Guides

1. Outline the factors that would be included in explaining to the patient the rationale for concurrent use of heparin sodium and warfarin sodium.
2. Formulate a plan for assessing the effects of therapy with an oral anticoagulant.
3. Outline the factors that would be included in a teaching plan when the patient is to administer subcutaneous heparin at home.
4. Describe the effects of protamine sulfate and vitamin K_1 on an ongoing anticoagulant therapy plan.
5. Explain the reason that patients are cautioned against use of over-the-counter products containing aspirin when they are taking an oral anticoagulant.
6. Formulate a plan for preparing the patient for continuing the use of warfarin sodium at home.
7. Describe the differences in the teaching plan for a patient taking warfarin sodium at home when the patient is (a) a 65-year-old man with chronic heart failure; (b) a 24-year-old mother of four children.

Additional Readings

Babcock, Robert B.; Dumper, C. Wesley; and Scharfman, William B.: Heparin-induced immune thrombocytopenia. *N. Engl. J. Med.*, **295**:237, July 29, 1976.

Bassan, Mayer, M., and Rogel, Shlomo: Current practice in the use of anticoagulants for ischemic heart disease: a survey of 200 hospitals. *Heart Lung*, **5**:742, September–October, 1976.

Bjerkelund, Christopher: Anticoagulant therapy in myocardial infarction. *Heart Lung*, **4**:61, January–February, 1975.

Brill, Winston J.: Biologic nitrogen fixation. *Sci. Am.*, **236**:68, March, 1977.

Caprini, Joseph A.; Zoellner, Judith L.; and Weisman, Marcia: Heparin therapy—part 1. *Cardiovasc. Nurs.*, **13**:13, May–June, 1977.

Coon, William W.: Anticoagulant therapy for venous thromboembolism. *Postgrad. Med.*, **63**:157, April, 1978.

Couch, Nathan P.: Axioms on venous thrombosis. *Hosp. Med.*, **13**:68, June, 1977.

Cudkowicz, Leon, and Sherry, Sol: Current status of thrombolytic therapy. *Heart Lung*, **7**:97, January–February, 1978.

Durkin, Deborah M.: Pulmonary fat embolism: a complication of fracture. *Heart Lung*, **5**:477, May–June, 1976.

Fitzmaurice, Joan B.: Venous thromboembolic disease: current thoughts. *Cardiovasc. Nurs.*, **14**:1, January–February, 1978.

Hirsh, Jack: Venous thromboembolism: diagnosis, treatment, prevention. *Hosp. Pract.* **10**:53, August, 1975.

Johnson, Colleen F., and Convery, F. Richard: Preventing emboli after total hip replacement. *Am. J. Nurs.*, **75**:804, May, 1975.

Kelly, Patricia, and Penner, John A.: Antihemophilic factor inhibitors. *J.A.M.A.*, **236**:2061, November 1, 1976.

King, C. Richard, and Daly, James W.: The prevention of postoperative pulmonary emboli with low-molecular-weight dextran. *Am. J. Obstet. Gynecol.*, **123**:46, September 1, 1975.

Maki, Dennis G.: Septic thrombophlebitis (part 2). *Hosp. Med.*, **13**:6, January, 1977.

Matseoane, Stephen; Butts, James A., Jr.; and Mandeville, Edgar O.: Ovarian hemorrhage complicating warfarin sodium anticoagulant therapy. *Am. J. Obstet. Gynecol.*, **124**:766, April 1, 1976.

Moore, Karen, and Maschak, Barbara J.: How patient education can reduce the hazards of anticoagulation. *Nursing '77,* **7:**24, September, 1977.

Moroz, Leonard A.: Increased blood fibrinolytic activity after aspirin ingestion. *N. Engl. J. Med.,* **296:** 525, March 10, 1977.

Newman, Robert L.; Sirridge, Marjorie; Brinkman, Margaret; Shannon, Reaner: A study of blood coagulation parameters. *Am. J. Obstet. Gynecol.,* **125:**108, May 1, 1976.

Roberts, Brooke: The acutely ischemic limb. *Heart Lung,* **5:**273, March–April, 1976.

Rosenberg, Robert D.: Actions and interactions of antithrombin and heparin. *N. Engl. J. Med.,* **292:** 146, January 16, 1975.

Ryan, Rosemary: Thrombophlebitis: assessment and prevention. *Am. J. Nurs.,* **76:**1634, October, 1976.

Salzman, Edwin W.; Deykin, Daniel; Shapiro, Ruth Mayer; and Rosenberg, Robert: Management of heparin therapy. *N. Engl. J. Med.,* **292:**1046, May 15, 1975.

Sasahara, Arthur A.; Stengle, James M.; and Sherry, Sol: Urokinase in thromboembolic disease: pulmonary embolism. *Am. Heart J.,* **89:**403, March, 1975.

Sherry, Sol: Preventing pulmonary embolism with heparin in low doses. *Postgrad. Med.,* **59:**80, May, 1976.

Udall, John A.: Patient selection for anticoagulation therapy in coronary heart disease. *Postgrad. Med.,* **60:**65, August, 1976.

Vera, Juan S.; Herzig, Edward B.; Sise, Herbert S.; and Brauer, Mark J.: Acquired circulating anticoagulant to factor VIII. *J.A.M.A.,* **232:**1038, June 9, 1975.

Vesell, Elliot S.; Passananti, Thomas; and Johnson, Alice O.: Failure of indomethacin and warfarin to interact in normal human volunteers. *J. Clin. Pharmacol.,* **456:**486, July, 1975.

Weiss, Harvey J.: Antiplatelet drugs—a new pharmacologic approach to the prevention of thrombosis. *Am. Heart J.,* **92:**86, July, 1976.

Wessler, Stanford: Heparin as an antithrombic agent. *J.A.M.A.,* **236:**389, July 26, 1976.

13

Decreased Tissue Perfusion

The adequacy of tissue perfusion is dependent on the integrity of the factors that control blood circulation. The balanced interaction of *cardiac output, blood volume,* and *vascular tone* maintains the transport system that supplies oxygen and nutrients to cells at organ sites. Disruption of any one of those parameters interferes with the supply of oxygen available to tissue for their normal physiologic processes. A complex *shock syndrome* can ensue when there is a prolonged disruption in the hemodynamic parameters.

Physiologic Correlations

The circulating blood is widely distributed throughout the body in the capillary beds. The narrow muscular arterioles deliver the blood to the capillary beds, or microcirculation, where oxygen and nutrients diffuse into the tissues and metabolic wastes diffuse into the blood in the microscopic vessels. Blood leaves the capillary beds through the venules.

Capillary Blood Flow

The microcirculation is the largest organic unit in the body, and it is estimated that it contains approximately 70 percent of the circulating blood at any given moment in time. The size of the capillary bed is the primary determinant of the quantity of blood in its network and the proportion of the cardiac output received each minute (Table 13–1). The most essential organs (i.e., brain, heart, hepatoportal, and kidney tissues) comprise only 7 percent of the total body weight, yet they receive 70 percent of the cardiac output each minute.

Oxygen Consumption

The metabolic activity of the organ is the determining factor in the oxygen uptake from blood

Table 13–1.
Relation Between Organ Size and Oxygen Uptake from Blood

Tissue	Percent of Total Body Weight	Percent of Cardiac Output Received/Minute	Percent Oxygen Uptake/Minute
Brain	2	14	23
Heart	0.5	5	12
Hepatoportal	4	28	20
Kidney	0.5	23	5
Skeletal muscle	49	16	20
Skin	6	8	5
Residual tissue	38	6	15

flowing through the microcirculation. The skeletal muscle, which comprises 49 percent of the total body weight, extracts an amount of oxygen roughly equivalent to the amount that is extracted by the brain or the hepatoportal tissues. The combined weight of those organs is only 6 percent of the total body weight, but their metabolic activities are essential to physiologic equilibrium.

Glycolysis can take place within the cell cytoplasm and the process produces energy without using oxygen. The high-energy-producing processes of the mitochondria (i.e., Krebs' cycle) require a continuous supply of oxygen for the cyclic conversions that release energy. The oxygen needs of the cell control the amount of blood that flows through the capillaries. The accumulation of metabolic products causes dilation of the precapillary sphincters. The dilation increases the blood flow to the level that is required to supply adequate oxygen to the cells.

Cerebral Autoregulation

Cerebral tissues also have the capacity to regulate blood flow. Elevated levels of carbon dioxide and pH of the blood at cerebral tissue sites cause dilation of the cerebral vessels. The autoregulation of the circulation is effective when there is an adequate carotid artery pressure. The quantity of blood flowing through cerebral tissues is reduced when the mean arterial pressure is low, and the tissues extract more oxygen from the circulating blood to compensate for the reduction in the flow

volume. When the mean systemic blood pressure drops below 60 mm Hg, the decrease in cerebral blood flow reduces the oxygen available. Below that level the hypoxic state of the cerebral tissues becomes evident in the patient's level of consciousness or in behavioral changes.

Compensatory Responses

The decreased arterial pressure at the carotid and aortic baroreceptors induces the transmission of impulses to the cardiovascular control centers in the medulla. The efferent sympathetic nerve impulses produce cardioacceleration and vasoconstriction.

The cardiovascular system has alpha, beta$_1$, and beta$_2$ adrenergic receptors and dopaminergic receptors. The specificity of the receptor determines which hormone will affect the target cell and the response that will occur after its binding with the receptor. The binding activates the enzyme *adenyl cyclase*, which causes conversion of intracellular *adenosine triphosphate* (ATP) to *cyclic adenosine-3′, 5′-monophosphate* (cAMP). The conversion releases energy that initiates cellular responses (i.e., smooth muscle relaxation or contraction) before the cAMP is inactivated. The responses that occur are determined by the characteristics of the cell.

Stimulation of cardiac *beta$_1$-adrenergic receptors* increases the sinus rate (positive chronotropic action), the force of contraction (positive inotropic action), and the rate of conduction through the atrioventricular node. *Beta₂-adrenergic-receptor* stimulation produces vasodilation (i.e., in skeletal muscles). *Alpha-adrenergic-receptor* stimulation causes vasoconstriction of almost all arteries and veins. *Dopaminergic receptor* stimulation causes vasodilation in the renal, mesenteric, coronary, and cerebral arteries.

Pathophysiologic Correlations

The sympathetic vasoconstriction is somewhat selective. When there is a need for blood for vital organ function, alpha-adrenergic stimulation at receptors in the skin, mucosa, intestine, and kidneys constricts the arterioles, venules, and capillary sphincters. The process reduces the blood flow through the metarterioles of the capillary beds. Most of the blood that enters the capillary

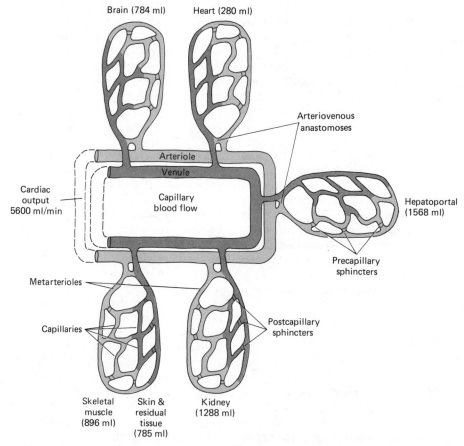

Fig. 13–1. The cardiac output each minute is circulated through tissue capillary beds. Sympathetic nerve–induced vasoconstriction shunts the blood through arteriovenous anastomoses at nonessential tissue sites (skeletal, skin, kidney) to provide the blood flow required at essential tissue sites.

bed is shunted through the arteriovenous anastomoses, and there is minimal perfusion of the microcirculation (Fig. 13–1). The selective vasoconstriction at the least essential tissues maximizes the effectiveness of the cardiac output by augmenting the blood flow to essential tissues. About 3 liters of blood flow per minute can become available to nourish the brain, heart, and hepatoportal tissues when there is an adequate blood volume.

Tissue Metabolism

The blood flowing through the organs in which vasoconstriction is highest gradually is deprived of the oxygen required for metabolic processes. The lack of oxygen shifts energy production to the less efficient anaerobic metabolism within the cells. The increased production and accumulation of metabolic products (i.e., lactate, pyruvate, adenosine, potassium and hydrogen ions) cause dilation of the precapillary sphincters.

The capillary dilation, during the time when postcapillary sphincters and venules are constricted, causes blood to pool in the microcirculation, and the systemic blood pressure is reduced. The stasis of blood in the capillaries promotes intravascular coagulation. The occlusion of the tiny capillaries by clots further contributes to the anaerobic metabolism and metabolic waste accumulation.

Cellular Injury

Irreversible injury to the cells can result from prolonged oxygen deprivation. The liberation of acidic products into the plasma causes metabolic acidosis that cannot be physiologically reversed while renal blood flow is compromised.

The release of proteolytic enzymes from the cellular lysosomes also may occur when anoxia exists at the tissue level. The liberated enzymes that escape deactivation by proteases can destroy the protein matrix of the cells and travel with the plasma to adjacent tissues.

The vicious cycle of vasoconstriction, ischemia, and secondary vasoconstriction can irreversibly damage cells when the shock state and the factor that precipitated the events remain untreated (i.e., sepsis, blood loss, cardiac failure). The paradox of the initial shock state is that sympathetic nerve-induced cardiac stimulation and vasoconstriction can maintain the pulse and blood pressure at near-normal levels while vital tissues are underperfused.

Antihypotensive Drugs

A primary factor in establishing hemodynamic equilibrium is correction of the maldistribution of blood flow that deprives some body tissues of oxygen and increases the production of acidic products. The reinstitution of normal hemodynamics requires immediate correction of blood volume deficits and electrolyte or acid-base imbalances. Preliminary administration of fluids usually is planned at a level that raises the central venous pressure (CVP) to 10 to 15 cm H_2O or the pulmonary wedge pressure (PWP) to 14 to 18 mm Hg. The maintenance of an adequate circulating blood volume is essential throughout therapy that is directed at correction of the blood distribution patterns. Treatment of the basic etiologic problem also is an important aspect of the pharmacotherapy for reversal of the shock state.

A variety of disease states can cause the pathophysiologic changes that constitute the etiology of shock (i.e., hemorrhage, sepsis, cardiac failure, trauma). Shock crosses the lines of etiologic categories and there are commonalities in the hemodynamic imbalances manifested as *cardiac failure, peripheral vascular failure, hypovolemia,* or *vasodilation. The common denominator in shock is inadequate transport of blood to cells.*

DRUG THERAPY

Shock is an acute syndrome requiring prompt treatment to reestablish hemodynamic equilibrium. Patients with *cardiac failure* or *peripheral vascular failure* need emergency treatment to correct their hypotensive state. Therapy is directed at use of a drug that strengthens cardiac contraction and provides sufficient vasoconstriction to raise the blood pressure high enough to perfuse the brain and heart. The hemodynamic status of individuals with *hypovolemia* or *vasodilation* may be somewhat less acute because the blood pressure usually is at least adequate to perfuse the brain and heart. Therapy for those individuals includes the use of drugs to produce enough vasodilation to redistribute blood and improve the perfusion of the visceral organs.

The hemodynamic status of the patient in shock frequently changes during therapy, and continual assessment is required to determine the effectiveness of the drugs. The initial drug and dosage may not be appropriate as the patient's status changes.

The drugs employed for treatment of shock are described as *sympathomimetics* because their effects at the adrenergic receptors are similar to those of the natural endogenous catecholamines. The drug selected for treatment in any given situation is based on the hemodynamic status of the patient.

The antihypotensive drugs can be grouped according to their most prominent adrenergic effects on the cardiovascular system. *Ephedrine sulfate, epinephrine, levarterenol,* and *metaramininol* produce both alpha- and beta-adrenergic effects. *Isoproterenol* and *mephentermine* have predominantly beta-adrenergic effects. *Dopamine* has beta-adrenergic effects at low dosage levels and it also has dopaminergic effects. At higher dosage levels the effects of dopamine are primarily alpha-adrenergic in character. *Methoxamine* and *phenylephrine* primarily have alpha-adrenergic effects on the cardiovascular system.

The intravenous route usually is employed for administration of the antihypotensive drugs because the rate of absorption from intramuscular or subcutaneous sites is uncertain while the venous blood flow is reduced by shock. The general guideline for systolic blood pressure elevation during therapy is to raise the level for the previously normotensive patient to a systolic level of 80 to 100 mm Hg. The desirable systolic blood pressure level for previously hypertensive patients may be at 30 to 40 mm Hg below their usual blood pressure. It is usual for their maximum to be at 100 to 110 mm Hg to avoid the increased cardiac work natural to higher systolic pressure levels.

ALPHA- AND BETA-ADRENERGIC-RECEPTOR AGONISTS

Epinephrine

The hormone epinephrine is produced in the adrenal medulla and exogenous administration produces the same direct effects on the adrenergic receptors as those that are produced by the endogenous hormone. Epinephrine is described as a biphasic drug. At lower doses within the therapeutic range it causes dilation of the arteries and arterioles by acting at beta$_2$-receptors, but at the higher therapeutic dosage levels it produces alpha-adrenergic effects manifested as vasoconstriction.

Action Mode. Epinephrine has a direct action on the cardiac beta$_1$-receptors that produces a positive chronotropic effect by stimulation of the sinoatrial node and a positive inotropic effect on the myocardium. The increased cardiac output raises the systolic blood pressure. There is an increase in myocardial oxygen consumption consequent to the increased strength of contraction and tachycardia. The net effect of the increased work can be a decrease in cardiac efficiency as well as myocardial irritability. Epinephrine has a direct vasoconstricting effect on the coronary arteries, but the increase in cardiac output elevates the coronary artery blood flow sufficiently to indirectly improve myocardial perfusion.

Epinephrine at usual therapeutic dosage levels acts at the arterial beta$_2$-adrenergic receptors to produce vasodilation (i.e., in skeletal muscles) and the decreased peripheral resistance is reflected in a decrease in the systemic diastolic pressure (Table 13–2). The beta-adrenergic receptors are more sensitive than the alpha-adrenergic receptors to epinephrine. The pressor effect at therapeutic

Table 13–2.
Clinical Manifestations of Vasopressor Drug Action

Adrenergic-Receptor Agonist	Cardiac Contraction		Blood Pressure		Urine Output (Normovolemic)	Cutaneous Blood Flow	Body Temperature	Blood Glucose
	Strength	Rate	Systolic	Diastolic				
Alpha- and beta- agonists								
Ephedrine sulfate	↑	—	↑	↑	↓	↓	↑	—
Epinephrine (ADRENALIN)	↑	↑	↑	↓	↓	↓	↑	↑
Levarterenol bitartrate (LEVOPHED)	↑	↓ (reflex)	↑	↑	↑	↓	↑	↑
Metaraminol bitartrate (ARAMINE)	↑	↓ (reflex)	↑	↑	↑	↓	↑	↑
Beta-agonists								
Isoproterenol hydrochloride (ISUPREL)	↑	↑	↑	↓	— ↓	↑	—	↑
Mephentermine sulfate (WYAMINE)	↑	↓ (reflex)	↑	↑	↑	↓	↑	↑
Mixed agonist								
Dopamine (INTROPIN)	↑	—	↑	—/↑	↑/↓	↓	↑	—
Alpha-agonists								
Methoxamine (VASOXYL)	—	↓ (reflex)	↑	↑	↑	↓	↑	—
Phenylephrine hydrochloride (NEO-SYNEPHRINE)	—	↓ (reflex)	↑	↑	↑	↓	↑	—

↑ = increased   — = unchanged
↓ = decreased

dosage is primarily related to the effects of the drug on cardiac output.

The alpha-adrenergic action of epinephrine constricts the renal vasculature. The vasoconstriction occurs during the time when peripheral resistance in other vascular beds is decreased by vasodilation. Constriction of the renal blood vessels initially decreases the glomerular filtration rate. The output of urine and the excretion of electrolytes (i.e., sodium, chlorides, potassium) may be decreased. Renal filtration gradually improves when blood distribution is equalized by the hemodynamic effects of the drug.

The alpha-adrenergic effect also decreases blood flow by constriction of the arterioles in the skin, mucosa, and viscera. The surface of the extremities may be cold to touch, but the body temperature may be elevated toward normal levels as a consequence of the cutaneous vasoconstriction.

Epinephrine is useful for the treatment of patients with low-output cardiac failure. It also is particularly useful for treatment of the anaphylactic shock state that occurs with acute allergic reactions. The action of epinephrine at beta$_2$-adrenergic receptors in the bronchial smooth muscle dilates the bronchial structures and that action is of primary importance in relieving acute allergic bronchospasm. The drug also acts at alpha-receptors of the bronchial arterioles to produce constriction, and that action antagonizes the action of the potent vasoactive substance *histamine* that is released in allergic reactions.

Therapy Considerations. Epinephrine may be diluted (1 mg/250 ml) for intravenous infusion during therapy for shock. The usual infusion rate is regulated to administer from 0.5 to 5 mcg/minute. Intravenous administration produces an immediate effect on the cardiovascular system, but the effect lasts only as long as the infusion is running. Epinephrine is widely distributed in all body tissues except the brain. It crosses the placenta and appears in the milk of nursing mothers.

The action of epinephrine rapidly is terminated by its uptake and metabolism in the varicosities of the sympathetic postganglionic nerve endings. The circulating drug is metabolized in the blood, liver, nerve endings, and other body tissues by enzymes (i.e., monoamine oxidase, catechol-O-methyltransferase), and the inactive metabolites (i.e., metanephrine and vanillylmandelic acid, or VMA) are excreted in the urine.

Epinephrine may produce hyperglycemia by its action on glycogen stores. It increases glycogenolysis in the liver. The blood glucose levels also are affected by the concurrent action of the drug that reduces glucose uptake by tissues and inhibits the release of insulin from the pancreas. Blood and urine samples may show the presence of glucose during therapy. The drug also causes glycogenolysis in the muscle and lactic acid blood levels may be elevated. The metabolic processes may produce a transient hyperkalemia followed by a prolonged hypokalemia.

Epinephrine also has a calorigenic activity that can increase tissue oxygen consumption up to 30 percent. The metabolism of lipids in adipose tissue during prolonged therapy may cause elevation of blood levels of free fatty acids, cholesterol, phospholipids, and low-density phospholipids.

Adverse Effects. The most important adverse effects during therapy with epinephrine are the cardiac arrhythmias that are caused by the irritability induced by the drug (i.e., premature ventricular contractions, palpitations, sinus tachycardia). Anxiety, tremulousness, tenseness, excitability, or insomnia may occur during therapy. Nausea, vomiting, sweating, pallor, respiratory weakness, and transient apnea also have occurred during therapy with epinephrine.

Interactions. The beta-adrenergic effects on the cardiovascular system may be antagonized by beta-adrenergic-blocking drugs (i.e., propranolol). The tricyclic antidepressant drugs can potentiate the tachycardia induced by epinephrine. Thyroid preparations highly sensitize the heart to the effects of epinephrine.

Ephedrine Sulfate

The drug has effects that are similar to those of epinephrine but it is longer acting. It also has a more prominent central nervous system stimulant effect than does epinephrine.

Action Mode. Ephedrine sulfate stimulates the beta$_1$-adrenergic receptors of the heart to produce a positive inotropic effect. The drug increases the strength of contraction without increasing the cardiac rate. The effect on the heart may be the primary reason for the pressor effect of ephedrine when the venous return is adequate.

The vasoconstriction caused by the drug is due to a direct action on the alpha-adrenergic receptors and to an indirect action caused by release of norepinephrine from its storage sites. The combination of increased cardiac output and increased peripheral vascular resistance raises the systolic blood pressure and it usually raises the diastolic pressure (Table 13–2). The drug possesses some of the biphasic quality of epinephrine.

There can be vasodilation produced by its action at arterial beta$_2$-adrenergic receptors and a concurrent action at alpha-receptors that causes vasoconstriction in selected vascular sites.

Ephedrine acts at beta-receptors on the arterioles in the skeletal muscle to produce vasodilation. Concurrent alpha-adrenergic stimulation of the arterioles in the skin, mucosa, and viscera causes constriction of the capacitance and resistance vessels. The constriction of postcapillary sphincters holds fluid in the capillary beds, and the increase in interstitial fluid may be accompanied by a decrease in circulating plasma volume.

Constriction of the renal arteries decreases the blood flow and thereby slows the glomerular filtration rate. There is a consequent decrease in the amount of urine output and in the excretion of electrolytes.

Ephedrine sulfate is employed for the treatment of shock and is used intermittently during administration of spinal anesthesia. The alpha- and beta-adrenergic effects of ephedrine counteract the initial hypotension associated with the injection of the anesthetic. The temporary effects are useful until the circulating plasma volume can be augmented.

Therapy Considerations. Ephedrine sulfate usually is administered as a subcutaneous or intramuscular injection. It may be given slowly as an intravenous injection (10 to 25 mg), and an additional dose of the drug may be injected in five to ten minutes. A period of one hour is required for the pressor response to be at a peak level. The maximum dosage for a 24-hour period is 150 mg. The dosage for children is 3 mg/kg of body weight or 100 mg/M^2 of body surface area. That total calculated dosage is divided and administered at four-to-six-hour intervals. Tolerance to the cardiac and pressor effects can develop rapidly with frequent use of the drug. The indirect action of ephedrine depletes the sympathetic nerve endings of the norepinephrine that is required for the therapeutic effects.

Ephedrine relaxes the smooth muscle of the gastrointestinal tract, and constipation or gaseous distention may be problematic during therapy.

The drug also contracts the urinary bladder trigone and sphincter and it relaxes the detrusor muscle. Urinary retention can occur with continued administration of the drug. There is some hepatic glycogenolysis with ephedrine therapy. Although the metabolic activity is less than that of epinephrine, there may be some hyperglycemia.

The drug is metabolized in the liver, and the unchanged drug or its metabolites are excreted in the urine. The excretion is pH dependent and excretion is slower as the urine becomes more alkaline. The elimination half-life of the drug is three hours in a urine with pH 5, but the half-life is doubled (six hours) at pH 6.3.

Adverse Effects. Cardiac irritability is the most important adverse effect, and there may be palpitations, tachycardia, or extrasystoles. There also can be manifestations of central nervous system stimulation (i.e., nervousness, anxiety, tension, agitation, excitability, talkativeness, insomnia). The problems are more profound with large parenteral doses of the drug (i.e., confusion, delirium, euphoria, hallucinations).

Throbbing headache, respiratory distress, fever, feeling of warmth, dry mouth and throat, precordial pain, and gastric disturbances (i.e., mild epigastric distress, anorexia, nausea, vomiting) may occur during therapy with ephedrine. High doses of the drug can cause acute urinary retention in elderly patients.

Interactions. Concurrent use of alpha-adrenergic-blocking drugs (i.e., phentolamine mesylate) can antagonize the pressor effect and lead to vasodilation. Beta$_1$-adrenergic-blocking drugs (i.e., propranolol) interfere with the cardiac stimulation effects of ephedrine.

The increased levels of norepinephrine at sympathetic nerve endings that are caused by monoamine oxidase inhibitors or tricyclic antidepressants can potentiate the pressor effects of ephedrine. Conversely, drugs that decrease the amount of norepinephrine in nerve endings (i.e., reserpine, methyldopa) may antagonize the pressor effects of ephedrine. Concurrent use of oxytocic drugs may cause severe sustained hypertension, and intracranial hemorrhage may occur during the postpartum period.

Levarterenol Bitartrate

Action Mode. The drug is identical to the endogenous catecholamine *norepinephrine* that is the natural neurotransmitter substance released by the sympathetic postganglion neuron. The drug has a direct beta₁-adrenergic activity that causes cardiac stimulation. It has a potent positive inotropic effect on the myocardium, and its action on the sinoatrial node produces a positive chronotropic effect. The beta-adrenergic effects are less intense than those of epinephrine or isoproterenol. The increased strength and rate of myocardial contraction increase the cardiac work and oxygen consumption and may decrease its efficiency. The chronotropic effects can be overcome by the increased vagal activity that occurs as a reflex response when the arterial pressure is increased. When the blood pressure is elevated toward normal levels, a reflex bradycardia occurs. The slower heart rate counteracts the positive effects on stroke volume natural to an increased strength of cardiac contraction, and the cardiac output may remain unchanged.

Levarterenol is a potent constrictor of the capacitance and resistance vessels. It acts at alpha-adrenergic receptors to increase the total peripheral resistance. The combined cardiac and vascular effects increase the systemic systolic and diastolic blood pressure (Table 13–2). Alpha-adrenergic receptors are less numerous in cerebral and coronary blood vessels, and the generalized vasoconstriction shifts blood flow from the skin, muscle, splanchnic, and renal vascular beds to the heart and brain.

The vasoconstriction in surface tissues combined with the increased oxygen consumption caused by the drug elevates the body temperature toward normal levels. Constriction of the renal blood vessels decreases the glomerular filtration rate. There is an initial decrease in the production of urine and excretion of electrolytes, but the renal blood flow increases as the blood pressure

rises toward normal levels in the normovolemic patient.

Prolonged administration of levarterenol may maintain the peripheral resistance at a level that decreases venous return to the heart and lowers the cardiac output. The basic cause of the decrease in circulating volume is loss of fluid into the interstitial spaces as a consequence of postcapillary vasoconstriction.

Levarterenol is considered to be a reliable drug for altering the blood distribution to the heart and brain in the emergency treatment of severe hypotension. Individuals with low pressure as a consequence of *cardiac failure* or *peripheral vascular failure* are benefited by the rapid reestablishment of hemodynamic parameters effected by the drug.

Therapy Considerations. The drug usually is administered as a diluted solution (i.e., 4 mcg/ml) by intravenous infusion. An infusion pump often is employed to maintain the flow rate after the initial period of continual titration of the drug flow rate with the blood pressure levels. The drug is so potent that its pressor effects must be monitored continuously.

The initial dosage for adults is 8 to 12 mcg/minute and the pediatric dosage is 2 mcg/M²/minute. The patient's blood pressure is taken every two minutes until it is stabilized at the desired level (i.e., 80 to 100/mm/Hg systolic), and the pressure then is taken every five minutes. The effects of the drug are evident almost immediately, but the pressor effect ceases within one to two minutes after the infusion is discontinued. At termination of therapy the drug dosage is reduced gradually. The dilution of the drug may be increased or the infusion rate may be reduced while the patient's blood pressure is monitored closely. The intravenous setup usually is left at the bedside for a short period of time to allow restarting of the infusion if the systemic blood pressure drops to 70 to 80 mm Hg. The problems with "weaning" the patient from the drug may be related to the postcapillary constriction that retains fluid in the interstitial spaces and decreases the intravascular plasma volume.

Extravasation of levarterenol into the tissues causes a local alpha-adrenergic-receptor–mediated vasoconstriction, and tissue necrosis can occur. The seriousness of the problem makes it mandatory to inspect the infusion site frequently, and to use the larger deep veins for the infusion. In some clinical trials, phentolamine mesylate (10 mg) is being added to the intravenous infusion to provide alpha-adrenergic blocking and decrease the tissue sloughing when levarterenol inadvertently infiltrates into the perivenous tissues.

A diluted solution of phentolamine mesylate may be infiltrated liberally into the cold, hard, pallid subcutaneous tissues where levarterenol has caused vasoconstriction. The subcutaneous injection can reverse the adverse effects on the local tissues only if it is used within 12 hours after the incident.

The circulating levarterenol primarily is distributed in sympathetic nerve tissues. The drug crosses the placenta. The effects of the drug are terminated by its uptake in sympathetic nerve endings, but the circulating drug is metabolized in the liver and other tissues by enzymes (i.e., catechol-O-methyltransferase, monoamine oxidase). The inactive metabolites (i.e., normetanephrine and vanillylmandelic acid) are excreted in the urine.

Hyperglycemia occurs as a consequence of levarterenol-induced glycogenolysis and the inhibition of insulin release from the pancreas. The blood sugar levels are less affected than they are during therapy with epinephrine. Elevation of the blood level of lactic acid is associated with the direct metabolic effects of levarterenol and the glycogenolysis resulting from decreased tissue perfusion. Increased lipolysis in adipose tissue also may increase the blood levels of free fatty acids and cholesterol.

Adverse Effects.   Ventricular irritability is the primary problem during therapy (i.e., ventricular tachycardia, ventricular fibrillation, palpitations, bradycardia). Restlessness, headache, tremor, anxiety, and insomnia occur in some patients, but the incidence is less than during therapy with epinephrine. Some patients have symptoms of hyper-

sensitivity to the effects of the drug (i.e., photophobia, intense sweating, vomiting, retrosternal or pharyngeal pain, severe hypertension, convulsions).

Interactions.   Anticholinergic drugs (i.e., atropine sulfate) can block the reflex bradycardia and enhance the pressor effects of levarterenol. The effects of the drug can be potentiated by the tricyclic antidepressants (i.e., imipramine), antihistamines (i.e., diphenhydramine, tripelennamine, dexchlorpheniramine), parenteral ergot alkaloids, guanethidine, methyldopa, or monoamine oxidase inhibitors. Concurrent use of the drugs can cause severe prolonged hypertension.

Metaraminol Bitartrate

The drug is classified as a direct- and indirect-acting sympathomimetic. It releases norepinephrine from its storage sites and that action leads to drug effects similar to those of the natural endogenous catecholamine or to those of levarterenol bitartrate. Metaraminol bitartrate has a longer duration of action than levarterenol but it has a less potent vasoconstriction action.

Action Mode.   Metaraminol stimulation of the cardiac beta$_1$-adrenergic receptors produces a positive inotropic effect on the myocardium. The chronotropic effect that is mediated through its action on the sinoatrial node is overcome by the increased vagal activity that is associated with the increase in arterial blood pressure. Bradycardia occurs as the pressure rises toward normal levels (Table 13-2). The initial inotropic effect in the hypotensive patient may increase the cardiac output and contribute to the pressor effects of the drug. The positive inotropic effects increase cardiac oxygen consumption and it may decrease cardiac efficiency.

Metaraminol releases norepinephrine from its storage sites in the varicosities of the sympathetic postganglionic neuron. It also may replace norepinephrine in the nerve endings and function as a false neurotransmitter. The drug also acts directly on the alpha-adrenergic receptors to cause constriction of capacitance and resistance blood vessels. The total peripheral resistance is increased and the systolic and diastolic blood pressures are elevated.

The vasoconstriction reduces the blood flow to the vital organs, skeletal muscle, and skin. The constriction of the pulmonary vasculature causes an elevation of the pulmonary arterial pressure even when the cardiac output is unchanged. Constriction of the renal blood vessels decreases the glomerular filtration rate during the early period of drug administration. The renal blood flow increases when the systemic blood pressure is elevated toward the normal level, and the output of urine and excretion of electrolytes are increased.

Therapy Considerations. Metaraminol may be diluted in an intravenous solution (15 to 100 mg/500 ml solution) for continuous infusion. The larger veins of the antecubital fossa or the thigh were usually employed to decrease the hazard of infiltration from the smaller veins. Infusion of the drug produces an effect on the cardiovascular system in one to two minutes. The drug also may be administered slowly as a bolus intravenous injection. The adult dosage is 0.5 to 5 mg and that for children is 10 mcg/kg of body weight or 300 mcg/M^2 body surface area.

Subsequent dosage may be administered subcutaneously or intramuscularly to adults (2 to 10 mg) or to children (100 mcg/kg or 3 mg/M^2). The blood pressure is taken at least ten minutes before each dose is administered parenterally. The pressor effect of the subcutaneous drug occurs in about 5 to 20 minutes and that of the intramuscular drug in ten minutes. The pressor effects persist for 20 to 60 minutes.

The same problems with maintaining the blood pressure at termination of therapy that occur with levarterenol are found with metaraminol. It is usual for the drug to be withdrawn gradually to allow observation of the hemodynamic status. After long periods of therapy with metaraminol, the return of hemodynamic equilibrium may be adversely affected by the impaired function of the adrenergic nerve that is caused by the depletion of norepinephrine stores.

Metaraminol has an action on glycogen stores that is similar to that of levarterenol. Plasma levels of glucose may be elevated by glycogenolysis, and the lipid levels are elevated by the lipolysis caused by the drug.

Adverse Effects. Most of the adverse effects and the drug interactions that occur during therapy are similar to, but more persistent than, those occurring when levarterenol is administered. Metaraminol produces fewer signs of cardiac irritability than levarterenol, but palpitations and bradycardia can occur. Large doses of the drug may produce signs of cardiac irritability (i.e., sinus or ventricular tachycardia, premature contractions). Central nervous system stimulation is unusual during therapy, but there occasionally can be evidence of apprehension, tremor, or anxiety. Precordial pain, respiratory distress, flushing, pallor, sweating, and nausea also occur during therapy with metaraminol.

Prolonged administration may deplete plasma volume by the postcapillary vasoconstriction that causes fluid accumulation in the interstitial spaces. The decreased circulating plasma volume can perpetuate the shock state or cause the recurrence of hypotension at termination of therapy. The depletion of norepinephrine in the sympathetic nerve endings also can cause tachycardia during prolonged therapy with metaraminol.

BETA-ADRENERGIC-RECEPTOR AGONISTS

Isoproterenol Hydrochloride

The drug is a synthetic sympathomimetic with strong specificity for beta-adrenergic receptors. It is one of the least potent vasoconstrictors. Isoproterenol produces an increase in cardiac output and peripheral dilation that is useful in redistributing the blood flow of patients with an adequate plasma volume.

Action Mode. Isoproterenol has a direct effect on the cardiac beta$_1$-adrenergic receptors of the sinoatrial and atrioventricular node that produces a positive chronotropic effect. The drug also produces an inotropic effect through its action on the myocardial tissue. The increased strength and rate of cardiac contraction increase myocardial oxygen consumption and decrease cardiac efficiency. The increase in coronary blood flow that is caused by the vasodilating action of the drug may not increase the blood supply to a level adequate for the increased oxygen demands. The drug is used with discrimination for individuals with known coronary artery insufficiency or myocardial hypoxia.

The drug has a direct beta$_2$-adrenergic action that dilates arteries and arterioles in skeletal, mesenteric, intestinal, pulmonary, and femoral vascular beds. That increased perfusion rate reduces the size of the capacitance bed and increases the venous blood flow to the heart. The combined effects of increased venous flow (preload), inotropic and chronotropic effects, and reduced arterial resistance (afterload) contribute to an increased cardiac output. Isoproterenol increases the arteriovenous shunting at the capillary beds and that effect may somewhat lessen the positive effects of the blood flow which has been increased to tissues.

The beta$_2$-adrenergic action is particularly prominent in the mesenteric and skeletal muscle beds, and that widespread dilation accounts for much of the decrease in peripheral resistance that is reflected in the lower diastolic blood pressure (Table 13–2). The drug also relaxes the smooth muscle of the bronchus, gastrointestinal tract, and uterus. Tolerance to both the cardiac and bronchodilator effects occurs with prolonged use of the drug. The vasodilation at renal sites usually has little effect on urine production. The generalized vasodilation and increased cardiac work increase the metabolic rate and raise the tissue oxygen requirements during therapy.

The drug is employed as an intravenous infusion to treat patients with sufficient blood flow to perfuse the brain and heart but insufficient flow to adequately perfuse visceral organs. Improvement in the blood circulation can decrease the central venous pressure enough to allow the addition of fluids to augment the circulating plasma volume.

Therapy Considerations. The usual initial intravenous dosage of isoproterenol is 0.5 to 5 mcg/minute, but in acute situations up to 30 mcg/minute may be infused. The infusion solution usually contains an adequate amount of the drug (i.e., 2 mcg/ml) to allow regulation of the drip rate as the hemodynamic parameters change. The flow rate is titrated with changes in the electrocardiogram, heart rate, central venous pressure, systemic blood pressure, and urine flow. When the cardiac rate exceeds 110 beats/minute or premature ventricular contractions occur, the drip rate of the infusion is slowed.

The action of isoproterenol is terminated rapidly by its uptake in the terminal adrenergic nerve tissues. The circulating drug is metabolized by the enzymes (i.e., catechol-O-methyl transferase) in the liver, lungs, and other body tissues. The major metabolite (3-O-methylisoproterenol) has weak beta-adrenergic-blocking activity. That active metabolite and drug conjugates are eliminated in the urine.

Isoproterenol increases the rate of glycogenolysis at hepatic sites, and it stimulates insulin secretion from the pancreas. There is less hyperglycemia with the administration of isoproterenol than there is with epinephrine. There may be an increase in plasma levels of free fatty acids. The drug also has calorigenic activity, and the increased oxygen demands of the tissues may not be met by the increased blood flow. The increase in aerobic metabolism can cause elevation of the lactic acid levels in the plasma.

Adverse Effects. Isoproterenol accelerates the spontaneous depolarization of myocardial cells, and there may be evidence of ventricular irritability (i.e., ventricular tachycardia, ventricular fibrillation, palpitations). Serious adverse effects occur infrequently. Some patients may have symptoms of central nervous system stimulation (i.e., nervousness, excitability, insomnia, tremor).

Lowering of the blood pressure at the time when the heart is stimulated by isoproterenol action may increase myocardial ischemia. Arrhythmias occur frequently when the drug is administered to patients with myocardial damage.

Interactions. Concurrent administration of beta-adrenergic-blocking agents (i.e., propranolol) antagonizes the action of the drug. There may be a marked decrease in the cardiac stimulation, vasodilation, and bronchodilation effects of the drugs when the beta-blocking agents are administered to the patient receiving isoproterenol.

Mephentermine Sulfate

Action Mode. Mephentermine sulfate has an indirect adrenergic action by displacing the norepinephrine from storage sites in the varicosities of the sympathetic postganglionic neuron. The drug action produces cardiac stimulation and vasoconstriction. Its positive chronotropic effect on the heart raises the systolic blood pressure, and it produces enough vasoconstriction to raise the diastolic blood pressure (Table 13–2).

Therapy Considerations. Slow intravenous injection of a bolus of the drug solution (15 to 30 mg) produces an immediate pressor effect that lasts for 30 to 45 minutes. The drug is only one one-hundredth as potent as epinephrine, but it has three to five times the duration of action of that drug. The drug may initially be administered intravenously and subsequent doses may be injected intramuscularly. Injection by that route produces a pressor effect in 15 minutes that lasts for one to two hours.

Adverse Effects. The primary undesired effect is central nervous system stimulation. The problems range from anxiety and euphoria to convulsions.

MIXED-ADRENERGIC-RECEPTOR AGONIST

Dopamine

The drug is similar to the natural endogenous catecholamine that is the immediate precursor in the synthesis of norepinephrine. Dopamine is a biphasic drug that produces an increase in cardiac output and renal blood flow at low dosage levels. At higher dosage the effects of alpha-adrenergic action on the vasculature predominate and vasoconstriction occurs.

Action Mode. Dopamine primarily is a direct beta-adrenergic agonist. It acts at cardiac receptors to produce a positive inotropic action. The increase in myocardial contraction may produce a 200 percent increase in cardiac force, which is similar to that occurring during therapy with epinephrine, levarterenol, or isoproterenol. The greater cardiac output raises the systolic blood pressure level (Table 13–2).

Dopamine has a direct action on the adrenergic receptors and it also has an indirect effect by releasing norepinephrine from its storage sites. The administration of the drug at the low dosage level of 1 to 10 mcg stimulates the beta$_2$-adrenergic receptors, and there is dilation of the coronary and visceral blood vessels. Although the systolic and pulse pressures increase, the diastolic blood pressure may remain unchanged or only slightly elevated.

The drug acts at dopaminergic receptors in the mesenteric and renal vasculature to produce dilation of those blood vessels. The renal blood flow may increase to eight times the pretreatment level, with a commensurate increase in the glomerular filtration rate.

Dopamine acts on the arterial alpha-receptors when it is administered at dosage levels between 10 and 20 mcg. The higher drug level (20 mcg) produces vascular constriction and a consequent elevation of the diastolic blood pressure. The vasoconstriction affects the capacitance and resistance vessels in most peripheral vascular beds, but vasodilation occurs in the mesenteric and renal vasculature.

Therapy Considerations. Dopamine may be infused intravenously as a diluted solution (i.e., 400 to 800 mcg/ml). The initial dosage usually is 2 to 5 mcg/kg of body weight per minute. The dosage may be increased by 5 to 10 mcg/kg/minute at 10-to-30-minute intervals to attain the desired tissue perfusion. The decision to modify the intravenous flow rate is based on the amount of urine output and the systemic blood pressure level. The pressure can be maintained effectively on doses of 20 mcg/kg/min or less in 50 percent of the patients.

Dopamine is most effective when administered early in shock. The drug action may lead to the production of urine in patients who are oliguric or anuric. As therapy continues, the urine output may be raised to normal levels. The increase in urine output is accompanied by the excretion of sodium and that may reduce preexisting fluid accumulation. The urine output must be monitored closely to assure that the dosage of dopamine is below that causing renal vasoconstriction.

The onset of drug effect occurs within five minutes when the drug is administered intravenously and the effect lasts only ten minutes after the infusion is terminated. The drug is widely distributed in body tissues. Seventy-five percent of the drug is metabolized by enzymes (i.e., monoamine oxidase, catechol-O-methyltransferase) in the liver, kidneys, or plasma to inactive metabolites (i.e., homovanillic acid). The remainder of the drug is metabolized to norepinephrine within the adrenergic nerve varicosities. The inactive metabolites are excreted in the urine.

Adverse Effects. Tachyarrhythmias occur less frequently during administration of dopamine than with epinephrine, levarterenol, or isoproterenol. The most frequent adverse effects are ectopic beats, nausea, and vomiting. Anginal pain, palpitations, dyspnea, and headache also occur during therapy with dopamine. Extravasation of the drug from the vein can cause necrosis of the tissues. Phentolamine may be infiltrated, in the manner previously discussed, to prevent the tissue injury.

Interactions. Concurrent administration of a monoamine oxidase inhibitor may necessitate a 10 percent reduction in dosage. The increased norepinephrine that is available can intensify the dopamine effects and prolong the duration from ten minutes to one hour.

The cardiac effects of the drug are antagonized by beta-adrenergic-blocking drugs. The peripheral vasoconstriction can be antagonized by alpha-adrenergic-blocking drugs. The effects of the drug on dopaminergic receptors in the mesenteric, renal, coronary, and cerebral tissues are antagonized by haloperidol and the phenothiazines, which block the dopaminergic receptors in those tissues.

ALPHA-ADRENERGIC-RECEPTOR AGONISTS

Phenylephrine Hydrochloride

Action Mode. The drug is a specific alpha-adrenergic agonist without beta-adrenergic activity at therapeutic dosage levels. It also acts indirectly by releasing norepinephrine from storage sites. The primary effect of phenylephrine is vasoconstriction of resistance vessels. The drug has a lesser effect on the capacitance vessels. The increased total peripheral resistance elevates the systolic and diastolic blood pressures (Table 13–2).

The increased peripheral vascular resistance also provides the stimulus for increased vagus nerve activity. Bradycardia is associated with the reflex vagal stimulation, and while the stroke volume increases, the cardiac output may decrease slightly. The increase in peripheral arterial resistance in the absence of an increased contractile force increases the work of the left ventricle and there may be a consequent elevation of atrial pressures.

The arterial alpha-adrenergic stimulation causes vasoconstriction in the vascular beds of the vital organs, skin, and skeletal muscle. The constriction of renal arteries decreases the glomerular filtration rate, and the urine output volume is low during the initial hours of therapy. When the blood pressure levels are elevated toward normal in the normovolemic patient, the urine flow is greater.

Therapy Considerations. The drug may be diluted for intravenous infusion. The initial infusion rate ranges from 100 to 180 mcg/minute and adjustments are made as the desired pressor response occurs. The drug also is given by injection of an intravenous bolus (i.e., 100 to 500 mcg) and the dosage may be repeated every 15 minutes. Subsequent administration may be planned by the use of intramuscular injections (i.e., 1 to 10 mg). The dosage for children is based on the calculation of 100 mcg/kg of body weight or 3 mg/M² body surface area.

Intravenous infusion produces a pressor effect immediately, which lasts from 15 to 20 minutes after the infusion is discontinued. Intramuscular administration of 5 mg produces an effect in 10 to 15 minutes that lasts one or two hours.

The effects of the drug are terminated partially by tissue uptake. The circulating drug is metabolized by monoamine oxidase at hepatic sites.

Adverse Effects. Severe reflex bradycardia with transient heart block can occur as the blood pressure rises, and ventricular arrhythmias may be precipitated. Adverse effects also include precordial pain, respiratory distress, pallor, and pilomotor response. Paresthesias and coolness may occur in the extremities that are used for injection of the drug.

Interactions. The pressor effects of the drug may be antagonized by the prior use of alpha-adrenergic-blocking drugs (i.e., phentolamine mesylate) or by drugs with alpha-blocking properties (i.e., phenothiazines). Atropine sulfate blocks the reflex bradycardia and enhances the pressor effects of phenylephrine. The pressor effects may be potentiated by the concurrent use of monoamine oxidase inhibitors, tricyclic antidepressants, or guanethedine, or the parenteral administration of ergot alkaloids.

Methoxamine Hydrochloride

The action mode and effects of methoxamine are similar to those of phenylephrine. The drug action on alpha-adrenergic receptors also produces the same evidence of hemodynamic changes (Table 13–2).

Therapy Considerations. Methoxamine may be diluted and slowly injected as an intravenous bolus in emergency situations. The usual adult dosage ranges from 3 to 5 mg, and the dosage for children is 80 mcg/kg of body weight or 2.5 mg/M² body surface area. Intravenous infusion or intramuscular injection of methoxamine may be planned to maintain the pressor response after the initial intravenous injection.

The intramuscular dosage for adults ranges from 10 to 15 mg, and the dosage for children is based on the calculation of 250 mcg/kg or 7.5 mg/M². At termination of therapy the drug dosage is reduced gradually and the blood pressure is monitored to assure that the levels remain elevated. Drug administration may be resumed if the blood pressure falls to 70 or 80 mm Hg.

Adverse Effects. Most of the adverse effects and interactions during therapy with methoxamine are similar to those found with the administration of phenylephrine. Large doses of methoxamine can cause urinary frequency, pilomotor stimulation response, projectile vomiting, and headache associated with excess blood pressure elevation.

Hydroxyamphetamine Hydrobromide
(PAREDINE)

Action Mode. The drug is a sympathomimetic amine that indirectly stimulates both the alpha- and beta-adrenergic receptors by releasing the catecholamine stores. The pressor effect is useful for temporary relief of postural hypotension in selected situations. For example, it may be employed for the control of postural hypotension when patients have heart block that cannot be effectively treated with an electronic pacemaker.

Therapy Considerations. The drug is taken orally. The 20-to-60-mg dose may be repeated three or four times or more during a 24-hour period as it is required for the control of the postural hypotension. The person should be cautioned that the effective doses used in the standing position may produce excessive blood pressure elevation when in a recumbent position.

Adverse Effects. Ventricular arrhythmias, palpitation, precordial pain, and marked hypertension can occur. The central nervous system stimulation effects of the drug may produce dizziness, restlessness, tremor, and headache. Gastrointestinal disturbances (i.e., nausea, dryness of the mouth, diarrhea) have also been reported.

NURSING INTERVENTION

The recognition and interpretation of changes in the cardiovascular status of the patient are important in early identification of shock. The regularly planned assessment of the patient can provide the initial clues to the effects of circulatory changes on body systems.

Initial Status Assessment

The vital signs are taken on a regularly scheduled, round-the-clock basis for all acutely ill patients, and therapeutic measures are implemented when those measurements indicate that there is an intercurrent medical problem. The basic disease process provides the framework for the monitoring of specific body systems for changes. For example, the postoperative patient's surgical dressing is examined frequently for evidence of bleeding or the urine is tested regularly for glucose content when the patient is a diabetic.

The compensatory sympathetic nervous system activity may mask the initial changes in the cardiovascular status that occur in shock. The objective measurements usually employed in monitoring acutely ill patients can remain within normal limits in the presence of hemodynamic imbalance. For example, the heart rate and the systolic blood pressure may be maintained by the activity of the norepinephrine, released at cardiac receptors. The diastolic blood pressure also may be maintained by the neural activity that initially causes constriction of the blood vessels of the skin, mucosa, renal, and mesenteric tissues. Discernible changes in the cardiovascular parameters sometimes can be determined by careful comparison of the measurements with previous recordings of the patient's blood pressure and the rate, strength, and regularity of the pulse.

Recognition of the early signs of shock makes it necessary to add to the standardized monitoring guides the directives to observe the patient for the *existence of increased sympathetic nerve activity* and the *adequacy of tissue perfusion*. The earliest physiologic changes in shock can be insidious and vague.

The shock-monitoring guidelines should be prefaced with a suggestion that the nurse listen carefully to the patient's statement that "something is wrong but I can't quite explain it." The same uneasiness about an inexplicable and unmeasurable change can enter the nurse's perceptions as she interacts with the patient. It often has proven advantageous for the nurse, who has only an intuitive clue that something is awry, to share that concern with the staff. It is usual for the nurses then to intensify their monitoring of the patient. The frequent assessment has been a factor in the identification of subsequent measurable changes in the patient's status.

Prompt discussion of the changes in the patient's status with the physician can lead to institution of treatment before the hemodynamic imbalance jeopardizes tissue function. Shock is a complex phenomenon, and once it is established, the patient's life is threatened.

The decreased circulation of blood to the skin and mucous membranes may cause pallor of those tissues that sometimes is identifiable. Many acutely ill patients have some dryness and paleness of the skin, tongue, and buccal tissues and changes are difficult to quantify. Coolness of the skin surface may provide the clue to more extensive problems with the redistribution of blood flow. Palpitation of the large arteries (i.e., carotids, femorals) can provide a fairly reliable estimate of the volume and pressure of the blood in the circulation. The smaller radial artery is less reliable as an indicator of the mean arterial pressure.

The two organ systems allowing fairly reliable assessment of blood perfusion are the kidneys and the brain. A decreased urine output may be the earliest indicator of the redistribution of blood during the sympathetic nerve–induced compensatory phase of blood distribution problems. When the patient has a urinary catheter in place, the collection receptacle can be changed to a small graduated container that allows more accurate measurement of the hourly urine output. When renal perfusion is questionable, a urinary catheter provides the only method for accurately measuring the urine output, which is an indicator of that perfusion.

Changes in blood flow to cerebral tissues may occur after there is evidence of inadequate renal perfusion because cerebral autoregulation maintains the blood flow until pressures are relatively low. Renal perfusion is marginal when the blood pressure drops to 70 mm Hg, but cerebral tissues can maintain perfusion until the mean pressure drops below 60 mm Hg. Underperfusion of the cerebral tissues is manifested by confusion, slow responses to questions, disorientation, drowsiness, or anxiety.

Assessing Progress

The initial status assessment can provide information about the onset of preshock perfusion problems, and those same parameters are monitored during therapy for shock. The treatment of coexisting problems (i.e., electrolyte,

acid-base, or fluid imbalances) concurrent with the administration of antihypotensive drugs requires continual assessment of the patient's status. Changes in the patient's hemodynamic parameters may necessitate modifications in the pressor drug regimen or in other therapies.

The administration of antihypotensive drugs requires continual monitoring of the patient's heart rate and blood pressure levels. Each of the drugs that provide a positive inotropic or chronotropic effect on the heart as part of their therapeutic action also can cause cardiac irritability. A cardiac monitor usually is employed to monitor the rhythm patterns. Myocardial irritability is relatively common, and the onset of ventricular arrhythmias may necessitate discontinuing the use of the particular pressor drug.

The drugs that primarily affect alpha–adrenergic receptors at vascular sites can cause sudden, life-threatening hypertension if they inadvertently are infused rapidly. It is usual to use a reliable regulating pump to control the infusion rate. In the absence of such a devise, placing an extra screw-type clamp on the tubing provides a safety device to protect against rapid infusion of the drug during position changes or the loosening of a single clamp.

The intensity of therapy frequently requires the presence of several health team members (i.e., nurses, inhalation therapists, physicians, laboratory technicians, consultants). It is important to have their efforts coordinated to provide an optimal amount of contact time, but it also is important to provide for the comfort and rest needs of the patient. The simplest position changes will require the assistance of at least one other person when the machines and other life support equipment are utilized for treatment of the patient in shock.

Review Guides

1. Formulate a plan for monitoring the status of a patient in shock who is receiving (1) *epinephrine*, (2) *levarterenol*, (3) *isoproterenol*, (4) *dopamine*.
2. On each of the four nursing plans identify the following:
   a. How the drug acts to produce the planned therapeutic effect.
   b. Specific measures that would be employed to monitor the therapeutic effects on the patient's hemodynamic status.
   c. Adverse effects that are related to the adrenergic action of the drug.
   d. Drug interactions that are related to the adrenergic action of the drug.

Additional Readings

Adams, Nancy R.: Reducing the perils of intracardiac monitoring. *Nursing 76,* **6:**66, April, 1976.

Ahlquist, Raymond P.: Present state of alpha- and beta-adrenergic drugs. 1. The adrenergic receptor. *Am. Heart J.,* **92:**661, November, 1976.

Alexander, Carl S.: Sako, Yoshio; and Mikulic, Esteban: Pedal gangrene associated with the use of dopamine. *N. Engl. J. Med.,* **293:**591, September 18, 1975.

Begley, Linda A.: External counterpulsation in cardiogenic shock. *Am. J. Nurs.,* **75:**967, June, 1975.

Boyd, Jeanette M. Loughrie: Understanding and treating cardiogenic shock. *R.N.,* **38:**53, April, 1975.

Dipalma, Joseph R.: Dopamine: new uses for an old drug. *Am. Fam. Physician,* **11:**149, April, 1975.

Eckhardt, Erica: Intra-aortic balloon counterpulsation in cardiogenic shock. *Heart Lung,* **6:**93, January–February, 1977.

Evans, Roger W.: Cardiogenic shock: can the prognosis be improved? *Postgrad. Med.,* **58:**79, December, 1975.

Forrester, James S.; Diamond, George; Chatterjee, Kanu; and Swan, H. J. C.: Hemodynamic therapy of myocardial infarction. *N. Engl. J. Med.,* **295:**1356, December 9, 1976.

Fritz, S. Delbert: Energy metabolism in shock. *Heart Lung,* **4:**615, July–August, 1975.

Ibrahim, M. Mohsen; Tarazi, Robert C.; and Dustan, Harriet P.: Orthostatic hypotension: mechanisms and management. *Am. Heart J.,* **90:**513, October, 1975.

Jahre, Jeffrey A.; Grace, William J.; Greenbaum, Dennis M.; and Sarg, Michael J., Jr.: Medical approach to the hypotensive patient and the patient in shock. *Heart Lung,* **4:**577, July–August, 1975.

Moyer, John H., and Mills, Lewis C.: Vasopressor agents in shock. *Am. J. Nurs.,* **75:**620, April, 1975.

Niazi, Ziad; Beckman, Charles; Shatney, Clayton; and Lillehei, Richard C.: Use of monitoring to improve survival in shock. *Geriatrics,* **30:**93, July, 1975.

Pawlik, Wieslaw; Mailman, David; Shanbour, Linda L.; and Jacobson, Eugene D.: Dopamine effects on the intestinal circulation. *Am. Heart J.,* **91:**325, March, 1976.

Roach, Lora B.: Color changes in dark skin. *Nursing 77,* **7:**48, January, 1977.

Roberts, Sharon L.: Skin assessment for color and temperature. *Am. J. Nurs.,* **75:**610, April, 1975.

Robie, Norman W., and Goldberg, Leon I.: Comparative systemic and regional hemodynamic effects of dopamine and dobutamine. *Am. Heart J.,* **90:**340, September, 1975.

Schumer, William: Metabolism during shock and sepsis. *Heart Lung,* **5:**416, May–June, 1976.

Shubin, Herbert, and Weil, Max Harry: Bacterial shock. *J.A.M.A.,* **235:**421, January 26, 1976.

Théroux, P.; Mizgala, H. F.; and Bourassa, M. G.: Hemodynamics and therapeutics of intravenous dopamine. *Can. Med. Assoc. J.,* **116:**645, March 19, 1977.

Weil, Max H.; Shubin, Herbert; and Carlson, Richard: Treatment of circulatory shock. *J.A.M.A.,* **231:**1280, March 24, 1975.

Wilson, Robert F.: Endocrine changes in sepsis. *Heart Lung,* **5:**411, May–June, 1976.

Wilson, Robert F.: The diagnosis and management of severe sepsis and septic shock. *Heart Lung,* **5:**422, May–June, 1976.

14

Sequestered Body Fluids

Intricate interactions between the hemodynamic, hormonal, and renal mechanisms maintain the physiologic fluid balance required for cellular function. Changes in the volume or electrolyte content of circulating plasma can be modified by the interacting factors that maintain fluid equilibrium.

Physiologic Correlations

FLUID EQUILIBRIUM

The normal hydrostatic colloidal osmotic pressures of the circulating plasma influence the outward movement of fluid at the tissue capillary beds. The pressure of the blood that enters the capillary circulation from the arterioles (25 mm Hg) provides a potential driving force for movement of fluids from the capillaries into the interstitial spaces. That "outward" driving force is modified by the "holding" pressure of the colloids (28 mm Hg) in the plasma (i.e., red and white blood cells, albumin, globulins).

The colloid and electrolyte content of the interstitial fluids is the factor that controls the natural movement of plasma fluid from the vasculature to maintain extracellular fluid equilibrium. Concurrent diffusion of solutes across the semipermeable membranes of the capillaries maintains the characteristic similarity between the electrolyte content of the intravascular and the interstitial fluids.

The occasional movement of colloids from the vasculature to the interstitial fluids can change the osmotic factors at the tissue level, but their removal by the lymphatic system maintains the osmotic equilibrium. At the venous end of the capillary beds, the intravascular colloidal content provides the inward force for fluid movement that causes the return of excess tissue fluid to the venous circulation.

Fluid exchange between the extracellular and intracellular compartments is maintained by the ratio of the solute concentration to the fluid volume. The osmotic pressure in the cells is stabilized by the presence of protein. The normal cell membrane is impermeable to protein passage and the negatively charged intracellular proteins maintain a constant cellular content of positively charged potassium and magnesium ions. The same relationship exists between the positively charged sodium ions and the electronegative chloride, bicarbonate, and proteins in the extracellular fluids.

FACTORS CONTROLLING SERUM OSMOLALITY

Changes in the electrolyte content of the extracellular fluid affect its osmolality, and fluid can be exchanged between the intracellular and the extracellular compartments to maintain equilibrium. Because sodium is the principal cation in the extracellular fluids, changes in the serum sodium level can be used as a guide to the osmolality of the body fluids. A slight deviation (1 to 2 percent) from the normal serum sodium level (136 to 145 mEg/ml) mobilizes the physiologic mechanisms for maintaining the fluid and sodium balance.

The initial response to a change in the osmolality of the extracellular fluids is the movement of intracellular fluid. For example, an elevated serum sodium ion level causes outward movement of the fluid from body cells into the extracellular spaces and then into the vascular system, this leads to some cellular dehydration. Slight shrinking of cells is a generalized process that occurs in all of the cells that are bathed by the interstitial fluids.

One of the earliest signs of the increased osmolality of blood is thirst. The dehydration of the cells of the hypothalamic thirst center provides the stimulus that causes the person to drink fluids.

Antidiuretic Hormone Activity

The elevated osmolality of the fluids bathing the cells of the hypothalamic osmoreceptors provides the stimulus for release of antidiuretic hormone (ADH) from the secretory storage granules of the posterior pituitary gland. The antidiuretic hormone is transported in the circulating plasma to the renal medulla where the ADH binds to the cell membranes of the collecting duct of the nephron (Fig. 14–1). The cell-bound hormone activates the enzyme *adenylate cyclase,* which then generates formation of *cyclic 3'-'5 adenosine monophosphate* (cAMP) from *adenosine triphosphate.* The cAMP mediates the hormone-induced increase in water permeability of the membranes in the collecting duct. The consequent acceleration of water reabsorption from the tubules can provide adequate amounts of fluid to decrease the extracellular osmolality to a normal level. When normal osmolality is reestablished, the circulation of plasma at the hypothalamic centers no longer stimulates the release of ADH.

Aldosterone Activity

A reduction in the osmolality of the circulating fluids can occur when there is an excessive extracellular loss of sodium (i.e., profuse diaphoresis). Hyponatremia usually is accompanied by a decrease in the arterial fluid volume. The decreased blood volume, which is reflected in a reduced blood flow or pulse pressure in the afferent renal arterioles, can precipitate the release of *renin* from the renal juxtaglomerular cells. The renin catalyzes the conversion of the renin substrate *angiotensin I,* which then is converted to *angiotensin II* by a converting enzyme from the lung tissues. *Angiotensin II* then stimulates the release of the mineralocorticoid *aldosterone* from the adrenocortical cells. In addition to the renin-angiotensin-aldosterone mechanism, decreased arterial volume can directly stimulate the release of aldosterone from the adrenal glands.

Aldosterone activity at the nephron distal tubules influences the exchange of sodium for potassium or hydrogen ions. The aldosterone-mediated exchange returns sodium ions to the extracellular fluids and the exchanged ions (hydrogen or potassium ions) are secreted into the distal tubular fluids. The return of the cation increases the osmolality of the extracellular fluids toward normal levels.

Nephron Activity

The nephrons are the functional units of the kidneys, and the movement of fluid and electrolytes across their membranes is a major factor in maintaining equilibrium between the solutes and solvents of the extracellular fluids throughout the body. The glomerulus acts as an ultrafilter permitting passage of approximately 130 ml of

plasma into the renal tubules each minute. An effective hydrostatic pressure of the blood in the afferent glomerular arteriole causes the movement of plasma outward from the glomerular capillary bed, through the glomerular membranes, and into Bowman's capsule (Fig. 14–1). The filtered plasma rapidly moves to the proximal tubule sites where up to 85 percent of the filtered content is reabsorbed (i.e., sodium, chloride, water, urea,

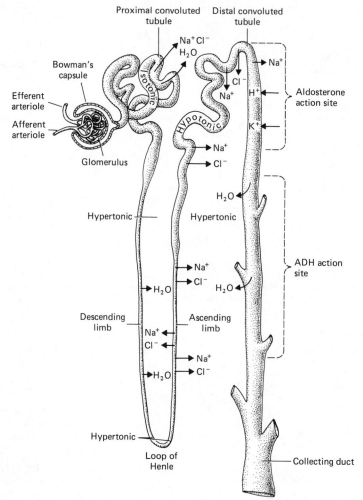

Fig. 14–1. The transfer of water and electrolytes across the nephron membranes influences the volume and composition of the extracellular fluids and the urine that is excreted.

uric acid, amino acids, bicarbonate, calcium, phosphorus, and glucose). Additional amounts of the solutes and fluid are reabsorbed as the remaining tubule content moves through the nephron unit. The final renal urine volume is excreted at the rate of only 1 ml/min.

Sodium is actively reabsorbed from the proximal tubule fluid, and its entry into the peritubular capillaries returns it to the circulation. The sodium reabsorption causes the obligatory reabsorption of chloride and bicarbonate ions with a sufficient amount of water to retain the osmotic proportions between the solutes and the solvent. In addition to the filtered bicarbonate, the tubule cells have a mechanism for converting carbonic acid to bicarbonate that is a vital part of the acid-base buffer system:

$$CO_2 + H_2O \rightleftharpoons H_2CO_3 \text{ (+ Carbonic anhydrase)} \rightleftharpoons$$
$$\text{(Carbonic acid)}$$
$$HCO_3 + H$$
$$\text{(Bicarbonate)}$$

The exchange of the hydrogen ions for the sodium ions returns additional sodium bicarbonate to the extracellular fluids, and the hydrogen ions enter the tubule fluid to increase its acidity.

The hypertonicity of the interstitial fluids in the renal medulla affects the movement of sodium, chloride, and water across the membranes of the loop of Henle, which projects into the renal medulla. The hypertonicity of the tissues is the osmotic factor that causes movement of fluid from the descending limb of the loop of Henle. The exodus of water from the tubule lumen increases the osmolality of the tubule content at the base of the loop. The thick ascending limb of the loop is relatively impermeable to the passage of water, and the active transport of chlorides is accompanied by movement of sodium ions without the movement of water (Fig. 14–1).

The tubule fluid that enters the distal convoluted tubule is hypotonic. Additional sodium is reabsorbed from the distal convoluted tubule in the presence of aldosterone, and water is reabsorbed in the presence of ADH. The final urine product is a concentrated solution containing only those constituents that are not required to maintain fluid and electrolyte equilibrium in the body.

Pathophysiologic Correlations

Disruption of the normal physiologic controls can expand the circulating plasma volume or allow accumulation of fluid in tissues. There are six generally accepted broad classifications of the physiologic problems leading to sequestration of fluids in body tissues. The pathophysiologic problems and their manifestations include:

1. Elevated capillary pressure resulting from peripheral, pulmonary, or portal venous hypertension (i.e., ascites, peripheral edema, pulmonary congestion, or edema).
2. Decreased plasma protein levels resulting from burns, ascites, or malnutrition (i.e., ascites, generalized edema, decreased total body protein).
3. Lymphatic blockage resulting from lymph node obstruction or excision (i.e., nonpitting edema, elephantiasis).
4. Increased capillary permeability resulting from tissue trauma, burns, or allergic reactions (i.e., edema, pruritic rash).
5. Increased quantity of chamber fluid resulting from the blocking of natural fluid flow routes (i.e., glaucoma, increased intracranial pressure).
6. Elevated serum sodium levels resulting from changes in nephron function, aldosterone, or antidiuretic hormone activity (i.e., generalized edema).

Each of the foregoing problems causes fluid accumulation that interferes with organ or tissue function. For example, the elevation of the pulmonary venous and capillary pressures that is associated with left ventricular failure interferes with the exchange of oxygen and carbon dioxide across the capillary membranes. When the total outward pressure at the pulmonary capillary membranes exceeds the colloidal osmotic pressure of the plasma proteins and cations (28 mm Hg), fluid seeps out of the distended capillaries into the alveolar spaces. The effect on respiration is directly related to the quantity of fluid that seeps into the alveoli and the ability of the lymphatics to remove the added fluid.

Fluid in the interstitial spaces, or edema, occurs when there is a marked elevation of the effective filtration pressure or a reduction in the colloidal osmotic pressure at the capillary membranes. For example, the edema that occurs consequent to the loss of protein from the plasma represents a reduction of the plasma colloidal osmotic pressure to approximately 15 mm Hg below the normal level. The replacement of protein is a necessary step in returning the "holding" pressure of colloids in the vasculature that counteracts the factors that contribute to an effective filtration pressure at the capillary beds. Conversely, the effective capillary filtration pressure must rise to a level approximately 15 mm Hg above the normal level before the hydrostatic force is great enough to override the intravascular colloidal osmotic pressure and cause the outward movement of plasma fluid.

Edema is graded on a 1+ to 4+ scale that describes the overt evidence of fluid accumulation in tissues. At least a 30 percent rise in the total interstitial fluid volume (normal = 12 liters) is present before there is outward evidence of a generalized increased in interstitial fluid content. A 1+ edema status exists when the accumulation of fluid in the extremities is at approximately the level that would cause slight tightness in the fit of shoes. The 1+ level of edematous fluid represents an increase in the extracellular fluid volume to approximately 15 to 30 liters. Distention of the same tissues to about two times their normal size represents a 4+ edema level, and the interstitial fluid reflects approximately a 60-liter fluid volume.

A more specific and objective evaluation of the change in the size of edematous tissues and estimation of the quantity of fluid in them can be made by measurement of the affected limbs or the abdomen. The most definitive measurement of the changes can be obtained by weighing the patient. A gain in weight of 2.2 kg (1 lb) is approximately equivalent to a 500-ml (1-pt) gain in the body fluid content on a day-to-day weight comparison. Changes in body weight can provide evidence of fluid shifts before they are evident by overt measurement or disruption in physiologic function.

The manifestations of edema are affected by the natural diurnal shift in extracellular fluid distribution. Several hours after awakening, a large percentage of the extracellular fluid migrates to the lower extremities and abdomen. The primary factor in the fluid shift is the effect of gravitational forces. The fluid shifting is most evident in the ankle and tibial areas of the ambulatory patient with excess interstitial fluid, but the gluteal area may also be edematous in patients who are bedridden. The fluid shifting is reversed by the recumbent position. Fluid from the lower extremities leaves the dependent portions of the body, and there is a more equal distribution of the fluid throughout the body.

The diurnal pattern is basic to the nocturia that occurs when there is an expanded extracellular fluid volume. For example, patients with edema secondary to cardiac problems may waken to go to the toilet several times during the night. The improved blood flow to the kidneys increases urine production during the hours that the person is recumbent.

Diuretics

The sequestration of fluids that is associated with diverse physiologic problems can be self-perpetuating until the physical limits for holding the excess fluid are exceeded in the tissues or body cavities. Correction of the pathophysiologic problem and the concurrent therapy to reinstitute osmotic equilibrium are essential to control the shifting of body fluids. The urgency for therapy is related to the extent of the disruptive effects of the accumulated fluid on physiologic function.

DRUG THERAPY

Sodium retention and the concurrent accumulation of fluid that maintains the osmotic equilibrium are the primary factors in the sequestration of fluids in body tissues. It is estimated that the average person has a sodium chloride intake of 10 gm/day. A reduction of that sodium intake level can somewhat decrease the imbalance that is attributable to the excess serum levels of the electrolyte. A severe sodium restriction can provide the stimulus for increased activity of aldosterone, and most or all of the sodium intake is avidly reabsorbed at the distal tubule sites in exchange for potassium or hydrogen ions. The renal threshold for sodium excretion becomes increased to a level that prevents urinary sodium output even when the daily intake of sodium is at the minimal level of 500 mg/day. The use of a diuretic promotes the renal excretion of sodium while allowing a moderate dietary sodium intake (i.e., 2 to 4 gm/day).

The six classes of diuretics commonly employed for control of edema are *thiazide diuretics and related derivatives, "high-ceiling" diuretics, potassium-sparing diuretics, osmotic diuretics, mercurial diuretics,* and the *carbonic anhydrase inhibitors.* Each of the drugs promotes diuresis by interfering with the processes by which the renal tubule cells reabsorb the filtered sodium from the tubule fluid. Each class of diuretics has a particular mode of action and characteristic effects on the transfer of sodium and other electrolytes from the tubule fluid. The resulting electrolyte and acid-base imbalances are predictable and they are generally controllable consequences of the diuretic drug action. Some modification of the imbalances is possible by utilizing the lowest effective dosage of the drug and an intermittent or alternate-day schedule for use of the drug.

The aim of diuretic drug therapy is to decrease the extracellular fluid volume by causing a net loss of sodium from the body. The patient is monitored closely during initial intensive therapy to ascertain the effectiveness of the drugs on sodium and fluid removal. The daily laboratory assays allow evaluation of the serum electrolyte and osmolality levels.

The comatose or acutely ill patient usually has an indwelling urinary catheter inserted to allow accurate measurement of the urine output. Early-morning weighing of the patient usually is planned to objectively evaluate the changes in fluid accumulation. During the initial days of diuretic therapy the urine output is high. When the excess plasma volume reaches a near-normal level, the drugs maintain a slightly low plasma volume without an appreciable day-to-day increase in the urine volume. Diuretics usually are administered early in the day to allow diuresis during the waking hours when the person is on a maintenance therapy plan.

The monitoring of serum values may be done frequently (i.e., daily, weekly) during the early phase of diuretic therapy, but the laboratory tests usually are spaced at three-month intervals after the electrolyte responses are stabilized. During interim periods the patient usually is examined in the home, office, or clinic for evidence of improvement in the fluid status or problems related to the diuretic therapy plan. It is important that the patient be instructed about assessments that must be made while taking the drugs to assure that there will be ongoing monitoring while the person is responsible for the unsupervised maintenance of the therapy plan.

Monitoring of the effects of the diuretic therapy includes careful observation for evidence of diuretic-induced dehydration or sodium depletion. When laboratory tests are being performed regularly, the decreased circulating plasma volume will be reflected in an elevated hematocrit level, and in elevation of the serum sodium and osmolality levels. Additional evidence can be obtained by taking the blood pressure and observing the person for signs of dehydration (i.e., marked thirst, excess dryness of the mucous membranes, decreased salivation, decreased urine output, increased concentration of the urine).

The monitoring plan also includes observations for evidence of sodium depletion (i.e., anorexia, nausea, vomiting, diarrhea, fatigue, dulled mental faculties, dizziness, lassitude, muscle cramps). Temporarily withholding the diuretic and increasing the sodium intake usually lead to the reversal of the low-salt syndrome.

THIAZIDE DIURETICS AND RELATED DERIVATIVES

The thiazides are sulfonamides, and *quinethazone, metolazone,* and *chlorthalidone* are pharmacologically and structurally similar drugs. The group of diuretics represents the most widely used drugs for the control of fluid accumulation or for hypertension control. Each of the drugs is well tolerated by the vast majority of persons using them. The major difference between the drugs is the therapeutic dosage level and the duration of action.

Action Mode. The thiazide group of drugs enhance the excretion of sodium, chloride, and water by interfering with the transport of sodium ions across the renal tubule epithelium. They inhibit the tubular reabsorption of sodium in the cortical portions of the ascending limb of the loop of Henle and at the distal tubules. By their action they interfere with the dilution of tubule fluid (Fig. 14–2).

The elevated tubule fluid content of sodium ions that is associated with the action of the diuretics increases the excretion of bicarbonate ions. The excretion rate of those anions is lower than that of chloride ions, and there is a negligible change in the pH of the urine consequent to their excretion. The elevated tubule content of sodium ions also causes a significant increase in the excretion of potassium ions consequent to the higher rate at which it is exchanged for sodium at the distal tubule sites. The mechanism returns a small amount of the sodium ions to the circulating fluids.

The thiazides also increase the excretion of magnesium and phosphate ions. There is some decrease in the excretion of calcium ions and ammonia. Their retention may be reflected in a slight increase in the plasma electrolyte levels. The

Table 14–1.
Orally Administered Thiazide Diuretics and Related Derivatives: Dosage-Action Duration

	Daily Dosage Range		
	Adult	Child (per kg body weight)	Action Duration (hr)
Bendroflumethiazide (BENURON, NATURETIN)	5–20 mg	50–100 mcg/kg	18–24
Benzthiazide (AQUATAG, EXNA)	5–200 mg	1–4 mg/kg	12–18
Chlorothiazide (DIURIL)	0.5–2 gm	10–15 mg/kg	6–12
Chlorthalidone (HYGROTON)	5–100 mg	2 mg/kg	48–72
Cyclothiazide (ANHYDRON)	2–6 mg	20–40 mcg/kg	18–24
Hydrochlorothiazide (ESIDREX, HYDRODIURIL)	25–200 mg	2–2.2 mg/kg	6–12
Hydroflumethiazide (SALURON)	50–200 mg	1 mg/kg	18–24
Methyclothiazide (ENDURON)	2.5–10 mg	50–200 mcg/kg	24
Metolazone (ZAROXOLONE)	2.5–200 mg	—*	12–24
Polythiazide (RENESE)	2–4 mg	20–80 mcg/kg	24–36
Quinethazone (HYDROMOX)	50–200 mg	—*	18–24
Trichlormethiazide (METAHYDRIN, NAQUA)	2–4 mg	70 mcg/kg	24

* Child dosage not established.

thiazide diuretics also decrease the rate of uric acid excretion.

Therapy Considerations. The differences in dosage levels reflect, at least in part, the variations in the gastrointestinal absorption of the thiazide group of diuretics (Table 14–1). The absorbed drugs are widely distributed in the extracellular fluids and they cross the placental barrier.

The diuretic action of the drugs is evident within two hours after their absorption from the gastrointestinal tract, and a peak effect occurs from three to six hours after the drugs are administered. *Chlorothiazide sodium* may be admin-

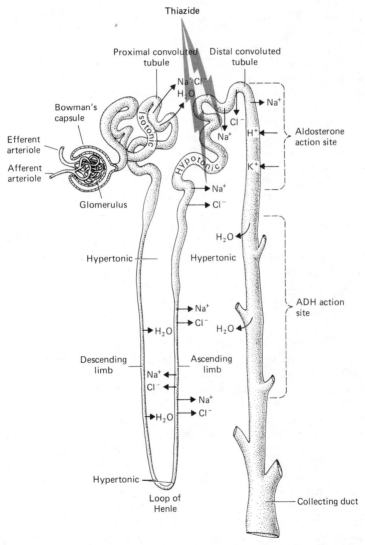

Fig. 14–2. The thiazide diuretics inhibit the reabsorption of sodium from the cortical segment of the ascending limb and from the distal convoluted tubule.

istered intravenously, and its diuretic effect occurs within 15 minutes of administration. The intravenous route of administration generally is reserved for emergencies or for persons who are unable to take oral medications.

The unchanged drugs are excreted by glomerular filtration and by active secretion from the proximal tubule cells of the nephron. The drugs with the lowest renal clearance rate generally are those requiring the lowest dosage for therapeutic effect and the least frequent intervals for administration. Insignificant amounts of the drugs are excreted in the milk of nursing mothers. The thiazides are reducing agents, and TES-TAPE rather than clinitest tablets should be employed when testing the urine for glucose content.

The sodium intake is seldom rigidly restricted during therapy with the thiazides. The general guidelines are usually described to the patient as a "no-added-salt" regimen, which includes the avoidance of highly salted foods (i.e., luncheon meats, smoked meats, commercially prepared dishes, seafood, snacks with a high salt content). The patient is given explicit instructions about foods to be avoided because a daily sodium chloride intake of 20 to 25 gm provides an overload that can counteract the diuretic effect of the drugs.

Adverse Effects. Dehydration and hyponatremia are concerns during therapy with the thiazides. Dehydration most frequently is seen in elderly patients, but it can occur in other patients during therapy. The patients are told to be alert for signs of decreased plasma volume during long periods of hot weather when the losses of fluids and sodium chloride through perspiration may potentiate the effects of the drugs.

"Dilutional" hyponatremia also may occur when large quantities of water are ingested to satisfy the thirst that occurs in hot weather. The correction of the problem requires temporarily withholding the drug and a severe restriction in the intake of fluids (<500 ml/day).

Plasma renin activity is considerably elevated during thiazide therapy, and the consequent increase in aldosterone secretion contributes to the incidence of hypokalemia caused by the thiazide diuretics. Potassium depletion occurs in approximately one third of the patients on a daily dosage regimen, but symptoms related to the hypokalemia rarely occur. Concurrent losses of potassium ions during episodes of diarrhea or vomiting and with overuse of laxatives or excess drainage from an ileostomy can precipitate signs of a potassium deficit.

Potassium losses are particularly significant when the person is receiving a digitalis glycoside. The dosage of digitalis is calculated on the basis of a normal level of potassium in the myocardial cells, and a decrease in the potassium level potentiates the effect of digitalis. Serious arrhythmias may occur as manifestations of digitalis toxicity.

Most of the patients who are on a daily schedule for thiazide use are advised to increase their intake of potassium-rich foods (i.e., bananas, citrus fruits, melons, dried fruits) to maintain a normal serum potassium level during thiazide therapy. Many patients find it difficult to ingest enough of the potassium-rich foods to influence the serum levels significantly.

When the serum potassium level is below 3 mEq/liter, weakness and muscle cramping may occur. Therapies that may be employed for maintenance of the serum potassium level include use of supplemental potassium (i.e., potassium chloride), the addition of a potassium-sparing diuretic to the therapy regimen (i.e., spironolactone, triamterene), and the restriction of the sodium intake to decrease the sodium-potassium ion-exchange rate in the distal tubules.

A potassium supplement frequently is employed for prophylactic or maintenance therapy when persons are receiving the thiazide diuretics. The liquid forms of the drug have an unpleasant taste, which can be partially disguised by mixing the drug with a small amount of citrus fruit juice. The electrolyte is freely secreted in exchange for sodium ions in the distal tubules, and that mechanism prevents hyperkalemia during oral therapy.

Hyperkalemia can occur when *potassium chloride* is administered intravenously at a rapid rate. The solution is very irritating and the conscious patient will complain of pain and a burning sensation along the course of the vein when the solution is infused rapidly. In some instances dilution of the solution is necessary to decrease the venous irritation.

There are several oral forms of potassium supplements. Each of the drugs has a bitter metallic taste, and patients are reluctant to take the drug. It is important that the person understand the rationale for using the drug and the necessity for taking it regularly. The most commonly used potassium supplements are *potassium chloride* (KAY CIEL ELIXIR, KLORVESS EFFERVESCENT), *potassium bicarbonate and citrate* (K-LYTE), *potassium gluconate* (KAON), and *potassium triplex*.

Hypochloremic-hypokalemic alkalosis may occur consequent to the renal losses of chloride and potassium ions. The problem occurs most frequently when there are concurrent losses of potassium chloride from the gastrointestinal tract (i.e., vomiting, diarrhea).

At the low dosage levels the thiazide diuretics enhance the proximal tubule reabsorption of uric acid and also inhibit its secretion from tubule cells by competing for the secretion sites. Although hyperuricemia is evident soon after the initiation of thiazide therapy, most patients remain asymptomatic. Persons who have a history of gout or a familial predisposition to the problem may have the painful joints common to the disease process. Some physicians add *allopurinol* to the therapy regimen to increase uric acid excretion when the patient has an elevated uric acid level (above 10 mg/100 ml), and the drug usually is employed when patients become symptomatic. At high dosage levels the thiazides act as *uricosuric agents* and they then facilitate the secretion of uric acid.

The thiazides can induce hyperglycemia, precipitate diabetes in prediabetics, or exacerbate preexisting diabetes. The problems are an indirect effect of the drugs that occurs as a consequence of the drug-induced potassium depletion. The cation is the natural companion of glucose in its movement into the intracellular content, and hypokalemia reduces the cellular transfer. Although significant hyperglycemia is rare, the fasting blood sugar level can be markedly elevated (i.e., 400 to 600/100 ml). The elevated blood glucose levels increase the osmolality of the extracellular fluids, and this can cause dehydration. The administration of thiazides to diabetics necessitates modification of their insulin or oral hypoglycemic drug dosage to levels allowing utilization of the higher blood glucose content. Correction of the hypokalemia usually improves the glucose tolerance level.

The foregoing metabolic problems are the adverse effects that occur most frequently during therapy with thiazide diuretics. Most of the other effects represent minor or infrequent problems (i.e., gastrointestinal irritation, weakness, pancreatitis, dryness, or a "bad taste" in the mouth).

Persons who have a history of an allergic reaction to a sulfonamide may have an allergic reaction while taking the thiazides. The appearance of a skin rash is carefully evaluated, and the drug therapy may be discontinued when it is considered to be drug related. Photosensitivity also can occur as an allergic response to the drugs. The skin becomes sensitized to ultraviolet rays (phototoxicity) and minimal exposure to the rays of the sun can cause an acute inflammatory reaction. Blood dyscrasias (i.e., leukopenia, thrombocytopenia, purpura) have occurred in a few patients during thiazide therapy.

Thiazide Toxicity. Toxic effects of the thiazides most frequently are a concern when children inadvertently ingest a large quantity of the drug tablets. Prompt administration of *ipecac syrup* will induce vomiting and remove the drug from the stomach. Gastric irrigation may be required to remove the drug from the stomach of an unconscious patient.

Absorption of a large quantity of the drug produces lethargy, which can progress to coma within a few hours. Gastrointestinal irritation and hypermotility of the digestive tract also may be present. Although there may be a temporary elevation of the blood urea nitrogen level, there seldom are serious changes in the serum electrolyte levels. The person is monitored regularly for a period of time that correlates with the action duration of the drug ingested, and treatment is planned for those symptoms that appear during the observation period.

Interactions. The drug interaction of primary concern during therapy with the thiazide diuretics is the potential for digitalis toxicity as a consequence of the drug-induced hypokalemia. Changes in the serum calcium or magnesium levels can also cause adverse effects when patients concurrently are receiving a digitalis glycoside. The person's electrolyte levels are carefully monitored for evidence of hypokalemia, hypomagnesemia, or hypercalcemia when both drugs are employed. Concurrent therapy with drugs known to cause excess excretion of potassium (i.e., corticosteroids, corticotropin, amphotericin B) can precipitate the symptoms associated with hypokalemia, and serious cardiac arrhythmias may occur when the individual also is taking digitalis.

The thiazide-induced potassium depletion can increase the responsiveness to nonpolarizing neuromuscular blocking agents (i.e., tubocurarine chloride, gallamine triethiodide). When patients are affected by the interaction, there is a prolongation of the neuromuscular blockade action that can depress the respiratory rate and cause periods of apnea.

The thiazides decrease renal clearance of *lithium carbonate.* The patient who is receiving the drug for control of an emotional problem may require reduction in the drug dosage to maintain the serum lithium levels within the therapeutic range.

The hyperglycemic effect of the thiazides may antagonize the hypoglycemic effect of insulin and the sulfonylurea drugs. A dosage adjustment may be required to maintain control of glucose utilization.

The thiazides potentiate the hypotensive effects of most of the agents employed for control of hypertension. The drug interaction provides a therapeutic advantage in the control of blood pressure levels, and the thiazides often are part of the hypertension control plan. The thiazide-induced plasma volume reduction may cause severe postural hypotension when the drug is added to a therapeutic regimen that includes any of the potent antihypertensive drugs. The thiazides can potentiate the hyperglycemic and hyperuricemic effects of the antihypertensive drug *diazoxide.* The incidence of postural hypotension also may be increased when alcohol, barbiturates, or narcotics are used during thiazide therapy.

Cholestyramine resin may bind thiazides and prevent absorption of the drug from the gastrointestinal tract. The drug interaction can be avoided by administering the thiazide one hour before giving the oral resin.

Probenecid blocks the thiazide-induced uric acid retention, and it may be utilized to therapeutic advantage when patients have symptoms of gout consequent to the retention of uric acid. The competition for the tubule secretion sites could block the secretion of thiazides when probenecid is administered, but there are no clinical studies indicating a significant effect on the duration of action of the thiazides.

"HIGH-CEILING" DIURETICS

The term *high ceiling* describes the potent diuretic effect of *furosemide* and *ethacrynic acid.* The peak diuretic effect is greater than that occurring with the use of any other diuretic. Although the drugs are chemically dissimilar, they have a similar mode of action at renal tubule sites.

Furosemide is more commonly employed than ethacrynic acid for control of acute problems of fluid accumulation (i.e., pulmonary edema) and for long-term therapy. Furosemide is easier to administer in emergency situations, has a broader dose-response ratio, and less frequently causes the adverse effects common to the use of ethacrynic acid (i.e., alkalosis, ototoxicity, gastrointestinal disturbances).

Action Mode. Furosemide and ethacrynic acid are thought to inhibit the outward active transport of chloride in the medullary portion of the ascending limb of the loop of Henle. Because the transport of chloride passively carries sodium into the interstitium, the drug action decreases the movement of sodium from the tubular fluid. The action of the drugs interferes with the concentrating and diluting mechanism in the descending and ascending limbs and with the concentrating mechanism in the collecting duct (Fig. 14–3). Their potent effect on the loop of Henle has popularized the term *loop diuretics*. The drugs also have a direct effect on electrolyte transport at proximal tubule sites. Their natriuretic and diuretic effects lead to excretion of 25 to 30 percent of the filtered sodium load.

The diuretic action of furosemide and ethacrynic acid produces copious quantities of a dilute urine containing high levels of chloride, sodium, potassium, hydrogen, calcium, magnesium, ammonium, and bicarbonate ions. The urine may

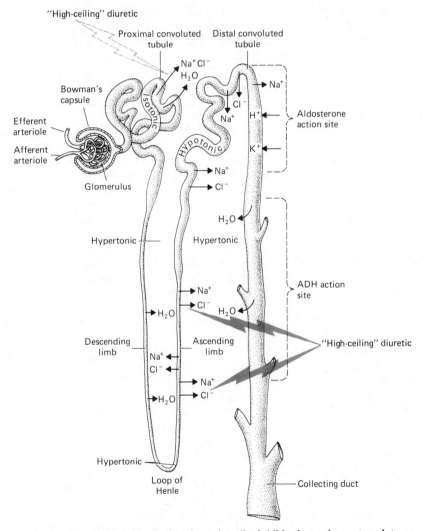

Fig. 14–3. The "high-ceiling" diuretics primarily inhibit the active outward transport of chloride ions in the medullary segment of the ascending limb, and the passive movement of sodium ions is reduced. The diuretics also have a limited effect on the reabsorption of electrolytes at proximal tubule sites.

show a lower pH level immediately after administration of either of the drugs. The diuretic effect and the electrolyte losses are greater with the "high-ceiling" drugs than with other diuretics. Like the thiazides, at low dosage levels the drugs cause uric acid retention, but at high dosage they have a uricosuric action.

The drugs have some renal vasodilator action that increases blood flow through the afferent arteriole. The improved perfusion is significant in averting the loss of renal function when diuretics are used for the control of chronic renal disease.

Adverse Effects. Many of the adverse effects of furosemide and ethacrynic acid are similar to those of the thiazide diuretics, but the incidence and severity of the problems are greater with the more potent diuretics. Initially the excretion of chloride, sodium, and potassium ions is approximately equal. The excess losses of potassium, hydrogen, and chloride ions can result in metabolic alkalosis. During prolonged administration the excretion of sodium and chloride ions declines and there is an increase in the excretion rate of potassium and hydrogen ions.

The profound diuresis that is produced by the drugs can cause fluid depletion severe enough to cause symptomatic orthostatic hypotension, and a wide variety of electrolyte imbalances. During the early adjustment phase of therapy the patient is observed closely for evidence of hypovolemia, hyponatremia, hypokalemia, hypochloremia, hypocalcemia, and hypomagnesemia. The patient who is being prepared for maintenance of the drug therapy plan is told to inform the physician if there is evidence of weakness, dizziness, fatigue, faintness, mental confusion, lassitude, muscle cramps, headache, paresthesias, thirst, anorexia, nausea, or vomiting that is not attributable to other clearly defined causes. Many patients are placed on an intermittent schedule for use of the drug to limit the incidence of adverse effects due to electrolyte imbalance. The intake of salt may be less restricted with the "high-ceiling" drugs than with most other diuretics, and that decreases the incidence of hyponatremia and hypochloremia.

Hypokalemia is the most serious electrolyte imbalance when patients concurrently are receiving a digitalis glycoside. The aldosterone-mediated exchange of potassium ions for sodium ions proceeds at a steady rate and may contribute to the problems related to hypokalemia. The diuretics have less effect on carbohydrate metabolism and blood glucose levels than that which occurs with the thiazide diuretics. The other adverse metabolic effect that the drugs have in common with the thiazide diuretics is hyperuricemia.

Rapid administration of large intravenous doses of either drug has caused vertigo, tinnitus, reversible or permanent hearing loss, and permanent deafness. The incidence of the problems has led to the practice of very slow intravenous injection to reduce the sudden peak in plasma drug levels that is known to be ototoxic.

Blood dyscrasias that have occurred during therapy include anemia, leukopenia, neutropenia, aplastic anemia, and thrombocytopenic purpura. Although the incidence of gastrointestinal disturbances is considerably higher during therapy with ethacrynic acid, either drug may cause problems with anorexia, nausea, vomiting, or diarrhea. The problems are more prevalent when large doses of the drugs are administered or when therapy continues on a daily schedule over a period of months. Reduction of dosage or an intermittent schedule for use of the drug usually lessens the gastrointestinal disturbances.

Interactions. Most of the drug interactions occurring during therapy with the "high-ceiling" diuretics are similar to those previously discussed as occurring during thiazide therapy (i.e., decreasing the elimination of lithium carbonate, potentiating the hypoglycemic effects of insulin and the sulfylureas, enhancing the hypotensive effects of antihypertensive drugs, prolonging the effects of the nonpolarizing neuromuscular blocking agents, interfering with the uricosuric effects of probenecid or sulfinpyrazone, and increasing the incidence of digitalis toxicity).

Administration of the drugs to a patient receiving one of the aminoglycoside antibiotics (i.e., kanamycin) known to have a high ototoxic potential can increase the incidence of hearing loss and deafness. The nephrotoxicity of the antibiotics *cephaloridine* and *neomycin* may be enhanced by concurrent administration of either ethacrynic acid or furosemide.

Ethacrynic acid can displace warfarin from its protein-binding sites and that action can potentiate the anticoagulant effect of the *coumarin* and *indandione* groups of anticoagulants. A reduction in the anticoagulant dosage may be required to prevent bleeding consequent to the decreased activity of the clotting factors.

Furosemide administration to patients receiving chloral hydrate has precipitated a brief sharp systolic blood pressure elevation. The problem is thought to result from the furosemide-induced displacement of the active metabolite of chloral hydrate *trichloroacetic acid* from its protein-binding sites. The metabolite in turn prevents the protein binding of thyroxine or displaces it from its protein-binding sites. The free thyroxine causes a brief hypermetabolic state.

Because furosemide is a sulfonamide derivative it also can cause skin rashes and photosensitivity reactions similar to those produced by the thiazides. It also competes for the same renal excretion sites as are employed by the salicylates. Concurrent administration of the drugs can cause the onset of salicylate toxicity when plasma drug levels are below those usually causing the problem.

Furosemide (LASIX)

Therapy Considerations. Furosemide is available in forms for oral and parenteral administration. The usual initial intravenous or intramuscular dosage in acute situations is 20 to 40 mg. The intravenous dosage is injected slowly over a period of one to two minutes. Intravenous administration usually produces diuresis within five minutes and a potent diuretic effect is fully evident within 15 to 30 minutes. The duration of the diuretic response persists for approximately two hours. When the response is inadequate in an acute situation, subsequent doses of the drug may be injected at two-hour intervals, and the dosage usually is 20 mg higher than the initial dose. Intramuscular administration follows the same dosage range but the onset of diuresis is slower.

The initial single parenteral dosage level for infants and children usually is calculated on the basis of 1 mg/kg of body weight, and the dosage may be increased in increments of 1 mg/kg when subsequent doses are given at two-hour intervals. The maximum daily parenteral dosage is 6 mg/kg of body weight. Furosemide usually is given orally after the acute situation is reversed.

Furosemide usually is administered orally in nonacute situations. The usual initial oral adult dosage is 20 to 80 mg, and that dosage level may be increased in 20- to 40-mg increments at six- or eight-hour intervals until the diuretic response is adequate. The maximum oral daily dosage level is 600 mg.

The initial oral dosage for infants and children is 2 mg/kg of body weight, and that dosage may be increased in increments of 1 to 2 mg/kg at six- to eight-hour intervals. The dosage maximum for infants and children is 6 mg/kg/day. Maintenance dosage usually represents a lower range after the excess plasma volume is reduced.

Sixty percent of the orally administered drug is absorbed from the gastrointestinal tract. The onset of action is evident from 30 minutes to one hour after the drug is administered. The maximal diuretic effect occurs in the first or second hour after administration of the drug, and the urine output remains relatively high for six to eight hours.

Ninety-five percent of the drug in the circulation is bound to plasma proteins. Furosemide crosses the placental barrier. After hepatic metabolism, the unchanged drug and the metabolites are rapidly excreted in the urine. Glomerular filtration and secretion from the proximal tubules can remove up to 50 percent of the orally administered drug within 24 hours. Hepatic degradation and excretion in the feces are nonrenal mechanisms that can remove up to 98 percent of the drug from the circulation within 24 hours when renal impairment prevents glomerular passage or tubular secretion.

Ethacrynic Acid (EDECRIN)

Therapy Considerations. The parenteral form of the drug is *ethacrynate sodium* (SODIUM EDECRIN). The reconstituted drug usually is injected as a single direct, or bolus, intravenous dose. The drug is injected slowly over a period of several minutes. The usual adult or children's dosage ranges from 0.5 to 1 mg/kg of body weight. Usually only one intravenous injection is required to produce a potent diuretic effect. The onset of diuresis occurs in five minutes and the peak effect occurs within 15 to 30 minutes. The duration of the diuretic action is approximately two hours.

The oral dosage of ethacrynic acid is planned to produce a gradual weight loss of 0.5 to 1 kg (1 to 2.2 lb) daily until the "ideal" weight for the person is reached. The usual initial therapeutic dosage for an adult is 50 to 100 mg given after breakfast on the first day. The dosage may be increased in 25- to 50-mg increments during the next two days; the total daily dosage is divided into two or three doses. The initial dosage for children is 25 mg, which may be increased in 25-mg increments until the desired diuretic response is attained. The dosage usually is reduced for maintenance therapy after the initial rapid decrease in plasma volume has subsided.

The orally administered drug is rapidly absorbed from the gastrointestinal tract. After absorption, the diuretic effect occurs in 30 minutes and it lasts for six to eight hours. The drug is distributed in body fluids but the liver is the only organ that contains significant quantities of the drug. Ethacrynic acid is metabolized to the active *cysteine conjugate,* which increases the diuretic effect of the drug. The unchanged drug and its metabolites are secreted into the tubular fluid at the proximal nephron sites (30 to 65 percent) and about one third (35 to 40 percent) of the cysteine conjugate is excreted with the bile. The drug is more rapidly excreted when the urine is slightly alkaline.

POTASSIUM SPARING DIURETICS

Spironolactone and *triamterene* act by differing mechanisms at the renal distal tubule sites to interfere with the exchange of sodium and potassium ions. The drugs are often employed conjointly with a thiazide or a "high-ceiling" diuretic to minimize the potassium losses when those losses are considered to jeopardize the health of the person. The distal tubular sodium exodus constitutes only a small fraction of the total reabsorption of the filtered sodium in the nephron (approximately 2 percent), and use of the drugs as the sole diuretic agent generally provides inadequate control of sodium and fluid accumulation. When used with another diuretic, the drugs have an additive or synergistic diuretic effect.

Spironolactone (ALDACTONE)

Action Mode. Spironolactone is a true competitive inhibitor of aldosterone at its renal sites of action in the distal tubules. The drug action produces an increased rate of excretion of sodium and chloride ions and water and concurrently decreases the excretion of potassium, ammonium, and phosphate ions.

Therapy Considerations. Spironolactone is administered orally. The usual daily dosage for adults is 50 to 100 mg, and that dose may be divided for use two times per day. The initial daily dosage for children is calculated on the basis of 3.3 mg/kg of body weight. Maintenance dosage may be at the same level or dosage reduction may be planned when the drug is used with another diuretic.

The absorption of the drug from the gastrointestinal tract varies with differing formulations. The microcrystalline product is the most completely absorbed drug form. When the drug is used as the sole diuretic agent, up to three days are required before diuretic effects are observed, and continued treatment for two weeks may be needed to produce maximal effects. The diuresis persists for a comparable time period after drug therapy is discontinued.

The drug is rapidly metabolized to the active metabolite *canrenone,* which has a serum half-life of 13 to 24 hours. The initial time lag in response is related to the relatively long half-life of the active metabolite and the time required for its attainment of a therapeutic plasma concentration. The serum half-life of the active metabolite also allows the spacing of dosage to a once-or-twice-a-day schedule. The metabolite is excreted in the urine and feces.

Adverse Effects. Hyperkalemia is the major adverse effect of the drug and the incidence is highest when the patient has compromised renal function. Hyperkalemia seldom is problematic unless the renal impairment is sufficient to cause a sharp elevation of the blood urea nitrogen (> 40 mg percent). Persons who are taking the drug should be informed that the potassium-containing salt substitutes, potassium supplements, or excess ingestion of potassium-rich foods should be avoided.

The steroid-like structure of the drug can cause painful gynecomastia in males. Animal studies have revealed a tumorigenic potential in the endocrine organs and the liver. The Food and Drug Administration regulations require labeling that indicates that the drug may be "a tumorigen."

Impotence also occurs in males and women sometimes have menstrual irregularities, vaginal spotting, and soreness of the breasts. Spironolactone can also produce androgen-like effects in females (i.e., hirsutism, deepening of the voice). Gastrointestinal disturbances (i.e., anorexia, nausea, vomiting, diarrhea), drowsiness, lethargy, and skin rashes also occur during therapy with spironolactone.

Interactions. The action of hypotensive agents may be potentiated when spironolactone is added to an antihypertensive drug regimen. The dosage of the hypotensive drug may be reduced to avoid the excess effects.

Salicylates inhibit the natriuresis of the drug. The interaction may be a consequence of competition for shared receptor sites in the renal tubules.

Triamterene (DYRENIUM)

Action Mode. Triamterene acts directly on the renal distal tubules to depress reabsorption of sodium and the excretion of potassium and hydrogen ions. Although it inhibits the same electrolyte-exchange process as that mediated by aldosterone, the drug acts independently of aldosterone action at the tubule sites.

The action of triamterene increases the excretion of sodium, chloride, calcium, magnesium, and bicarbonate ions. The excretion rate of chlorides is relatively low, and the concurrent inhibition of potassium excretion is reflected in an elevation of the serum potassium and chloride levels. The excretion of bicarbonate may be reflected in a slight rise in the pH of the urine.

Therapy Considerations. Triamterene is administered orally. The initial adult daily dosage is 200 mg, and the dosage is divided for administration after two meals. Maintenance therapy may be at one half that dosage level. The dosage for children ranges from 4 to 6 mg/kg of body weight. The daily dosage maximum for adults and children is 300 mg/day.

The drug is rapidly absorbed from the gastrointestinal tract, but there is considerable individual variation in the rate of absorption. Diuresis usually occurs within two to four hours after the drug is administered. The maximum therapeutic effect occurs several days after initiation of therapy.

The absorbed drug is distributed in the brain, heart, ocular fluid, fat, liver, and skeletal muscles. It crosses the placental barrier. Approximately 67 percent of the drug is bound to plasma proteins. The serum half-life of triamterene is quite short (100 to 120 minutes).

Adverse Effects. Like spironolactone, triamterene may cause retention of potassium ions at a level that causes symptomatic hyperkalemia (i.e., cardiac irregularities). The consistent excretion of bicarbonate ions coupled with the decreased excretion of hydrogen ions can increase the potential for metabolic acidosis.

At the termination of therapy, the daily drug dosage is gradually reduced because a rebound kaliuresis can occur when use of the drug is abruptly terminated. The serum creatinine levels are moderately elevated during therapy, but they return to pretreatment levels approximately 7 to 14 days after therapy is terminated.

Most of the other adverse effects are mild and respond promptly to a dosage decrease or to the change from a daily to an intermittent schedule for use of the drug. The problems are primarily gastrointestinal disturbances (i.e., nausea, vomiting, diarrhea).

OSMOTIC DIURETICS

Mannitol, urea, and *glycerin* are the osmotic agents employed for the control of fluid accumulation. Glycerin is an oral osmotic agent used primarily for consistent control of persistent fluid accumulation at selected body sites (i.e., intraocular, cerebral).

Mannitol and urea are employed parenterally for short-term control of fluid accumulation. Mannitol is the preferred drug because it is easier to prepare for administration in emergency situations. It also is preferred for the treatment of increased intraocular pressure because it does not enter the eye chamber and can be employed when inflammation is present. The potent diuresis that occurs following infusion of the drugs necessitates the insertion of a urinary catheter at the time of drug administration when the patient is unconscious or acutely ill.

Action Mode. The osmotic effect of the drugs at tissue sites causes fluid to move from the cells, body cavities, and interstitial spaces into the vasculature. Delivery of the expanded intravascular volume to the kidneys leads to the excretion of the excess fluid load.

The osmotic diuretics act as nonreabsorbable solutes in the renal tubule lumen, and the ensuing high osmolality of the tubular fluid interferes with sodium and water reabsorption. The elevated osmolality of the tubule fluid affects electrolyte and water movement throughout the renal tubule. By preventing the obligatory reabsorption of the filtrate from the proximal tubules, the medullary interstitium becomes less hypertonic. The hyperosmolality of the descending limb limits the outward movement of water into the interstitium, and more fluid is delivered to the distal tubule and the collecting duct. Proportionately more water than sodium is excreted in the urine.

The drug action increases the excretion rate of potassium, chlorides, calcium, phosphorus, magnesium, urea, and uric acid. The drugs are useful for reducing an edematous brain mass, for decreasing an elevated cerebrospinal fluid pressure, and for reducing intraocular pressure. When either mannitol or urea is administered parenterally, the patient with increased intracranial pressure may show remarkable improvement, but a rebound increase in pressure elevation often occurs about 12 hours after the drug is administered.

Mannitol (OSMITROL)

Therapy Considerations. The usual adult dosage for the reduction of increased intracranial or intraocular pressure is calculated on the basis of 1.5 to 2 gm/kg of body weight. The diluted drug solution is infused over a 30-to-60-minute period.

There usually is evidence of a reduction in the pressure at cerebral tissue sites within 15 minutes after the drug infusion is started. A reduction in intraocular pressure usually occurs within 30 to 60 minutes. Diuresis occurs from one to three hours after the infusion is started. The duration of effect after cessation of the intravenous infusion ranges from six to eight hours.

Mannitol sometimes is employed to promote urinary output when there is a marked oliguria or suspected inadequate renal function. The drug can prevent or reverse acute functional renal failure by reversing the sharp reduction in renal blood flow. It is usual for a test dose to be administered before therapy is initiated. The intravenous infusion test dose for adults is 200 mg/kg of body weight, and the diluted drug is infused over a three- to five-minute period. The pediatric test dose is calculated on the basis of 200 mg/kg. When the production of urine following the test dose is at the level of 30 to 50 ml/hour for two to three hours, a therapeutic infusion is started. The adult dosage ranges from 50 to 100 gm and the pediatric dosage is 2 gm/kg body weight. The diluted infusion is run over a two- to six-hour period.

Only a minimal amount of the drug is metabolized to glycogen in the liver. The unchanged drug is freely filtered by the glomeruli, and less than 10 percent of the drug is reabsorbed from the nephron unit. The major portion of the drug dosage (80 percent) is excreted within three hours after administration.

Adverse Effects.   The adverse effects of greatest concern are cellular dehydration and fluid or electrolyte imbalances. The use of a test dose is planned to prevent accumulation of the drug when renal function is impaired, but accumulation of mannitol may occur when the testing is not employed. Rapid administration of large doses of the drug can cause an overexpansion of the extracellular fluid and a resultant increase in the cardiac workload or the sequestration of fluid in vital body tissues (i.e., pulmonary edema). Mannitol almost always is administered to acutely ill patients who are hospitalized, and the facilities for monitoring those patients lessen the potential problems of sharp changes in fluid and electrolytes. Adverse effects of the drug also include headache, nausea, vomiting, chills, dizziness, polydipsia, lethargy, confusion, and angina-like chest pain.

Urea (UREVERT)

Therapy Considerations.   Urea is infrequently employed for the control of diuresis, but it may be employed for the control of life-threatening cerebral edema. The adult dosage is calculated on the basis of 1 to 1.5 gm/kg of body weight. The drug is infused intravenously over a one-to-three-hour period.

Urea is widely distributed in equal concentrations in the intracellular and extracellular fluids (i.e., lymph, bile, cerebrospinal fluids). The drug also crosses the placenta. The drug enters the eyeball, and its use is contraindicated when there is irritation or inflammation of the ophthalmic tissues. The presence of the drug in the ocular chambers can cause a rebound increase in intraocular pressure when the plasma drug concentration falls below that of the ocular chamber concentration. Intravenous administration produces a reduction in intraocular or cerebral pressure within one to two hours and the effect persists up to six hours after termination of the infusion.

The highest concentration of urea is present in the kidneys. A portion of the parenterally administered drug is hydrolyzed in the gastrointestinal tract by bacterial *urease*. The products of that hydrolysis are carbon dioxide and ammonia. The urea that is resynthesized from the ammonia is excreted by the kidneys. During therapy with urea, the kidney function is closely monitored to assure that there is adequate function to allow elimination of the infused drug and the endogenously produced urea.

Adverse Effects.   The high incidence of adverse effects has been a major factor in the decline in use of urea. Extravasation of the intravenous infusion can cause pain, phlebitis, venous thrombosis, and necrotic sloughing of the tissues at the site of the injection. The drug is infused into the larger veins of the upper extremities because thrombosis often occurs in the more tortuous superficial veins of the legs.

Urea can cause hypervolemia and electrolyte imbalances. The most frequent adverse effects include headache, nausea, and vomiting. Syncope, disorientation, dizziness, hypotension, tachycardia, and cardiac arrhythmias have occurred during therapy with the drug.

Glycerin (OPHTHALGAN, OSMOGLYN)

Therapy Considerations.   The drug is administered orally in a daily dosage of 120 ml that usually is divided for use in four equal doses. The oral liquid is flavored with a tart citrus base that is planned to disguise the unpalatability of the drug. Patients find the drug somewhat more palatable when it is poured over cracked ice immediately before it is taken. The use of a drinking straw also limits contact between the drug and the oral mucosa.

The drug is employed selectively to control intraocular or cerebrospinal fluid pressure elevations. The movement of fluid from the involved tissues occurs approximately ten minutes after the drug is administered, and a peak effect occurs from 30 minutes to two hours after the drug is ingested.

The usual adult daily dosage of the 50 percent glycerin solution provides slightly more than 300 kcal. Most of the drug is incorporated into the fatty tissues as triglycerides, and only a small amount (14 percent) of the drug is excreted by the kidneys.

Adverse Effects. The most frequent adverse effects are nausea and vomiting. The osmolality of the stomach content immediately after administration of the drug is the primary causative factor although most patients place the blame on the unpalatable taste of the drug. Headache results from cerebral tissue dehydration in many patients. The incidence of nausea, vomiting, and headache seems to decrease slightly when the patient remains recumbent for a short time after taking the drug.

MERCURIAL DIURETICS

The mercurial diuretics have a long history of use for control of fluid accumulation but they have been replaced by the newer "high-ceiling" diuretics. The only organic mercurial diuretic currently in clinical use is mercaptomerin sodium.

Mercaptomerin Sodium (THIOMERIN)

Action Mode. The drug depresses tubular mechanisms that are involved in the active reabsorption of sodium and chloride. The mercurial inactivates sulfhydryl-containing enzymes throughout the nephron units. The drug inhibits the active transport of chloride ions from the medullary and cortical segments of the ascending limb of the loop of Henle and that action prevents the passive movement of sodium ions into the medullary interstitium. Sodium reabsorption also is inhibited at the terminal portion of the proximal tubule and at distal tubule sites.

The action of the drug increases the excretion of sodium and chloride ions and water. Mercaptomerin sodium also depresses the active secretion of potassium from the distal tubules, but it does not affect the exchange mechanisms at that site. Because some sodium ions continue to be exchanged for potassium and hydrogen ions, there is a slightly higher excretion level of chloride ions than sodium ions. During therapy with mercaptomerin sodium, plasma bicarbonate levels are elevated, and the increased excretion of potassium, chloride, and hydrogen ions can cause a hypokalemic hypochloremic alkalosis. The mercurial is ineffective in an alkalotic state, and the diuretic effect is terminated.

Therapy Considerations. A hypersensitivity test usually is planned before therapy with the mercurial diuretic is initiated. A small dose of the drug (i.e., 62.5 mg) is injected approximately 24 hours before the start of therapy. When the test is negative, the diuretic therapy can be instituted.

The drug is administered either subcutaneously or intramuscularly. The adult dosage of 125 to 250 mg usually is administered once or twice a week.

The *sodium thioglycollate* of the drug molecule allows slow release of the mercurial ions from the injection site and interferes with the attachment of the mercurial ions to tissue proteins. The drug is rapidly absorbed after injection, and a diuretic effect becomes evident within one to three hours after it is administered. The diuretic effect lasts for 12 to 24 hours.

The circulating drug is extensively bound to plasma proteins. The drug molecules may localize in the liver, but the primary site of accumulation is in the renal cortex. The drug is metabolized to a monocysteine complex, and the released mercury recomplexes with cysteine at renal tissue sites. The urinary rate of excretion is so rapid that it begins before the diuretic effect is evident.

Adverse Effects. The profound diuresis produced by the drug can cause plasma volume depletion and dehydration or hypotension. Hypokalemia occurs less frequently with mercaptomerin than with the other diuretics. Metabolic alkalosis and hyponatremia are the electrolyte problems of greatest concern during therapy.

The test dose of the drug is planned to avoid the allergic reactions (i.e., anaphylaxis, fever, chills, gastrointestinal disturbances) that occur during the initial days of therapy. Mercury poisoning is the other major concern during mercaptomerin therapy. The initial signs of toxicity (stomatitis, metallic taste, gingivitis, gastritis, colitis, anemia, peripheral neuritis) are forewarnings of the devastating problems of renal and hepatic tissue destruction.

Interactions. Ammonium chloride counteracts the metabolic alkalosis caused by the mercurial diuretic. Administration of ammonium chloride may be planned for three to four days before initiation of the diuretic therapy to provide the advantage of the drug interaction during therapy with the mercurial diuretic.

CARBONIC ANHYDRASE INHIBITORS

Acetazolamide (DIAMOX), *dichlorphenamide* (DARANIDE, ORATROL), *ethoxzolamide* (CARDRASE) ETHAMIDE), and *methazolamide* (NEPTAZANE) are the carbonic anhydrase inhibitors currently used as adjunctive therapy in the control of acute glaucoma. The carbonic anhydrase inhibitors were the first oral diuretics, but they have been replaced by their sulfonamide relatives the thiazides. One reason for their limited use is the rapid onset of tolerance, and the drugs can become ineffective within 48 hours after therapy is initiated.

Action Mode. The drugs inhibit the generation of bicarbonate from carbon dioxide and water by inhibition of the enzyme carbonic anhydrase. The decreased availability of bicarbonate reduces the coupling with sodium ions, and larger amounts of that electrolyte are excreted. The carbonic anhydrase inhibition occurs primarily in the proximal and distal tubules, which retards sodium and hydrogen ion exchange throughout the nephron. Although they are relatively weak diuretics, their action promotes the excretion of a hypotonic urine. The diuresis consists of sodium bicarbonate rather than the sodium chloride that is excreted with most of the other diuretics. The higher rate of delivery of sodium ions at distal tubule sites increases the exchange of sodium ions for potassium ions rather than for hydrogen ions and there may be an associated hypokalemia. The retention of hydrogen ions causes a hyperchloremic acidosis that decreases the effectiveness of the drugs.

Therapy Considerations. The drugs may be employed with a diuretic that tends to cause metabolic alkalosis (i.e., thiazides, furosemide, ethacrynic acid) because of their ability to counteract that problem. When they are used for adjunctive therapy in the control of edema, the drugs are employed on an intermittent or alternate-day schedule to avert the development of tolerance to their action.

Adverse Effects. Metabolic acidosis, gastrointestinal disturbances, drowsiness, fatigue, transient myopia, and paresthesias in the extremities are the most frequent adverse effects during therapy. The allergic reactions common to the sulfonamides (urticaria, fever, blood dyscrasias) have occurred only rarely during therapy with the carbonic anhydrase inhibitors.

Plasma Volume Control

Albumin Replacement

A decrease in the level of plasma proteins lowers the intravascular colloidal osmotic factor that maintains the circulating plasma volume. Without the "holding" force of the plasma proteins, the hydrostatic pressure and negative interstitial pressure at the capillary membranes cause the intravascular fluid to move outward into the tissues. The process can produce tissue edema while the intravascular volume is low.

Intravenous infusion of *human albumin* (AL-BUMISOL, ALBUSPAN) replaces the serum albumin losses and restores the normal colloidal osmotic forces. The 5 percent albumin solution is administered without additional dilution to provide the concentration required for reversal of the osmotic pressures. The 25 percent solution may be diluted or it may be infused undiluted. It is usual for oral fluid to be restricted for several hours after the infusion of the parenteral albumin solution, and regularly scheduled intravenous maintenance therapy is interrupted whenever possible. The albumin is infused at the slow rate of 2 to 3 ml/minute to gradually reverse the hypoproteinemic status and avoid a sudden fluid shift from the tissues to the vasculature.

The sodium content of normal human serum albumin 25 percent has been standardized to 130 to 160 mEq per liter. Either the standardized serum albumin product or the older "salt-poor albumin" can be given to persons having a sodium-intake restriction. The intravenous infusion of a single 20-ml vial of human albumin (25 percent) can increase the blood volume by approximately 500 ml. The effect is evident in an elevation of the blood pressure and in a lowering of the hematocrit value. Those parameters and the plasma protein levels provide the basis for decisions about the additional albumin replacement requirements of the patient. Occasionally there are allergic reactions during therapy (i.e., chills, fever, anaphylaxis).

Antidiuretic Hormone Replacement

The absence of the antidiuretic hormone (ADH) can cause excretion of copious amounts of dilute urine. The hormone deficiency most frequently occurs as a consequence of compromised pituitary or hypothalamic gland function and it is known as *central diabetes insipidus.*

Patients with diabetes insipidus may excrete up to 200 ml of urine hourly, and the specific gravity of the urine is close to that of water (i.e., 1.005).

It becomes necessary for the person to drink amounts of fluid equal to the amount of urine excreted in an attempt to maintain the body fluid balance.

Purified extracts of pituitary gland are available for subcutaneous or intramuscular injection. *Vasopressin* (PITRESSIN) and *vasopressin tannate* provide pharmacologic substitutes for the natural antidiuretic hormone. *Lypressin* (DIAPID) is a synthetic agent that provides an ADH effect without the vasopressor effect. It is used as a nasal spray. An investigational drug known as DDAVP or *desmopressin* is used as an inhalant.

The parenteral forms of the antidiuretic hormone have concurrent effects on vascular smooth muscle and on the muscle of the abdominal organs (i.e., gastrointestinal tract, uterus, bladder). The effects are somewhat less evident with use of the drugs as a nasal spray or inhalant.

Each of the preparations can be employed on a long-term basis, and the patient or a family member is carefully instructed in proper use of the drug. The aspects that require particular emphasis are the measurement of fluid intake, avoidance of concentrated sweets, and measurement of the amount and specific gravity of the urine. A vital part of the instruction is related to the use of a chart format for recording the daily weight, the quantities of fluid ingested, and the quantity and specific gravity of voidings. That chart form is useful for periodically assessing the progress of therapy and for regulating the drug dosage. Supervised practice sessions are planned to assure that the patient and family member understand the specific therapy plan and the appropriate methods for using the drug.

Aldosterone Replacement

Persons with adrenocortical insufficiency, or hypoadrenal syndrome, have insufficient sodium in the body tissues to maintain normal function. Hypotension and fatigue are the most distressing overt signs of the problem. The extent of the adrenal gland insufficiency determines the level of cortical hormone replacement (glucocorticoid, androgen, mineralocorticoid). Replacement of the mineralocorticoid activity of aldosterone is a vital factor in maintaining the electrolyte and fluid balance at physiologic levels.

Desoxycorticosterone acetate (DOCA) and *fludrocortisone* (FLORINEF) are the mineralocorticoids employed to reinstitute the reabsorption of sodium ions from the distal tubules. The restoration of sodium and potassium ion balance improves the extracellular and intracellular fluid equilibrium. Those improvements in turn have a positive effect on hemodynamic function, nutrient utilization, and nitrogen excretion. The concurrent increase in glandular secretions (salivary, sweat, gastrointestinal glands) has a positive effect on their function.

During therapy the person is encouraged to increase the intake of salty snacks in an effort to lower the drug requirements. The adverse effects of the drugs that occur during therapy include edema associated with excessive retention of sodium and water, hypertension, cardiac hypertrophy, and hypokalemia.

NURSING INTERVENTION

The nurse plays a vital role in planning for the implementation of the diuretic therapy regimen and in preparing the patient for maintenance of the therapy plan. The following outline provides a guide for planning nursing intervention when the patient is receiving a diuretic for the control of sequestered fluid. The guidelines contain suggestions for approaches that can be used in the clinical setting *to establish base lines for assessing the effect of the diuretic on fluid accumulation, to plan measures to maximize the diuretic drug effect and maintain fluid balance, and to prepare the patient for assessing the progress of the diuretic drug therapy plan.*

Guidelines for Nursing Intervention

I. Establish base lines for assessing the effect of the diuretic on fluid accumulation.
  A. Obtain the patient's statement of the problem and the functional limits caused by the problem.
  B. Obtain information about the psychosocial factors affecting resolution of the problem (i.e., health history, health care practices, compliance with prescribed therapies, previous problems with drugs).
  C. Examine the patient for signs of excess tissue fluid in extremities, sacral and periorbital areas, lungs, and peritoneal cavity.
    1. Observe the skin for tension.
    2. Test distended tissues for rebound after digital compression (pitting).
    3. Compare the skin color and surface temperature with uninvolved surfaces.
    4. Observe the rate and pattern of breathing.
    5. Listen to the lung fields for areas of dullness or for fluid content (i.e., moist rales, wheezing).
    6. Palpate the abdomen for shifting of fluid content (ascites) or liver enlargement.
    7. Measure the sites of fluid accumulation (i.e., ankles, calves, abdominal girth).
    8. Define the effect of the fluid on body function (i.e., lung expansion, joint movement).
  D. Examine the patient for evidence of an excess circulating blood volume.
    1. Take the blood pressure and compare the current systolic pressure and pulse pressure levels with previous recordings.
    2. Count the pulse rate and note its strength and regularity.
    3. Examine the veins for pulsation or distention (i.e., jugular vein fullness when supine and with the head rest elevated to 30 degrees).
  E. Analyze the fluid requirements and the fluid losses.

1. Examine the mucous membranes and note the quantity of saliva present. Also note the moisture, color, size, and fullness of the tongue (including coating).
2. Note the amount and characteristics of fluid losses through the skin (diaphoresis) and body cavities (i.e., saturation of dressings, suction quantity).
3. Take the patient's temperature.
4. Measure the quantity and specific gravity of the urine.
5. Weigh the patient.

F. Examine the clinical record for relevant data. These include
   1. Daily fluid balance recordings.
   2. Serum albumin/globulin ratio.
   3. Serum sodium level.
   4. Serum osmolarity.
   5. Hematocrit level.
   6. Chest x-ray report.
   7. Central venous pressure (CVP) recordings.

II. Plan measures to maximize the diuretic drug effect and to maintain fluid balance.
   A. Explain to the patient the effects of the diuretic and of fluid and sodium restriction on fluid accumulation.
   B. Implement the prescribed fluid, drug, and sodium restriction schedule.
      1. Identify the fluid intake allowances (i.e., oral, parenteral, instillations) within the 24-hour restriction.
      2. Calculate the amount of fluid required for taking oral medications during the 24-hour period.
      3. Ascertain the patient's preferred distribution of fluid intake (i.e., mealtime fluids) and food preferences.
      4. Schedule the drug administration to allow for diuresis during the daytime hours.
      5. Include the patient in the health team planning for implementation of the prescribed restrictions.
   C. Assess the diuresis level and the changes in fluid accumulation.
      1. Maintain a record of the fluid intake and output.
      2. Teach the patient to measure and record the fluid intake.
      3. Analyze the relationship between changes in the daily fluid balance, changes in body weight, and tissue fluid accumulation.
   D. Employ measures to minimize the effects of accumulated fluid.
      1. Protect the edematous tissues from trauma.
      2. Mobilize the pooled fluid (i.e., positioning, controlled exercise, elastic stockings).
   E. Reassess the patient's physiologic status to define the effectiveness of the diuretic drug, changes in fluid accumulation, and the adverse effects of the diuretic drug.

III. Prepare the patient for assessing the progress of the diuretic drug therapy plan.
   A. Teach the patient how to assess changes in fluid accumulation. Measures include
      1. Keeping a record of the daily weight.
      2. Observing changes in the patterns of urination.
      3. Observing the concentration of the urine.
      4. Examining the fluid accumulation sites regularly.
   B. Review with the patient, and a family member, the plan for use of the diuretic, potassium supplements, and the sodium-fluid restriction.
      1. Plan with the patient for implementation of the specific drug therapy regimen within the usual schedule of daily activities.

2. Provide specific written instructions for the patient to use at home.

C. Explain to the patient the factors that may change the sodium requirements and fluid balance. These include

1. Increased or decreased fluid intake.
2. Persistent vomiting or diarrhea.
3. High environmental temperatures.
4. Elevation of the body temperature.

D. Describe to the patient the problems that require physician contact. These include

1. Signs of dehydration, including marked thirst, excess dryness of the skin and mucous membranes, de-creased urine output, and increased concentration of the urine.
2. Signs of the low-salt syndrome, including anorexia, nausea, vomiting, diarrhea, fatigue, dulled mental faculties, muscle cramps.
3. Adverse effects of the particular drug.

E. Describe to the patient the measures that can be employed to support the drug action (i.e., elevation of the extremities, foot exercises).

F. Reassess the patient's readiness to maintain the drug therapy plan at home.

Review Guides

1. Outline in detail the factors that would be included in explaining to the patient the rationale for use of hydrochlorothiazide and spironolactone for the control of edema.
2. Describe the measures that should be employed by the patient when assessing the effectiveness and the onset of adverse effects of hydrochlorothiazide and spironolactone.
3. Outline a plan for monitoring the status of a patient who is receiving furosemide for control of acute pulmonary edema.
4. Formulate a plan for instructing a clinic patient who has received an initial prescription for chlorthalidone and potassium chloride and directions that the patient interprets as being to "eat food without adding salt and get plenty of rest."
5. Describe in detail the measures that would be employed by the nurse when the unresponsive patient is receiving mannitol for control of increased intracranial pressure.

Additional Readings

Bay, William H., and Ferris, Thomas F.: Hypernatremia and hyponatremia: disorders of toxicity. *Geriatrics,* **31**:53, August, 1976.

Beerman, Björn; Groschensky-Grind, Margaretha; and Rosén, Anders: Absorption, metabolism, and excretion of hydrochlorothiazide. *Clin. Pharmacol. Ther.,* **19**:531, May, 1976.

Cannon, Paul J.: The kidney in heart failure. *N. Engl. J. Med.,* **296**:26, January 6, 1977.

Cunningham, Joseph H.; Richardson, Robert H.; and Smith, Jan D.: Interstitial pulmonary edema. *Heart Lung,* **6**:617, July–August, 1977.

Gardner, Kenneth D., Jr.: Potassium: the intracellular cation. *Primary Care,* **2**:161, March, 1975.

Gifford, Ray W., Jr.: A guide to the practical use of diuretics. *J.A.M.A.,* **235**:1890, April 26, 1976.

Goodlin, Robert C.: Severe pre-eclampsia: another great imitator. *J. Obstet. Gynecol.,* **125**:747, July 15, 1976.

Grant, Marcia M., and Kubo, Winifred M.: Assessing a patient's hydration status. *Am. J. Nurs.,* **75**:1306, August, 1975.

Haughey, Edmund J., Jr., and Sica, Frances M.: Diuretics. *Nursing 77,* **7**:34, February, 1977.

Hays, Robert M.: Antidiuretic hormone. *N. Engl. J. Med.,* **295**:659, September 16, 1976.

Isacson, Lauren Marie, and Schulz, Klaus: Treating pulmonary edema. *Nursing 78,* **8**:42, February, 1978.

Jamison, Rex L., and Maffley, Roy H.: The urinary concentrating mechanism. *N. Engl. J. Med.,* **295:** 1059, November 4, 1976.

Jones, Claudella, and Feller, Irving: Burns: what to do during the first crucial hours. *Nursing 77,* **7:**22, March, 1977.

Karim, A.; Zagrella, J.; Hribar, J.; and Dooley, M.: Spironolactone, 1. Disposition and metabolism. *Clin. Pharmacol. Ther.,* **19:**158, February, 1976.

Kemp, Ginny, and Kemp, Doug: Diuretics. *Am. J. Nurs.,* **78:**1006, June, 1978.

Keyes, Jack L.: Basic mechanisms involved in acid-based homeostasis. *Heart Lung,* **5:**239, March–April, 1976.

Krumloosky, Frank A., and del Greco, Francesco: Diuretic agents: mechanisms of action and clinical uses. *Postgrad. Med.,* **59:**105, April, 1976.

Lancour, Jane: ADH and aldosterone: how to recognize their effects. *Nursing 78,* **8:**36, September, 1978.

Lee, Wai-Nang P.; Lippe, Barbara M.; La Franchi, Stephen H.; and Kaplan, Solomon A.: Vasopressin analog DDAVP in the treatment of diabetes insipidus. *Am. J. Dis. Child.,* **130:**166. February, 1976.

Lewiston, Norman, J.; Theodore, James; and Robin, Eugene D.: Intracellular edema and hydration: effects on energy metabolism in alveolar macrophages. *Science,* **191:**403, January, 1976.

Ling, Gilbert N., and Walton, Cheryl L.: What retains water in living cells? *Science,* **191:**293, January, 1976.

Lohmöller, Georg; Lohmöller, Reinhilde; Pfeffer, Marc A.; Pfeffer, Janice M.; and Frohlich, Edward D.: Mechanism of immediate hemodynamic effects of chlorothiazide. *Am. Heart J.,* **89:**487, April, 1975.

McFarlane, Judith M.: The child with diabetes insipidus. *Pediatr. Nurs.,* **1:**20, December, 1975.

MacLeod, Stuart M.: The rational use of potassium supplements. *Postgrad. Med.,* **57:**123, February, 1975.

Maffly, Roy H.: How to avoid complications of potent diuretics. *J.A.M.A.,* **235:**2526, June 7, 1976.

Mariani, G.; Strober, W.; Keiser, H.; and Waldmann, T. A.: Pathophysiology of hypoalbuminemia associated with carcinoid tumor. *Cancer,* **38:**854, August, 1976.

Moses, Arnold M.: Diabetes insipidus and ADH regulation. *Hosp. Pract.,* **12:**37, July, 1977.

Priest, John N.; Ahmed, Mohammed; and Nuttall, Frank Q.: Pathologic hypofunction of the renin-angiotension-aldosterone system. *Postgrad. Med.,* **59:**86, February, 1976.

Ramsay, David J., and Ganong, William F.: CNS regulation of salt and water intake. *Hosp. Pract.,* **12:**63, March, 1977.

Renkin, Eugene M., and Robinson, Roscoe R.: Glomerular filtration. *N. Engl. J. Med.,* **290:**785, April 4, 1974.

Rogenes, Paula R., and Moylan, Joseph A.: Restoring fluid balance in the patient with severe burns. *Am. J. Nurs.,* **76:**1953, December, 1976.

Schwartz, Allan B.: Therapy of hypokalemia. *Am. Fam. Physician,* **13:**148, April, 1976.

Seller, Robert H.; Banach, Stanley; Namey, Thomas; Neff, Martin; and Swartz, Charles: Cardiac effects of diuretic drugs. *Am. Heart J.,* **89:**493, April, 1975.

Tisher, C. Craig: Functional anatomy of the kidney. *Hosp. Pract.,* **13:**53, May, 1978.

Tullis, James L.: Albumin: Background and use. *J.A.M.A.,* **237:**355, January 24, 1977; 460, January 31, 1977.

Vidt, Donald G.: Diuretics: use and misuse. *Postgrad. Med.,* **59:**143, May, 1976.

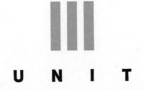

U N I T

Drugs Used to Maintain Cellular Reproduction and the Integrity of Tissues

15

Abnormal Cell Proliferation

There are more than one-half million new cases of cancer each year in the United States. Although that figure represents the incidence of cancer at the 12 commonly affected tissue sites, there are more than 100 different classifications of the malignant cells. The basic commonality in all cancer is the transformation of cells to more primitive and less well-differentiated cell types. The major outcome of the abnormal cell proliferation is disruption of physiologic function.

Physiologic Correlations

Cell Life-Cycle

The reproduction of cells is a cyclic process that provides for the growth, reparative, and replacement processes required for normal tissue function. The cell life-cycle begins with the phases of mitosis (interphase, prophase, metaphase, anaphase, telophase) that lead to cell division (Fig. 15–1). The mitotic phase, or "M" phase, is followed by clearly defined events in the cell life-cycle. The new cells continue through the three biochemically distinct phases that lead to their mitotic division. The G_1, or first gap after mitosis, is followed by the "S" phase during which *deoxy-ribonucleic acid* (DNA) directs the synthesis of protein. The synthesis phase is followed by a second gap, or G_2, during which *ribonucleic acid* (RNA) continues to produce cellular proteins as a preliminary to cellular reproduction. Some of the cells remain in a period of dormancy, or G_0, from which they later can move into the reproduction cycle.

Protein Synthesis

DNA is the genetic material of the cell that provides the selective template, or pattern, for formation of the ribosomal, messenger, and trans-

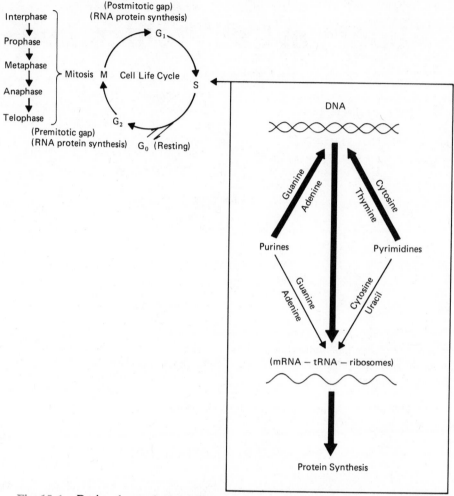

Fig. 15–1. During the synthesis phase of the cell life-cycle, deoxyribonucleic acid (DNA) directs the specific assembly pattern for the nucleic acids that are constructed on the ribonucleic acid (RNA) template for protein synthesis.

fer RNA that are involved in the synthesis of cellular proteins. The pattern, or specific sequences, of the long-chain nucleic acids determines the particular proteins, or enzymes, that will be synthesized on the ribosomal RNA templates.

The biosynthesis of proteins is dependent on the availability of enzymes that convert the purines and pyrimidines to the long-chain nucleic acids appropriate to the proteins being synthesized. The

purines (i.e., guanine, adenine) are utilized primarily in the synthesis of nucleotides by the DNA and they also are incorporated into the proteins that are structured by RNA.

The purines themselves utilize several enzymes and coenzymes in their assembly process. For example, endogenous folic acid is reduced by the enzyme *folic acid reductase* to *tetrahydrofolic acid*, which transports single-carbon fragments for the synthesis of the purine ring. The tetra-hydrofolic acid also is utilized in the methylation of *deoxyuridylic acid,* which forms the nucleotide *thymidylic acid* in preparation for its utilization by DNA.

The pyrimidines (i.e., cytosine, thymine, uracil) also provide nitrogenous bases for the formation of nucleotides required for the DNA-directed synthesis of proteins. The proteins or enzymes that are synthesized determine the structure, metabolic activity, proliferation rate, and function of the cell.

Cellular Reproduction Rates

The cellular reproduction rate varies in different body tissues. The *bone marrow, gastrointestinal epithelium, germinal epithelium of the gonads, epidermal tissues* (i.e., skin, hair follicles), and *embryonic structures* have a more rapid reproduction rate than most of the other body tissues. The high mitotic activity of the cells that line the gas-trointestinal tract provides replacement cells every one to eight days for those intraluminal cells that are damaged during the normal digestive processes.

The short 8-to-12-day lifespan of the platelets requires a rapid reproduction rate in the myelogenous tissues to maintain the number of platelets at the level required for the physiologic processes that control bleeding. The leukocytes have a lifespan in the circulation similar to that of the platelets. The granulocytes (neutrophils, eosinophils, basophils) regularly are reproduced in the bone marrow and the nongranular leukocytes (lymphocytes and monocytes) are reproduced primarily in the spleen. The rapid reproduction rate of those reticuloendothelial tissues provides the blood elements required for the control of infection and for the immunologic responses. The longer lifespan of the erythrocytes (120 days) in the circulation requires a much slower reproduction rate to maintain the red blood cell level necessary for oxygen transport.

Pathophysiologic Correlations

Cancer represents the proliferation of abnormal cells that can proceed at a rate rapid enough to deprive normal body tissues of the nutrients essential for their growth, function, repair, and reproduction. The mutant cells are relatives of normal body cells, and their rate of growth and reproduction are influenced by the characteristics of the tissues from which they originate.

Types of Cancer

The four major types of cancer are *carcinoma, sarcoma, lymphoma,* and *leukemia.* Each type of cancer has characteristics that facilitate understanding of the impact of the malignant neoplasm on physiologic function.

1. The *carcinomas* are solid neoplasms growing from derivatives of the embryonal *ectoderm* or *entoderm.* The epithelial tissue derivatives include neoplasms of tissues at internal and external body sites (i.e., skin, glands, nerves, breasts, linings of the respiratory, gastrointestinal, urinary, and genital systems). The carcinomas represent the most prevalent forms of cancer.

2. The *sarcomas* are solid neoplasms growing from derivatives of the embryonal *mesoderm* or *mesenchyme.* The group represents neoplasms in connective tissue, cartilage, bone, muscle, and adipose tissues. Although bone marrow and lymphoid tissues have the same embryonal origins as the sarcomas, the characteristics of the malignant cells arising from those tissues make it necessary to separate them from the solid neoplasms identified as sarcomas.

3. The *lymphomas* are characterized by the aggregation of large numbers of abnormal, nonfunctional lymphocytes in the lymphoid tissues. Hodgkin's disease is one of the more common types of the malignant lymphomas.

4. The *leukemias* include several blood dyscrasias that are characterized by a marked increase in the number of nonfunctional immature leuko-

cytes in the circulating peripheral blood. The overproduction of abnormal leukocytes crowds the bone marrow and suppresses erythrocyte and platelet production. The leukocytes also infiltrate and enlarge the liver, spleen, and lymph nodes. When the predominant leukocytes are the granulocytes that are produced in the bone marrow (neutrophils, eosinophils, or basophils), the disease is described as *myelocytic leukemia*. The name may include a specific designation of the particular granulocyte that is proliferating at an abnormal rate. The disease also is described as *acute myelogenous leukemia,* to describe the rapid progression of the disease that occurs in infants and children, or as *chronic myelogenous leukemia,* which has a slower onset and occurs in the older age groups.

When the predominant abnormal immature leukocytes are the agranular cells that are produced in the spleen (monocytes and lymphocytes), the designation includes the particular cellular type. *Acute lymphocytic leukemia* is a rapidly progressing disease of children. It also is a manifestation of an abnormality in the subgroup of lymphocytes known as the *T cell type* that are thymus dependent and differentiate in the thymus. *Chronic lymphocytic leukemia* progresses more slowly and it occurs in the older age groups. It is a manifestation of an abnormality in the subgroup of lymphocytes known as the *B cell type* that remains in the bloodstream as the primary producer of antibody. Both groups of lymphocytes are derived from the reticuloendothelial tissues. The difference in the age groups that develop the two types of lymphocytic leukemia may be an indication that an underlying immunologic maturity is a factor in the type of lymphocyte that becomes malignant.

Cancer Growth Characteristics

The major types of cancer share the two common characteristics of *anaplasia* and *metastasis.* Anaplasia describes the transformation of a cell to one with a structural abnormality. The neoplastic cell resembles a more primitive or embryonic cell, and there is an absence of the specialized functions that are common to the mature form of the cell. The abnormal cell has a greater ability to multiply than its parent cell.

Malignant neoplasms have an ability to infiltrate and invade surrounding tissues as they grow. Single cells or a small group of cells can separate from the malignant tissue and travel through the lymphatic system and bloodstream to distant sites within the host. The groups of transplanted cells, or *metastases,* lodge in favorable sites and multiply.

Common Physiologic Problems

Commonalities in the physiologic problems occur in association with cancer cell invasion of body tissues and with the metastatic dissemination of malignant cells throughout the body.

The problems that occur most frequently in patients with cancer are *edema, thrombophlebitis, elimination problems, hemorrhage, anemia, fractures, malnutrition,* and *infection.* Some of the physiologic problems relate to the pressure of the malignant growth on the vasculature (i.e., edema, thrombophlebitis) or to pressure on the gastrointestinal tract (i.e., nausea, anorexia, constipation). The infiltration of normal organs by cancer tissue, in addition to causing pressure that inhibits the natural organ function, can erode into the capillaries and cause hemorrhage. The decreased production of platelets and erythrocytes in the bone marrow of the patient with leukemia causes a high incidence of bleeding episodes and anemia. The displacement of normal structural components in the bones by a sarcoma can increase their fragility and cause spontaneous fractures.

The general health status of the person also is adversely affected by the continual diversion of the endogenous nutrient supplies to the malignant cells that are reproducing rapidly. The malnutrition of normal tissues predisposes the individual to infection and disability. The therapeutic plans for the patient have the dual purpose of restoring the general health status while arresting or eradicating the cancer tissue.

Antineoplastic Drugs

Surgery, radiation therapy, and antineoplastic drugs are the modalities currently employed for the treatment of cancer. The mode of therapy is selected on the basis of the unique characteristics of the particular type of cancer. Surgery is the primary treatment for many of the solid carcinomas and sarcomas; radiation therapy is the primary treatment for some of the lymphomas (i.e., Hodgkin's disease); and chemotherapy is the primary treatment for leukemia. Radiation therapy and chemotherapy may be employed as adjuncts to surgery in a multidimensional approach to control of malignant neoplasms.

Many times the goal of therapy is to extend the life expectancy and to improve the quality of the person's life (palliative therapy). Surgery, radiation therapy, or antineoplastic drugs may be employed to reduce the disruption of physiologic processes that is caused by the cancer tissue when the person has advanced, widely disseminated cancer.

Immunotherapy for the control of cancer is being investigated intensively. The current investigations involve the use of cancer cells and other antigens (i.e., *Corynebacterium parvum* and bacille Calmette Guérin, or BCG) to stimulate endogenous production of antibodies in quantities adequate to control the proliferation of cancer cells. Immunotherapy capitalizes on the body's natural immune mechanisms and is considered to be a method that can provide an added stimulus to the body's rejection of cancer cells before they proliferate and disseminate throughout the body.

DRUG THERAPY

Modern antineoplastic drug therapy represents a diversified biochemical approach to the control of cancer. Current knowledge of the growth characteristics of normal and malignant cells and of the action mode of the chemotherapeutic agents allows drug administration to exploit the vulnerability of cancer cells.

ADVERSE EFFECTS

The antineoplastic drugs are highly toxic agents with a low therapeutic index. There seldom is a therapeutic outcome without the incidence of some adverse effects.

Drug therapy usually is planned and directed by a specialist in chemotherapy, or oncologist. The patient is actively involved in all aspects of the therapy program, and the benefits, risks, and probable adverse effects are specifically discussed with the person and appropriate family members before therapy is initiated. Inclusion of the patient in the plan for monitoring the effects of therapy is a valuable adjunct to the monitoring done by the professional members of the health team.

The antineoplastic drugs are cytotoxic and they act on the biochemical pathways of normal and neoplastic cells. The cells are more vulnerable during active reproduction, and those cells that proliferate rapidly are the ones most likely to be destroyed. Although there is some variation in the time of onset, the duration, and the severity of toxic effects on normal rapidly proliferating tissues, it is predictable that the drugs will affect the bone marrow, gastrointestinal epithelium, germinal epithelium of the gonads, epidermal tissues, and embryonic structures.

Bone Marrow Depression

Depression of the bone marrow is the most frequent toxic effect of the chemotherapeutic drugs. Therapy may be interrupted when the leukocyte count reaches 3000/cu mm (normal = 5000 to 10,000/cu mm), and the patient's status and blood values are monitored closely until the count reaches its lowest point, or nadir. The patient may be placed in protective isolation when the residual drug continues to lower the leukocyte level (leukopenia). The patient's status is monitored regularly because infection can occur rapidly. The usual outward signs of infection are absent when leukocyte production is depressed.

The platelet count is also monitored closely during the period of bone marrow depression, and drug therapy may be interrupted when the platelet count drops (thrombocytopenia) to 100,000/cu mm (normal = 150,000 to 350,000/cu mm). Observations for bleeding are intensified until the nadir is reached and the platelet production slowly raises the level to the normal range.

Immunosuppression

Most of the antineoplastic drugs also have immunosuppressive properties. There is considerable variation in the intensity of the drug-induced suppression of the natural immune responses. Depression of the production of leukocytes in the bone marrow reduces the natural primary inflammatory reaction, and concurrent suppression of lymphocyte production in the lymphoid tissues (lymphocytopenia) reduces the production of antibodies. Debilitated cancer patients who are receiving antineoplastic drugs are very susceptible to the opportunist organisms that cause serious antibiotic-resistant infections.

Gastrointestinal Toxicity

Signs of gastrointestinal tissue toxicity also occur frequently during antineoplastic drug therapy. The earliest signs of the toxicity may be erythema and ulceration of the tissues of the oral mucosa, or *stomatitis,* with concurrent nausea, vomiting, or diarrhea. Therapy may be interrupted for a period of time long enough for the regeneration of the epithelial tissues.

Gonadal Toxicity

Some of the antineoplastic drugs cause sterility and testicular atrophy in males. Azoospermia or oligospermia has been observed in patients receiving the drugs over prolonged periods of time. Amenorrhea is the most frequently observed sequel in females on long-term therapy.

Embryonic Toxicity

The chemotherapeutic drugs also have mutagenic, carcinogenic, and teratogenic potentials. Administration of high therapeutic doses of the drugs during the first trimester of pregnancy could result in congenital anomalies in the fetus. Women of childbearing age are informed of the possible hazard to the fetus and advised to utilize measures for conception control while taking the drugs.

Epidermal Tissue Toxicity

Alopecia is the most common manifestation of epidermal tissue toxicity. Baldness may be partial or complete, and there may also be loss of axillary and pubic hair. Some patients purchase a wig to prepare for the time when the hair will be very thin or completely absent.

A tourniquet, which may be constructed of surgical stockinette or a similar material, may be placed around the head at a level just below the patient's hairline to obstruct the flow of blood containing the drug. That obstruction of the external carotid tributaries has decreased the alopecia by preventing the action of the drug on the hair follicles.

Hyperpigmentation of the nails, nailbeds, and dermal folds and photosensitization that causes intense erythema with minimal exposure to the ultraviolet sun rays and subsequent hyperpigmentation are also toxic epidermal reactions. There is sometimes a partial loss of fingernails but that seldom is upsetting to patients. The hair and fingernails usually regrow and that regrowth sometimes takes place during the course of drug therapy.

Uric Acid Retention

Hyperuricemia occurs as an indirect effect of the drugs. The problem represents an increase in uric acid that is associated with the rapid breakdown of large numbers of cancer cells. Patients usually are placed on a "force-fluids" schedule to assure that the renal blood flow is maintained at a level that will move the uric acid crystals rapidly through the nephrons. Accumulation of the crystals can cause renal stone formation. Many physicians prescribe intravenous administration of sodium bicarbonate concurrent with administration of the antineoplastic drug to alkalinize the urine thereby decreasing the aggregation of uric acid crystals. *Allopurinol* may also be employed to prevent formation of the uric acid.

Nausea and Vomiting

Nausea and vomiting are common problems during antineoplastic drug therapy. The greatest discomfort usually is evident in the hours immediately following administration of the drug. Antiemetic drugs sometimes are prescribed for administration prior to giving the drug. Administration of the antineoplastic drug at bedtime may lessen the discomfort of nausea and decrease its interference with eating at a time when good nutrition is a vital aspect of therapy.

Factors Affecting Toxicity

Adverse effects are most prevalent when the patient has recently received chemotherapeutic drugs or radiation therapy. Each course of therapy is planned at a time when physiologic function has returned to the level considered normal for the individual. An interval of one month may be required before such stability is reached. Chemotherapy usually is instituted approximately 30 days after surgery to allow time for wound healing before the use of the drugs that can inhibit the growth of new cells at the incision site.

Intermittent, high-dosage drug therapy causes fewer adverse effects than continuous therapy at a lower drug dosage level. The intermittent plan also allows time for normal cells to reproduce between the courses of therapy. Because normal cells have a greater capacity for repair and reproduction than cancer cells, they can utilize the intervals between courses of therapy for that regeneration. The drug-free period is a time interval specifically calculated to maintain suppression of cancer cell reproduction.

DRUG THERAPY REGIMENS

Antineoplastic drugs are administered on cyclic, sequential, or simultaneous patterns that al-low as many as five agents to be employed to induce or maintain remission. The maintenance of remission involves the use of one or more chemotherapeutic agents for a prolonged period of time. Throughout therapy the patient's status is monitored at regular intervals. Periodic physical examinations, x-rays, and hematologic evaluations are scheduled to monitor the effectiveness of therapy and to allow early identification of adverse effects of the drugs.

There is no panacea in drug therapy for cancer and no one drug is useful against a particular type of malignant neoplasm in all patients. Pretreatment evaluation of the patient's clinical status and a histologic diagnosis are prerequisites to individualized therapy. The final outcome of therapy is dependent on the interaction between the drug, the cancer, and the patient in each individual situation.

The dosage of the antineoplastic drug is individualized on the basis of the patient's physiologic status, therapeutic response, and the incidence of adverse effects of the drugs. Therapy frequently must be interrupted to allow adverse effects to subside. The therapeutic plans also may be modified as the effectiveness of the drug decreases. The problem of cancer tissue resistance to one or more of the drugs may necessitate utilization of alternate drugs.

Combination chemotherapy is widely employed in an attempt to delay the emergence of cancer tissue resistance to the drugs and the incidence of adverse effects. The use of drugs in combinations also provides an additive or synergistic effect on the eradication of cancer cells. The protocols for varying regimens usually include drugs that are effective individually for the particular type of cancer being treated. The regimens also utilize representatives from varied drug classes that act at differing phases of the cell life-cycle (Table 15–1). The multidimensional attack on the cancer cells is planned to kill the largest possible number of malignant cells in the vulnerable periods of their cell cycle. The various regimens are commonly referred to by the initials (acronyms) representing the drugs included in the protocol (i.e., COAP, POMP, MOPP). The initials generally

Table 15–1.

Drug Groups Represented in Commonly Used Antineoplastic Drug Protocols

Drug Therapy Combination	Drug Class	Drug Therapy Combination	Drug Class
Leukemia		*MOPP regimen:*	
COAP regimen:		Mechlorethamine	Alkylating agent
Cyclophosphamide	Alkylating agent	Vincristine*	Antimitotic
Vincristine*	Antimitotic	Procarbazine	Mixed action agent
Cytarabine	Pyridimine anti-metabolite†		
Prednisone	Glucocorticoid	Prednisone	Glucocorticoid
Cytarabine	Pyrimidine anti-metabolite†	*Gastrointestinal Neoplasm*	
		Cytarabine	Pyrimidine anti-metabolite†
Thioguanine	Purine anti-metabolite	Fluorouracil	Pyrimidine anti-metabolite§
		Mitomycin	Antibiotic
POMP regimen:		Carmustine	Alkylating agent
Mercaptopurine‡	Purine anti-metabolite	Fluorouracil	Pyrimidine anti-metabolite§
Vincristine*	Antimitotic		
Methotrexate	Folic acid anti-metabolite	Fluorouracil	Pyrimidine anti-metabolite§
Prednisone	Glucocorticoid	Semustine	Alkylating agent
VAMP regimen:		*Breast Carcinoma*	
Vincristine	Antimitotic	*CAF regimen:*	
Methotrexate	Folic acid anti-metabolite	Cyclophosphamide	Alkylating agent
		Doxorubicin‖	Antibiotic
Mercaptopurine	Purine anti-metabolite	Fluorouracil	Pyrimidine anti-metabolite§
Prednisone	Glucocorticoid		
Osteogenic Sarcoma		*CMF regimen:*	
Cyclophosphamide	Alkylating agent	Cyclophosphamide	Alkylating agent
Doxorubicin	Antibiotic	Methotrexate	Folic acid anti-metabolite
Melphalan	Alkylating agent		
Vincristine	Antimitotic	Fluorouracil	Pyrimidine anti-metabolite§
Cyclophosphamide	Alkylating agent		
Doxorubicin	Antibiotic	*CMFP regimen:*	
Methotrexate	Folic acid anti-metabolite	Cyclophosphamide	Alkylating agent
		Methotrexate	Folic acid anti-metabolite
Cyclophosphamide	Alkylating agent		
Doxorubicin	Antibiotic	Fluorouracil	Pyrimidine anti-metabolite§
Methotrexate	Folic acid anti-metabolite		
Vincristine	Antimitotic	Prednisone	Glucocorticoid
Lymphoma		*COOPER regimen:*	
Bleomycin	Antibiotic	Cyclophosphamide	Alkylating agent
Dacarbazine (DTIC)	Alkylating-like agent	Methotrexate	Folic acid anti-metabolite
Doxorubicin	Antibiotic	Vincristine*	Antimitotic
		Fluorouracil	Pyrimidine anti-metabolite§

Table 15-1—Continued

Drug Therapy Combination	Drug Class	Drug Therapy Combination	Drug Class
Vincristine	Antimitotic	Prednisone	Glucocorticoid
COP or CVP regimen:		*Testicular Carcinoma*	
Cyclophosphamide	Alkylating agent	Bleomycin	Antibiotic
Vincristine*	Antimitotic	Vinblastine	Antimitotic
Prednisone	Glucocorticoid	Chlorambucil	Alkylating agent
		Dactinomycin	Antibiotic
		Methotrexate	Folic acid antimetabolite

* Regimen title refers to trade name (ONCOVIN).
† Cystosine analog.
‡ Regimen title refers to trade name (PURINETHOL).
§ Thymine and uracil analog.
‖ Regimen title refers to trade name (ADRIAMYCIN).

designate the generic or trade name of the drug or the drug class that it represents.

Regional Drug Infusion

The myriad of adverse effects that occur during systemic drug therapy can be circumvented in selected situations by infusing the drug directly into the circulation to an involved organ or into a body cavity containing the malignant cells. *Isolated perfusion, arterial infusion,* and *intracavity instillation* are the administration methods utilized for nonsystemic treatment of neoplasms or their metastases. Isolated perfusion and arterial infusion allow the introduction of the antineoplastic drug at a high concentration that would be intolerable if the drug were administered orally or parenterally for systemic distribution. The cancer tissue assimilates the drug and a minimal amount of it is returned to the general circulation.

Isolated Perfusion. The drug administration method involves isolation of the vasculature of a regional arterial bed (i.e., an extremity). The isolated limb is shunted off from the circulation by the occlusion of the arterial and venous tributaries. The blood vessels are cannulated and the blood flow is circulated through the limb by an external pump. The pump provides the power for circulation of the drug through the extremity and also provides for oxygenation, filtering, and removal of carbon dioxide as blood passes continuously through it. Several hours of drug perfusion of the limb usually are planned to allow delivery of the drug at a high concentration for a period of time that is adequate to destroy a large number of cancer cells.

Arterial Infusion. The administration method involves placement of a catheter into a large artery that supplies the arterial bed at the tumor site. A clock-directed metric infusion pump (i.e., chronofusor) continuously delivers the drug to the target tissue at a precalculated infusion rate. The method of drug administration has been employed for treatment of metastatic lesions in the liver and for the treatment of head and neck cancer. The arterial catheter is sutured in place to assure integrity of the system during the period of drug infusion. Patients have been treated on an ambulatory basis in some of the clinical trials with the arterial infusion technique. The low incidence of systemic adverse effects due to the localized drug distribution has allowed continuance of therapy over periods ranging from several months to a year with minimum toxicity.

Intracavity Instillation. Cancer tissue often releases large quantities of fluid into adjacent body cavities (i.e., peritoneal, pleural) and the excess fluid impinges on organ function. Although simple aspiration can remove the fluid content from the body cavity, it is rapidly replaced by the malignant tissues. The administration of a drug (i.e., quinacrine hydrochloride) into the cavity, after aspiration of the excess fluid, inhibits fluid accumulation by inducing an inflammatory reaction. The cancer tissues within the cavity, and the vessels supplying blood to them, become fibrotic and the release of fluid from those tissues is inhibited. When the aspirate from the body cavity contains free cancer cells, an antineoplastic drug may be instilled (i.e., methotrexate). The uniform distribution of the drug throughout the cavity is improved by changing the patient's position every five to ten minutes for one hour after the drug instillation. At the end of 24 to 36 hours the remaining fluid may be removed by paracentesis. The major problem that occurs after intracavity instillation is the formation of adhesions that may interfere with organ function.

Cell Life-Cycle Effects

An antineoplastic drug usually is classified under the action mode that is common to the entire class of chemically related drugs. Their actions also can be defined in terms of their effect on cancer *cell life-cycle phases*. Although there is general agreement about those modes of action, it is probable that the current intensive clinical investigations will reveal new or mixed actions for many of the drugs.

The drugs that are identified as being *cell life-cycle phase specific* are the *antimetabolites* and the *antimitotics*. The drugs in those groups, or drug classes, usually are effective against the cancer cells with a rapid rate of reproduction. The *cell life-cycle phase-nonspecific* drugs include the *antineoplastic antibiotics* and the *alkylating agents*. The drugs in those groups, or drug classes, usually are effective against large-volume, slowly reproducing cancer tissues. A few of the drugs

have action modes that are somewhat characteristic of both groups. The designation of specific and nonspecific action on the cell life-cycle phases provides an additional frame of reference for understanding the action of the major classes of antineoplastic drugs. The *antineoplastic hormones* are not included in the cell life-cycle designation. Their action changes the hormonal stimulus to tissue growth.

ANTIMETABOLITES

The antimetabolites interfere with the synthesis, or S phase, of the cell life-cycle by inhibiting the enzymatic conversions required for nucleotide synthesis. The drugs are structural analogs of the *purines, pyrimidines,* or *folic acid,* and their competition with the natural metabolites inhibits the enzymatic processes required for the utilization or production of active vitamins (i.e., folic acid), nitrogenous bases, or nucleosides. The absence of the natural metabolic building blocks interferes with the DNA-directed biosynthesis of proteins. The action of the antimetabolites slows the entry of the cells into the S phase of protein building.

The antimetabolites are divided into subclasses that describe the particular cellular function that is inhibited. The drugs disrupt DNA activity by acting as *purine analogs, pyrimidine analogs,* or *folic acid analogs.* The analogs that are similar to the nucleosides, nitrogenous bases, or the percursors that are required for the functions of both DNA and RNA are capable of inhibiting synthesis at more than one phase of the cellular protein-building sequence (Fig. 15–2).

Purine Analogs

The purine analogs *mercaptopurine, thioguanine,* and *azathioprine* interfere with synthesis of the nucleotides *adenylic acid* and *guanylic acid* by providing substitute metabolites for the nitrogenous bases *adenine* or *guanine.* The analog substitution is the primary action of the drugs. Mercaptopurine and azathioprine are adenine analogs, and thioguanine is a guanine analog. The substi-

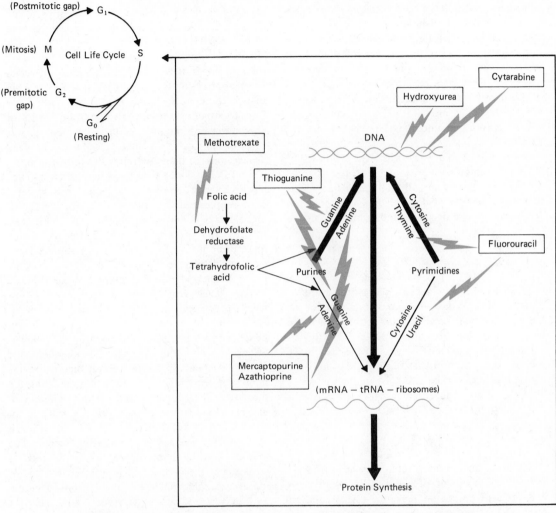

Fig. 15–2. The antimetabolites provide purine, pyrimidine, or folic acid analogs that interfere with the DNA-directed synthesis of cellular proteins.

tution of the analog delays the synthesis phase of the cell life-cycle.

Pyrimidine Analogs

The pyrimidine analogs *floxuridine* and *fluorouracil* interfere with the synthesis of the nucleotide *thymidylic acid* by providing a substitute metabolite for the nitrogenous base *thymine*. The analogs also provide a uracil analog that becomes incorporated in RNA and prevents the uptake of the preformed uracil. The process leads to the production of a fraudulent RNA and the synthesis of nonfunctional proteins. The pyrimidine analogs are an example of the drugs with diverse actions that can be described as having specific and nonspecific effects on the cell life-cycle. Their inhibition of DNA synthesis is S phase specific, but the interference with RNA construction of proteins can occur throughout the cell life-cycle.

Cytarabine interferes with the synthesis of DNA by acting as a substitute for the nucleoside *cytidine*. The analog substitution prevents the conversion of the nucleoside to the *deoxycytidine* that is required for the assembling of the DNA strand. Phosphorylated derivatives of the drug become incorporated into the RNA chain and inhibit its function.

Hydroxyurea interferes with the synthesis of DNA by inhibiting the activity of the enzyme *ribonucleotide reductase* that is required for incorporation of the nucleoside *thymidine* into the DNA strand. The drug also may directly damage DNA.

Folic Acid Analog

Methotrexate provides an analog for the natural vitamin *folic acid*. The competitive action of the drug inhibits the enzymatic conversion of the vitamin to *tetrahydrofolic acid*. The affinity of the enzyme *dihydrofolate reductase* for the drug is far greater than its affinity for folic acid. The drug action causes a marked reduction in the intracellular pool of the reduced folates that are required for the biosynthesis of purines.

Mercaptopurine (PURINETHOL)

The drug has produced complete or partial remissions in one half of the children who have been treated for acute leukemia. Although the response rate has been lower in the treatment of acute lymphocytic leukemia in adults, it is often the initial drug selected for therapy. Therapy with mercaptopurine has also produced remissions or improvement in patients with chronic granulocytic leukemia. The drug is used in combination with other drugs in the treatment of leukemia. (Table 15–1).

Therapy Considerations. Mercaptopurine is administered orally and the drug is readily absorbed from the gastrointestinal tract. The initial dosage for children and adults is based on the calculation of 2.5 mg/kg of body weight, and the drug is given in one daily dose up to a maximum of 150 mg. The drug may cause a rapid fall in the leukocyte count during the first or second week of therapy in adults who have a high total leukocyte count, but children seldom have a sharp drop in their blood counts.

A treatment course of two to four weeks or longer may be required to produce an improvement in the patient's hematologic status. The drug dosage may be increased after the fourth week to a level that is twice the initial dosage (5 mg/kg/day). When a remission occurs, the dosage level may be reduced to the initial dosage level (2.5 mg/kg/day) for maintenance therapy. Continued therapy is required to avoid a relapse that occurs quite promptly when therapy is interrupted. Drug therapy during the periods of remission may maintain the patient's hematologic status at near-normal levels for periods ranging from a few weeks to several months.

The maximum effect on the blood count may be delayed for periods as long as four to six weeks after the initiation of drug therapy, and the formed elements in the peripheral blood may remain low for a similar period of time after the therapy is interrupted or discontinued. The hemoglobin value and the white blood cell and thrombocyte counts are evaluated at least once each week during therapy with mercaptopurine. The therapy usually is interrupted when there is an abnormally rapid decline in the total number of mature granulocytes in the blood count. Therapy may be resumed when the blood count stabilizes and begins to rise from the nadir.

Adverse Effects. The primary toxic effect is bone marrow depression, which is manifested as leukopenia, anemia, or pancytopenia. At the high therapeutic drug dosage levels there is an increased incidence of thrombocytopenia, and the prolongation of the clotting time predisposes the person to bleeding episodes (Table 15–2).

Anorexia, nausea, and vomiting occasionally occur during therapy. The problems occur more frequently in adults than they do in children. Diarrhea occurs infrequently.

Table 15–2.
Selected Patient Care Problems During Antimetabolite Drug Therapy

Antimetabolite	Nausea and Vomiting	Stomatitis	Thrombo-cytopenia (Bleeding Potential)	Leukopenia (Infection Potential)	Lympho-cytopenia (Immuno-suppression)	Alopecia
Azathioprine	Occ.	0	+	+	+	+
Cytarabine	.+	+	+	+	+	+
Fluorouracil	+	+	+	+	+	+
Hydroxyurea	Mild	+	+	+	+	Rare
Mercaptopurine	Occ.	0	+	+	+	+
Methotrexate	Nausea only	+	+	+	+	Occ.
Thioguanine	Occ.	+	+	+	+	0

The drug causes less gastrointestinal toxicity than the folic acid analog *methotrexate*. Stomatitis and esophageal or intestinal ulceration have occurred in some patients receiving mercaptopurine. Alopecia and skin eruptions are the manifestations of epidermal tissue toxicity that occur during the drug therapy period.

The drug has immunosuppression properties, and infections (i.e., fungal, protozoal, viral, and uncommon types of bacterial infections) have occurred. Allergic reactions have included drug fever, serum sickness, joint pains, and eosinophilia. Jaundice with an associated high alkaline phosphatase level and a slight elevation of the bilirubin level has occurred in a number of patients during therapy with mercaptopurine.

Thioguanine

Thioguanine is metabolized to the ribonucleotide, which provides its antineoplastic activity. The drug has a slight structural difference from that of mercaptopurine and it has similar therapeutic effects. It sometimes is employed when patients have adverse effects during therapy with mercaptopurine.

Thioguanine is employed for the treatment of patients with acute leukemia and it has produced temporary remissions in patients with chronic myelocytic leukemia. The drug has produced remissions more frequently when used for the treatment of children with acute leukemia than when used in the treatment of adults with leukemia. Thioguanine has also been employed in combination with cytarabine for the treatment of leukemia.

Therapy Considerations. Thioguanine is administered orally, and the dosage level is planned to compensate for the fact that the drug is only partially absorbed from the gastrointestinal tract. The absorbed drug rapidly enters into the anabolic and catabolic pathways of purines and little of the drug remains in the circulation. A minimal amount of the drug crosses the blood-brain barrier. Detoxification of the drug occurs in the liver and the drug metabolites are excreted in the urine and feces.

The usual dosage for children and adults is calculated on the basis of 2 mg/kg of body weight and the drug is taken as a single dose daily. Some adults who have an initially high total leukocyte count have a rapid fall in the leukocyte count within a few days, but the problem seldom occurs in children. Therapy may be continued for a period ranging from two to four or more weeks before improvement in the hematologic status is evident. At the end of the fourth week, the dosage level may be increased to 3 mg/kg/day. Maintenance therapy is planned after a remission occurs, and the drug dosage level usually is 2 mg/kg/day.

The hemoglobin value and the white blood cell and thrombocyte counts are evaluated at least once each week during therapy. The drug therapy usually is interrupted immediately when the hematologic evaluation reveals an initial change that indicates an abnormal depression of the bone marrow because the drug continues to affect the blood levels for several days after the last dose of the drug is given. Therapy may be resumed when the nadir is reached and the blood values indicate that the bone marrow has resumed the production of blood cells. Blood counts usually are evaluated daily when there is an indication of a changing hematologic status.

Adverse Effects. The principal toxic effect is bone marrow depression, which is manifested as leukopenia, reticulopenia, anemia, and thrombocytopenia (Table 12–2). The reversible bone marrow depression is rather prolonged and the aplasia is similar in character to that caused by ionizing radiation.

Some adults have problems with nausea, vomiting, anorexia, and diarrhea but those problems occur less frequently in children. Stomatitis occurs in some patients as an early indication of gastrointestinal tissue toxicity.

The hyperuricemia and hyperuricosuria that occur during therapy are indicators that the person should have a high fluid intake to assure excretion of the uric acid crystals. Other problems that may occur during therapy with thioguanine include photosensitivity, skin rash, jaundice, loss of the vibration sense, and an unsteadiness of gait. The adverse effects occur infrequently and they subside when therapy is discontinued.

Azathioprine (IMURAN)

The drug is a derivative of *mercaptopurine* and it has pharmacologic actions that are similar to those of that drug. Azathioprine seldom is employed for the treatment of cancer but is frequently employed for the prevention of rejection responses after renal homotransplants. It has been a valuable agent when utilized in conjunction with other immunosuppressive agents (i.e., local irradiation, corticosteroids, other cytotoxic drugs) for the treatment of patients in the early postoperative period.

Therapy Considerations. The drug is most effective when it is administered during the induction period of the posttransplant antibody response. Administration of the drug usually is initiated 24 hours after the surgery or within 48 hours following the initial antigenic stimulation. The effects of the drug and its active metabolite *mercaptopurine* may not become evident for several days after the initiation of the drug therapy, and the effects of the drug may persist for a similar period of time after the drug therapy is discontinued.

The drug usually is administered orally and it is readily absorbed from the gastrointestinal tract. The absorbed drug rapidly enters the anabolic and catabolic pathways of the purines, and the plasma levels of the drug may be relatively low. Thirty percent of the drug is bound to plasma proteins. The drug is split by enzymes in the body tissues to the active metabolite *mercaptopurine*. The unchanged drug and the metabolites are excreted by the kidneys.

The usual oral or intravenous initial dosage for children or adults is calculated on the basis of 3 to 5 mg/kg of body weight, given as a single dose daily. Schedules for use of azathioprine vary according to the patient's status and the protocols in varying renal transplantation centers. The drug therapy may be initiated a few days prior to the surgery or it may begin within 24 to 48 hours after the renal transplant surgery. The intravenous route is used for therapy until the patient is able to take the drug orally. The dosage may be reduced to 1 to 2 mg/kg daily for maintenance therapy after the initial intense antibody response period.

Adverse Effects. The adverse effects of azathioprine are the same as those previously presented for *mercaptopurine* (Table 15–2). The use of the drug with other immunosuppressive therapies may increase the toxic potential that is common to all of the antineoplastic drugs.

Fluorouracil and Floxuridine

Floxuridine is catabolized to fluorouracil, and systemic levels of the drug produce the same metabolic effects as those of fluorouracil (5-FU). Floxuridine is employed primarily for continuous regional intra-arterial infusion in the palliative treatment of patients with carcinomas. The daily dosage of the infused drug is 100 to 600 mcg/kg of body weight and the drug dosage delivery rate is controlled by a pump regulator device to provide a uniform rate of infusion.

Fluorouracil is employed for the palliative treatment of solid tumors that have metastasized extensively and are not amenable to surgery or radiation therapy. The drug has produced temporary improvement in a relatively large number of patients with advanced carcinoma of the gastrointestinal tract. From 10 to 40 percent of the patients with cancer of the rectum and colon have had remissions lasting from five months to five years. A similar temporary remission rate (10 to 35 percent) has been obtained in patients with metastatic breast cancer who were treated with fluorouracil. The drug frequently is employed in combination with other drugs for the treatment of patients with gastrointestinal neoplasms or breast carcinoma (Table 15–1).

Therapy Considerations. The primary method for administration of fluorouracil is intravenous injection of the drug, but the same solution may be diluted in prune juice or ginger ale and administered orally. The drug is distributed in the bone marrow, liver, and other body tissues. The highest concentration of the drug is found in the malignant tissues, and those levels persist for longer periods of time than the concentration of the drug in the normal tissues. A minimal amount of the drug is present in the plasma three hours after it is administered. Fluorouracil is metabolized primarily in the liver, and a small portion of the drug is anabolized in body tissues to an active metabolite. Approximately 60 to 80 percent of the drug is excreted from the lungs as carbon dioxide. The metabolite *urea* is excreted in the urine. Within six hours after the drug is administered intravenously, 15 percent of the unchanged drug is excreted in the urine.

The drug is irritating to the veins, and the use of a small-gauge needle (i.e., 25 gauge) lessens the hazard of extravasation from the vein during administration of the drug. The dosage of fluorouracil is calculated on the basis of the person's weight in the absence of edema or obesity (lean body weight).

The initial dosage for the course of therapy usually is calculated on the basis of 12 mg/kg of body weight, given as a single daily dose for four days. Subsequent doses may be given every other day at a lower dosage range (i.e., 2 to 6 mg/kg) for a period of 12 days.

Many of the patients who receive the drug as palliative treatment are debilitated. Their dosage maximum usually is lower (i.e., 400 mg) because there is a higher risk of drug toxicity when the person has a marginal physiologic or nutritional status.

The initial course of therapy may be repeated at 30-day intervals or a weekly maintenance dosage (i.e., 10 to 15 mg/kg) may be given. The usual weekly dosage maximum for maintenance therapy is 1 gm of fluorouracil per week.

Adverse Effects. White blood counts usually are evaluated before each dose of fluorouracil is administered because the drug frequently causes granulocytopenia, thrombocytopenia, and anemia (Table 15–2). The nadir of the white blood count usually occurs from 9 to 14 days after the initiation of therapy but it may occur as late as the twenty-fifth day. The maximum depression of the bone marrow production of thrombocytes may become evident during the seventh to the seventeenth days of therapy. The occurrence of bone marrow depression necessitates interruption of the drug therapy, and the hematologic recovery usually is complete within 30 days after the administration of the drug is discontinued.

The toxic effects of fluorouracil on the gastrointestinal tissues can be so severe that there is hemorrhage from the affected tissues. Anorexia and nausea commonly occur during the first week of therapy and vomiting also occurs frequently. The administration of antiemetics may increase the patient's ability to continue therapy, but the occurrence of intractable vomiting necessitates interruption of the drug therapy. The problems usually subside within two to three days after the administration of the drug is discontinued.

Stomatitis frequently occurs and may be the earliest sign of gastrointestinal tissue toxicity. It frequently occurs during the fifth to eighth day of therapy but it may appear as early as the fourth day after the initiation of drug administration. The occurrence of stomatitis or other evidence of gastrointestinal tissue toxicity (i.e., diarrhea) necessitates interruption of the therapy to halt the progression of the tissue destruction and to allow time for tissue repair.

Significant loss of hair or alopecia frequently occurs as a manifestation of epidermal tissue toxicity. A few patients have a partial loss of the fingernails. The appearance of a maculopapular rash on the extremities also is a relatively common manifestation of the tissue toxicity. Some persons have erythema, scaling, or increased pigmentation of the skin, and the skin reactions may be intensified by exposure to strong sunlight. The skin reactions generally are reversible when therapy is terminated.

After a period of two weeks of therapy, some patients have a fever without concurrent evidence of infection. Other problems that sometimes occur during therapy with fluorouracil are epistaxis, photophobia, euphoria, and cerebellar-related neurologic problems (i.e., ataxia). Angina pectoris has also been precipitated in some patients during therapy with fluorouracil.

Cytarabine (CYTOSAR)

The drug is employed primarily for the treatment of granulocytic leukemia in adults, and it is also used for treatment of other acute leukemias in children and adults. The drug has produced complete or partial remissions with a duration of a few days to several months in 20 to 25 percent of the adults with acute leukemia who were treated with cytarabine. Maintenance therapy is continued during periods of remission because relapse promptly occurs when therapy is discontinued.

Therapy Considerations. The drug usually is administered by intravenous injection or infusion during the initial period of therapy. The subcutaneous route may be employed for administration of the drug during maintenance therapy.

Cytarabine is widely distributed in the body tissues and it crosses the blood-brain barrier. Only a minimal quantity of the drug can be found in the blood within 5 to 20 minutes after it is administered intravenously. The drug is metabolized in the liver and the kidneys. Most of the drug (89 to 94 percent) is excreted in the urine as the inactive metabolite within 24 hours after intravenous administration.

The initial daily dosage of cytarabine is calculated on the basis of 2 mg/kg of body weight, and the drug may be administered as an intravenous injection for a period of ten days. At the end of the ten-day period, the dosage may be increased to two times the initial level and it may be administered as a single daily intravenous injection.

When the drug is administered by intravenous infusion, the dosage level is lower (i.e., 0.5 to 1 mg/kg) and the intravenous flow rate may be prescribed at a level that requires from 1 to 24 hours for administration of the drug. At the end of the ten-day course of therapy the intravenous infusion dosage may be increased (i.e., 2 mg/kg daily). After a remission has occurred, the maintenance dose (i.e., 1 mg/kg) may be administered once or twice each week. The injection sites are alternated and the tissues are examined carefully because the injections can cause pain and cellulitis.

Adverse Effects. Bone marrow depression results in peripheral leukopenia, thrombocytopenia, and anemia in most of the patients who are treated with cytarabine (Table 15–2). Megaloblastosis occurs in almost all patients, and it may be evident in examination of the blood samples during the first 24 hours of therapy. Daily blood cell evaluations may be planned to monitor the progress of the bone marrow depression. The drug therapy usually is interrupted when the white blood cell count has decreased to 3000/cu mm or the platelet count has decreased to a level below 100,000/cu mm. The blood values continue to fall after the drug therapy is interrupted, and their nadir occurs approximately five to seven days after the cessation of therapy. The leukopenia and thrombocytopenia increase the potential for infection (i.e., pneumonia) or bleeding episodes, and observation of the patient is intensified to identify the earliest signs of the problems.

Nausea and vomiting occur frequently during therapy with cytarabine; the incidence seems to be slightly higher when the patient receives the drug by intravenous infusion than with intravenous injections. Evidence of gastrointestinal tract tissue toxicity includes diarrhea, stomatitis, and esophagitis, which necessitate the interruption of the drug therapy.

Alopecia, dermatitis, skin rash, keratitis, and conjunctivitis are the most frequent indications of toxicity of the superficial tissues. Hyperuricemia often is associated with an accelerated lysis of the leukemic cells during therapy. Other adverse effects that may occur during therapy with cytarabine include neuritis, lethargy, confusion, dizziness, chest pain, joint pain, urinary retention, renal dysfunction, and hepatoxicity.

Hydroxyurea (HYDREA)

The drug has produced a positive response in 20 percent of the patients with resistant chronic myelocytic leukemia. Hydroxyurea has a more rapid onset of leukopenic activity than mercaptopurine or thioguanine. The drug has also been employed for the treatment of patients with recurrent, metastatic, or inoperable ovarian carcinoma.

Therapy Considerations. Hydroxyurea is administered orally and it is readily absorbed from the gastrointestinal tissues. After absorption of the drug, peak serum concentrations occur in two hours but the serum levels decline rapidly. The drug readily crosses the blood-brain barrier, and there are peak cerebrospinal fluid concentrations of the drug within three hours after it is administered. One half of the drug is degraded in the liver, and the metabolites are excreted from the respiratory tract or as *urea* in the urine. The re-

mainder is excreted in the urine as the unchanged drug.

The adult dosage for the intermittent method of treatment of solid tumors is calculated on the basis of 80 mg/kg of body weight, usually administered as a single dose every three days. The dosage for the continuous method of treatment of adults who have leukemia is 20 to 30 mg/kg, administered orally as a single daily dose.

Adverse Effects. Megaloblastosis often occurs within the first 24 hours after initiation of therapy. The problem is self-limiting, the red blood cells gradually becoming more normal as therapy progresses.

Leukopenia is the earliest and most frequent manifestation of the depression of bone marrow function during therapy with hydroxyurea (Table 15–2). Thrombocytopenia and anemia occur less frequently than leukopenia. Interruption of therapy leads to rapid recovery of the blood cell production by the bone marrow. The omission of only a few of the drug doses may be sufficient to allow adequate improvement in the patient's hematologic status.

The red blood cell, white blood cell, and platelet counts are evaluated at least weekly during therapy with hydroxyurea. The hemoglobin value is also monitored closely because the drug may reduce iron utilization by erythrocytes.

Nausea, vomiting, and anorexia occur but the symptoms are relatively mild. Constipation can be a problem in some patients. The occurrence of stomatitis, ulceration of the gastrointestinal tissues, or diarrhea necessitates interruption of the drug therapy to allow the regeneration and repair of the damaged epithelium.

Epidermal toxicity is usually mild; the problems include maculopapular skin rash, facial erythema, pruritus, hyperkeratosis, and hyperpigmentation. The problems subside when therapy is terminated.

Alopecia, dysuria, and hyperuricemia rarely occur. A few patients have a transient elevation of the blood urea nitrogen, serum uric acid, and creatinine levels that indicates decreased renal tubule function.

Methotrexate (AMETHOPTERIN)

The drug has produced remissions in more than 75 percent of the patients who were treated for trophoblastic tumors. The most positive results are obtained when therapy is started early in the disease, and the remission rate is slightly lower when the cancer has metastasized. Methotrexate frequently is employed in combination with other drugs for the treatment of leukemia, osteogenic sarcoma, breast carcinoma, or testicular carcinoma (Table 15–1).

When methotrexate is used in combination with other antineoplastic drugs for treatment of metatastic tumors of the testes, there is a decrease in the size of the metastases and in the tumor mass in approximately one third to one half of the patients. The courses of therapy usually are repeated at one-to-three-month intervals for several years to maintain the suppression of tumor growth.

Methotrexate in combination with other chemotherapeutic drugs has produced remissions in 90 percent of the patients treated for acute lymphocytic leukemia. The drugs of the combination are given during the remissions to maintain the control of the leukemia.

Therapy Considerations. The drug inhibits the enzyme *dehydrofolate reductase,* which converts folic acid to tetrahydrofolic acid. *Calcium leucovorin,* a derivative of tetrahydrofolic acid, is used during high-dose methotrexate therapy to block the effects of the antineoplastic drug on the normal body tissues. The plan is popularly called "leucovorin rescue." The calcium leucovorin may be administered intramuscularly at the time the methotrexate is administered intrathecally. It may also be administered several hours after intravenous administration of high-dose methotrexate sodium to control the duration of the exposure of the normal rapidly proliferating cells to the destructive effects of the drug.

Sodium methotrexate, the parenteral form of the drug, may be administered as an intramuscular, intravenous, intrathecal, or intra-arterial injection. Methotrexate is administered orally.

The drug is completely absorbed from the gastrointestinal tract at the usual therapeutic dosage levels. Peak serum levels of the drug are attained within one to two hours after oral administration. The serum half-life of the orally administered drug ranges from two to four hours, but the half-life is lengthened to a range of eight to ten hours when the drug is given orally at high dosage levels.

Up to 50 percent of the drug in the circulation is bound to serum proteins. Methotrexate is actively transported across the cell membranes. It is widely distributed in the body tissues and it crosses the placental barrier. The highest concentrations of the drug are found in the kidneys, gallbladder, spleen, liver, and skin. Methotrexate may be retained in the kidneys for several weeks and is retained in the liver tissues for several months after the termination of therapy. A regular daily dosage schedule can cause high levels of the drug to accumulate in body tissues.

An insufficient amount of the drug crosses the blood-brain barrier to provide therapeutic concentrations, but the drug that is injected into the cerebrospinal fluid passes into the systemic circulation. Peak serum concentrations of the drug may be attained within two hours after it is injected into the cerebrospinal fluid.

Most of the drug is excreted in the urine unchanged. Glomerular filtration and active tubular secretion move the drug from the plasma into the tubular urine. A small amount of the drug enters the intestinal tract with the bile and is eliminated with the feces. Up to 92 percent of an intravenous dose of methotrexate sodium is excreted in the urine within 24 hours after it is administered. The excretion rate is reduced when the urine is alkaline.

The dosage and the length of each course vary with the particular type of malignant tissue being treated. The dosage for the treatment of trophoblastic tumors (i.e., 15 to 30 mg/day) may be continued for five days and three to five courses of therapy may be planned. A one- to two-week drug-free period is planned between the courses of therapy.

The daily dosage of methotrexate that is employed alone for the treatment of lymphoblastic leukemia or in combination with other drugs is based on the calculation of 3.3 mg/M² of body surface area. During periods of remission, the maintenance dosage of the drug (20 to 30 mg/M³) may be administered orally or intramuscularly two times each week, or it may be administered intravenously (2.5 mg/kg) every 14 days.

When there is meningeal leukemia, intrathecal administration (200 to 500 mcg/kg) may be planned at two-to-five-day intervals. After the cerebrospinal fluid cell count returns to a normal level, one additional dose of the drug may be injected.

Adverse Effects. Since methotrexate has immunosuppressive activity, the lymphocyte levels may be low during therapy. The drug has been employed for control of the kidney rejection response after renal transplantation because of its ability to control the immune response.

The use of methotrexate at high dosage levels in combination with other cytotoxic drugs increases the potential for toxicity in the rapidly proliferating normal body tissues. Leukopenia, thrombocytopenia, and anemia may develop rapidly (Table 15–2).

The leukocytes generally have two periods of depression. The first decrease in the leukocyte levels occurs four to seven days, and the second occurs 12 to 21 days, after the initiation of therapy. Each decrease in the leukocyte levels is followed by a 6-to-14-day recovery period during which the cell count gradually rises. The platelet count may reach its nadir in 5 to 12 days, and the recovery of platelet production occurs over a period of approximately 12 days. The nadir of the hemoglobin value occurs 6 to 13 days, and that of the reticulocytes occurs two to seven days, after the initiation of therapy. Each of those values recovers gradually from its low point.

The hematologic values are evaluated frequently during the predictable periods of blood cell depression, and they are evaluated at least once each week throughout therapy. Drug therapy is interrupted when there is a sharp drop in the blood cell counts. The drug dosage may be decreased when the hematologic changes are less profound.

Stomatitis usually is the earliest sign of the toxicity of methotrexate. There may be erythema, ulceration, and bleeding at several sites in the gastrointestinal tissues. Drug therapy is interrupted when there is ulcerative stomatitis or diarrhea because those problems are forewarnings of the enteric tissue erosion that can cause hemorrhagic enteritis or intestinal perforation.

Toxic effects of methotrexate on epidermal tissues may cause erythematous rashes, pruritus, urticaria, folliculitis, photosensitivity, depigmentation, hyperpigmentation, acne, or furunculosis. The other dermatologic problems that may occur are petechiae, ecchymoses, and telangiectasia. Alopecia occurs occasionally. The regrowth of hair may not be complete for several months after therapy is discontinued.

A rapid destruction of the cancer cells may cause an elevation in the serum uric acid levels. Severe uric acid nephropathy and acute renal failure may occur as a consequence of the increased levels of the uric acid in the kidneys. Sodium bicarbonate often is prescribed to alkalinize the urine. The dosage is described as that amount that will maintain the urine pH at 7 to 7.2, and the pH of each voiding governs the frequency of sodium bicarbonate administration. A "force-fluids" level of intake is part of the therapeutic plan for flushing the uric acid crystals through the nephrons.

Hepatotoxicity occurs when the drug is administered at high dosage or in small frequent doses and also occurs during prolonged therapy with the drug. The liver function tests may be abnormal within one to three days after drug administration is started, but they return to normal levels in a few days. The tests show a poor correlation with the hepatotoxicity that is found with liver biopsy (i.e., atrophy, necrosis, fatty changes, fibrosis, cirrhosis).

Methotrexate has caused infertility in both males and females. Menstrual dysfunction may occur in female patients and the sperm counts in males may be low. The drug may cause pulmonary infiltration, headache, drowsiness, blurred vision, malaise, dizziness, or osteoporosis (i.e., aseptic necrosis of the head of the femur).

Interactions. Concurrent administration of weak organic acids (i.e., salicylates, sulfonamides) may decrease the renal tubule secretion of methotrexate and slow its elimination. The drug may be displaced from its protein-binding sites by salicylates, sulfonamides, phenytoin, tetracyclines, chloramphenicol, or aminobenzoic acid. The increased levels of the methotrexate that can occur as a consequence of the drug interactions increase its toxicity potential. Vitamin preparations containing folic acid may alter the response to methotrexate.

ANTIMITOTICS

Vinblastine sulfate and *vincristine sulfate* are the cell cycle phase-specific vinca plant alkaloids that are employed for antineoplastic drug therapy. Although the primary action mode of the drugs is simliar, their toxic effects on normal body tissues are different. The absence of cross-resistance between the drugs is an indication of their pharmacologic differences.

Action Mode

The vinca plant alkaloids are known to interrupt the mitotic phase of the cancer cell lifecycle by binding to the mitotic spindle or by crystallizing the spindle proteins. The effects of the drugs during clinical therapy indicate that other complex actions on intracellular protein synthesis are attributable to each of the drugs.

Vinblastine Sulfate (VELBAN)

The drug inhibits purine synthesis and the formation of urea by interfering with the cellular utilization of glutamic acid. Vinblastine also has some immunosuppressive activity.

The drug is employed for treatment or palliation of lymphomas, lymphosarcoma, neuroblastoma, testicular carcinoma, and advanced mycosis fungoides. It has produced complete remissions in 10 to 30 percent of the patients, who were treated for lymphoma, after four to six weeks of therapy, and improvement (i.e., decreased size of lymph nodes, liver, spleen) in 50 to 90 percent of the patients. Vinblastine is also employed in combination with other drugs in varying cancer therapy regimens (i.e., treatment of testicular carcinoma).

Therapy Considerations. Vinblastine is administered intravenously. The solution is rapidly cleared from the blood and becomes localized in body tissues. It is metabolized in the liver to the metabolite *desacetylvinblastine,* which has a higher antineoplastic activity than the parent drug. The drug metabolite is slowly excreted in the urine and also enters the intestinal tract with the bile.

The reconstituted solution may be injected slowly into the vein (i.e., over a one-minute period) or may be injected into the tubing of a running intravenous infusion. Vinblastine is a tissue irritant, and its extravasation into the perivenous tissues can cause pain, cellulitis, thrombosis, phlebitis, and necrosis. When leakage does occur, the application of cold compresses may prevent the interstitial spread of the drug solution. The area sometimes is infiltrated with isotonic sodium chloride solution as a means of diluting the irritating solution. Care should also be taken when preparing the solution to avoid contact with the tissues. Washing the hands thoroughly can avoid the transfer of the irritating drug solution to other body tissues (i.e., the eyes).

The initial drug dosage is calculated on the basis of 100 mcg/kg of body weight, and the dose is administered at intervals of seven days. Weekly increments in the dosage (i.e., 50 mcg/kg) may be made until the maximum dosage is reached (500 mcg/kg) or until there is evidence of toxicity. The maintenance dosage of the drug usually is defined as the level that is 50 mcg less than the dosage that leads to a decrease in the leukocyte count to 3000/cu mm. That dosage is administered at one-to-two-week intervals during the remission of cancer cell growth. Leukocyte counts are evaluated before the drug is administered throughout the period of therapy with vinblastine.

Adverse Effects.   Bone marrow depression occurs more frequently during therapy with vinblastine than it does with vincristine. The nadir of the leukocyte count usually is evident within four to ten days after initiation of therapy with vinblastine. The recovery of leukocyte production usually occurs within 7 to 14 days after the initial rise from the nadir, but a longer period of time elapses (i.e., 21 days) when the drug is administered at the high dosage levels. The drug effect on the production of thrombocytes is usually minimal, with only a transient drop in the platelet count (Table 15–3).

Nausea, vomiting, headache, and paresthesias may occur within four to six hours after the administration of the drug, and the problems sometimes last up to ten hours. Antiemetics often are given to control the nausea and vomiting. The headache and paresthesias and the constipation, adynamic ileus, and abdominal pain that occur during therapy with vinblastine are related to the neurotoxicity of the drug. Although other neurologic problems occasionally occur during ther-

apy with vinblastine, they appear less frequently and are less severe than the disruptive problems that occur with vincristine administration.

The toxic effects of vinblastine on the gastrointestinal tissues may cause stomatitis and diarrhea. The occurrence of epithelial tissue ulceration necessitates interruption of the drug therapy to prevent the extension of the tissue damage.

Epidermal tissue toxicity occurs only infrequently, and the problems generally are limited to dermatitis, skin vesiculation, alopecia, and phototoxicity. Aspermia occasionally occurs in male patients. The extensive tissue catabolism associated with leukemia or lymphoma may cause hyperuricemia or hyperuricuria.

Vincristine Sulfate (ONCOVIN)

The drug is frequently employed for the treatment of children wth acute leukemia. It has produced partial or complete remissions in a high percentage of patients who were treated for acute lymphocytic or undifferentiated stem cell leukemia. Vincristine is employed in combination with other drugs for the treatment of leukemia, lymphoma, osteogenic sarcoma, and breast carcinoma.

Therapy Considerations.   Vincristine is administered intravenously. The drug is very irritating to tissues. It may cause localized thrombo-

Table 15–3.

Selected Patient Care Problems During Antimitotic and Antiobiotic Drug Therapy

Drug	Nausea and Vomiting	Stomatitis	Thrombo-cytopenia (Bleeding Potential)	Leukopenia (Infection Potential)	Lympho-cytopenia (Immuno-suppression)	Alopecia
Antimitotics						
Vinblastine	+	+	Slight	+	+	+
Vincristine	—	—	+	+	+	+
Antibiotics						
Bleomycin	+	+	—	—	+	+
Dactinomycin	+	+	+	+	+	+
Doxorubicin	+	+	+	+	+	+
Mithramycin	+	+	+	Mild	+	
Mitomycin	+	+	+	+	±	+

phlebitis and it causes local irritation and cellulitis when it extravasates into the tissues. Intense jaw pain sometimes occurs 20 to 30 minutes after the drug is injected into the bracheal vein.

The diluted drug may be slowly injected directly into a vein (i.e., over a one-minute period) or it may be injected into the tubing of a running intravenous infusion. The usual dosage for children is calculated on the basis of 0.05 to 0.15 mg/kg of body weight and the dose is administered at weekly intervals. The dosage may be increased at weekly intervals in increments ranging from 0.025 to 0.15 mg/kg until there is evidence of toxicity. The usual maintenance dosage ranges from 0.05 to 0.075 mg/kg and the dose is administered at weekly intervals.

Adverse Effects. Vincristine is less toxic to the bone marrow than vinblastine (Table 15–3). When the drug is administered to children with acute leukemia, the nadir of the leukocyte count usually occurs on the fourth day of therapy and it begins to rise on the fifth day. The thrombocyte counts are also decreased and they gradually rise during the first weeks of therapy. The hemoglobin value recovers more slowly.

Neurotoxicity occurs frequently during therapy with vincristine, and the effects include many neurologic and neuromuscular problems. Headache, constipation, abdominal pain, paresthesias of the extremities, and depression of the deep tendon reflexes occur frequently. Neuritis, joint pain, foot drop, slapping gait, ptosis, vocal cord paralysis, weakness of the hand muscles, adynamic ileus, ataxia, confusion, weakness, nervousness, amnesia, coma, psychosis, and mental confusion are some of the disruptive problems that may occur during therapy with vincristine. The drug dosage may be reduced or therapy may be interrupted when reflexes are diminished or paresthesias are present.

Many patients have alopecia and some degree of hair loss occurs frequently. Epidermal tissue toxicity may also include urticaria or a maculopapular skin rash. Hyperuricemia occurs when there is rapid lysis of the malignant cells. Other problems that sometimes occur during therapy include weight loss, hypertension, fever, and transient urinary symptoms (i.e., frequency, dysuria).

ANTINEOPLASTIC ANTIBIOTICS

The antibiotics employed for treatment of cancer have a cytotoxic potential that precludes their use for treatment of infections. The antibiotics generally are cancer cell cycle phase-nonspecific agents. The antibiotics *bleomycin* and *mithramycin* have some actions similar to those of the drugs in the cell cycle phase-specific groups of drugs, but *dactinomycin, doxorubicin,* and *mitomycin* are considered to be entirely cell cycle phase-nonspecific drugs.

Action Mode

The antineoplastic antibiotics inhibit protein synthesis throughout the cell life-cycle by interfering with protein synthesis. They complex with DNA and that action inhibits the DNA-directed RNA synthesis. *Bleomycin* also acts in the G_2 premitotic phase of the cell life-cycle by inhibiting incorporation of *thymidine* into the DNA strand. *Mithramycin,* in addition to the cell phase-nonspecific action of the antibiotics, interferes with DNA-directed synthesis of RNA by complexing with the nitrogenous base *guanine*.

Bleomycin Sulfate (BLENOXANE)

Bleomycin frequently is employed as an adjunct to surgery in the treatment of carcinoma. It is used alone or in combination with other drugs in the treatment of lymphomas and testicular carcinoma. A 50 percent regression in lymphoma tissue has occurred in 25 percent of the patients treated with bleomycin. Control of the malignant tissue has lasted from a few months to two years.

Therapy Considerations. Bleomycin is administered by subcutaneous, intramuscular, intravenous, intrapleural, or intra-arterial injection. The drug is absorbed systemically following injection into the pleural, peritoneal, or pericardial cavities. The highest concentrations of the drug are found in the skin, lungs, kidneys, peritoneum, and lymphatics. The drug concentration is also high in tumor cells of the skin and lungs. From 20 to 40 percent of the unchanged drug is excreted in the urine in 24 hours.

The initial two doses of bleomycin usually consist of a minimal amount of the drug (i.e., 2 units or less) that is used as a test dose to determine whether the patient is allergic to the drug. Subsequent dosage levels are based on the calculation of 0.25 to 0.50 units/kg of body weight and the dose is administered intravenously, intramuscularly, or subcutaneously one or two times a week. Maintenance therapy is planned when approximately 50 percent of the desired response is attained. A daily 1-unit dose or a weekly 5-unit dose of the drug may be administered intravenously or intramuscularly to maintain the control of the malignant growth. The total dosage maximum of 400 units limits the duration of therapy, but that limitation has decreased the incidence of toxicity that is related to high drug dosage.

Adverse Effects. Unlike other antineoplastic drugs, bleomycin seldom causes serious bone marrow toxicity (Table 15–3). Leukopenia, thrombocytopenia, and a slight depression of the hemoglobin values usually reach their nadir by the twelfth day of therapy. The blood values return to their pretreatment levels by the seventeenth day after initiation of therapy.

The most serious adverse effect during therapy with bleomycin is interstitial pneumonitis, which occurs in 10 percent of the patients treated. The incidence of the pneumonitis is highest when the drug is used to treat elderly (>70 years old) patients. The clinical findings are similar to those that occur with infectious pneumonia. Dyspnea and fine rales provide the earliest evidence of the problem. Pulmonary function tests and chest x-rays usually are evaluated at one-to-three-week intervals throughout therapy. The drug therapy is interrupted if there is a rapid decline in the forced vital capacity. The pulmonary involvement can progress from pneumonitis to pulmonary fibrosis

and death has occurred in approximately 1 percent of the patients.

Epidermal toxicity usually occurs within two to three weeks after the initiation of therapy in 50 percent of the patients treated. The problems reflect the high uptake and cumulation of the drug by the normal skin. The earliest manifestations are urticaria or erythematous swelling, and the affected tissues gradually become tender and pruritic. Hyperpigmentation frequently occurs in the pressure areas and in the nail cuticles, on the scalp, and at injection sites. Hyperkeratosis, nail changes, alopecia, and mucosal lesions (i.e., stomatitis, tongue ulceration, lip lesions) can occur. In approximately 2 percent of the patients the reactions are serious and the drug therapy is terminated.

Fever occurs within one hour after the injection of the drug in 25 percent of the patients treated and it occurs in 90 percent of the patients who receive bleomycin for the treatment of lymphoma. The temperature rises slowly and may remain elevated for 4 to 12 hours. The fever may be accompanied by chills. The fever and chills may occur sporadically rather than occurring with each adminstration of the drug.

Anaphylactoid reactions and other manifestations of allergic reactions (i.e., hypotension, wheezing) have occurred in a small number of patients (1 percent). Patients with lymphoma frequently have immediate allergic reactions or delayed reactions may occur several hours after the first or second dose of the drug is administered. Observation of the patient at five-minute intervals for 15 minutes and at 15-minute intervals for the following hour usually is planned to assure that any allergic reaction is detected immediately in patients with lymphoma. Other adverse reactions that may occur during therapy with bleomycin include nausea, vomiting, general weakness, hypotension, and pain at the tumor site.

Dactinomycin (COSMEGEN)

The drug is employed principally in combination with surgery or radiation therapy for the treatment of nephroblastoma (Wilms' tumor) and its metastases. The survival rate of children with nephroblastoma has been increased to two years as a result of the combination therapy.

Dactinomycin is also used in combination with other antineoplastic drugs for the treatment of testicular or uterine carcinoma. That drug therapy has produced a decrease in the malignant tissue masses in one third to one half of the patients treated. The drug therapy is continued at one-to-three-month intervals to suppress the growth of the cancer tissue.

Therapy Considerations. Dactinomycin is administered in short courses by intravenous injection. There is a high concentration of the drug in the kidneys, liver, and spleen after parenteral administration. Approximately 50 to 90 percent of the drug is excreted with the bile and 12 to 20 percent is excreted in the urine in 24 hours. There is minimal drug biotransformation.

The drug is very irritating to the soft tissues, and severe local reactions may occur when it extravasates into the tissues. The reconstituted solution usually is introduced into the tubing of a running intravenous infusion to avoid damage to the vein (i.e., phlebitis). The daily dosage level for adults is 500 mcg. The total five-day dosage for children is calculated on the basis of 15 mcg/kg of body weight. The drug is administered in five-day courses that may be repeated at two-week intervals.

Adverse Effects. Leukopenia, agranulocytosis, anemia, thrombocytopenia, and pancytopenia may occur soon after therapy is initiated (Table 15–3). The depressed blood levels also can occur one to two weeks after the completion of a course of drug therapy. The leukocyte counts are evaluated daily and the platelet count may be evaluated every three days during therapy with dactinomycin. A marked drop in the blood cell counts necessitates the interruption of therapy.

Nausea and vomiting may occur from four to five hours after the drug is administered. Anorexia, abdominal pain, and diarrhea also occur frequently. Inflammation may occur in almost all of the gastrointestinal tract tissues. The occurrence of ulcerative stomatitis is an indication of extensive damage to the tract tissues. The short courses of therapy allow time for their regeneration and repair during the drug-free intervals.

Epidermal toxicity usually appears as dermatitis, acne, erythema, or folliculitis. Some patients have alopecia during therapy with dactinomycin. The rapid lysis of cancer cells may increase the quantity of uric acid that is excreted in the urine. Other problems that may occur during therapy with dactinomycin include malaise, fatigue, lethargy, fever, myalgia, and epistaxis. Because the drug is an antibiotic, allergic reactions are potential problems.

Doxorubicin Hydrochloride (ADRIAMYCIN)

The drug is employed for the treatment of sarcomas, carcinomas in most body tissues, malignant lymphomas, and acute lymphoblastic or acute myeloblastic leukemias. The drug is used in combination with other antineoplastic agents in the treatment of lymphoma, osteogenic sarcoma, and breast carcinoma.

Therapy Considerations. Doxorubicin is administered intravenously. Thirty seconds after intravenous administration, the drug is present in the tissues of the liver, lungs, heart, and kidneys, where it binds to the intracellular nucleic acids. The drug is metabolized in the liver and by the enzymes at tissue sites to the active metabolite *adriamycinol,* which has antineoplastic activity. The other drug metabolites are therapeutically inactive. The metabolism of the drug is rapid and up to 70 percent of the drug appears as the metabolites in the plasma within 30 minutes after the dose is administered.

Most of the drug (80 percent) is excreted with the bile and 10 to 20 percent may be excreted within 24 hours. A small amount of the unchanged drug (5 percent) is excreted in the urine. The presence of the drug in the urine imparts a red color for one to two days after the drug dose is given. Patients should be informed of the urine discoloration to avoid the anxiety that may be associated with their interpretation that it is blood in the urine.

Since the drug is extremely irritating to the tissues, the intravenous dosage usually is injected into the tubing of a running intravenous to decrease the concentration of the drug that comes in contact with the vein. Extravasation into the tissues can cause cellulitis, lymphangitis, or necrosis.

The adult dosage level is calculated on the basis of 60 to 75 mg/M^2 of body surface area, usually administered in a single dose at 21-day intervals. An alternate plan involves administration of the drug dosage (30 mg/M^2) for three days and that course is repeated at four-week intervals. The maximum total dosage recommended over a lifetime is 550 mg/M^2 because cumulation can cause a fatal form of cardiotoxicity.

Adverse Effects. Leukopenia occurs in approximately 60 to 75 percent of the individuals who are treated with doxorubicin (Table 15–3). Thrombocytopenia and anemia also occur frequently. The maximum effect on the bone marrow production of the blood cells occurs during the second week after the drug is administered. The blood cell counts generally return to the normal level within a week.

Up to 80 percent of the patients have stomatitis during the second week followng administration of doxorubicin, and it may progress to ulceration of the sublingual and lateral tongue margins and the palate within a period of two to three days. The acute period of discomfort may last for three to seven days.

Vomiting occurs in from 20 to 55 percent of the patients on the day that the drug is administered and occasionally is accompanied by nausea. Some patients also have diarrhea on the day that the drug is administered.

The cardiotoxicity that occurs in patients receiving doxorubicin is of two types. Electrocardiograms are evaluated at regularly scheduled 30-day intervals during the entire period of therapy. Cardiotoxic effects can be of an acute transient type in 30 percent of the patients. There are abnormalities in the cardiac conduction patterns, and the problems gradually subside. The second type is a chronic cardiotoxicity that is dose dependent. The seriousness of the problem is the rationale for the recommended maximum lifetime dosage. The cardiotoxicity can result in a rapidly progressing syndrome of congestive heart failure and cardiorespiratory decompensation that is irreversible and unresponsive to therapy. The outcome of the acute episode is fatal.

Almost all patients have alopecia during therapy. Regrowth of the hair may begin two to three months after the drug administration is terminated. Other evidence of epidermal tissue toxicity includes hyperpigmentation of the skin folds or the nailbeds and pigmented banding of the fingernails, which may occur more than six weeks after therapy is initiated.

Mithramycin (MITHRACIN)

The drug, in addition to its action on cancer cells, inhibits the synthesis of DNA and RNA in the osteoclasts. That action reduces the responsiveness of the osteoclasts to the stimulus of parathyroid hormone. The bone calcium pool, which normally is broken down by the osteoclasts to maintain the serum calcium ion level at normal values, is unavailable. During therapy with mithramycin the serum calcium levels are low.

The drug is employed for the treatment of hypercalcemia and of the hypercalciuria associated with some advanced neoplasms. The administration of a single intravenous dose of the drug results in reduction of the serum calcium levels within 24 to 48 hours, and the beneficial effects last from 3 to 15 days. The drug has also produced complete or partial remissions in patients with malignant testicular tumors that had metastasized beyond the regional lymph nodes.

Therapy Considerations. The drug is administered intravenously. The circulating drug moves readily into the hepatic cells and the renal tubular cells, and it clusters along the bone surfaces. Mithramycin crosses the blood-brain barrier and the cerebrospinal fluid concentration equilibrates with plasma levels within four to six hours after the drug is administered. Up to 40 percent of the drug is excreted in the urine within 15 hours.

Mithramycin is given slowly by intravenous injection or may be infused intravenously over a period of four to six hours. Extravasation of the drug may cause cellulitis and local irritation. The dosage usually is calculated on the basis of 25 to 30 mcg/kg of body weight, and the drug is administered daily for a period of eight to ten days. Added courses of therapy may be planned at monthly intervals to achieve or maintain regression of the cancer tissue.

Adverse Effects. Leukopenia occurs in a small number of patients (Table 15–3). Thrombocytopenia may be rapid in onset and may occur during therapy or the onset may be delayed until several days after the last dose is administered. The most serious effects are the hemorrhagic episodes that occur in approximately 5 percent of the patients. They represent a drug-induced suppression of the clotting factors (i.e., prolonged prothrombin time, increased fibrinolytic activity) in addition to depression of the platelet count. The prothrombin time, bleeding time, and platelet count are evaluated before each dose of the drug is administered. The hemorrhage can occur in most of the body tissues and there can be external evidence of bleeding (i.e., hematemesis, epistaxis, ecchymosis) or there may be internal hemorrhage (i.e., into the gastrointestinal tract).

Nausea, vomiting, and anorexia are the most common adverse effects. The problems are more frequent and more severe when the drug is administered rapidly. Stomatitis and diarrhea also occur during therapy with mithramycin.

Mitomycin (MUTAMYCIN)

The drug, in addition to its cancer cell cycle phase-nonspecific activity, interferes with DNA activity by causing cross-linking of the DNA strands in a manner somewhat comparable to the action of the alkylating drugs.

Mitomycin is employed as an adjunct to surgery or radiation therapy and is used for the palliative treatment of carcinoma in many body tissues. It is used primarily for the treatment of advanced metastatic disease when the cancer tissue is resistant to the action of other antineoplastic drugs. Mitomycin is used in combination with cytarabine and fluorouracil for treatment of gastrointestinal neoplasms.

Therapy Considerations. Mitomycin is administered intravenously. The drug rapidly is distributed in the body tissues where it is reduced by enzymes. The enzymatic reduction of the drug within susceptible cells is necessary for its antineoplastic activity. The highest concentrations of the drug are in kidneys, muscles, eyes, lungs, intestines, and the stomach. The microsomal enzymes in the liver and the enzymes in the kidney, spleen, and brain rapidly reduce the drug. Less than 10 percent of the unchanged drug is excreted in the urine.

The reconstituted drug usually is administered by injection into the tubing of a freely running intravenous infusion. The drug is very irritating to the tissues and its introduction into the vein may cause pain and thrombophlebitis. Extravasation can cause cellulitis and tissue breakdown.

The total course dosage is calculated on the basis of 20 mg/M² of body surface area. The dosage may be given as a single intravenous dose or it may be divided for the administration of one half of the dosage daily for five consecutive days. The remainder of the drug is given for a second period of five days following a two-day drug-free period. That plan of therapy may be repeated after a two-to-three-week drug-free period. Longer intervals may be necessary when the cumulative drug levels cause bone marrow depression.

Weekly hematologic evaluations during therapy include the platelet count, prothrombin time, bleeding time, white blood cell count and differential analysis, and hemoglobin determinations. The evaluations are continued weekly for up to eight weeks after the therapy is discontinued because there is frequently a delayed depression of the hematologic values.

Adverse Effects. Thrombocytopenia and leukopenia may occur up to eight weeks after therapy is started, and they are the most frequent (64 percent of the patients) toxic effects (Table 15–3). The bone marrow production of the blood cells usually produces normal blood cell levels within three months after the therapy is discontinued. About 25 percent of the patients have persistently low blood cell counts for several months. Serious thrombocytopenia occurs two to four weeks after the initiation of therapy in approximately 40 percent of the patients who are treated (platelets <10,000/cu mm). That nadir may last for a very short period of time. After the recovery of the cell count there may be another depression to the same nadir.

Up to 50 percent of the patients who receive mitomycin have severe leukopenia, and the leukocyte count may decrease during the second to the fourth week of therapy. The leukocyte nadir may occur during the sixth week.

Nausea and vomiting occur in many patients (14 percent) within one to two hours after the drug is administered, and the nausea may continue for two to three days. The other common patient problems are fever, anorexia, and malaise. Epidermal tissue toxicity occurs in a small number of patients, and it usually consists of mouth ulcers, desquamation, and pruritus of the skin or alopecia.

ALKYLATING AGENTS

The drugs in the group, or class, that are identified as the alkylating agents are commonly employed for the treatment of cancer. Most combination drug therapy regimens include an alkylating agent in the protocol.

Action Mode

The alkylating agents are cancer cell life-cycle nonspecific drugs that can act at any time in the cell life-cycle. They form linkages with guanine causing purination. That action interferes with the utilization of purines in the assembling of the DNA strand. The miscoding of DNA interferes with its replication and with the transcription of RNA. The alkylating agents may also have some effects on proteins during their intracellular synthesis. The action of the drugs slows the progression of the cell life-cycle by acting in the postmitotic (G_1) synthesis (S), and mitotic (M) phases of its growth and reproduction sequences. The interference with the cell phases disrupts the synthesis of proteins and also, by preventing the cellular reproduction, causes the cells to become large masses of the ineffective proteins that gradually die.

The alkylating agents consist of six groups of pharmacologic agents. *Chlorambucil, cyclophosphamide, mechlorethamine, melphalan,* and *uracil mustard* are the *nitrogen mustards. Thiotepa* is an *ethylenimine; busulfan* is an *alkylsulfonate; darcarbazine* and *procarbazine* are *triazenes;* and *pipobroman* is a *piperazine derivative. Carmustine, lomustine,* and *semustine* are the *nitrosoureas,* the newest of the alkylating agents. The similarities and differences between the drugs when they are employed clinically for treatment are related in part to their pharmacologic groupings.

Busulfan (MYLERAN)

The drug has produced remissions in 80 to 90 percent of the patients who were treated for chronic myelocytic leukemia. More than half of the patients had an initial remission of 9 to 12 months' duration. Subsequent remissions lasted for longer periods of time.

Therapy Considerations. Busulfan is administered orally. The drug is rapidly absorbed from the gastrointestinal tract and it appears in the plasma within 0.5 to 2 hours after administration. The drug is metabolized extensively and 10 to 50 percent of the metabolites are slowly excreted in the urine over a 24-hour period.

The adult daily oral dosage ranges from 1 to 12 mg. The daily pediatric dosage is calculated on the basis of 60 to 120 mcg/kg of body weight. Therapy for children is titrated to maintain the leukocyte count at the level of 20,000/mm³. Maintenance may be continued at dosage levels of 1 to 4 mg/day to prevent rapid relapses. Intensive therapy usually is reinstituted when the leukocyte count reaches 50,000/mm³. Continuous therapy may be required to reduce the leukocyte count to the desired level. Blood cell counts are evaluated at least once each week during the periods when the drug is being taken.

Adverse Effects. Some patients are extremely sensitive to the drug and hematologic toxic effects may occur abruptly. In some of those patients the effects have been irreversible.

Severe leukopenia, anemia, and thrombocytopenia occur during therapy with busulfan (Table 15–2). The bone marrow depression is the major toxic effect. It generally is reversible when the drug therapy is discontinued.

The drug seldom causes gastointestinal toxicity, but nausea, vomiting, anorexia, or diarrhea may occur during therapy. The toxic effects of the drug on epidermal tissues may be manifested as urticaria, rashes, dryness of the skin, or alopecia. The extensive purine catabolism that occurs in patients with leukemia may cause hyperuricemia and elevation of the uric acid excretion rate.

In rare instances the long-term use of the drug causes diffuse interstitial pulmonary fibrosis, which is popularly called "busulfan lung." The syndrome can progress to respiratory insufficiency and death has occurred. A wasting syndrome that is described as being "Addison-like" without the adrenocorticoid insufficiency may occur. The syndome includes melanoderma, hypotension, gastrointestinal disturbances, weight loss, fatigue, and confusion. Long-term therapy has also caused aspermia, testicular atrophy, impotence, sterility, and mild gynecomastia in male patients and amenorrhea or ovarian fibrosis in females.

Chlorambucil (LEUKERAN)

The drug has produced remissions in a large number of patients with chronic lymphocytic leukemia or malignant lymphoma. It also has been employed with dactinomycin and methotrexate in the treatment of testicular carcinomas.

Therapy Considerations. The drug is administered orally. The usual daily dosage is calculated on the basis of 100 to 200 mcg/kg of body weight and the course of therapy usually lasts three to six weeks. The maintenance dosage is calculated on the basis of 30 mcg/kg/day. Weekly evaluations of the blood hemoglobin values and the total and differential white blood cell counts are planned during therapy with chlorambucil.

Adverse Effects. Anorexia, nausea, and vomiting may occur at high drug dosage levels but they seldom are problems at the therapeutic dosage levels. Chlorambucil produces few side effects. Excessive dosage or prolonged treatment may produce severe bone marrow depression.

Cyclophosphamide (CYTOXAN)

The drug has produced remissions or regressions in lymphoma, acute leukemias, and chronic lymphatic leukemia. The effectiveness of the drug is related to its chemical structure. It is a phosphamide ester of the antineoplastic drug mechlorethamine. The enzymes *phosphoramidase* and *phosphatase* are very active in cancer cells, and they rapidly liberate the active drug from its inactive form. The drug is also used investigationally at lower dosage for suppression of the immune response in some of the chronic autoimmune diseases (i.e., nephrotic syndrome, rheumatoid arthritis).

Therapy Considerations. The drug is administered orally or as intravenous, intramuscular, intraperitoneal, intrapleural, or intratumor injections. The initial daily intravenous dosage is calculated on the basis of 2 to 8 mg/kg of body weight and the dosage is administered for six days. When the leukocyte count begins to rise from the nadir, therapy may be resumed. It is usual for the oral route to be used for administration as soon as the patient can take the drug by that route. The dosage for maintenance therapy (50 to 200 mg) is administered in a single daily dose. The white blood cell and thrombocyte counts usually are evaluated daily, and the maximum period between the evaluations is four days during therapy with cyclophosphamide.

Adverse Effects. Marked leukopenia may occur during therapy with cyclophosphamide. The leukocyte count nadir usually occurs between the ninth and fourteenth days but the response may be delayed up to 30 days after the initiation of therapy (Table 15–4). When therapy is interrupted, the leukocyte count returns to the normal level in 7 to 14 days. Thrombocytopenia may occur in some patients, but it occurs less frequently than in patients who are treated with mechlorethamine.

Transient alopecia occurs more frequently (20 to 30 percent of the patients) during treatment with cyclophosphamide than it does with the other alkylating drugs. The hair loss generally occurs three weeks after initiation of therapy, and regrowth of the hair may start five to eight weeks after drug therapy is terminated. The new hair may differ in color and texture from previous hair and the color of new skin and nails may be darker.

Mild nausea and vomiting occur frequently.

Anorexia, weight loss, diarrhea, and mucosal ulceration occur in some patients who receive high doses of the drug.

The use of the drug in young people with autoimmune diseases has caused irreversible sterility. Low sperm counts or reversible ovarian suppression has occurred after 1 to 18 months of therapy.

Hemorrhagic cystitis has been reported as occurring in some patients. The incidence of the problem has resulted in the practice of administering the drug in the early morning to avoid having the drug in the bladder overnight. The person is also encouraged to maintain a relatively high intake of fluids. Other problems that can occur include fatigue, transient dizziness, blurring of vision, and clouding of the thought processes.

Darcarbazine (DTIC)

The drug has produced remissions or reduction of the malignant tissue in 20 to 50 percent of the patients treated for disseminated malignant melanoma. Although the median duration of the remissions is only four months, some patients have been in remission for up to three years. Darcarbazine has also been employed with immunotherapy (i.e., BCG) effectively. The drug is employed in combination with other antineoplastic drugs for treatment of lymphomas and soft tissue sarcomas.

Table 15–4.
Selected Patient Care Problems During Alkylating Drug Therapy

Alkylating Drug	Nausea and Vomiting	Stomatitis	Thrombo-cytopenia (Bleeding Potential)	Leukopenia (Infection Potential)	Lympho-cytopenia (Immuno-suppression)	Alopecia
Busulfan	+	0	+	+	+	+
Chlorambucil	0	0	0	0	+	0
Cyclophosphamide	+	+	+	+	+	+
Darcarbazine	Severe	0	+	+	+	Rare
Mechlorethamine	Severe	0	+	+	+	Rare
Melphalan	Mild	0	+	+	+	0
Pipobroman	Mild	0	+	+	+	Rare
Procarbazine	Severe	+	+	+	+	0
Thiotepa	Mild	0	+	+	+	0
Uracil mustard	+	0	+	+	+	+

Therapy Considerations. The drug is administered intravenously. Darcarbazine is distributed in the plasma, and peak levels are reached immediately after the intravenous injection. The plasma half-life is 35 to 75 minutes. A limited amount of the drug crosses the blood-brain barrier and cerebrospinal fluid drug levels may be 14 percent of the plasma drug levels.

Darcarbazine is metabolized in the liver by the microsomal enzymes, and some of the metabolites contribute to the antineoplastic activity of the drug. Within six hours 30 to 45 percent of the unchanged drug or its metabolites is excreted in the urine by tubular secretion.

The diluted drug may be administered slowly (i.e., over a one-minute period) by intravenous injection or by intravenous infusion over a 15-to-30-minute period. The drug is very irritating to the tissues and can cause severe pain and tissue damage when it extravasates from the vein.

The usual daily adult dosage is calculated on the basis of 2 to 4.5 mg/kg of body weight and the dosage is given for ten days. The course of therapy may be repeated at three-to-four-week intervals. The leukocyte, erythrocyte, and platelet counts are evaluated prior to therapy and at regular intervals during therapy with darcarbazine.

Adverse Effects. Leukopenia and thrombocytopenia are the most common manifestations of the bone marrow toxicity (Table 15–4). The blood cell depression occurs in only 20 percent of the patients treated at the lower level of the therapeutic dosage range. Depression of the erythrocytes occurs frequently but it usually produces only a mild anemia. The blood cell changes appear gradually within two to four weeks after the course of therapy is completed. A sharp drop in the hematologic status may necessitate interruption of therapy, but the problems usually are less severe than those that are produced by the other antineoplastic drugs.

Up to 90 percent of the patients have nausea, severe vomiting, and anorexia that occurs within an hour after the initial dose is administered. The problems may persist for up to 12 hours. Patients seem to develop a rapid tolerance, and the problems generally subside within one or two days of therapy. Foods and fluids may be restricted for one hour or more prior to administration to avoid the discomfort and the dehydrating effects of vomiting. Epithelial tissue toxicity causes alopecia and erythematous, macular, or papular rashes.

Interactions. The metabolism of darcarbazine may be enhanced when it is administered concurrently with phenobarbital or the phenytoins. The more rapid rate of metabolism can decrease the effectiveness of the drug.

Mechlorethamine Hydrochloride
(MUSTARGEN)

The drug has produced improvement in 60 to 65 percent and complete remissions in 15 percent of the patients with Hodgkin's disease. It has also been employed for palliative treatment of bronchogenic carcinoma. Mechlorethamine has produced improvement in 25 to 50 percent of the patients when it was injected into the pleural, peritoneal, or pericardial cavity to control effusions that contained malignant cells. It has also been used for intra-arterial or regional perfusion of malignant tissues. Mechlorethamine may be employed in combinations with other drugs for the treatment of lymphoma. The MOPP regimen has produced a 60 to 88 percent positive response, and one third of the patients have a ten-year remission, or "cure."

Therapy Considerations. The intravenous solution usually is injected into a running intravenous infusion to lessen the tissue irritation. The drug is a powerful vesicant, and contact with the patient's tissues or those of the nurse preparing the drug can cause an allergic contact dermatitis with inflammation and exudation. When the drug extravasates into the tissues, the area may be infiltrated with *sodium thiosulfate solution* and an ice pack may be applied for 6 to 12 hours to decrease the pain and limit the travel of the drug in the interstitial fluids.

The usual course of therapy consists of a single dose of the drug calculated on the basis of 400 mcg/kg of body weight. The rationale for the single-dose administration is to limit the incidence of the severe vomiting to one day. The course of therapy may be repeated at three-to-six-week intervals. Frequent blood counts are done, and the evaluation of the hematologic status affects the intervals between the therapeutic courses.

Adverse Effects. Lymphocytopenia generally occurs within 24 hours after the drug is administered. The nadir of the granulocytopenia is evident in six to eight days, and the recovery of leukocyte production occurs within ten days to three weeks. The occurrence of the nadir and recovery of platelet production parallels that of the granulocytes. The decline of erythrocytes that occurs over the first two-week period usually does not cause significant anemia.

Up to 90 percent of the patients have major episodes of nausea and vomiting, which are attributable to drug-induced stimulation of the medullary vomiting centers. Vomiting usually occurs from one to three hours after the drug is given and subsides in eight hours. Anorexia and nausea may persist for a 24-hour period. Administration of antiemetics or sedatives before the intravenous injection modifies the problems.

Epidermal tissue toxicity rarely causes alopecia or serious skin rashes. The immunosuppressive effects may precipitate the herpes zoster that commonly occurs in patients with lymphoma. Occurrence of the acute phase necessitates interruption of therapy to avoid its dissemination.

Impaired spermatogenesis and amenorrhea are manifestations of the toxic effect of the drug on germinal tissues. Rapid catabolism of cancer cells may cause hyperuricemia and nephropathy can occur.

Mechlorethamine causes central nervous system depression in some patients. The problems may include weakness, headache, vertigo, drowsiness, progressive muscle paralysis, convulsions, and psychosis.

Melphalan (ALKERAN)

The drug has produced an objective response in one third to one half of the patients who were treated for multiple myeloma. Pain relief occurred rapidly but the general improvement occurred very gradually over a period of several weeks to many months. The drug has also been used with other drugs in the treatment of osteogenic sarcoma.

Therapy Considerations. The drug is administered orally as a 6-mg daily dose for two to three weeks. When the leukocyte and platelet counts indicate recovery of the blood cell production, maintenance therapy at a dosage of 2 mg/day may be instituted. Leukocyte and platelet counts are evaluated two to three times a week during intensive therapy and at one-to-three-week intervals during maintenance therapy.

Adverse Effects. Anemia, neutropenia, and thrombocytopenia reach their nadirs within a few weeks and recovery from that low level is fairly rapid. Nausea and vomiting occur primarily when the drug is administered in a single dose to patients who have fasted. Alopecia rarely occurs during therapy with melphalan.

Pipobroman (VERCYTE)

The drug is employed primarily for the treatment of polycythemia vera. It is also employed for the treatment of chronic granulocytic leukemia.

Therapy Considerations. The drug is administered orally and is well absorbed from the gastrointestinal tract. The initial daily dosage is based on the calculation of 1 to 2.5 mg/kg of body weight. When it is used for the treatment of polycythemia vera, the maintenance dosage (100 to 200 mcg/kg/day) may be started when the hematocrit is reduced to 50 to 55 percent. The maintenance dosage for patients with leukemia (7 to 175 mg/day) may be started when the leukocyte count reaches 10,000/cu mm. Bone marrow studies may be performed at the time of the maximum hematologic response. Leukocyte and platelet counts are evaluated every other day and complete blood counts may be evaluated weekly during intensive therapy.

Adverse Effects. The bone marrow depression that usually occurs four weeks after the patient receives the initial dose of the drug causes leukopenia, thrombocytopenia, and anemia. When there is a sharp drop in the leukocyte or platelet counts, therapy may be interrupted to allow recovery of the blood cell production.

The rapid lysis of leukemic cells may cause hyperuricemia. The rapid lysis of red blood cells in polycythemia vera may cause an increase in the bilirubin levels and reticulocytosis. The other problems that occur during therapy include gastrointestinal disturbances (i.e., nausea, vomiting, abdominal cramping, diarrhea, anorexia), which usually are transient. When the problems persist, therapy may be terminated.

Procarbazine Hydrochloride (MATULANE)

The drug is employed as palliative treatment of patients with generalized Hodgkin's disease. It is also used in combination with other antineoplastic drugs in the treatment of lymphoma.

Therapy Considerations. The drug is administered orally and is well absorbed from the gastrointestinal tract. The highest concentrations of the drug are present in the liver, kidneys, intestinal tissues, and skin. It is metabolized rapidly in the liver. Approximately 25 percent of the metabolites and the unchanged drug are excreted in the urine within 24 hours.

The initial daily oral dosage range for adults is 100 to 200 mg during the first week. The dosage may then be increased to 300 mg/day. The maintenance dosage is given (50 to 100 mg/day) after a remission has occurred. The pediatric dosage is usually 50 mg/day for the first week and it may be increased after that period of time. The pediatric maintenance dosage is 50 mg/day. Bone marrow studies and blood cell evaluations usually are done before initiation of therapy and they are repeated when the maximum hematologic response is attained. The hemoglobin, hematocrit, white blood cell and leukocyte differential, reticulocyte, and platelet counts usually are repeated at three-to-four-week intervals throughout therapy.

Adverse Effects. Leukopenia, thrombocytopenia, and anemia are the manifestations of bone marrow depression during therapy with procarbazine (Table 15–4). Severe nausea and vomiting frequently occur. Therapy is interrupted when stomatitis or diarrhea occurs. Other gastrointestinal problems are anorexia, dryness of the mouth, and constipation. A few patients have epidermal tissue toxicity that produces dermatitis, alopecia, pruritus, or hyperpigmentation.

The drug can cause central nervous system toxicity. Drug therapy is interrupted when there are neuropathies, paresthesias, or confusion. The neural toxicity of the drug produces neurologic and neuromuscular dysfunction (i.e., mental depression, acute psychosis, headache, dizziness, nervousness, insomnia, unsteadiness, ataxia, decreased reflexes, tremors, convulsions, myalgia, arthralgia).

Interactions. Procarbazine has monoamine oxidase activity, and the concurrent administration of sympathomimetic drugs, tricyclic antidepressants, local anesthetics, and drugs or foods with a high tyramine content can cause an exaggerated sympathetic nerve-related response (i.e., marked hypertension). Concurrent use of central nervous system depressants may produce effects that are synergistic with those that are caused by procarbazine.

Thiotepa

The drug has produced remissions in patients who were treated for advanced or metastatic carcinoma of the lung, breast, and ovary. Thiotepa has also produced remissions in patients with chronic granulocytic or lymphocytic leukemia and malignant lymphoma. It has been used for pleural, peritoneal, intra-arterial, and intracerebral injections for the treatment of metastases. The topical solution has produced positive effects in the treatment of bladder carcinoma.

Therapy Considerations. The drug is usually administered topically or by intramuscular or intravenous injection. Although the drug is rapidly distributed in body tissues, the onset of action is slow and the therapeutic effects may not be apparent for several weeks. Most of the drug is excreted in the urine in 24 to 48 hours.

The initial daily dose is usually 30 mg, administered intravenously for five days. The maintenance dose is administered at weekly intervals. The leukocyte and platelet counts and the hemoglobin value may be evaluated daily for the first seven to ten days. Weekly evaluations then are planned until at least four weeks after therapy is terminated.

Adverse Effects.   The initial evidence of hematopoietic depression is lymphopenia, which may be followed by neutropenia, thrombocytopenia, and mild erythrocyte depression. The maximum leukopenia may occur from two to four weeks after therapy is discontinued.

The nausea, vomiting, and anorexia with thiotepa therapy are less severe than with the other alkylating drugs. Other problems that may occur during therapy include headache, fever, amenorrhea, decreased spermatogenesis, and allergic responses.

Uracil Mustard

The drug is employed primarily for the palliative treatment of neoplasms of the reticuloendothelial system. It has produced improvement in patients with chronic myelocytic or lymphocytic leukemias or lymphomas.

Therapy Considerations.   The drug is administered orally. The initial daily dosage is 1 to 2 mg and it is administered for seven days. The maximum dosage level for initial therapy is 500 mcg/kg of body weight. Maintenance therapy at a dosage level of 1 mg/day is continued for three months. When a remission is attained, the same dosage may be given daily for three out of every four weeks. The hematologic status is evaluated one to two times a week, and those evaluations may be continued for at least two to four weeks after termination of therapy to monitor the delayed bone marrow depression period.

Adverse Effects.   Leukopenia, thrombocytopenia, and anemia occur frequently. The depression of the platelet counts may be greater than that of the leukocyte counts. Recovery of blood cell production usually occurs within two to three weeks after therapy is terminated.

Anorexia, epigastric distress, abdominal pain, nausea, vomiting, and diarrhea occur frequently. The problems may become severe enough to necessitate interruption of the drug therapy. Other drug-related problems that may occur include amenorrhea, oligospermia, and hyperuricemia.

Carmustine (BICNU)

The drug has been employed in clinical trials for the treatment of glioma, lymphoma, melanoma, and myeloma, and for lung, breast, and gastrointestinal tract carcinomas. It has been used in combination with fluorouracil in the treatment of gastrointestinal neoplasms.

Therapy Considerations.   The drug is administered intravenously. It is rapidly distributed in body tissues and there is a minimal amount of the drug in the plasma within five minutes after it is administered, which suggests that the metabolites provide its activity. The high lipid solubility of the drug allows its rapid entry into the cerebrospinal fluid, and the drug levels may be 50 percent higher than those of the plasma. Up to 70 percent of the drug metabolites are excreted in the urine within 96 hours. Approximately 10 percent is excreted as carbon dioxide from the lungs.

Care must be taken when preparing the drug to avoid contact with the skin because it causes a brown staining of the tissues. The dosage and frequency of administration differ in the study protocols. The drug is infused slowly over a 30-to-60-minute period. Rapid infusion can cause local burning along the vein route.

The intravenous dosage of 200 mg/M^2 of body surface area may be administered as a single dose or it may be divided and administered over a two-to-five-day period. The course of therapy may be repeated at six-to-eight-week intervals.

Adverse Effects. Nausea and vomiting may occur within two hours after the drug is infused. Pretreatment with antiemetics modifies the problems.

Thrombocytopenia generally occurs on the thirtieth day of therapy, and the platelet count rises more rapidly than the leukocyte count. The mean nadir of the white blood cell count occurs on day 34 and recovery of the leukocyte production occurs over the following eight to ten days.

Pigmentation has occurred along the vein of injection. Hepatotoxicity occurs in some patients. The toxic effects generally are mild and reversible when therapy is terminated. The hepatotoxicity is more prevalent during therapy with carmustine than with the other nitrosoureas.

Lomustine (CEENU)

The drug has been employed in clinical trials for the palliative treatment of epidermoid carcinoma of the lungs, malignant melanoma, and brain tumors. One third of the patients treated for malignant and metastatic brain lesions showed improvement that lasted from 44 to 50 weeks. Seventy-five percent of the patients with Hodgkin's disease who were treated had short periods of remission (i.e., 71 days).

Therapy Considerations. The drug is administered orally and is readily absorbed from the gastrointestinal tract. The dosage of the drug is calculated on the basis of 130 mg/M^2 of body surface area, given as a single oral dose every six to eight weeks. Blood counts are evaluated before each dose and at weekly intervals.

Adverse Effects. Nausea and vomiting occur in 45 to 75 percent of the patients. The problems begin within two to six hours after the dose is administered and they persist for less than 24 hours. Pretreatment with antiemetics or administration of the drug early in the morning before food is taken may alleviate the problems.

Thrombocytopenia generally occurs approximately four weeks after the drug is given and persists for a period of one to two weeks. Leukopenia

may occur six weeks after the drug is administered and lasts for one to two weeks.

Toxic manifestations include the appearance of stomatitis and alopecia. The problems seldom necessitate the interruption of therapy.

Semustine (Methyl CCNU)

The drug has been employed in clinical situations similar to those of lomustine. It has also been employed investigationally in combination with fluorouracil for the treatment of gastrointestinal malignancies.

Adverse Effects. The drug produces bone marrow depression that results in thrombocytopenia, leukopenia, and some decreased red blood cell production. Thrombocytopenia is more frequent and more severe than leukopenia.

ANTINEOPLASTIC HORMONES

The hormones that are employed specifically for therapy of malignancies of the endocrine glands include *calusterone, megestrol, testolactone, methoxyprogesterone, polyestradiol, diethylstilbestrol, tamoxifen citrate,* and *mitotane.* The hormones are employed to decrease the activity of the natural body hormones that stimulate tissue growth or release excess levels of hormones from the endocrine glands.

Calusterone (METHOSARB)

The drug is structurally and pharmacologically related to the natural male hormone testosterone. It is used in the palliative treatment of advanced widely disseminated carcinoma of the breast in postmenopausal women. Treatment of premenopausal women may follow suppression of ovarian function by surgical removal or by radiation therapy to the ovaries. About 25 percent of the patients treated with calusterone have a decrease in the size of cancer tissues in involved organs.

Action Mode. The androgenic hormone changes the hormonal balance in receptive tissues.

The androgen protects the cell surface from the natural hormones progesterone and the estrogens that can stimulate the growth of malignant tissue in the reproductive organs of the female.

Therapy Considerations. The drug is administered orally and is well absorbed from the gastrointestinal tract. The daily dosage (150 to 300 mg) is administered over a period of three months. Initially there is an increase in the serum alkaline phosphatase, which indicates improvement in the lesions in the bones.

Adverse Effects. The drug causes less viralization in the female patients than that produced by testosterone. Hirsutism frequently occurs. Approximately 25 percent of the patients have a deepening of the voice, acne, and the growth of facial hair. The hormone therapy may also cause oiliness of the skin, some loss of the scalp hair, clitoral enlargement, or increased libido.

Edema may occur during therapy, but it usually is mild. Hypercalcemia occurs as a manifestation of the hormonal stimulation of calcium release from the bony metastases. Other problems related to the drug therapy include fever, mild nausea, and vomiting.

Testolactone (TESLAC)

The drug is similar to calusterone. It is employed for the palliative treatment of advanced or widely disseminated mammary carcinoma in postmenopausal women. It is effective when the metastases are in the soft, nonvisceral tissue and bone.

Therapy Considerations. Testolactone may be administered orally or intramuscularly. The oral drug is well absorbed from the gastrointestinal tract. The drug is metabolized in the liver and the unchanged drug or the glucuronide metabolite is excreted in the urine.

The daily oral dosage of the drug is 250 mg, administered four times a day for three months. The intramuscular dosage is 100 mg, injected deeply into the upper outer quadrant of the glu-

teal region three times each week. The injection may cause pain, local irritation, and inflammation.

Adverse Effects. The drug lacks the virilizing effects common to testosterone. The anabolic effects of the drug may cause retention of nitrogen, potassium, and phosphorus.

Megestrol Acetate (MEGACE)

The drug is a progestational substance that is employed for the palliative treatment of recurrent or metastatic endometrial or breast carcinoma. Up to 50 percent of the patients had improvement and regression of cancer tissue growth that was maintained for six months.

Action Mode. The effect of the drug on cancer tissue may be a consequence of the inhibition of the pituitary production of luteinizing hormone. The drug may also convert the actively growing stroma into decidua.

Therapy Considerations. The drug is administered orally and is well absorbed from the gastrointestinal tract. The peak plasma levels are attained within one to three hours. Megestrol is metabolized in the liver and the metabolites are excreted in the urine over a period of ten days. The drug causes insignificant adverse effects.

Methoxyprogesterone Acetate (DEPO-PROVERA)

The drug is a progesterone derivative employed for adjunctive and palliative treatment of patients with recurrent, inoperable, and metastatic endometrial carcinoma. The effects of the drug are usually evident a few weeks to several months after therapy is instituted.

The initial adult dose is 0.4 to 1 gm/week, administered intramuscularly. The maintenance dose of 400 mg/month may be started after there is an indication of the therapeutic effect.

The adverse effects, which occur infrequently, are nervousness, insomnia, fatigue, and dizziness. There have been reports of allergic reactions (i.e., pruritus, urticaria, angioedema, anaphylaxis).

Polyestradiol Phosphate (ESTRADURIN)

The drug is employed for palliative treatment of patients with advanced prostatic carcinoma. It is an estrogenic drug that stimulates the action of estrogen as estradiol units split from the molecule. The therapeutic effect usually occurs within three months.

Therapy Considerations. The dosage of the drug is 40 to 80 mg, given every two to four weeks as a deep intramuscular injection. The initial injection may cause a burning sensation, but subsequent injections often are less uncomfortable. The drug therapy usually is terminated at the end of three months. Approximately 30 percent of the patients who are benefited by the therapy have a period of improvement after the course of therapy, which is known as "rebound regression" of the malignant tissue.

Approximately 90 percent of the intramuscular dosage leaves the circulating blood within 24 hours and is stored in the reticuloendothelial system. When the level of free plasma estradiol drops, more of the drug is released from the storage sites and that process provides a continuous drug effect. Larger doses prolong the drug activity rather than increasing the plasma levels of the drug. There have been reports of thrombotic episodes that may be attributable to the effects of the drug.

Diethylstilbestrol Diphosphate (STILPHOSTROL)

The drug, like polyestriadiol, is an estrogenic substance. It is employed for the palliative treatment of patients with advanced prostatic carcinoma.

The initial oral dosage is 50 to 200 mg, administered three times a day. Therapy may be changed from oral administration to intravenous infusion when there is no therapeutic response. The initial intravenous dose is 0.5 gm. On subsequent days the dosage may be increased to 1 gm and that dosage may be given for five or more days. The drug may be given intravenously (i.e.,

0.25 to 0.50 gm) one or two times a week as a maintenance dosage or it may be given orally.

Tamoxifen Citrate (NOLVADEX)

The drug is a nonsteroidal oral antiestrogen that is used for the palliative treatment of disseminated breast cancer in postmenopausal women. Tamoxifen competes with estrogen for binding sites in the cytoplasm and it enters the cell nucleus where it remains bound to nuclear chromatin for prolonged periods of time.

The drug is administered orally and the usual dosage is 10 to 20 mg two times/day. The oral drug is well absorbed and peak serum concentrations are attained within 4 to 7 hours. The drug metabolites enter the feces with the bile and most of the dosage is excreted in the feces.

The most frequent adverse effects are transient episodes of hot flashes, nausea, and vomiting. Less frequent problems are vaginal bleeding and discharge, skin rashes, and transient leukopenia or thrombocytopenia. Problems that occur infrequently include severe hypercalcemia in patients with bone metastases, and tumor or bone pain associated with sudden transient enlargement of the tissue lesions during the initial days of treatment.

Mitotane (LYSODREN)

The drug is employed for the palliative treatment of inoperable adrenocortical carcinoma. Prior to the drug therapy the accessible cancer tissue and metastases are removed surgically. The mean duration of cancer cell regression following therapy with mitotane has been ten months. Some improvement is evident within six weeks after therapy is initiated.

Action Mode. The drug suppresses the function of adrenal tissues. It also inhibits the action of the hormones that are released from the adrenocortical tissues.

Therapy Considerations. The drug is administered orally and the dosage is calculated to allow for the low rate of gastrointestinal absorption of the drug (35 to 40 percent). The drug may remain in the blood for approximately two months after therapy is discontinued. The adipose tissues are the primary storage site of the drug, but it is distributed in most of the body tissues. The drug is metabolized in the liver and the kidneys to the metabolite, which is excreted with the bile and urine.

The initial dosage range is from 9 to 10 gm daily, and that dose is divided for administration three to four times a day. The dosage may be increased above the initial level to a maximum dosage range of 2 to 16 gm/day until improvement or adverse effects occur. A decrease in the 17-hydroxycorticoid levels usually becomes apparent within two to three days after therapy is initiated.

Adverse Effects. The most frequent adverse effects (80 percent of patients) are anorexia, nausea, vomiting, and diarrhea. Central nervous system depression (i.e., lethargy, somnolence, dizziness, vertigo) and skin reactions also occur frequently. The adrenal insufficiency that occurs may be treated by the administration of corticosteroids. A few patients have had hypersensitivity reactions to the drug.

NURSING INTERVENTION

Care of the patient who has cancer is probably one of the most challenging aspects of nursing. The multiplicity of problems that are directly related to the effects of the malignant growth on body function are only a small part of the overall problem. During drug therapy the highly toxic agents cause additional problems for the patient.

The presentation of antineoplastic drugs has included many factors about the drugs that have implications for nursing care. The following guide for planning nursing intervention is intended for use in utilizing the information about the drugs when preparing an individualized plan of nursing care for the patient who has cancer.

Guidelines for Nursing Intervention

I. Establish base lines for assessing the effect of the antineoplastic drug on malignant tissue.
 A. Obtain the patient's statement of the problem and the functional limits caused by the problem.
  1. Analyze the patient's statement for clues to the emotional and physical problems common to patients with cancer. These include
   a. Fear, anxiety, psychologic distress.
   b. Tolerating pain and discomfort because of concern about narcotic addition.
   c. Lack of information affecting the person's perception of the planned diagnostic tests or the therapy plan.
 B. Obtain information about the psychosocial factors contributing to the problem (i.e., health history, health care practices, compliance with prescribed therapies).
 C. Examine the patient for the signs of the physical problems that are commonly present in patients with cancer. These include
  1. Malnutrition, anorexia, tissue breakdown.
   a. Weigh the patient.
   b. Test muscle tone and strength.
   c. Examine the body structure, presence of fat padding, skin turgor.
  2. External and internal bleeding.
   a. Test the stools, urine, sputum, vomitus for occult blood content.
   b. Examine the oral mucosa, nasal passages, and skin surfaces (i.e., wounds, incisions, injection sites) for petechial hemorrhage or bleeding.

c. Take the pulse and blood pressure.

d. Evaluate the person's tolerance to activity.

3. Infection and fever with malaise.

a. Check the vital signs and skin surface for evidence of increased metabolic activity (temperature, pulse, respiratory rate, skin flushed and warm).

b. Examine surface tissues for lesions and the body orifices and wounds for drainage.

4. Edema.

a. Listen to the lung fields for fluid content.

b. Measure the abdominal girth, calves, and ankles.

c. Test surface tissues for distention (rebound after digital pressure).

5. Elimination problems (i.e., constipation, which is commonly associated with gastrointestinal or widespread pelvic cancer).

a. Palpate the abdominal margins for large-bowel distention.

b. Use the stethoscope to assess the level of peristalsis.

D. Determine the individual's ideal nutrient and fluid intake for maintenance of healthy tissue and for elimination of fecal wastes and compare the calculated amount with the person's intake patterns (i.e., frequency, amount, preferences).

E. Examine the clinical record for relevant data. These include

1. Progression and forms of therapy for the malignancy.

2. Functional and performance problems.

3. Biopsy reports indicating primary and metastatic sites.

4. X-ray study reports.

5. Hematologic studies (i.e., red blood cell count, white blood cell count and leukocyte distribution, hematocrit, hemoglobin, prothrombin level, platelet count).

6. Weight profiles.

7. Graphic records of temperature and vital signs.

F. Select an objective parameter that can be used for evaluating the person's progress during the drug therapy period.

II. Plan measures to maximize the antineoplastic drug effect and to maintain or restore normal tissue function.

A. Clarify for the patient the effect of the antineoplastic drug and the rationale for the drug therapy.

B. Implement the prescribed activity, nutrient, and fluid intake plan.

1. Provide foods based on the patient's tolerance and nutrient needs (i.e., high-protein diet or small, spaced meals).

2. Encourage nutritious snacks at the person's prime tolerance times.

C. Schedule administration of the drug to allow minimal adverse effects on the patient's ability to function (i.e., give it at bedtime with the prescribed sedative or hypnotic to decrease nausea and interference with eating meals).

D. Implement the prescribed measures to maintain comfort and modify the adverse effects of the prescribed antineoplastic drug (i.e., antiemetics, analgesics, fluids, and alkylating drugs to increase excretion of uric acid).

E. Reassess the patient's status to define the effects and adverse effects of the drug.

1. Observe changes in the functioning of the target tissues (i.e., decreased pain, increased mobility).

2. Observe the patient for evidence of toxic effects of the drug on nontarget, rapidly proliferating tissues.

These include

a. Bone marrow tissue: leukopenia-infection potential; thrombocytopenia-bleeding potential; erythrocytopenia-anemia potential; lymphocytopenia-infection potential (decreased immune response).

b. Gastrointestinal tissues: stomatitis (i.e., burning sensation when drinking citrus juices, lesions at lip and tongue margins), diarrhea.

c. Epidermal tissues: alopecia, loss of axillary or pubic hair; pigmentation of nails or skin folds; photosensitivity.

d. Gonadal tissues: changes in menstruation or libido.

3. Obtain the patient's statement of the drug effect on the tissues (i.e., bleeding gums when brushing teeth, excess fatigue).

4. Maintain a record of the objective and subjective changes for their evaluation by the health team.

III. Prepare the patient and a family member for assessing the progress of the antineoplastic drug therapy plan.

A. Review with the patient and a family member the plan for use of the drug, nutrient intake, activity progression.

B. Plan with the patient for implementing the specific drug therapy plan within the usual schedule of daily activities.

1. Remind the patient to *keep the drugs out of the reach of children.*

2. Provide specific written instruction for the patient to use at home.

C. Teach the patient how to assess changes in tissue status and body function.

D. Describe to the patient the problems that require physician contact. These include changes in function related to

1. Growth of the malignant tissues.

2. Toxic effects of the drugs on normal body tissues (i.e., sore throat, fever, excess fatigue, bleeding, infections).

3. Adverse effects of the specific drugs being utilized for therapy.

E. Describe to the patient the measures that can be employed to modify the adverse effects of the drugs. These include the measures utilized during therapy and

1. Maintaining nutritional intake.

2. Avoiding exposure to individuals with infections (i.e., colds).

F. Reassess the person's readiness to maintain the drug therapy plan at home.

Review Guides

1. Formulate a plan for monitoring the patient's status for evidence of the toxic effects of an antineoplastic drug. Include in the plan

a. The specific body tissues that should be examined.

b. The tissue changes that indicate toxicity.

c. The measures that can be employed to modify the problems.

d. The measures that can be employed to protect the person from potential problems.

2. For each of the following groups of drugs, identify those effects of the therapy that should be discussed with the individual who is receiving the drugs:

a. Mechlorethamine
   Procarbazine
   Vincristine

b. Bleomycin
   Darcarbazine
   Doxorubicin

c. Cytarabine
   Fluorouracil
   Mitomycin

d. Cyclophosphamide
   Methotrexate
   Fluorouracil
e. Mercaptopurine
   Methotrexate

   Vincristine
f. Chlorambucil
   Dactinomycin
   Methotrexate

Additional Readings

Bingham, Carol Ann: The cell cycle and cancer chemotherapy. *Am. J. Nurs.,* **78:**1200, July, 1978.

Bruya, Margaret Auld, and Madeira, Nancy Powell: Stomatitis after chemotherapy. *Am. J. Nurs.,* **75:** 1349, August, 1975.

Chabner, Bruce A.; Myers, Charles E.; Coleman, C. Norman; and Johns, David G.: Medical progress: the clinical pharmacology of antineoplastic agents. *N. Engl. J. Med.,* **292:**1107, May 22, 1975; **292:** 1159, May 29, 1975.

Crist, William M.; Ragab, Abdelsalam H.; and Vietti, Teresa J.: Chemotherapy of childhood medulloblastoma. *Am. J. Dis. Child.,* **130:**639, June, 1976.

Dreizen, Samuel; Bodey, Gerald P.; and Rodriquez, Victorio: Oral complications of cancer chemotherapy. *Postgrad. Med.,* **58:**75, August, 1975.

Dreizen, Samuel; Bodey, Gerald P.; Rodriquez, Victorio; and McCredie, Kenneth B.: Cutaneous complications of cancer chemotherapy. *Postgrad. Med.,* **58:**150, November, 1975.

Desotell, Susan: A brighter future for leukemia patients. *Nursing 77,* **7:**18, January, 1977.

Fochtman, Dianne: Malignant solid tumors in children. *Pediatr. Nurs.,* **2:**11, November–December, 1976.

Gee, Timothy G.; Haghbin, Mahroo; Dowling, Monroe D., Jr.; Cunningham, Isabel; Middleman, Mary P.; and Clarkson, Bayard D.: Acute lymphoblastic leukemia in adults and children—differences in response with similar therapeutic regimens. *Cancer,* **37:**1256, March, 1976.

Gilladoga, Angela C.; Manuel, Corazon; Tan, Charlotte T. C.; Wollner, Norma; Sternberg, Stephen S.; and Murphy, M. Lois: The cardiotoxicity of adriamycin and daunomycin in children. *Cancer* (Conference Suppl.), **37:**1070, February, 1976.

Greene, Trish: Current therapy for acute leukemia in childhood. *Nurs. Clin. North Am.,* **11:**3, March, 1976.

Harris, Curtis C.: The carcinogenicity of anticancer drugs—a hazard in man. *Cancer* (Conference Suppl.), **37:**1014, February, 1976.

Harris, Jules; Sengar, Dharmendia; Stewart, Thomas; and Hyslop, Daphne: The effects of immunosuppressive chemotherapy on immune function in patients with malignant disease. *Cancer* (Conference Suppl.), **37:**1058, February, 1976.

Jones, Stephen E.; Durie, Brian G. M.; and Salmon, Sydney E.: Combination chemotherapy with adriamycin and cyclophosphamide for advanced breast cancer. *Cancer,* **36:**90, July, 1975.

Komp, Diane M.; George, Stephen L.; Falletta, John; Land, Vita J.; Starling, Kenneth A.; Humphrey, G. Bennett; and Lowman, James: Cyclophosphamide-asparaginase-vincristine-prednisone induction therapy in childhood acute lymphocytic and nonlymphocytic leukemia. *Cancer,* **37:**1243, March, 1976.

Kopersztych, Samuel; Rezkallah, Maria Thereza; Miki, Silvia S.; Naspitz, Charles K.; and Mendes, Nelson F.: Cell-mediated immunity in patients with carcinoma—correlation between clinical stage and immunocompetence. *Cancer,* **38:**1149, September, 1976.

Lauter, Carl B.: Opportunistic infections. *Heart Lung,* **5:**601, July–August, 1976.

Lawrence, H. J.; Simone, Joseph; and Aur, R. J. A.: Cyclophosphamide-induced hemorrhagic cystitis in children with leukemia. *Cancer,* **36:**1572, November, 1975.

Levine, Myra E.: Cancer chemotherapy—a nursing model. *Nurs. Clin. North Am.,* **13:**271, June, 1978.

Livingston, Robert B.; Fee, William H.; Einhorn, Lawrence H.; Burgess, Michael A.; Freireich, Emil J.; Gottlieb, Jeffrey A.; and Farber, Mark O.: BACON (bleomycin, adriamycin, CCNU, oncovin, and nitrogen mustard) in squamous lung cancer—experience in fifty patients. *Cancer,* **37:**1237, March, 1976.

Lokich, Jacob J.: Managing chemotherapy-induced bone marrow suppression in cancer. *Hosp. Pract.,* **11:**61, August, 1976.

Lokich, Jacob J.; Frei, Emil, III; Jaffe, Norman; and Tullis, James: New multiple-agent chemotherapy (B-DOPA) for advanced Hodgkin's disease. *Cancer,* **38**:667, August, 1976.

Miller, Suzanne A.: Oncology nurse and chemotherapy. *Am. J. Nurs.,* **77**:989, June, 1977.

Morgenfeld, Marcos E.; Pavlavsky, Alfredo; Suarez, Argimiro; Somoza, Nilda; Pavlovsky, Santiago; Palau, Marcio; and Barros, Carlos A.: Combined cyclophosphamide, vincristine, procarbazine and prednisone (COPP) therapy of malignant lymphoma-evaluation of 190 patients. *Cancer,* **36**:1241, October, 1975.

Nesbit, Mark; Krivit, William; Heyn, Ruth; and Sharp, Harvey: Acute and chronic effects of methotrexate on hepatic, pulmonary and skeletal systems. *Cancer* (Conference Suppl.), **37**:1048, February, 1976.

Nirenberg, Anita: High-dose methotrexate. *Am. J. Nurs.,* **76**:1776, November, 1976.

North, Carolyn, and Weinstein, Gerald D.: Treatment of psoriasis. *Am. J. Nurs.,* **76**:410, March, 1976.

Old, Lloyd J.: Cancer immunology. *Sci. Am.,* **236**:62, May, 1977.

Pochedly, Carl: How does leukemia invade the central nervous system? *Postgrad. Med.,* **59**:101, January, 1976.

Richert-Boe, Kathryn E., and Bagley, Grover, Jr.: Treating acute nonlymphocytic leukemia. *Geriatrics,* **33**:50, February, 1978.

Rudolph, Ross; Stein, Richard S.; and Pattillo, Roland A.: Skin ulcers due to adriamycin. *Cancer,* **38**:1087, September, 1976.

Santorelli, Alan C.; Shansky, Charles W.; and Rosman, Martin: Biochemical approaches to the combination chemotherapy of colon cancer. *Cancer* (Conference Suppl.), **36**:2445, December, 1975.

Scharf, Jehuda; Nakir, Menachem; Eidelman, Shmuel; Jacobs, Richard; and Levin, Dan: Carcinoma of the bladder with azathioprine therapy. *J.A.M.A.,* **237**:152, January 10, 1977.

Segaloff, Albert: Appraising current therapy for breast cancer. 3. Hormonal manipulation and chemotherapy. *Postgrad. Med.,* **60**:191, September, 1976.

Serpeck, Arthur A.: Cancer in the elderly, *Hosp. Pract.,* **13**:101, February, 1978.

Shoss, Robert G., and Lumpkin, Lee R.: Current therapy of psoriasis. *Am. Fam. Physician,* **15**:114, January, 1977.

Sinkovics, Joseph G.: Progress in clinical immunotherapy for tumors. *Postgrad. Med.,* **59**:110, February, 1976.

Smyth, A. Collier, and Wiernik, Peter H.: Combination chemotherapy of adult acute lymphocytic leukemia. *Clin. Pharmacol. Ther.,* **19**:240, February, 1976.

Theologides, Athansios: Why cancer patients have anorexia. *Geriatrics,* **31**:69, June, 1976.

Ugoretz, Richard J.: Cardiac effects of doxorubicin therapy of neoplasms. *J.A.M.A.,* **236**:295, July 19, 1976.

Vinciguerra, Vincent; Coleman, Morton; Jarowski, Charles I.; Degnan, Thomas J.; and Silver, Richard T.: A new combination chemotherapy for resistant Hodgkin's disease. *J.A.M.A.,* **237**:33, January 3, 1977.

Von Hoff, Daniel D.; Rozencweig, Marcel; Layard, Maxwell; Slavik, Milan; and Muggia, Franco M.: Daunomycin-induced cardiotoxicity in children and adults. *Am. J. Med.,* **62**:200, February, 1977.

Wahl, Theresa Pretti, and Glythe, James G.: Chemotherapy in gynecological malignancies—and its nursing aspects. *J. Obs. Gyn. Neonatal Nurs.,* **5**:9. September–October, 1976.

Wasserman, Todd H.; Slavik, Milan; and Carter, Stephen K.: Clinical comparison of the nitrosoureas. *Cancer,* **36**:1258, October, 1975.

Wolk, Joel A.; Stuart, Marie J.; Stockman, James A.; and Oski, Frank A.: Neutropenia, fever and infection in children with acute lymphocytic leukemia. *Am. J. Dis. Child.,* **131**:157, February, 1977.

Wood, Robert E.: Pseudomonas: the compromised host. *Hosp. Pract.,* **11**:91, August, 1976.

16

Bacterial Infection

Exposure to microorganisms that can cause infection is an everyday occurrence in the life of humans. Complex and interrelated factors determine whether an exposure to pathologic organisms will lead to an infectious process. The outcome is influenced by changes in the agent-host-environment interaction and their effect on the physiologic processes that control the invasion of pathogens.

Physiologic Correlations

The intact skin and mucous membranes provide a widespread anatomic barrier to environmental pathogens. Microorganisms that enter the body orifices can be destroyed by the natural protective mechanisms of those open tracts.

Barriers to Pathogens

The hydrochloric acid and the proteolytic enzymes in the stomach kill all but the most resistant organisms. The mycobacteria (i.e., *Mycobacterium tuberculosis*) have thick cell walls that allow their survival. The organisms that survive gastric destruction and traverse the intestinal wall are exposed to enzymatic destruction by proteins (i.e., properdin) and globulins (i.e., complement) in the circulation.

The organisms that enter the respiratory passages are exposed to destruction by the lysosomes of the mucus. Bacterial debris or surviving bacteria remain trapped in the mucus and gradually move toward the oral exit as the cilia sweep them upward. Only those organisms less than 2 microns in size can traverse the narrow branchings of the terminal bronchi. The organisms that are small enough to reach the lung tissues are exposed to the alveolar macrophages that readily ingest foreign matter.

Subclinical Infection

The body maintains a state of physiologic readiness to abort an invasion by pathogens. Subclinical infection probably occurs frequently, its progress being halted by the activity of the leukocytes. The white blood cells are maintained at the level of 5000 to 10,000/cu mm in the circulation. The total leukocyte count represents a percent distribution of the *neutrophils, eosinophils,* and *basophils,* which are produced primarily by the bone marrow, and the *lymphocytes* and *monocytes,* which are produced in the lymphatic tissues of the lymph nodes, tonsils, spleen, thymus, and mucosa of the intestine (Fig. 16–1).

Subclinical infections involve a local tissue response and a response by the white blood cells that phagocytize the bacteria. The initial granulocyte activity may proceed without overt evidence of the pathogen invasion within the host tissues. Lymphatic drainage from the site may remove the surviving bacteria and deliver them to the lymph node tissue where they are destroyed. The swelling of lymph nodes near the surface

(i.e., submaxillary nodes) may be the initial or the only evidence of the pathogen presence.

Physiologic Defense Mechanisms

The normal physiologic response to an invasion by numerous virulent microorganisms represents an attempt to isolate or destroy the pathogens. The *histocytes* in the tissues that are sensitized by the invading bacteria are transformed into *mast cells* that engulf the organisms. The simultaneous release of *leukocytosis-promoting factor* and *necrosin* from the sensitized tissues elicits the responses of the initial defense against infection (Fig. 16–2).

Rupture of the mast cells releases the vaso-active substance that cause an elevation of the capilliary pressure and a subsequent release of fluid, protein, histamine, and the irritating substance *bradykinin* into the tissues. The activity of necrosin is additive to the capillary effects of the vasoactive substances. Necrosin also acts co-jointly with fibrinogen to clot the fluid in the sensitized tissues. That action isolates the area and prevents the movement of pathogens and fluid from the attack site. The elevated osmolality of the sensitized tissues also causes the movement of fluid from the cells and capillaries, and the tissues gradually become swollen.

The leukocytosis-promoting factor travels with the blood to the bone marrow. Neutrophils that are liberated from the marrow stores rapidly travel to the sensitized tissue to phagocytize the invading bacteria. The neutrophils move the

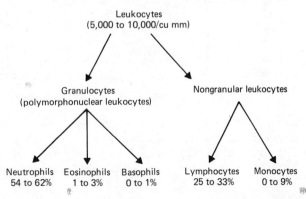

Fig. 16–1. The total number of leukocytes represents a percent distribution of granulocytes and nongranular leukocytes.

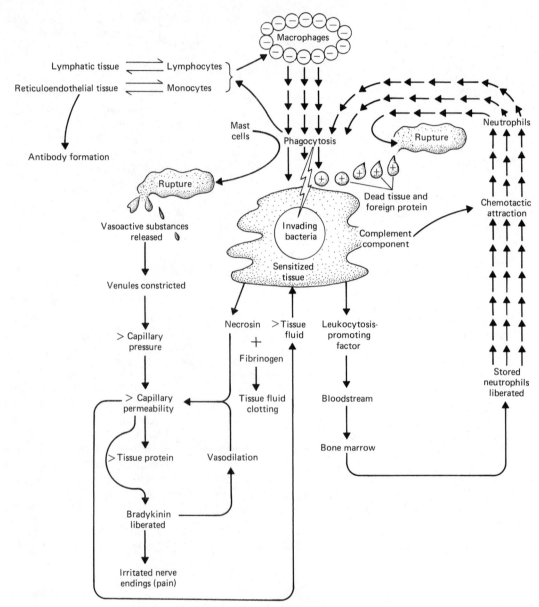

Fig. 16–2. Physiologic responses to bacterial invasion.

bacteria into their vacuoles where they are destroyed by enzymes and hydrogen peroxide. The distention of the neutrophils by the ingested bacterial debris causes their cell membranes to rupture, and they spew dead tissue and foreign protein into the tissues. The debris provides the electropositive chemotactic force that attracts the lymphocytes and monocytes to the site.

The macrophage activity of the lymphocytes and monocytes is a slower process than that of the neutrophils, but they have a larger capacity for ingestion of bacteria and protein products from the area. Bactericidal enzymes within the macrophages destroy most of the bacteria. At the completion of their activity at the tissue sites, the lymphocytes return to the tissues of their origin. Some of the material contained in the lymphocytes provides the memory pattern for the formation of antibodies in the reticulendothelial tissues subsequent to the pathogen invasion period.

Pathophysiologic Correlations

The individual characteristics of microorganisms influence the effectiveness of the physiologic mechanisms for the control of infection. Reproductive processes of the pathogens are the same as those of normal body cells. They follow the same *deoxyribonucleic acid* (DNA)–directed, *ribonucleic acid* (RNA) synthesis of proteins for cellular structures and enzymes. One of the most important structures synthesized by the enzymes of bacteria is the cell membrane.

Bacterial Cell Membrane

The interwoven strands of the thick cell wall are constructed from the intermediates *polysaccharides* or *glycopeptides*. The final bacterial cell wall is a three-dimensional, tightly cross-linked structure consisting of an inner layer of *mucopeptides,* a middle layer of *polysaccharides,* and an outer layer of *peptidoglycan strands*. The intracellular content is maintained at an osmolality level higher than that of the body fluids, and the cell wall forms an impermeable barrier against the entry of fluids from the surrounding environment. The cell wall actively transports supplies to the cytoplasm and controls the inward and outward movement of nutrients.

Bacterial Biologic Characteristics

The site of the invasion and the characteristics of the microorganism determine the course of the infection. The following descriptions of pathogen characteristics are examples of the factors affecting their virulence and invasiveness:

1. *Staphylococci* can reproduce in an aerobic or an anaerobic environment. The pathogens liberate a cellular toxin that accelerates the release of necrosin, and the infected area more rapidly is walled off from the surrounding tissues. Staphylococcal invasion can cause pockets of infection at widely separated sites in the body tissues.

2. The cell walls of some *streptococci* and *pneumococci* contain antigenic proteins and they also secrete *hyaluronic acid*. Those biologic products increase the pathogens' virulence by inhibiting phagocytosis by the white blood cells. The hyaluronic acid also increases the permeability of surrounding tissues and allows the pathogens to travel as they increase in number.

3. The *exotoxins* of *streptococci* and the *endotoxins* of the gram-negative organisms are cytotoxic and they enhance the invasiveness of the pathogens.

Infection in Body Tissues

Staphylococcus infections are common in the bladder, blood, eyes, intestines, lungs, meninges, skin, mucous membranes, and subcutaneous tissues. The other pathogens that cause infections in the major body systems include

Bladder: *Enterobacter, Escherichia coli, Klebsiella, Proteus, Pseudomonas aeruginosa.*

Blood: *Escherichia, Haemophilus, Pneumococcus, Pseudomonas aeruginosa, Streptococcus.*

Ears: *Haemophilus, Pneumococcus, Streptococcus.*

Eyes: *Pseudomonas, Streptococcus.*
Intestines: *Bacteroides, Enterobacter, Escherichia coli, Klebsiella, Proteus, Salmonella, Shigella.*
Lungs: *Escherichia, Haemophilus, Klebsiella, Mycoplasma, Pneumococcus, Pseudomonas aeruginosa, Streptococcus.*
Meninges: *Escherichia, Haemophilus, Klebsiella, Meningococcus, Mycobacterium, Pneumococcus.*

Host Responses

In addition to the characteristics of the pathogens and their prime sites for growth and multiplication when they become entrenched in tissues, the condition of the host is an important variable in the progression of the infection. For example, anemic patients frequently have bladder infections, and the problem is thought to relate to the iron deficiency. In the individual with malnutrition the leukocytes are more slowly mobilized in response to stimuli during a pathogen invasion. In those patients there may be a direct relationship with the depletion of protein stores for the formation of leukocytes.

A minor infection may become a major problem when the defense mechanisms are impaired in the acutely ill or debilitated patient. The normal flora of body tissues may be transferred to sites that are not resistant to the organisms.

For example, burns or wounds may become contaminated with strains of *Enterobacter, Escherichia, Proteus,* or *Pseudomona* that are natural inhabitants of the intestine.

Infection is associated with a local response in the involved tissues that causes inflammation, swelling, pain, and disruption of normal tissue function. There are diverse problems related to the direct effect of the infection at particular tissue sites. The generalized responses are manifestations of the increased metabolic activity that is directly related to the precipitation of the defense mechanisms (i.e., elevated body temperature, acceleration of heart and respiratory rates, chills, malaise, weakness, fatigue).

Laboratory tests provide information about the extent of the infection. The elevation of the leukocyte count and the differential, or percent, distribution of the white blood cells vary during the phases of the infectious process. The initial phase of the infection is accompanied by a rise in the quantity of circulating neutrophils, and the subsequent activity of nongranular leukocytes raises the lymphocyte and monocyte levels of the blood samples.

The level of leukocytes remains consistently elevated while the defense mechanisms are active. When an infection persists for a protracted period of time, the levels of monocytes may remain elevated. There is some indication that lymphocytes can change characteristics and become monocytes when they travel in the circulating blood.

Anti-infective Drug Therapy

Drugs frequently are employed to control an infection, hasten recovery, and decrease the effect of the infection on the person's living patterns. The widespread use of anti-infective drugs has led to the emergence of some microorganism strains that are resistant to the drugs previously controlling their growth and reproduction. The problem is particularly prevalent in the hospital environment. The occurrence of a hospital acquired, or *nosocomial,* infection, which often is

resistant to the usual drugs, frequently lengthens the period of hospitalization and interferes with the recovery of the patient.

PATHOGEN SUSCEPTIBILITY

The anti-infective drug that is selected for control of an infection is chosen on the basis of the susceptibility of the pathogen. Samples of the fluids containing the organism are cultured and the growth is subjected to tests of drug susceptibility. The laboratory reports identify the rank order of the drugs that inhibit the growth of the pathogen. After the susceptibility of the organism is identified, the selection of a particular drug for the treatment is based on the clinical situation and the pharmacologic properties of the drug.

In acute or life-threatening situations, the drug therapy may be instituted immediately after the culture is obtained. There is some predictability in the pathogens that will grow in various body tissues, as was described earlier in the chapter. Interim therapy is based on the known drug susceptibility of the particular pathogens. The therapy may be modified when the results of susceptibility are available, but the patient has some protection against the devastating effects of the infection in the 48-hour interval before the final reports are obtained.

PATHOGEN RESISTANCE

The susceptibility cultures are an essential aspect of drug therapy because microorganism strains can develop resistance to drugs. The organisms that are most notorious for developing resistance to drugs are the gram-positive *Staphylococcus,* and the gram-negative *Enterococcus, Enterobacter, Klebsiella, Proteus, Pseudomonas,* and *Escherichia.*

One of the factors that causes the resistance of those organisms is the emergence of mutants as a result of frequent exposure of the organism to anti-infective drugs. The strain of *Staphylococcus* commonly described as *penicillinase producing* is able to enzymatically inactivate the natural penicillin and some semisynthetic forms of the drug. The problem of *Staphylococcus* resistance was identified several years ago when there was a widespread hospital inpatient problem with penicillin-resistant *Staphylococcus* infections. There is increasing evidence that the same penicillinase-producing strains now are emerging as resistant organisms in the community. Although alternate drugs can be employed for treatment (i.e., semisynthetic penicillinase-resistant penicillins, erythromycin), the cost to the

patient is considerably higher when those drugs are used.

The resistance of many gram-negative pathogens has recently been described as a transfer of genetic determinants of resistance (R factor). The offending organisms acquire genetic material called *R factors* that mediate the drug resistance. The *R factors* can be transferred from one pathogen to another of the same species or to one or more organisms of a different species. The transfer confers resistance to pathogens previously susceptible to the action of a drug. For example, the semisynthetic penicillin *ampicillin* has been employed universally for the treatment of children with *Haemophilus influenzae meningitis* for several years, but there is an increasing incidence of ampicillin-resistant organisms in many European countries. The problem is somewhat insidious and gradually emerges when a drug is utilized specifically for the control of an organism. The first report of the ampicillin resistance occurred in 1972, but it only recently has become a fairly common problem in several countries.

DRUG ACTION

Antibacterial Spectrum

The terms *broad spectrum* and *narrow spectrum* are employed to describe the range of activity of drugs in the control of pathogens. Those drugs capable of limiting the growth and reproduction of a wide variety of organisms are described as broad-spectrum drugs and those drugs with a high degree of specificity for only a few drugs are described as having a narrow spectrum of activity.

Bacteriostatic Activity

The primary barrier to pathogen eradication is the thick cell wall of the organisms. The vulnerable phases of cell division are the principal targets for eradication of the pathogens during drug therapy. The mechanisms of action of the anti-infective drugs can be categorized as *blocking the synthesis of DNA, inhibiting protein synthesis, inducing defective protein synthesis, interfering with cell wall construction,* or *interfering with the permeability of the cell membrane.*

All of the anti-infective drugs are bacteriostatic agents. Those drugs that cause irreparable damage to the cell by interfering with its growth and reproduction are idenitfied as *bactericidal* drugs. For example, the induction of defective protein synthesis that is caused by some drugs (i.e., the aminoglycosides) prevents the intracellular production of enzymes and inhibits the metabolic processes of the cell. The penicillins interfere with cell wall construction, and that action allows leaking of the intracellular contents and the consequent death of the organism (Fig. 16–3). The bactericidal drugs may be bacteriostatic at low dosage levels that disrupt cell building without destroying the pathogen.

Drugs that block DNA synthesis, inhibit protein synthesis, or interfere with the permeability of the cell membrane can limit the cellular development and halt the progression of the infection.

That process allows the natural defense mechanisms to participate in the destruction of the pathogens.

An important aspect of therapy with bacteriostatic drugs is the continuance of therapy for a period adequate for elimination of the organisms. Early interruption of therapy can allow the emergence of mutant strains that are resistant to subsequent therapy. The patient who is being treated for an infection must be informed of the rationale for continuing uninterrupted therapy to the planned end point of that therapy because many persons discontinue taking the drugs when the overt symptoms subside. There are many infections with indeterminate end points, but the prescribed course of penicillin therapy for a streptococcal pharyngeal infection or treatment for uncomplicated urinary tract infections is continued for a period of ten days. The end point of many infections may be defined as the occurrence of two negative organism cultures.

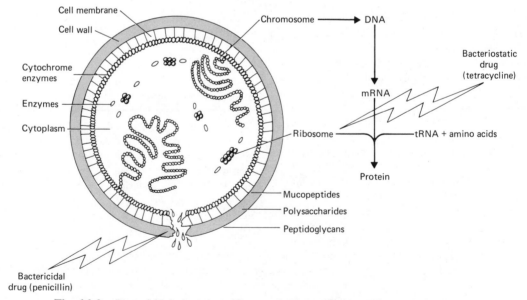

Fig. 16–3. Bactericidal drugs can disrupt the interdigiting of the mucopeptides, polysaccharides, and peptidoglycans that are required for bacterial cell wall construction. The subsequent leaking of the cytoplasmic content destroys the pathogen. Bacteriostatic drugs can interfere with protein building during the reproduction cycle of the bacterium.

Antibiotics

The term *antibiotic* describes the product of an organism that is utilized to destroy another organism. The term is also employed to describe the semisynthetic or synthetic drugs that have a chemical structure based on that of the original natural drug from which they are derived.

The antibiotics are classified in pharmacologic groups that have similar clinical applications and properties that influence patient care plans during therapy. The individual drugs within each group have some similarities and differences that are considered when the drugs are employed for infection control. The groups of antibiotics include the *penicillins, cephalosporins, erythromycins* (and drugs with a similar action), *tetracyclines, polymyxins, aminoglycosides, chloromycetin,* and *miscellaneous antibiotics.*

DRUG THERAPY

There are numerous antibiotic drugs and their availability makes it possible to control some of the most resistant, persistent, or life-threatening infections. Although susceptibility testing is essential to assure the selection of the drug that predictably will be effective, there are drugs that have proven dependable for the control of selected important pathogens (Table 16–1). The

Table 16–1.

Drugs Employed for Control of Selected Important Pathogens

| Pathogen | Antibiotic Drug Therapy | |
	Primary Drug	Alternate Drug
Gram-positive pathogens		
Staphylococcus aureus	Penicillin G	Cephalosporins, clindamycin, or vancomycin
Staphylococcus aureus (penicillinase producing)	Cloxacillin, methicillin, nafcillin, or oxacillin	Cephalosporins, clindamycin, or vancomycin
Streptococcus (Diplococcus) pneumoniae	Penicillin G	Cephalosporins, chloramphenicol, or erythromycins
Streptococcus pyogenes	Penicillin G	Erythromycins
Gram-negative pathogens		
Escherichia coli	Gentamicin with penicillin G or ampicillin	Ampicillin, carbenicillin, cephalosporins, chloramphenicol, kanamycin, tetracyclines, or tobramycin
Haemophilus influenzae	Amoxicillin or ampicillin	Tetracyclines
Klebsiella pneumoniae	Gentamicin (may be given with cepholosporins)	Cephalosporins, chloramphenicol, kanamycin, tetracyclines, or tobramycin
Neisseria gonorrhoeae	Penicillin G	Ampicillin, chloramphenicol, spectinomycin, or tetracyclines
Proteus mirabilis and others	Ampicillin or gentamicin	Amoxicillin and tobramycin, cephalosporins, chloramphenicol, gentamicin, kanamycin, tetracyclines, or tobramycin
Pseudomonas aeruginosa and others	Carbenicillin or gentamicin	Polymyxins, tobramycin, or gentamicin
Shigella	Ampicillin	Chloramphenicol

choice between a primary drug and an alternate drug is influenced by the circumstances in the clinical situation. One of the most important factors is the patient's history of an allergic reaction to a drug. For example, when the patient has a *Staphylococcus aureus* infection and a history of an allergic response (i.e., rash) to penicillin, the alternate drugs (cephalosporins, clindamycin, vancomycin) may be employed for therapy. The decision to use a particular alternate drug will depend on the results of the organism susceptibility tests.

Suprainfection

Antibiotic drug therapy may change the balance in the normal microbial relationships within the body and allow dominance of an organism that usually is suppressed by other organisms in the tissues. The suppressing, or controlling, organisms may be absent as a result of their susceptibility to the drug being employed for control of a pathogen.

The suprainfection may also represent the growth of an organism that is derived from the environment. Those infections usually are *Candida albicans* infections in the mouth, anus, or vagina that appear following antibiotic therapy at high dosage or for prolonged periods of time.

The respiratory and intestinal tracts are the most common sites of suprainfections. The dominance of the organisms in the intestine (i.e., *Bacteroides,* coliform bacilli) may cause black hairy tongue, diarrhea, abdominal cramps, and pruritus in the anal region. The infection in the respiratory tract may cause pneumonia or thick, yellowish mucus that is difficult to remove by coughing or suction. The infection may not be evident until the precipitating antibiotic therapy has been terminated. Treatment of suprainfections usually involves measures to relieve the symptoms and to control the pathogen involved in the suprainfection.

PENICILLINS

The natural penicillins and the semisynthetic derivatives each have the same basic *6-aminopeni-cillanic acid* chemical structure that is composed of a *thiazolidine ring* and a *beta-lactam ring*. The derivatives of penicillin are synthesized by the addition of various side chains.

Penicillin G and *penicillin V* are the natural penicillins. Their spectrum of activity is limited to the control of gram-positive organisms and *Neisseria*. They are ineffective in the control of the penicillinase-producing strains of *Staphylococcus aureus*. The semisynthetic penicillins that share that limitation are *amoxicillin, ampicillin, carbenicillin, hetacillin, phenethicillin,* and *ticarcillin*. Those semisynthetic penicillins are more effective than the natural penicillins in controlling some of the important gram-negative pathogens (i.e., *Haemophilus influenzae, Escherichia coli, Proteus mirabilis*).

The semisynthetic penicillins that are effective in the control of penicillinase-producing *Staphylococcus aureus* are *cloxacillin, dicloxacillin, methicillin, nafcillin,* and *oxacillin*. Those penicillin derivatives, like the natural penicillins, have no significant activity against gram-negative organisms.

Action Mode

The concentration of penicillin at the site of infected tissues determines whether the drug will be bacteriostatic or bactericidal in action. The penicillins interfere with the enzymatic activity required for cell wall synthesis during the time that the pathogens are dividing. The inhibition of the enzyme *transpeptidase* prevents the cross-linking of the outer layer of peptidoglycan strands of the cell wall. That action causes a defect in the structure that can allow the intracellular content to leak outward. The loss of integrity lessens the hyperosmolality of the cellular fluid, which normally is maintained at a level roughly equivalent to a 10 to 20 percent glucose concentration.

Therapy Considerations

Penicillin therapy may be instituted after the collection of a specimen of the organism in acutely ill patients, but the results of the pathogen susceptibility are particularly important during therapy. There is evidence that *R factor* has transferred the resistance of previously susceptible pathogens (i.e., *Enterobacteria*) to some of the semisynthetic penicillins.

The penicillins may be administered by the oral or parenteral route. Some of the oral forms are unstable in the gastric acid, and food in the stomach may adsorb some of the drug. Because the quantity of the drug that is absorbed from the duodenum varies, the dosages are adjusted to allow for those differences (Table 16–2).

The absorbed drug is widely distributed in body fluids and tissues. Its ability to enter collections of blood or purulent fluids is an important advantage in the eradication of bacteria. The highest concentrations of the drug are found in the lungs, intestines, liver, and skin. The drugs pass into inflamed synovial fluids and attain drug concentrations similar to those of the serum. The passage of the drugs into the cerebral spinal fluid is also increased when the tissues are inflamed, and the drug concentrations may rise to a level that is 30 to 65 percent of the serum levels with some forms of penicillin (i.e., ampicillin). The small amount of the drug that crosses the normal blood-brain

barrier is actively transported out of the cerebrospinal fluid. The drug crosses the placental barrier, and small amounts appear in the saliva and in the milk of nursing mothers.

The protein binding of the penicillins varies (Table 16–2). The drug readily dissociates from the protein binding when serum or tissue drug levels are reduced. The serum half-life of each of the penicillins is lower than that of most other drugs. Renal tubular secretion readily moves the unchanged drug toward the urine excretion route. Some of the drug is metabolized in the liver and the degradation products are excreted with the bile.

The short elimination half-lives of the penicillins necessitate closely scheduled times for administration. The addition of procaine to penicillin G aqueous suspension slows the absorption rate from the intramuscular tissues, and the serum drug levels are maintained for a 24-hour period. The penicillin G procaine formulation in oil with aluminum stearate produces therapeutic serum levels for 72 to 96 hours, and the penicillin G benzathine formulation provides two-to-three-week drug levels. Serum drug levels that are attained with the formulations are lower than those

Table 16–2,
Penicillin: Selected Dose-Response Factors

Drug	Usual Adult Oral Dosage	Effect of Food on Absorption	Plasma Protein Binding (%)	Serum Half-Life (Minutes)
Penicillin G, potassium	0.6–3 million u	↓	65	30
Amoxicillin	250–500 mg q8h	—	17	60
Ampicillin	250–500 mg q6h	↓	23	50 to 110
Carbenicillin indanyl sodium	382–764 mg q6h	—	50	60
Cloxacillin sodium	500 mg–1 gm q6h	↓	95	30
Dicloxacillin sodium	125–250 mg q6h	↓	96–98	40
Hetacillin	225–450 mg q4h	↓	20 to 25	50 to 110
Methicillin sodium	Parenteral only	—	35 to 40	30
Nafcillin sodium	500 mg–1 gm q6h	↓	90	60
Oxacillin sodium	500 mg–1 gm q6h	↓	94	30
Phenethicillin potassium	125–250 mg q6h	—	75 to 80	30
Ticarcillin disodium	Parenteral only	—	60–65	70
Penicillin V	125–500 mg q6h	↓	79	30

↓ = Decreased absorption, drug administered one hour before or two hours after meals.
— = Absorption unaffected.

required for intensive therapy, but the prolonged therapy they provide is effective for the control of susceptible pathogens in many ambulatory patients.

Allergic Reactions

History taking is particularly important during antibiotic therapy. Any previous drug allergy or recurrent allergic responses to other substances are important in the planning of the drug therapy.

The principal allergic responses during penicillin therapy are an immediate anaphylactic reaction, which can be fatal, and a delayed serum sickness reaction that is associated with rash, urticaria, fever, and pain and swelling of the joints. The allergic responses are estimated to occur in approximately 5 percent of the patients receiving the drug, and anaphylaxis occurs in 0.04 percent of those persons.

The anaphylactic reactions, which involve laryngeal edema and circulatory failure, occur more frequently with parenteral administration of penicillin but they can occur when the drug is administered orally. Equipment for cardiopulmonary emergency treatment should always be on hand when penicillin is administered parenterally.

The primary allergens are the degradation products *penicilloic acid* and *penicilloyl* compounds, which may form haptens with body proteins to produce the devastating allergic reaction. The *penicilloyl polylysine* (PPL) product is considered to be the major determinant of the allergic responses, and it has been employed by intradermal injection for sensitivity testing in selected situations when the patient has a history of an allergic response. The test is employed only when penicillin is the most effective drug for eradication of a life-threatening pathogen (i.e., beta-hemolytic streptococcal endocarditis).

The penicillins have produced blood dyscrasias that are considered to be hypersensitivity, or allergic, reactions. The responses include thrombocytopenia, thrombocytopenic purpura, eosinophilia, leukopenia, and agranulocytosis. The hematologic problems are reversible when drug therapy is terminated.

Adverse Effects

The gastrointestinal irritation of oral forms of penicillin can cause nausea, vomiting, or epigastric distress. The other problems that occur (i.e., diarrhea, black hairy tongue) are related to supra-infections.

Intramuscular injections of the penicillins cause pain at the injection site, and there have been sterile abscesses. Deep injections into the gluteal muscle may cause painful sciatic nerve irritation with paralysis of the extremity. Intravenous therapy can cause phlebitis and thrombophlebitis.

The elevated serum drug levels that can occur when there is poor renal function can cause convulsions. The central nervous system toxicity is thought to occur as a consequence of drug interference with the inhibitory function of the neurotransmitter *gamma-aminobutyric acid*.

Interactions

Probenecid competes with penicillin for renal tubular sites for secretion. Concurrent administration slows the excretion rate of penicillin and prolongs the serum penicillin levels. The interaction is employed to therapeutic advantage. Administration of probenecid (i.e., 500 mg q6h) increases the antibiotic serum level up to 300 percent, and the serum half-life is elevated to more than three times the usual level (i.e., 100 minutes). The therapeutic plan is employed primarily when the pathogen is only moderately susceptible to penicillin (i.e., staphylococci and gonococci) and sustained high plasma concentrations are desired to assure effectiveness.

Phenylbutazone, indomethacin, aspirin, and sulfinpyrazone increase the half-life of penicillin by competing for the renal tubular transport mechanisms when the drugs are employed concurrently. Phenylbutazone also inhibits the hepatic penicillin-metabolizing enzymes. Both aspirin and sulfinpyrazone can displace penicillin from its serum protein-binding sites. That displacement becomes clinically significant when the drugs are used with penicillin forms that are more than 92 percent plasma protein bound.

Both penicillin G and ampicillin act synergistically with aminoglycoside antibiotics when they are administered concurrently. The cell wall defect caused by penicillin allows the entry of the aminoglycoside (i.e., streptomycin), which interferes with intracellular protein synthesis.

Parenteral solutions of penicillin, which are acid, can be inactivated by many antibiotics that are basic when they are admixed in the same solutions. Antacids (i.e., aluminum hydroxide gel) may delay the absorption of oral penicillins by adsorbing the drug.

Preparations Available

Penicillin G. The drug is commonly employed parenterally for the control of virulent pathogens. It is the primary antibiotic used for the control of the gram-positive organisms *Actinomyces israelii; Bacillus anthracis; Clostridium tetani; Streptococcus (Diplococcus) pneumoniae; Staphylococcus aureus* (nonpenicillinase producing); *Streptococcus, Enterococcus* group; *Streptococcus pyogenes;* and *Streptococcus viridans* group (with streptomycin) and of the gram-negative organisms *Neisseria gonorrhoeae; Neisseria meningitidis;* and *Treponema pallidum;* and of oropharyngeal strains of *Bacteroides.*

Approximately one third of the oral formulation is absorbed, and the dosage (Table 16–2) is adjusted to a level that is four to five times the parenteral dosage to provide a sufficient amount of the drug to attain the therapeutic serum level required for treatment. Peak serum drug levels are reached within one hour after oral administration. Children over 12 years of age receive the same oral dosage as that of adults. The daily dosage for children under 12 years of age is calculated on the basis of 25,000 to 90,000 units/kg of body weight, divided for administration three to six times per day, for the treatment of most infections.

Intravenous therapy may be a continuous infusion of the drug (i.e., 5,000 to 100,000 units/ hour) or it may be planned as intermittent therapy. The large dosages employed for intravenous administration may cause the urine tests for gly-

cosuria to show a false positive reaction when the cupric sulfate (Benedict's) solution is used. When the daily dosage levels reach the higher levels (i.e., 8 million units), cupric sulfate tablets (CLINITEST) or the glucose oxidase reagents (CLINISTIX, TES-TAPE) should be utilized for the urine tests. The potassium and sodium content of the penicillin solutions is also considered when the total daily intravenous electrolyte intake reaches high levels. For example, the oral sodium intake may be adjusted to allow for the increased infusion of that electrolyte.

Penicillin G sodium is available in solutions with and without buffers for parenteral infusion. *Penicillin G potassium* is available in capsules, tablets, or solutions for oral administration (GENE-CILLIN G-RECILLIN, K-CILLIN, SUGRACILLIN, PEN-TIDS, PFIZERPEN G), and it is also available in solutions for parenteral administration. *Penicillin G procaine* (CRYSTICILLIN, DIURNAL-PENICILLIN, DURACILLIN, PFIZERPEN, WYCILLIN) is available in solutions for intramuscular injection when a prolonged but lower serum drug level is desirable for pathogen control. *Penicillin G benzathine* (BI-CILLIN, PERMAPEN) is available as suspensions or tablets for oral use, and it is available in suspensions for deep intramuscular injection for prolonged (two to three weeks) control of infections susceptible to lower levels of penicillin.

Penicillin V. The drug is the primary antibiotic for the control of infection caused by *Streptococcus aureus* (nonpenicillinase producing), *Streptococcus (Diplococcus) pneumoniae,* and *Streptococcus pyogenes.* The dosage level for children over 12 years of age is the same as that for adults (Table 16–2). The dosage for younger children is calculated on the basis of 15 to 50 mg kg of body weight and that dosage is divided for administration three to six times a day. *Penicillin V* (PEN-VEE, V-CILLIN), *penicillin V benzathine* (PEN-VEE SUSPENSION), *penicillin V hydrabamine* (COMPOCILLIN-VK), and *penicillin V potassium* (LEDERCILLIN-VK, ROBICILLIN VK, VEE-TIDS) are available in capsules, solutions, suspensions, chewable wafers, or tablets for oral administration.

Amoxicillin (AMOXIL, LAROTID, POLYMOX). The semisynthetic drug has a spectrum of antibiotic activity similar to that of ampicillin. It may be the primary drug employed for the treatment of infections caused by *Haemophilus influenzae,* and it is also used as an alternate drug for infections caused by *Proteus mirabilis,* or *Salmonella.* The drug capsules and the suspension are administered orally, and the presence of food in the stomach seems to have no effect on absorption. Children weighing more than 20 kg receive the same dosage of amoxicillin as that given to adults (Table 16–2). Children weighing from 9 to 20 kg are given a dosage calculated on the basis of 20 to 40 mg/kg of body weight, and those weighing less than 8 kg are given 25 to 50 mg of amoxicillin at eight-hour intervals.

Ampicillin. Anhydrous ampicillin (OMNIPEN, PENBRITIN) and the *ampicillin trihydrate* (ALPEN, AMCILL, POLYCILLIN, PRINCIPEN) are available as capsules, suspensions, and tablets for oral administration. Ampicillin trihydrate is also available in solution for intramuscular administration. *Ampicillin sodium* (AMCILL-S, ALPEN-N, OMNIPEN-N, POLYCILLIN-N, PRINCIPEN/N) is available in vials of solution for administration by intramuscular or slow intravenous injection or by intravenous infusion.

Ampicillin has a broad spectrum of antibiotic activity, and it may be the primary drug employed for treatment of infections caused by *Eschericia coli, Haemophilus influenzae, Proteus mirabilis, Shigella,* and *Treponema pallidum.* It is also used as an alternate drug for the treatment of *Bordetella pertussis,* hospital-acquired *Escherichia coli, Neisseria gonorrhoeae, Salmonella,* and *Bacteroides* infections. The drug is also employed in combination with *streptomycin, kanamycin,* or *gentamicin* for the control of infections caused by the *Streptococcus* and *Enterococcus* groups, and it may be employed alone or in combination with streptomycin for the control of infections caused by *Listeria monocytogenes.*

The recommended oral dosages are the same for adults and for children weighing more than 20 kg (Table 16–2). That dosage range also is em-

ployed for the parenteral administration of ampicillin sodium. The parenteral dosage for adults with severe infection (i.e., septicemia) may be calculated on the basis of 150 to 200 mg/kg of body weight. The parenteral dosage for children under 20 kg in weight is calculated on the basis of 50 to 200 mg/kg. The dosage may be divided and administered every six or eight hours.

Carbenicillin. Carbenicillin disodium (GEOPEN, PYOPEN) is administered by intramuscular or intravenous injection or by intravenous infusion. *Carbenicillin indanyl sodium* (GEOCILLIN) is available as tablets for oral administration. The nausea and unpleasant aftertaste caused by the drug have, in a few instances, caused extreme discomfort for the patients and the drug therapy was discontinued.

Although serum drug levels are low with the use of *carbenicillin,* the drug attains a high concentration in the urine. It is particularly useful for treatment of *Pseudomona aeruginosa* infections in the urinary tract. The drug is also employed as an alternate therapeutic agent for infections caused by *Enterobacter aerogenes* or hospital-acquired *Escherichia coli.* It is used in conjunction with *tobramycin* for infections caused by *Proteus.*

There is a wide range in the parenteral dosage of carbenicillin, and the level administered is directly related to the severity and location of the infection being treated. The adult parenteral dosage is based on the calculation of 400 to 500 mg/kg/day to a maximum dosage of 40 gm/day. The parenteral dosage for pediatric patients ranges from 50 to 500 mg/kg/day, and the drug may be administered by slow intravenous infusion.

Cloxacillin (TEGOPEN, CLOXAPEN). The drug is primarily used for the control of infections caused by penicillinase-producing *Staphylococcus aureus.* It is available in capsules and solution for oral administration. The dosage for children weighing 20 kg or more is the same as the adult dosage (Table 16–2). Children weighing less than 20 kg may receive a dosage based on the calculation of 50 to 100 mg/kg of body weight and that dosage is divided for administration at six-hour intervals. Daytime doses should be given one to two hours before meals.

Dicloxacillin (DYANPEN, PATHOCIL, VERACILLIN). The drug is employed primarily for the control of infections caused by penicillinase-producing *Staphylococcus aureus*. The oral dosage for children weighing 40 kg or more is the same as the adult dosage (Table 16–2). Those children and adults may receive dicloxacillin intramuscularly at a dosage range of 250 to 500 mg every six hours. Children weighing less than 40 kg are given a daily oral dosage based on the calculation of 25 mg/kg of body weight or daily intramuscular dosages based on 25 to 50 mg/kg of body weight. The dosage is divided for administration at six-hour intervals.

Hetacillin. Hetacillin (VERSAPEN) and *potassium hetacillin* (VERSAPEN-K) are rapidly hydrolyzed to ampicillin and share the same antibiotic activity and dosages as ampicillin (Table 16–2). Hetacillin is available as a suspension or chewable tablets for oral administration; potassium hetacillin is available in capsules administered orally or as solutions for intramuscular or slow intravenous injection.

Methicillin Sodium (CELBENIN, STAPHCILLIN, AZAPEN). The drug is employed for the control of severe infections caused by penicillinase-producing *Staphylococcus aureus*. The usual daily intramuscular dosage range for adults is 4 to 6 gm, which may be divided for administration at four-to-six-hour intervals. The daily dosage for infants and children is based on the calculation of 25 mg/kg of body weight, which may be divided for administration at six-hour intervals.

The usual adult intravenous dosage is 1 to 2 gm. The drug may be infused at a rate of 10 ml/minute, or it may be administered at four-to-six-hour intervals. In severe infections the adult intravenous dosage may be as high as 12 gm daily.

Nafcillin Sodium (UNIPEN). The drug is employed primarily for the control of severe infections caused by penicillinase-producing *Staphylococcus aureus*. Because the drug is irregularly absorbed from the duodenum, another semisynthetic penicillin may be employed when oral drug therapy is indicated.

The adult dosage for intramuscular injection is 500 mg every six hours, which may be given at four-hour intervals when the infection is severe. The pediatric dosage is calculated on the basis of 25 mg/kg of body weight, injected intramuscularly twice each day. The daily dosage for neonates is based on 20 mg/kg of body weight, which may be divided for administration two times a day. The usual adult intravenous dose is 500 mg to 1 gm every four hours, and the drug may be given as a slow injection over a five- or ten-minute period.

Oxacillin Sodium (BACTOCILL, PROSTAPHLIN). The drug is employed primarily for the control of severe infections caused by penicillinase-producing *Staphylococcus aureus*. There have been a few reports of hepatic dysfunction in patients receiving oxacillin sodium. The serum *glutamic oxaloacetic transaminase* (SGOT) levels were elevated and there were symptoms similar to those of viral hepatitis (fever, nausea, vomiting). The symptoms abated when drug therapy was discontinued.

Oxacillin sodium is available as capsules or suspensions for oral administration. Children who weigh 40 kg or more may receive the same dosage as that of adults (Table 16–2). Children weighing less than 40 kg may receive a daily dosage based on the calculation of 50 mg/kg of body weight, which may be divided for administration at six-hour intervals.

The parenteral dosage may be administered intramuscularly or as an intravenous injection that is infused over a five-or-ten-minute period. The parenteral dosage for children weighing more than 40 kg and for adults is 250 to 500 mg, administered every four to six hours. Children weighing less than 40 kg are given a daily dosage based on the calculation of 50 mg/kg of body weight, which may be divided and administered at four-to-six-hour intervals.

Phenethicillin Potassium (MAXIPEN, SYNCIL-LIN). The drug is a semisynthetic homolog of penicillin V, and it has an antibiotic spectrum of activity similar to that of both of the natural penicillins. Children over 12 years old are given the same oral dosage as adults (Table 16–2). Younger children may receive a daily dosage based on the calculation of 12.5 to 50 mg/kg of body weight, which may be divided for administration at four-to-eight-hour intervals.

Ticarcillin Disodium (TICAR). The antibiotic activity of ticarcillin is similar to that of carbenicillin disodium. Its primary use is for the treatment of infections caused by *Pseudomonas aeruginosa.* The drug is administered as a deep intramuscular injection, a well-diluted intravenous injection, or an intravenous infusion. The maximum dosage for each intramuscular injection is 2 gm, and *lidocaine hydrochloride* may be added to decrease the pain of the injection.

The parenteral dosage for children weighing over 40 kg and for adults is based on the calculation of 200 to 300 mg/kg/day, which is divided for injection every three to six hours. Children weighing less than 40 kg may receive a daily dosage based on 50 to 100 mg/kg of body weight.

CEPHALOSPORINS

The cephalosporins are semisynthetic antibiotics with a structure and pharmacologic actions similar to those of the penicillins. The basic structure of the cephalosporins is a *7-aminocephalosporanic acid.* Additions to the nucleus provide the various agents in the group of drugs.

Action Mode

The cephalosporins are bactericidal drugs, and they act in a manner similar to that of the penicillins to interfere with the synthesis of the cell wall during the period when the organisms are dividing. The drugs inhibit the activity of the enzyme *transpeptidase,* which is required for the *transpeptidization* necessary for the final cross-linking of the peptidoglycan strands of the outer cell wall.

Cephalosporins have a broad spectrum of activity and are effective against many gram-positive organisms and some gram-negative organisms. They are employed clinically primarily as alternate drugs for the control of infections caused by the gram-positive pathogens *Streptococcus* (*Diplococcus*) *pneumoniae;* nonpenicillinase-producing *Staphylococcus aureus;* and *Streptococcus viridans* group; and for the control of infections caused by the gram-negative pathogens *Escherichia coli* (hospital-acquired or community-acquired infections); *Klebsiella pneumoniae;* and *Proteus mirabilis.*

The cephalosporins differ in their resistance to the *cephalosporinase* that is produced by some gram-negative pathogens (i.e., *Escherichia coli, Enterobacter, Proteus, Pseudomonas*). Many of the enterococci strains that are resistant to the usual therapeutic levels of the cephalosporins attained in the serum are susceptible to the higher levels of the drug that accumulate in the urine.

Therapy Considerations

The absorption of *cephaloglycin* from the gastrointestinal tract is less than that of *cephalexin* and *cephradine,* but dosage adjustments provide adequate cephaloglycin levels (Table 16–3). The presence of food in the stomach delays absorption but does not affect the total quantity of the drug that enters the serum.

There is considerable variation in the serum protein binding of the drug that enters the serum. The circulating drug is widely distributed in body tissues and fluids. Unlike the penicillins, the drugs do not pass into the cerebral tissues when the meninges are inflamed. Cephalosporins cross the placenta. *Cephaloglycin, cephalothin,* and *cephapirin* are partially metabolized in the liver to metabolites that have less antibiotic activity than the parent compounds.

The drugs are excreted by glomerular filtration and renal tubule secretion. The primary mode of excretion of *cephalothin* and *cephapirin* is tubular secretion. Small amounts of the drug are secreted into the milk of nursing mothers.

Tests for glycosuria may show a false-positive

Table 16–3.
Cephalosporins: Selected Dose-Response Factors

| Drug | Route | Usual Daily Dosage Range | | Plasma Protein Binding (%) | Serum Half-Life (Minutes) |
		Adult (gm)	Child (mg/kg BW)		
Cefazolin sodium	IM/IV	0.75–2	25–50	60–86	69–132
Cephalexin	Oral	1–4	25–100	10–20	36–72
Cephaloglycin	Oral	1.5–3	25–50	0–30	>40
Cephaloridine	IM/IV	1.5–3	30–50	0–31	60–96
Cephalothin sodium	IM/IV	2–6	80–160	65–79	30–60
Cephapirin sodium	IM/IV	2–6	40–80	44–50	30
Cephradine	IM/IV	2–4	50–100	0–20	60–120
	Oral	1–2	25–100		

reaction during therapy with the cephalosporins when the cupric sulfate reagents (Benedict's, CLINITEST, or Fehling's solution) are used. The urine glucose tests can be performed by using the glucose oxidase reagents (CLINISTIX, TES-TAPE).

The irritating effects of the drugs on tissues causes phlebitis or thrombophlebitis when the drugs are injected intravenously. Those problems are somewhat lessened by adequate dilution of the drug and slowing of the injection to a rate that requires from three to five minutes to infuse the solution. The injection should be made with a small-gauge needle into the largest available vein. When the person has a running intravenous, injection of the drug into the tubing provides adequate dilution to lessen the irritation. Injection of the drug into the intramuscular tissues may cause pain and an induration that can progress to a sterile abscess or tissue necrosis.

Adverse Effects

Allergic reactions have occurred in 5 percent of the patients receiving the cephalosporins. Anaphylactic reactions have occurred rarely. The delayed reactions have included mild urticaria, pruritus, erythematous skin rashes, fever, and serum sickness. Persons who have a history of an allergic reaction during therapy with penicillin also may have a reaction to the cephalosporins. Although one of the cephalosporins may be given to a patient with a history of a delayed-type reaction to

penicillin, a previous penicillin-induced anaphylactic reaction is considered to be a contraindication to the use of the drugs.

Nephrotoxicity has occurred with the use of the cephalosporins, and the patient's renal status is evaluated throughout therapy. The evidence of the renal toxicity includes the presence of casts, red blood cells, or protein in the urine and a decrease in the quantity of the urine output. The decrease in renal tubular function causes an elevation of the blood urea nitrogen (BUN) and creatinine levels.

Gastrointestinal disturbances are relatively common during therapy with the cephalosporins and they can occur with oral or parenteral therapy. Oral therapy commonly causes nausea, vomiting, and diarrhea. The disturbances also include glossitis, dyspepsia, heartburn, and abdominal cramping. Some central nervous system depression (i.e., dizziness, headache, malaise, fatigue) has occurred with cephalosporin drug therapy.

Interactions

Probenecid blocks the renal tubule secretion of the cephalosporins by its competitive action at the tubule sites. The drug interaction has been employed to elevate and prolong the serum drug levels during therapy.

Concurrent administration of potent diuretics or drugs with a high nephrotoxic potential increases the incidence of toxicity during therapy with the cephalosporins. Although the risk is greater during therapy with cephaloridine, the concurrent use of the drugs with any of the cephalosporins usually is avoided.

Preparations Available

Cefazolin sodium (ANCEF, KEFZOL) is administered parenterally. The dosage is the same for the deep intramuscular injection and for the intravenous injection (Table 16–3). The schedule for adults and children is three or four times a day.

Cefadroxil monohydrate (DURICEF) capsules are employed at a dosage of 1 gm twice per day for treatment of adults with urinary tract infections caused by *E. coli, P. mirabilis,* or *Klebsiella.*

Cephalexin monohydrate (KEFLEX) is available as capsules, suspensions, and tablets for oral administration. The daily dosage (Table 16–3) is divided into four equal doses and administered four times a day.

Cephaloglycin (KAFOCIN) is available as capsules for oral administration. The dosage (Table 16–3) is adjusted to allow for the low gastrointestinal absorption (25 percent) of the drug. Cephaloglycin is rapidly metabolized to *desacetylcephaloglycin,* which has approximately one half the antibacterial activity of the parent drug against gram-positive organisms and less antibiotic effect on gram-negative organisms. Up to 98 percent of the activity of the drug in the serum and urine is related to the action of the metabolite. Cephaloglycin produces a high incidence of severe, persistent diarrhea, and it has caused gastrointestinal bleeding and severe enterocolitis that necessitated discontinuation of therapy. Other oral cephalosporins are more frequently employed for the treatment of urinary tract infections.

Cephaloridine (LORIDINE) is administered parenterally (Table 16–3). The daily dosage of the drug usually is divided and administered two to four times a day. The drug causes a higher incidence of nephrotoxicity than the other cephalosporins and acute tubular necrosis has occurred. The nephrotoxicity occurs less frequently when administered as a maximum level of 4 gm/day.

Cephalothin sodium (KEFLIN) is usually administered intravenously because the large doses of the drug are very irritating to the tissues. Approximately 20 to 40 percent of the drug is metabolized to *desacetylcephalothin,* which has 20 to 25 percent of the antibiotic activity of the parent drug.

Cephapirin sodium (CEFADYL) is administered parenterally. In severe infections the drug may be administered in dosages as high as 12 gm/day. The total dosage (Table 16–3) usually is divided for administration four to six times a day. Cephapirin sodium is partially metabolized to *desacetylcephapirin,* which has 50 percent of the antibiotic activity of the parent drug.

Cephradine (ANSPOR, VELOSEF) is administered orally or parenterally, and the total daily dosage (Table 16–3) usually is divided for administration at four-to-six-hour intervals. The maximum daily dosage for adults is 8 gm/day and for children it is 4 gm/day.

ERYTHROMYCINS (AND SIMILAR DRUGS)

The *erythromycins* and *troleandomycin* are structurally similar drugs that are classified as *macrolide* antibiotics (Table 16–4). *Clindamycin* and *lincomycin* are structurally different but they have a similar mode of action and antibiotic spectrum of activity. The differing aspects of the drugs will follow the description of erythromycin.

Action Mode

The drugs interfere with the reproductive processes of pathogens by competing for receptor sites on the ribosomal units. That action disrupts the synthesis of intracellular proteins. The drugs generally are bacteriostatic, but at high dosage levels they may be bactericidal. Erythromycin readily penetrates the wall structure of dividing gram-positive organisms and those pathogens may contain up to 100 times more of the drug than that contained in the gram-negative microbes.

Erythromycin is considered to be the primary antibiotic for the control of infections caused by the gram-positive pathogen *Corynebacterium*

Table 16–4.

Dosage Ranges of Macrolide and Similar Antibiotics

Drug	Route	Daily Dosage Range		Number of Divided Doses
		Adult (gm)	Child (mg/kg BW)	
Erythromycin *(E-MYCIN, ERYTHROMYCIN, ILOTYCIN, ROBIMYCIN)	Oral	1–4	30–100	4
Erythromycin estolate* (ILOSONE)	Oral	1–4	10–20	4
Erythromycin ethylsuccinate*	Oral	1.6–6.4	48–160	4
(EES 400, PEDIAMYCIN)	IM	0.3–0.6	3–12	3–6
Erythromycin gluceptate*	IV	2–4	15–20	4
(ILOTYCIN GLUCEPTATE)				
Erythromycin lactobionate*	IV	2–4	15–20	4
(ERYTHROCIN LACTOBIONATE)				
Erythromycin stearate*	Oral	1–4	30–100	2–4
(BRISTAMYCIN, ERYPAB, ETHRIL, PFIZER-E)				
Clindamycin hydrochloride (CLEOCIN)	Oral	0.6–1.8	8–20	4
Clindamycin palmitate hydrochloride	Oral	0.6–1.8	8–25	3–4
Clindamycin phosphate	IM/IV	0.6–2.7	15–40	2–4
Lincomycin hydrochloride	Oral	1.5–2	30–60	3–4
(LINCOCIN)	IM	0.6–1.2	10–20	1–2
	IV	1.2–3	10–20	2–3
Troleandomycin (TAO)	Oral	1–2	6.6–11	4

* Macrolide antibiotics.

diphtheriae and the gram-negative pathogen *Bordetella pertussis*. It is also used as an alternate to penicillin G in the treatment of syphilis. It is considered to be an alternate drug for the control of gram-positive infections caused by *Bacillus anthracis; Clostridium perfringens (welchii); Streptococcus (Diplococcus) pneumoniae; Streptococcus pyogenes;* and *Listeria monocytogenes;* and it is used with streptomycin in the control of infections caused by *Streptococcus viridans.*

Therapy Considerations

The gastric acids may inactivate some of the oral drug, and several oral formulations are buffered or coated to prevent their destruction in the acids. The absorption of the drugs occurs in the duodenum. Approximately 18 percent of the absorbed drug is bound to serum proteins. The amount of the drug bound may be 73 percent for some formulations (i.e., erythromycin base).

The elimination half-life of the drug ranges from one to three hours, and the dosage usually is administered at regular six-hour intervals to maintain the antibacterial serum levels of the drug. The absorbed drug is widely distributed in body tissues and fluids with the exception of the cerebrospinal fluids. Most tissues have concentrations of the drug that are higher than those of the serum. The drug crosses the placental barrier.

One of the distinct advantages of the drug is that it is metabolized in the liver, and the drug and its metabolites are excreted with the bile. That property makes the drug useful for persons with compromised renal function. Some reabsorption from the bile occurs during enterohepatic recycling, and small amounts of the drug are excreted in the urine. The drug is also excreted in the milk of nursing mothers.

The parenteral solutions are very irritating to the veins and may cause phlebitis or thrombophlebitis. Well-diluted solutions can be injected slowly (over 20 to 60 minutes) into a large vein, or the solution may be injected into the tubing of a running intravenous solution.

There is a local anesthetic in the erythromycin ethylsuccinate for intramuscular administration. The additive modifies the discomfort, but patients complain of pain at the injection site and sterile abscesses and necrosis can occur.

Erythromycin is also available as a rectal suppository. The drug causes local irritation, burning, and mild hyperemia, and it may cause irregularities in the bowel movements.

Adverse Effects

The most frequent adverse effects are minor gastrointestinal irritations; the problems occur more frequently at high dosage levels. Stimulation of the smooth muscle by the drug induces hypermotility of the intestines, which may cause diarrhea and abdominal cramping. Other problems include nausea and vomiting, and occasionally there may be stomatitis, heartburn, anorexia, melena, or pruritus in the anal region.

Mild allergic reactions may occur during therapy with the erythromycins. Anaphylaxis has occurred rarely. Hepatotoxicity occurs in adults during prolonged (one to two weeks +) therapy with *erythromycin estolate*. The problem is thought to be a hypersensitivity to the particular formulation rather than to the erythromycin. The toxicity is manifested as a reversible cholestatic hepatitis that is preceded by abdominal cramping, nausea, and vomiting. Discontinuance of the drug therapy may provide some relief, but several weeks may be required for the symptoms to subside.

Clindamycin Hydrochloride

The drug is a semisynthetic derivative of lincomycin. *Clindamycin palmitate hydrochloride* and *clindamycin phosphate* (Table 16–4) are inactive until they are hydrolyzed to the base, and that metabolic effect occurs rapidly after the drugs are absorbed. Clindamycin has the same inhibitory action on the bacterial synthesis of proteins as the erythromycins, and its spectrum of antibiotic ac-

tivity is also similar. It is employed as a primary drug for the treatment of infections caused by *Bacteroides* in the gastrointestinal tract and as an alternate drug in the treatment of infections caused by nonpenicillinase-producing *Staphylococcus aureus* and anaerobic *Streptococcus*.

Therapy Considerations. The drug is well absorbed from all administration routes. It is 94 percent bound to serum proteins. The drug is widely distributed in body tissues and fluids, with the exception of cerebrospinal fluid. It crosses the placental barrier. The drug is metabolized in the liver, and two of the metabolites, *clindamycin sulfoxide* and N-*dimethylclindamycin*, have antibiotic activity. The drug and metabolites are excreted in the urine, bile, and feces. The secretion of the drug in the saliva causes an unpleasant or bitter taste in the mouth.

The intramuscular injections are painful and the drug can cause induration or sterile abscesses. Deep injection into the muscle minimizes the problems. The irritating effects of the drug may cause thrombophlebitis, erythema, pain, and localized swelling.

Adverse Effects. Gastrointestinal disturbances (i.e., abdominal pain, diarrhea, anorexia, nausea, vomiting, melena, flatulence) may be severe enough to necessitate cessation of the drug therapy. Diarrhea may persist for several days after therapy is terminated, and there have been many reports of pseudomembranous colitis directly related to the effects of the drug.

Anaphylactic reactions rarely occur, but there may be a skin rash or urticaria. There are fewer adverse effects with clindamycin than with lincomycin therapy.

Lincomycin Hydrochloride

The drug has a mode of action and spectrum of antibacterial activity similar to those of the erythromycins. The drug is available in formulations for oral, intramuscular, or intravenous administration (Table 16–4).

Therapy Considerations. The absorbed drug is loosely bound to serum proteins (72 percent). The drug is widely distributed in body tissues and fluids. It crosses the placental barrier. The elimination half-life is 4.6 to 5.6 hours. The drug or its active metabolite is excreted in the urine, bile, breast milk, and feces.

Adverse Effects. The major problem is a severe and persistent diarrhea, which may be accompanied by blood and mucus in the stools. The problem occurs frequently and necessitates termination of the drug therapy. It occurs more commonly when the drug is administered orally, but it can occur with parenteral drug administration. Other problems indicative of gastrointestinal irritation include nausea, vomiting, abdominal cramps, heartburn, and glossitis.

Allergic responses occur in only a small number of patients. The reactions may include skin rash, dermatitis, urticaria, pruritus, or serum sickness. Anaphylaxis may also occur.

Troleandomycin

The mode of action of the drug is similar to that of the erythromycins, and the spectrum of antibacterial activity includes the same gram-positive organisms. The drug is employed primarily for the control of severe infections caused by susceptible staphylococci, streptococci, or pneumococci that are resistant to less toxic drugs.

Adverse Effects. The major adverse effect is an allergic type of hepatotoxicity. The effects on the hepatic tissues appear after a period of two weeks of therapy, and that limits the use of the drug for the control of the severe infections, which tend to persist or require treatment for periods of six weeks or more. The effects on the hepatic tissues include both cholestatic and hepatocellular changes. Drug therapy is usually restricted to a period of ten days to reduce the risk of liver damage, and therapy is terminated when any symptoms of hepatotoxicity appear.

The drugs may cause nausea, vomiting, or diarrhea. Anaphylactic reactions are rare, but there may be varying skin rashes as manifestations of an allergic reaction.

TETRACYCLINES

Chlortetracycline, demeclocycline, and *oxytetracycline* are natural antibiotics, and *doxycycline, methacycline, minocycline,* and *tetracycline* are semisynthetic antibiotics. There are differences in their clinical effectiveness, but the drugs have the same action mode, antibiotic spectrum, and pharmacologic properties.

Action Mode

The tetracyclines have a bacteriostatic action and a broad spectrum of antibacterial activity. They interfere with the growth of pathogens by binding to the ribosomes and interfering with the synthesis of intracellular proteins.

The drugs are employed clinically for the control of infections caused by the gram-positive *Bacillus anthracis, Clostridium perfringens* (*welchii*), *Clostridium tetani,* and *Listeria monocytogenes* and the gram-negative *Enterobacter, Escherichia coli* (hospital or community acquired), *Neiserria gonorrhoeae, Haemophilus influenzae, Klebsiella pneumoniae, Proteus, Treponema pallidum,* and *Bacteroides* (oropharyngeal and gastrointestinal strains). The tetracyclines may also be employed alone or with *streptomycin* in the control of infections caused by the gram-negative *Brucella.*

Therapy Considerations

The tetracyclines are well absorbed from the gastrointestinal tract. The drugs are administered one hour before or two hours after meals to avoid the interference of food with absorption. The absorption of the drugs is also delayed by the presence of milk, iron, or sodium bicarbonate, or by antacids containing aluminum, calcium, or magnesium. Withholding the antacid until one hour after the administration of the tetracycline improves absorption. Gastric disturbances (i.e., nausea, dyspepsia) occasionally are severe enough to necessitate administration of the drug with milk or a snack.

Effective serum drug levels are attained within one to two hours after administration of the oral preparations and those levels are maintained for six hours. The parenteral drug is rapidly absorbed and the peak serum levels may be maintained for 12 hours.

The drugs differ in their plasma protein-binding capacity (Table 16–5). Those drugs with a high binding level also have longer serum half-lives. The drugs are widely distributed in body tissues and fluids. The highest concentrations appear in the bone marrow, spleen, lymph nodes, liver, lungs, and kidneys. Minocycline may pass the blood-brain barrier, and each of the drugs crosses the placental barrier.

There is little metabolism of the tetracyclines. The drugs are concentrated in the liver and excreted primarily in the bile. Some of the unchanged drug is excreted in the urine. The drug is also secreted in the milk of nursing mothers.

Tetracyclines may produce a false positive result when the urine is tested for glucose content using a cupric sulfate reagent (Benedict's Qualitative Reagent, CLINITEST). The false positive result may be due to the ascorbic acid in the parenteral tetracyclines rather than a problem related to the testing method.

Adverse Effects

Suprainfections of the gastrointestinal and urinary tract are quite frequent and they can be severe. Although the infections in the intestines can represent growth of fungi or yeast, they frequently are caused by *Staphylococcus aureus*. The occurrence of *staphylococcal enterocolitis* necessitates cessation of therapy with the drug and prompt treatment of the infection. Suprainfections of the urinary tract usually are caused by *Staphylococcus*, *Proteus*, or *Pseudomonas*.

The gastric disturbances that occur during therapy include anorexia, epigastric distress, nau-

Table 16–5.

Tetracyclines: Selected Dose-Response Factors

Drug	Route	Daily Dosage Levels		Plasma Protein Binding (%)	Average Serum Half-Life (hr)
		Adult (gm)	Child (mg/kg BW)		
Chlortetracycline hydrochloride (AUREOMYCIN)	Oral	1–2	25–50	45–70	5.6
	IV	0.5–2	10–20		
Demeclocycline hydrochloride (DECLOMYCIN)	Oral	0.6	7.5–15	40–90	12.3
Doxycycline hyclate (VIBRAMYCIN)	Oral	0.1–0.3	2.5–5	25–93	17.8
	IV	0.1–0.2	2.5–5		
Methacycline hydrochloride (RONDOMYCIN)	Oral	0.6–1.2	7.5–15	80–90	14.3
Minocycline hydrochloride (MINOCIN)	Oral	0.1–0.2	2–4	70–76	14.8
	IV	0.2–0.4	2–4		
Oxytetracycline hydrochloride (TERRABON, TERRAMYCIN)	Oral	1–2	25–50	20–35	9.6
	IM	0.25–0.8	15–25		
	IV	0.5–2	10–20		
Tetracycline hydrochloride (ACHROMYCIN V, PANMYCIN, ROBITET, SK-TETRACYCLINE, SUMYCIN, TETRACYN, TETREX-S)	Oral	1–2	25–50	25–65	8.5
	IM	0.25–0.8	15–25		
	IV	0.5–2	10–20		

sea, vomiting, bulky loose stools, and diarrhea. There have been reported instances of an increase in the intracranial pressure in infants that caused a bulging of the fontanels.

There is cross-sensitivity to the tetracyclines, and patients having an allergic response to one of the drugs probably will be allergic to all of the drugs in the group. Although an anaphylactic reaction can occur during therapy with the tetracyclines, the allergic reactions more frequently are delayed reactions, which include skin rashes, urticaria, dermatitis, and angioedema. Photosensitivity occurs most frequently with *demeclocycline* and to a lesser extent with *chlortetracycline*, *oxytetracycline*, or *tetracycline*. The photosensitivity reaction may cause pigmentation of the skin, nails, and dermal folds. Patients receiving the drugs should be cautioned against exposure to intense ultraviolet light sources or sunlight.

The tetracyclines are deposited with calcium in the bones and teeth during their calcification. Administration of the drugs to pregnant women after the fourth month of gestation may allow the drug to be deposited in the deciduous teeth and bones of the fetus. The drugs also cause permanent discoloration, enamel defects, and dental caries in children receiving the drug before they are eight years old.

Rapid intravenous administration or high drug dosage has been associated with a high incidence of nausea, vomiting, chills, fever, and hypotention. The drug is very irritating to the veins and causes a high incidence of phlebitis. The drug solution for intramuscular administration has a local anesthetic additive. The formulation reduces the severe pain of the injection, but the drug must be injected deep into the muscle to avoid damage to the tissues.

Long-term therapy can cause hematologic changes that are manifested as leukocytosis, thrombocytopenic purpura, neutropenia, and abnormalities in the granulocytes or lymphocytes. An increase in ascorbic acid excretion and a decrease in the content of that vitamin in the leukocytes of elderly patients suggest that the drug may have an adverse effect on the vitamin status in the elderly.

Preparations Available

Chlortetracycline hydrochloride (Table 16–5) is infrequently employed for therapy since other tetracyclines that are more effective have been developed. The drug is available as capsules for oral administration and as a sterile solution for intravenous therapy.

Demeclocycline is available as an oral suspension. *Demeclocycline hydrochloride* is available as capsules and film-coated tablets for oral administration (Table 16–5).

Doxycycline hyclate is available as capsules for oral administration and as solutions for intravenous administration. *Doxycycline monohydrate* is available as a suspension for oral administration (Table 16–5).

Methacycline hydrochloride is available as capsules and as a suspension for oral administration (Table 16–5).

Minocycline hydrochloride is available as capsules, as tablets, and as a syrup for oral administration. It is also available as a solution for intravenous injection (Table 16–5).

Oxytetracycline, oxytetracycline hydrochloride, and *calcium oxytetracycline* are available as suspensions for oral administration. Oxytetracycline and oxytetracycline hydrochloride are also available in capsules for oral administration or as solutions for parenteral injection (Table 16–5).

Tetracycline is available as capsules and suspensions, *tetracycline hydrochloride* as capsules and tablets, and *tetracycline phosphate complex* as capsules for oral use. Tetracycline hydrochloride and tetracycline phosphate complex are also available in solutions for parenteral administration (Table 16–5). Tetracycline hydrochloride (TOPICYCLINE) powder, with a special diluent, is available for topical application in the treatment of acne vulgaris.

POLYMYXINS

Polymyxin B sulfate, colistimethate sodium, and *colistin sulfate* are the natural antibiotic representatives of the polymyxin group. The drugs are bactericidal agents that are utilized primarily for their effectiveness in the control of infections caused by *Pseudomonas aeruginosa* in the urinary tract and other body sites.

Action Mode

The drugs bind with the phospholipids of the bacterial cell membrane. That action produces a detergent-like effect that decreases the natural impermeability of the membrane. Leaking of the intracellular fluid changes the osmolality of the cell content and leads to the death of the pathogen.

Polymyxins are utilized for the control of infections caused by *Enterobacter aerogenes*, *Escherichia coli*, *Haemophilus influenzae*, *Klebsiella pneumoniae*, and *Pseudomonas aeruginosa*. Polymyxin B commonly is used prophylactically with neomycin as a bladder irrigant for patients with indwelling catheters.

Polymyxin B Sulfate (AEROSPORIN)

Therapy Considerations. The drug is administered by intramuscular and intrathecal injection and intravenous infusion. It is also used as an inhalant, irrigant (bladder), or ocular antibiotic. The intramuscular dosage of the drug for adults and children is based on the calculation of 25,000 to 30,000 units/kg of body weight. The drug is highly irritating to the muscle tissues; so the intravenous route is more commonly employed. The calculation for intravenous infusion is based on 215 mg/kg/day, which is given in one or two equally divided doses.

The absorbed drug is readily distributed in body tissues. Serum protein binding is low, but 50 percent of the drug does bind reversibly with phospholipids of the cell membranes in the liver, kidneys, heart, muscle, and brain. The serum half-life ranges from 4.3 to 6 hours and most of the unchanged drug (60 percent) is excreted in the urine.

Adverse Effects. The frequent occurrence of nephrotoxicity and neurotoxicity has limited the use of the drug. The manifestations of the nephro-

toxicity include diminished urine output, elevation of the blood urea nitrogen and creatinine levels, and the appearance of red and white blood cells, casts, or albumin in the urine. The neurotoxicity can cause a neuromuscular blockade that is difficult to reverse. Transient neurologic problems include ataxia, blurred vision, flushing of the face, circumoral paresthesias, slurred speech, numbness of the extremities, and mental confusion. Drug therapy is terminated when symptoms appear. Serum creatinine levels may remain elevated or become higher for one to two weeks after the therapy is discontinued.

Interactions. The neuromuscular blocking properties of other drugs (i.e., tubocurarine) may be potentiated by polymyxin B. Concurrent administration of other drugs that produce nephrotoxic effects increases the incidence and severity of renal damage.

Colistimethate Sodium and Colistin Sulfate

Therapy Considerations. Colistimethate sodium (COLY-MYCIN) is administered by intramuscular or intravenous injection and *colistin sulfate* is given orally. The daily intramuscular and intravenous dosage for adults and children is based on the calculation of 2.5 to 5 mg/kg of body weight. The daily dosage usually is divided and administered in two to four doses. The intravenous solution is injected slowly over a three-to-five-minute period or it may be given as an infusion.

The daily oral dosage of colistin sulfate for infants and children is based on 5 to 15 mg/kg of body weight and is divided for administration three times a day. The oral drug is used primarily for the treatment of acute bacterial diarrheas in infants and children. The drug is poorly absorbed from the intestine, and its intraluminal retention and concentration are the rationale for use of the oral drug.

Adverse Effects. The nephrotoxicity and neurotoxicity caused by polymyxin B also occur with colistimethate sodium. The drug therapy is discontinued at the earliest evidence of the problems. Febrile reactions, gastrointestinal disturbances, or skin rashes may occur with colistimethate sodium therapy. The low absorption rate of colistine limits the incidence of adverse effects during therapy.

AMINOGLYCOSIDE ANTIBIOTICS

The aminoglycoside antibiotics include *amikacin sulfate, gentamicin sulfate, kanamycin sulfate, neomycin sulfate, paromomycin, spectinomycin dihydrochloride, streptomycin sulfate,* and *tobramycin sulfate* (Table 16–6). The classification *aminoglycoside* describes the common chemical structure of the drugs. The antibiotics have a similar mode of action, antibiotic spectrum of activity, and toxic effects.

Action Mode

The aminoglycosides have a bactericidal effect that results from their disruption of protein synthesis by the organism. Their interference with ribosomes in the reproduction processes causes the synthesis of defective nonfunctional proteins.

The drugs are employed for the control of serious systemic infections caused by gram-negative pathogens. They are also used to treat urinary tract infections.

Adverse Effects

The aminoglycosides produce a high incidence of *ototoxicity* and *nephrotoxicity*. The drug dosage, frequency of administration, duration of therapy, and renal status of the individual all affect the incidence of toxicity.

Ototoxicity. The neurotoxic effects of the drugs affect the function of the *auditory branch* and *vestibular branch* of the *eighth cranial nerve*. Vestibular nerve damage usually is preceded by severe headache, nausea, vomiting, and vertigo. Damage to the auditory branch causes loss of the ability to hear high-frequency sounds. The nerve damage may occur several days after therapy is instituted or it may appear several months after therapy is terminated.

Audiometric studies are usually planned during therapy to allow early identification of the nerve injury. The patient may not be aware of the hearing loss, but any indication from the patient that there is a loss of equilibrium, ringing in the ears (tinnitus), dizziness, or vertigo should be discussed with the physician promptly. The drug dos-

Table 16–6.

Aminoglycoside Antibiotics

Drug	Route	Daily Dosage Adult	Child (mg/kg BW)	Number of Divided Doses
Amikacin sulfate (AMIKIN)	IM/IV	15 mg/kg	10–15	2–3
Gentamicin sulfate (GARAMYCIN)	IM/IV	3–5 mg/kg	6–7.5	3
Kanamycin sulfate (KANTREX)	Oral	8–12 gm	50	4
	IM/IV	15 mg/kg	15	
Neomycin sulfate (MYCIFRADIN)	Oral	3–12 gm	50–100	4
	IM	0.6–1 gm	—	2–4
Paromomycin (HUMATIN)	Oral	4 gm	25–35	4
Spectinomycin dihydrochloride (TROBICIN)	IM	2–4 gm	—	—
Streptomycin sulfate (STRYCIN)	IM	2–4 gm	10–40	2–4
Tobramycin sulfate (NEBCIN)	IM/IV	3–5 mg/kg	3	3

age is reduced when the therapy is essential to the life of the patient or drug therapy may be discontinued. Vestibular nerve damage usually is reversible when therapy is terminated but symptoms may continue for a year or more. Loss of hearing may be permanent when the nerve damage is extensive.

The problems occur less frequently in well-hydrated patients with adequate renal function. Previous or concurrent therapy with drugs that have an ototoxic potential (i.e., furosemide, ethacrynic acid) increases the incidence of the eighth cranial nerve damage. Drug dosage levels usually are reduced for individuals with a creatinine clearance level lower than 70 ml/minute/1.73 M^2 of body surface area. The reduced dosage decreases the hazard of ototoxicity due to cumulative serum drug levels.

Nephrotoxicity. The irritating effects of the drugs can damage the renal tubules. Nephrotoxic effects are seldom serious but they can cause retention of nitrogenous breakdown products. The blood urea nitrogen (BUN) and creatinine levels may be elevated and those levels usually are evaluated frequently during therapy. Increasing the fluid intake and alkalinizing the urine may minimize the tubule irritation.

Amikacin

The drug is a semisynthetic derivative of kanamycin. It is employed for the control of infections caused by the gram-negative organisms *Acinetobacter, Enterobacter, Escherichia coli, Klebsiella, Proteus, Providencia, Pseudomonas,* and *Serratia.* It may also be employed with carbenicillin in the treatment of infections caused by *Pseudomonas aeruginosa.* Because the drug is relatively new, there are fewer pathogen strains that are resistant to amikacin than to the other aminoglycosides. The therapeutic considerations, dosage (Table 16–6), and adverse effects of the drug are identical to those of kanamycin sulfate. Amikacin is used primarily for the control of pathogens that are resistant to other aminoglycosides.

Gentamicin Sulfate

The drug is the primary agent employed for the control of infections caused by *Acinetobacter, Enterobacter aerogenes, Proteus, Pseudomonas,* and *Serratia.* It is frequently used with penicillin G or ampicillin in the control of *Streptococcus, Enterococcus* group, and hospital-acquired *Escherichia coli* infections. It is a primary drug for the control of infections caused by *Klebsiella pneumoniae* and may be used in combination with cephalosporins for those infections. It is also considered to be an alternate drug for the control of infections caused by *Proteus mirabilis* and *Pseudomonas aeruginosa.*

Therapy Considerations. Gentamicin sulfate is rapidly absorbed after intramuscular administration and peak serum levels are attained within 30 to 90 minutes. The therapeutic blood levels range from 5 to 7 mcg/ml, and the dosage (Table 16–6) may be adjusted to maintain that range. Approximately 20 to 30 percent of the circulating drug is bound to plasma proteins. The serum half-life is 2.3 hours. The drug is usually administered at six- or eight-hour intervals to provide a relatively consistent antibacterial activity. The serum antibiotic levels are diminished by the seventh hour after administration of the drug.

The circulating drug is widely distributed in body tissues and fluids and it crosses the placental barrier. When the meninges are inflamed, the drug crosses the blood-brain barrier and the cerebrospinal fluid drug levels may be two thirds those of the plasma. The unchanged drug is excreted in the urine by glomerular filtration.

Adverse Effects. Gentamicin sulfate more frequently causes vestibular nerve damage than auditory nerve damage, and it may cause complete loss of vestibular function. Nephrotoxicity also occurs, and evaluation of the blood urea nitrogen and creatinine levels and of the quantity and constituents of the urine is a routine aspect of the therapy plan. Signs of impaired renal function are evaluated carefully, and the drug dosage is often adjusted downward to lessen the hazard of toxicity.

Other evidence of neural toxicity includes the occurrence of numbness, skin tingling, or peripheral paresthesias. There have also been infrequent reports of gastrointestinal problems (i.e., nausea, vomiting, diarrhea, decreased appetite), anemia, and a depressed production of leukocytes.

Kanamycin Sulfate

The drug is considered to be an alternate drug for the control of infections caused by *Enterobacter aerogenes,* community- or hospital-acquired *Escherichia coli, Klebsiella pneumoniae, Serratia, Proteus mirabilis,* and other *Proteus* strains. It is also used with penicillin G or ampicillin for infections caused by the gram-positive *Streptococcus, Enterococcus* group.

Therapy Considerations. Kanamycin sulfate is employed orally for the treatment of intestinal infections (Table 16–6). It is also used to diminish the bacterial flora prior to intestinal surgery. The drug is poorly absorbed from the intestinal tract.

The intramuscular drug may cause pain and nodule formation at the injection site. The drug is rapidly absorbed and peak serum levels are attained within an hour. The serum half-life is three hours. The drug is administered at six-hour intervals to maintain the antibiotic levels, which are low by the sixth to eighth hour. Approximately 90 percent of the unchanged drug is excreted in the urine by glomerular filtration.

Adverse Effects. Damage to the auditory branch of the eighth cranial nerve is somewhat more frequent than the toxic effects on the vestibular branch. The high serum drug levels that occur with renal dysfunction can cause permanent damage to these nerves. The dosage maximum (15 mg/kg BW) is planned to lessen the nerve toxicity.

Nephrotoxicity is also a major problem during therapy with kanamycin sulfate. The problem may

be limited to mild renal tubule irritation with the appearance of casts, albumin, or red blood cells in the urine. Drug therapy may be continued when there is no further evidence of impaired renal function. Therapy is terminated when the blood urea nitrogen (BUN) and creatinine levels are elevated sufficiently to indicate tubular necrosis. The return of renal tubule function is slow when nephrotoxicity has occurred.

The parenterally administered drug may produce gastrointestinal problems (i.e., nausea, vomiting, abdominal distress, diarrhea), headache, fever, general weakness, or paresthesias. Suprainfections are side effects of the orally administered drug.

Neomycin Sulfate

The drug is employed primarily as an oral agent for the control of intestinal infections caused by *Escherichia coli.* Some strains of the organism are resistant to the drug, and therapy usually is instituted after stool cultures and pathogen susceptibility results are obtained.

The drug is also used for intestinal antisepsis prior to surgery. It is administered orally or as a retention enema to destroy the nitrogen-fixing bacteria when the patient's blood ammonia levels are elevated (i.e., liver disease). The drug is also used as a bladder irrigant and as a prophylactic agent at the insertion sites of catheters.

Therapy Considerations. Approximately 3 percent of the orally administered drug is absorbed from the intact intestine. Higher levels of the drug (10 percent) may be absorbed from the intestines of neonates or from the hypomobile or diseased intestine (i.e., colitis, ulceration). Absorbed drug may produce the same toxic effects as the other aminoglycosides. One of the reasons that parenteral administration of the drug has become obsolete is the high incidence of neuromuscular blockade caused by the systemic drug.

Adverse Effects. The oral drug may cause nausea, vomiting, and diarrhea. The increased intestinal motility may decrease the absorption of nutrients or vitamins and may increase the fecal elimination of bile and electrolytes. The short-term therapy that usually is planned (i.e., three to six days) prevents excess physiologic disruption from the intestinal losses of essential nutrients and fluids. Suprainfections representing the overgrowth of the natural intestinal microorganisms can occur with prolonged oral drug therapy. The effect of the decreased absorption of vitamin K on the coagulation processes is evaluated when oral therapy must be continued for more than a few days.

Paromomycin

The drug is employed primarily for the control of intestinal infections caused by *Escherichia coli*. Like neomycin, it is also used to decrease the bacterial flora prior to intestinal surgery or for the control of the nitrogen-fixing bacteria when the patient has elevated blood ammonia levels. It is also effective in the control of *Entamoeba histolytica*.

Adverse Effects. The major adverse effect is diarrhea. The usual six-day course of oral drug therapy (Table 16–6) usually limits the effects of the drug on electrolyte, nutrient, or fluid requirements.

Spectinomycin Dihydrochloride

The drug is employed primarily for the control of gonorrhea when the organism (*Neisseria gonorrhoeae*) is resistant to penicillin G. The therapy consists of a single injection of the drug. The lower dosage (Table 16–6) produces bactericidal concentrations in the serum within one hour, and that level is maintained for eight hours. The unchanged drug and its active metabolite are excreted in the urine.

The single-dose therapy limits the incidence of adverse effects common to the aminoglycosides. A decrease in the quantity of urine output, dizziness, nausea, fever, urticaria, or insomnia may occur.

Streptomycin Sulfate

The drug is employed with other antibiotics for the control of severe infections. It is used with penicillin G or ampicillin for control of the *Streptococcus, Enterococcus* group; with penicillin G or erythromycin for control of the *Streptococcus viridans* group; and with tetracycline or chloramphenicol for control of *Brucella* infections. The combination therapy delays the onset of resistance, which decreases the effectiveness of streptomycin when it is used alone. The resistance of most organisms occurs in two to five days and that of the *Mycobacterium tuberculosis* occurs in four to six weeks.

Therapy Considerations. The intramuscular drug (Table 16–6) is readily absorbed, and the peak serum drug levels that are attained in 30 minutes remain elevated up to 12 hours. Approximately 34 percent of the drug is bound to serum proteins. The serum half-life of streptomycin is 2.4 to 2.7 hours.

The drug is widely distributed in body tissues and fluids and it crosses the placental barrier. Highest concentrations of the drug are found in the ears and kidneys early in therapy, and the drug is slowly released from those depots. The drug penetrates tuberculosis cavities and caseous tissues. About 30 to 90 percent of the drug is excreted by glomerular filtration within 24 hours. Small quantities of the drug are excreted in the milk of nursing mothers, saliva, bile, sweat, and tears.

Pain and irritation occur at the intramuscular injection site. Alternating the sites and injecting the drug deeply into a large muscle reduces the discomfort for the patient. Contact with the drug during preparation of the injection can cause sensitization of the person handling the drug.

Streptomycin may cause a false positive urine glucose result when cupric sulfate reagents (Benedict's Reagent, CLINITEST) are utilized. The glucose oxidase reagents (CLINISTIX, TES-TAPE) can be used as an alternate method because they are unaffected by the drug.

Adverse Effects. Ototoxicity may occur four weeks after therapy is instituted. It is the most common and serious adverse effect. The incidence is higher when the drug is given for prolonged periods or at daily dosage levels in excess of 1.8 to 2 gm. Injury to the vestibular branch of the eighth cranial nerve is more common than injury to the auditory branch.

The neurotoxicity also may cause blurred vision or amblyopia associated with optic nerve toxicity; drowsiness or irritability associated with encephalopathy; and transient circumoral, facial, and peripheral paresthesias. Neuromuscular blockade also can occur, and it may affect the depth of respirations in debilitated patients.

Allergic reactions include skin rashes, fever, urticaria, pruritus, joint pains, and angioedema. Anaphylactic reactions occur rarely. Hematologic changes may include neutropenia, leukopenia, pancytopenia, or hemolytic anemia.

Nephrotoxicity occurs less frequently with streptomycin than with the other aminoglycosides. Hepatotoxicity may occur when the patient receives large doses of the drug. Other adverse effects include central nervous system depression (i.e., lassitude, lack of concentration, muscle weakness).

Tobramycin Sulfate

The drug is employed as an alternate drug for the control of infections caused by *Acinetobacter, Enterobacter aerogenes,* hospital-acquired *Escherichia coli, Klebsiella pneumoniae, Proteus mirabilis* and other species, and *Pseudonomas aeroginosa* and other species. Tobramycin sulfate is closely related to gentamicin sulfate and has a similar antibiotic spectrum and pharmacologic properties.

Therapy Considerations. The drug is readily absorbed from the intramuscular injection site, and peak serum levels (4 mcg/ml) are attained within 30 to 90 minutes. The serum levels persist for eight hours, and the administration schedule is planned to correlate with that time span (Table 16–6). The serum half-life of the drug is two hours.

The absorbed drug is widely distributed in body tissues and fluids and it crosses the placental barrier. The unchanged drug is excreted in the urine by glomerular filtration; the urine has high antibiotic levels for three to six hours after the drug is administered. Approximately 84 percent of the drug is excreted within the first eight hours, and urine levels of the drug remain elevated for that time period.

The drug is irritating to the tissues. Pain may occur at the intramuscular injection site and thrombophlebitis can occur at the intravenous injection site. The problems are decreased by injection of the drug deep into the muscles or the intravenous dose can be infused over a period of 30 to 60 minutes by injecting the drug into the tubing of a freely running intravenous setup.

Adverse Effects. The incidence of ototoxicity and nephrotoxicity during therapy with tobramycin is slightly lower than with gentamicin. The difference may reflect the more recent availability of tobramycin for therapy. Other adverse effects of the drug include hematologic changes (i.e., decreased hematocrit and hemoglobin levels, granulocytopenia, thrombocytopenia), nausea, vomiting, fatigue, lethargy, and headache.

CHLORAMPHENICOL

The drug is an effective broad-spectrum antibiotic, but it is reserved for treatment of serious infections because it is potentially highly toxic to the bone marrow. Susceptibility tests are employed as the basis for selecting the drug for therapy.

Action Mode

Chloramphenicol is a bacteriostatic drug. It acts primarily by interfering with the synthesis of protein in the pathogen. By substituting for the essential amino acid *phenylalanine* at ribosomal binding sites, it inhibits the development of the polypeptides in the reproducing organisms. A concurrent interference with the synthesis of proteins in the normal rapidly proliferating cells of the host can cause disruption of physiologic processes (i.e., bone marrow toxicity).

The drug is a primary agent for the control of acute serious infections caused by *Haemophilus influenzae* (i.e., meningitis) or *Salmonella*. It is used as an alternate drug for control of infections caused by *Acinobacter, Bacteroides, Brucella, Enterobacter, Escherichia coli, Francisella tularensis, Klebsiella pneumoniae, Neisseria gonorrhoeae, Proteus mirabilis* and other *Proteus, Salmonella, Serratia, Shigella,* and *Streptococcus (Diplococcus) pneumoniae.*

Therapy Considerations

Chloramphenicol (CHLOROMYCETIN, AMPHICOL, MYCHEL) may be administered orally or by intravenous injection at a daily dosage that is based on the calculation of 50 mg/kg for adults and children. The dosage initially may be double that level in meningeal infections. The dosage level for infants under two weeks of age is lower (i.e., 25 mg/kg of body weight) because the infants have poorly developed mechanisms for hepatic *glucuronide conjugation* and renal excretion. *Chloramphenicol palmitate* is the suspension that is administered orally and *chloramphenicol sodium succinate* is administered intravenously. The drug is administered at four regularly spaced intervals during the 24-hour period.

Chloramphenicol is well absorbed from the intestinal tract. The circulating drug is 25 to 60 percent bound to plasma proteins and has a serum half-life that ranges from 1.6 to 3.3 hours. The drug is widely distributed in body tissues and fluids, and the highest drug concentrations are in the liver and kidneys. The elevated serum drug concentrations that are attained with high dosage provide therapeutic cerebrospinal fluid drug concentrations. The drug crosses the placental barrier.

The drug is conjugated to the inactive metabolite by *glucuronyl transferase* in the liver, and the unchanged drug and its inactive metabolites are excreted in the urine by glomerular filtration or tubular secretion. Small amounts of the drug are secreted in the milk of nursing mothers and in the saliva and bile.

Adverse Effects

The most serious adverse effect of chloramphenicol is bone marrow depression. Although the problem occurs infrequently, it can be life threatening. There is a relationship between the incidence of the hematologic changes and the rapid rate of blood cell proliferation in children and premenopausal women.

The risk-to-benefit ratio is carefully assessed before therapy with the drug is instituted, and the serum drug concentrations and hematologic status are evaluated regularly (i.e., every two days) throughout the period of therapy. There is a reversible and irreversible type of bone marrow depression.

The more common reversible type can occur during short-term therapy. The bone marrow depression is characterized by vacuolization of the erythroid precursors, depressed production of reticulocytes, anemia, leukopenia, and thrombocytopenia. Blood cell production recovers when the drug therapy is terminated.

The more serious and irreversible type of bone marrow depression is characterized by aplastic or hypoplastic anemia. There may also be thrombocytopenia, granulocytopenia, or erythrocytopenia. The rare hematologic problem may occur as a delayed response several weeks after termination of therapy in susceptible patients.

Administration of chloramphenicol to premature infants or neonates less than two weeks old is individualized and closely supervised. The immature hepatic mechanisms for metabolic inactivation of the drug can cause toxic drug concentrations that can result in a fatal gray syndrome. The toxic reaction is characterized by abdominal distention, progressive pallid cyanosis, and acute circulatory collapse.

The bone marrow toxicity has made long-term therapy with chloramphenicol obsolete. There is almost always some decrease in red blood cell maturation during therapy with the drug. Other problems that can occur during short-term therapy include gastrointestinal disturbances (i.e., nausea, vomiting, diarrhea, unpleasant taste in the mouth, stomatitis), neurotoxic effects (i.e., headache, confusion), and allergic reactions (i.e., fever, skin rashes, angioedema, urticaria).

Interactions

The effect of chloramphenicol on the hepatic microsomal enzymes may decrease the metabolism of coumarin, tolbutamide, or phenytoin. The orally administered drug may reduce the number of intestinal bacteria that are required for the synthesis of vitamin K and that action may enhance the effects of oral anticoagulants.

MISCELLANEOUS ANTIBIOTICS

Vancomycin Hydrochloride (VANCOCIN)

The drug is a bactericidal antibiotic. It has a different chemical structure than most other antibiotics.

Action Mode. The drug interferes with the synthesis of the bacterial cell wall in a manner different from that of the penicillins. It binds to the wall to block the glycopeptide polymerization that is required for union of the peptidoglycan strands.

Vancomycin hydrochloride is employed as an alternate drug in the control of infections caused by *Staphylococcus aureus; Streptococcus viridans* group; and *Streptococcus, Enterococcus* group. Its antibiotic spectrum includes most of the gram-positive pathogens.

Therapy Considerations. Vancomycin may be utilized orally for the control of *Staphylococcus* enterocolitis. The adult dosage is 2 gm/day and the dosage for children is based on the calculation of 44 mg/kg of body weight. The total daily dosage usually is divided for administration four times a day. The orally administered drug is poorly absorbed from the intestine and there seldom is evidence of systemic effects.

The well-diluted intravenous solution may be infused over a period of 20 to 30 minutes. The dilution reduces the severe pain and the risk of thrombophlebitis, which are associated with the irritation of the drug. The daily intravenous dosage (1 gm) for adults usually is divided and administered two or four times a day. The daily intravenous dosage for children is based on the same calculation as the oral dosage (44 mg/kg of body weight) and that dosage may be divided for administration every six hours. There is usually a measurable therapeutic response within 48 to 72 hours after therapy is instituted.

Approximately 10 percent of the circulating drug is bound to plasma proteins. The serum half-life of the drug is six hours. Vancomycin is widely distributed in body tissues and fluids, and it crosses the placental barrier. Most of the unchanged drug is excreted in the urine by glomerular filtration.

Adverse Effects. Like the aminoglycosides, vancomycin hydrochloride causes ototoxicity and nephrotoxicity. The drug-induced damage to the auditory branch of the eighth cranial nerve can cause permanent deafness. The drug therapy usually is terminated when the patient complains of tinnitus, but there may be a progressive hearing loss after therapy is discontinued.

Allergic reactions occur in 10 percent of the patients receiving the drug. Anaphylaxis may occur and there can also be delayed allergic responses (i.e., fever, urticaria, skin rashes).

Bacitracin (BACIQUENT)

The drug inhibits bacterial cell wall synthesis in reproducing pathogens by preventing the transfer of the mucopeptide to the cell wall during its construction. Use of the drug systemically is obsolete but it is frequently utilized in ointments for the prevention or control of topical infections. The potential for nephrotoxicity and allergic reactions must be considered when superficial lesions allow absorption of the drug.

Novobiocin Calcium (ALBAMYCIN) and Novobiocin Sodium

The drug is occasionally employed for the control of gram-positive pathogens or *Proteus* and *Pseudomonas pseudomallei*. Up to 20 percent of the patients receiving the drug have adverse effects that represent allergic reactions, bone marrow depression, intrahepatic biliary obstruction, or pneumonitis. The high incidence of adverse effects has limited the use of the drug. It is used infrequently for the treatment of infections caused by pathogens resistant to other antibiotics.

Synthetic Antimicrobials

Many chemical preparations have some specificity for pathogens in particular organ sites. The drugs include the *sulfonamides, urinary tract–specific agents,* and *antimycobacterial drugs* that are employed for the control of tuberculosis or leprosy. The drugs may be utilized in varying combinations and may be used with antibiotics in the control of susceptible pathogens.

SULFONAMIDES

The sulfonamides are derivatives of sulfanilamide. Although the sulfonamides have a broad antibacterial spectrum and a long history of effective control of pathogens, many organisms have developed resistance. The drugs remain the agents of choice for the control of urinary tract infections, but newer anti-infective drugs have generally replaced the sulfonamides in the control of systemic infections. The similarities between the sulfonamides allow a general description of the group, and differences between the drugs are presented separately.

Action Mode

The drugs act as antimetabolites and block the synthesis of tetrahydrofolic acid from aminobenzoic acid. That action interferes with the bacterial synthesis of intracellular proteins. Many bacteria utilize preformed folic acid to build proteins, but those pathogens that synthesize the vitamin integrate the drug metabolite (Fig. 16–4).

The sulfonamides may be administered parenterally (i.e., sulfisoxazole) for control of *Actinomyces israelii* or *Haemophilus influenzae*. The high concentrations of the sulfonamides that are attained in the urinary tract make them the agents of choice for the control of pathogens in that tract. Their mode of action produces a bacteriostatic effect.

Therapy Considerations

The sulfonamides are administered orally, parenterally, or topically for the control of infections. The drugs included on Table 16–7 are administered orally for their systemic effects in the control

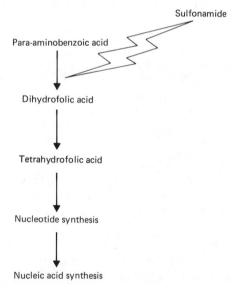

Fig. 16–4. Sulfonamides inhibit nucleic acid synthesis in bacteria by substituting for the aminobenzoic acid that is required for their protein synthesis.

Table 16–7.
Sulfonamide Drug Dosage

Drug	Adult Initial Maintenance (gm)		Child Initial Maintenance (mg/kg BW)		Number of Divided Doses	Peak Blood Level (hr)
Sulfachlorpyridazine (SONILYN)	2–4	2–4	75	150	3–6	2–4
Sulfacytine (RENOQUID)	0.5	1	—*	—*	4	2–3
Sulfadiazine (COCODIAZINE)	2–4	2–4	75	150	3–6	2–4
Sulfameter (SULLA)	1.5	0.5	—*	—*	1	4–8
Sulfamethizole (THIOSULFIL)		1.5–4		30–45	3–4	2–3
Sulfamethoxazole (GANTANOL)	2	2–3	50–60	50–75	2–3	4–8
Sulfamethoxypyridazine (MEDICEL)	1	0.5	30	15	1	4–8
Sulfapyridine		2		—*	4	4–8
Sulfisoxazole (GANTRISIN)	4	4–8	75	15	4–6	2–4

* Dosage not established.

of infections. The drugs are well absorbed from the small intestine (70 to 90 percent), and small amounts of the drug may be absorbed from the stomach. The rate of absorption varies between the sulfonamides. Those drugs with a more rapid absorption rate produce peak circulating drug concentrations within two to four hours. Intervals between administration generally are shorter for those drugs. The more slowly absorbed drugs often are given as a single daily dose or they may be given at 12-hour intervals.

An initial loading dose that is double the maintenance dosage may be given to raise the blood drug concentration to the desired therapeutic level (i.e., 12 to 15 mg/100 ml). The blood levels are evaluated frequently to assure maintenance of the therapeutic concentration. The absorbed drug is widely distributed in the body fluids and it appears in the glandular secretions (i.e., saliva, sweat, tears). The drugs readily cross the placental barrier.

The liver is the primary site of drug metabolism and some of the drug may be metabolized in other body tissues. Most of the sulfonamides are inactivated by acetylation and some are conjugated with glucuronic acid at hepatic sites. The N^4-*acetyl* metabolite is less soluble in acid urine than the unchanged drug or the conjugate. The daily fluid intake should be increased to an amount that is adequate to maintain a 24-hour urine output of 1500 ml during therapy with the sulfonamides. Alkalinization of the urine may also be planned to increase the solubility of the unchanged drug and its metabolites. This measure is important to prevent the accumulation of crystals during therapy. Raising the pH of the renal tubular fluids and the urine accelerates the drug excretion rate and increases the concentration of the drug in the urine while the blood levels of the drug are decreased. Monitoring of the quantity and the acidity of urine is an essential aspect of the drug therapy.

Adverse Effects

Many adverse effects can occur during therapy with the sulfonamides. The shorter-acting drugs are often preferred because their rapid elimination is an advantage when drug-related problems occur.

Allergic responses, which occur in approximately 5 percent of the patients taking the drugs, may include fever, maculopapular rashes, urticaria, pruritus, or joint pain. Prior use of a sulfonamide orally, parenterally, or topically may have sensitized the individual, and an allergic reaction can be precipitated when the drug is administered.

The appearance of a skin rash should be discussed immediately with the physician. Drug therapy is terminated when a rash appears during sulfonamide therapy because it is one of the forerunners of the Stevens-Johnson syndrome, which involves destructive lesions of the skin and mucous membranes. Other early indications are fever, severe headache, stomatitis, conjunctivitis, and rhinitis. The syndrome is fatal in approximately 25 percent of the individuals unless therapy is terminated at the presyndrome phase.

Gastric irritation frequently causes anorexia, nausea, and vomiting during therapy. The problems arise when the drugs are administered orally or parenterally and that is an indication that the drugs are also irritating to the medullary vomiting center. Administering the drug with food may decrease the gastric irritation. An antiemetic may be prescribed to allow continuation of therapy if the problems are persistent.

Depression of the central nervous system may cause headache, lethargy, dizziness, drowsiness, or ataxia. Blood dyscrasias occur infrequently with the usual maximum ten-day course of therapy, but they can include a decrease in the production of the granulocytes and platelets or hemolytic anemia in individuals with a *glucose-6-phosphate dehydrogenase (G-6-PD) deficiency*. The drugs can displace protein-bound bilirubin, and there have been reports of kernicterus and death in infants.

High concentrations of the drug metabolites in the nephrons may precipitate crystal formation that blocks or damages the tubules. The newer sulfonamides and the sulfonamide combinations have a greater solubility than the original formulations, and precipitation of crystals occurs less frequently with their use. When the urinalysis shows crystals, or red blood cells, alkalinization of the urine usually is planned. The alkalinization will produce an orange-yellow urine and may cause a similar discoloration of the skin. The primary preventive measure is to increase the intake of fluids to a level that readily moves the crystals through the tubules.

Interactions

The sulfonamides may potentiate the effects of anticoagulants, methotrexate, or sulfonylurea hypoglycemic agents by displacing them from their plasma protein-binding sites. The competition with sulfonamides for renal tubule secretion sites may decrease the excretion rate of salicylates or the thiazides and other drugs with a sulfonamide component in their structure.

Preparations Available

Each of the drugs in Table 16–7, with the exception of sulfapyridine, is employed primarily for the treatment of urinary tract infections caused by susceptible pathogens that are identified in a culture of the urine. The frequency of administration is an indicator of the duration of the effect of each drug in the table. *Sulfisoxazole* and *sulfacytine* generally are the drugs of choice for therapy.

Sulfapyridine is employed primarily for the suppression of *dermatitis herpetiformis*. The drug is administered orally. Alkalinization of the urine is usually planned during therapy with the poorly soluble drug and fluid intake should also be encouraged. Sulfapyridine usually produces relief of symptoms, but the exact mode of action is unknown.

Sulfamethoxazole is available in a combination with *trimethoprin*, which blocks the synthesis of folic acid at a later stage than the sulfonamide. The product (BACTRIM, SEPTRA) is commonly used for the treatment of urinary tract infections or acute otitis media in children over two months of age. The drug combination provides an antibacterial effect by the synergistic action of the two drugs.

Sulfadiazine sodium is administered intravenously. The solution is administered as a well-diluted, short-term infusion because the alkaline solution is irritating to the tissues. *Sulfisoxazole diolamine* is the parenteral drug form most frequently utilized for administration. It is also used orally for the treatment of otitis media and topically for susceptible infections in the eye. In general, topical application of the sulfonamides is avoided because there is a high incidence of sensitization by that route.

Topical Sulfonamides. *Mafenide acetate* and *silver sulfadiazine* are the sulfonamides that are employed for the prevention or control of infections in patients who have extensive second- and third-degree burns. The drugs are effective in the control of *Candida albicans, Enterobacter, Escherichia coli, Klebsiella, Staphylococcus,* and *Streptococcus* infections. The drugs, unlike other sulfonamides, are able to penetrate collections of purulent material. They are available as creams, which soften the eschar and allow penetration of the drug.

Mafenide acetate (SULFAMYLON ACETATE) diffuses into the interstitial fluids at the site of application, but little of the drug is absorbed into the systemic circulation. The application of the cream causes some pain, and premedication of the patient with a mild sedative may be planned to decrease the discomfort. Allergic responses may occur during therapy. Mafenide and its metabolites inhibit carbonic anhydrase and can cause metabolic acidosis in the presence of impaired pulmonary or renal function or extensive burns.

Silver sulfadiazine (SILVADENE) causes little pain at the site of application. The drug is absorbed from the topical sites during prolonged therapy. Blood drug levels may attain the same range as those occurring with oral drug administration, and the patient is observed for evidence of the adverse effects common to systemic sulfonamides.

Intraintestinal Sulfonamides. *Phthalylsulfathiazole* (CREMOTHALIDINE, ROTHALID, SULFATHALIDINE) and *sulfasalazine* (AZULFIDINE, RORASUL) are the oral sulfonamides employed for the control of infections caused by susceptible organisms within the intestinal lumen. Only small quantities of the drug are absorbed from the intestine.

Phthalylsulfathiazole is administered at a daily dosage range of 50 to 100 mg/kg of body weight.

That dosage is divided and administered three, four, or six times a day. The maximum daily dosage is 8 gm. The drug produces a tenacious, stringy stool that is difficult to evacuate. Suprainfection by the intestinal bacteria that are resistant or by organisms from the environment (i.e., *Candida albicans*) can result from the suppression of intestinal bacteria. Prolonged therapy can also interfere with the synthesis of vitamin K and potentiate the effects of oral anticoagulants when the drugs are used concurrently.

Sulfasalazine is initially administered to adults at a dosage of 3 to 4 gm/day. The dosage may be reduced to 2 gm/day for maintenance therapy. The initial daily dosage for children is calculated on the basis of 40 to 60 mg/kg of body weight. The maintenance dosage is calculated at the lower level of 30 mg/kg. The total daily dosage for adults or children is divided into four to six equal doses.

The drug is partially metabolized in the connective tissues of the colon. The metabolism releases sulfapyridine to act in the intestine, and some of the drug is absorbed. The action of the drug in the treatment of intraluminal disease (i.e., ulcerative colitis) probably is other than bacterial suppression because the drug has little effect on the natural bacterial flora.

URINARY TRACT–SPECIFIC AGENTS

The *methenamines, nalidixic acid, oxolinic acid,* and *nitrofurantoin* are employed for the treatment of infections in the urinary tract. The drugs may be used alone or in combination with other drugs in the control of acute or chronic urinary tract infections.

Methenamine

The drug is a nonspecific antibacterial agent effective in the control of chronic urinary tract infections caused by *Enterobacter, Escherichia coli, Pseudomonas, Proteus,* and *Staphylococcus.* The drug frequently is employed for the treatment of patients with indwelling catheters who have bladder infections.

Methenamine provides an antimicrobial effect

by liberation of ammonia and formaldehyde in the bladder, renal tubule, or urine. The activity of the drug is dependent on the acidity of the urine, and acidifying agents may be given to maintain the urine at pH 5.5 or lower. The drug can act as a bactericidal agent when the quantity of formaldehyde in the urine is high. The urea-splitting activity of some species of *Proteus* and *Pseudomonas* necessitates a marked increase in the intake of natural acidifying agents (i.e., cranberry juice) or of drugs (i.e., ascorbic acid) to maintain an acid medium for the drug effect. Milk products and systemic antacids (i.e., sodium bicarbonate) should be avoided during therapy with methenamine. The drug may be given with other antimicrobial agents except sulfonamides, which form insoluble precipitates with the formaldehyde.

Persons taking the drug sometimes have minor gastrointestinal problems (i.e., nausea, vomiting), which may result from the liberation of small amounts of formaldehyde in the stomach. Allergic reactions are rare and are usually limited to dermatologic responses (i.e., pruritus, rash, urticaria).

The methenamine preparations, with the exception of the parent compound *methenamine* (URITONE), provide an acid portion that has antiseptic properties and they contribute to urine acidification. *Methenamine mandelate* (MANDELAMINE) is the most frequently used form of the drug. The formulation contains 48 percent methenamine and 52 percent mandelic acid. *Methenamine hippurate* (HIPREX) contains approximately 44 percent methenamine and 56 percent hippuric acid. *Methenamine sulfosalicylate* (HEXALET) contains 39 percent methenamine and 61 percent sulfosalicylic acid. The usual oral dosage for each of the drugs is 4 gm/day for adults and 0.5 gm/day for children over 12 years old. That dosage is divided for administration four times during the person's waking hours (i.e., after meals and at bedtime).

Nalidixic Acid

The drug is employed to treat infections caused by susceptible strains of *Enterobacter, Escherichia coli, Klebsiella, Proteus, Pseudomonas,* and *Streptococcus* that are resistant to other drugs. During therapy urine cultures are evaluated frequently. Resistance to the drug may develop within 48 hours after institution of therapy, and positive cultures of the urine after that period of time indicate bacterial resistance to the drug.

Nalidixic acid produces an antibacterial effect by interfering with the DNA-directed synthesis of proteins. It inhibits the incorporation of the nucleotide thymidine by DNA.

Nalidixic acid (NEG-GRAM) is administered orally. The adult dosage is 4 gm/day and the daily dosage for children is calculated on the basis of 50 mg/kg of body weight. The daily dosage is divided for administration four times a day. Peak urine drug levels are attained within three to four hours. Approximately 80 percent of the drug is excreted in 24 hours and the antibacterial levels of the drug in the urine are maintained throughout that period.

The most common adverse effects are gastrointestinal disturbances (i.e., nausea, vomiting). Skin rash and urticaria also appear frequently. The neurologic problems, which occur infrequently, may include dizziness, diplopia, weakness, headache, drowsiness, or paresthesias.

The drug may cause a false positive reaction for glycosuria when the cupric sulfate reagents (i.e., Benedict's qualitative solution, CLINITEST) are employed for the test.

Oxolinic Acid

The drug is structurally related to nalidixic acid, and it has the same mode of action and antibacterial spectrum of activity. Its effectiveness in control of *Enterobacter, Escherichia coli, Klebsiella,* and *Proteus* is well established. Therapy may be instituted after a urine specimen has been obtained for culture when the patient's urinary tract infection requires immediate therapy.

Antibacterial drug levels are present in the urinary tract within two to four hours after the oral drug is administered and those levels persist for about 12 hours. The drug is metabolized in the liver and kidneys, and some of the antibacterial activity in the urinary tract is related to the presence of the drug and the active metabolites. Bacterial resistance to the drug develops rapidly, and positive urine cultures may reappear 48 to 72 hours after therapy is instituted. Patients should be cautioned to continue therapy without interruption to decrease the incidence of resistance.

The most common adverse effect is central nervous system stimulation, which may be manifested as insomnia, dizziness, nervousness, or headache. The problems arise more frequently in elderly patients. Gastrointestinal disturbances occur less frequently and usually include anorexia, vomiting, diarrhea, or constipation. Pruritus is the most frequent sign of allergy to the drug.

The daily dosage of *oxolinic acid* (UTIBID) for adults is 1.5 gm, divided for administration twice each day for two to four weeks. The dosage for pediatric patients has not been established.

Nitrofurantoin

The drug is employed for control of susceptible strains of *Enterobacter, Escherichia coli, Klebsiella, Proteus, Staphylococcus aureus,* and *Streptococcus faecalis.* It is seldom utilized as a primary drug, but it may be employed for prophylaxis or for the control of chronic infections. The drug is thought to interfere with several enzyme systems to interrupt the synthesis of proteins during reproduction of the pathogens.

Approximately 40 percent of the unchanged drug is found in the urine within 12 hours after administration of the oral drug. Retention of the drug in the urinary tract is highest when the tubule urine is acid. When the urine pH is low, there is greater renal tubule back diffusion that recycles the drug and maintains a high concentration in the tubule fluid. The excretion rate is higher when the urine is neutral or alkaline. The metabolites of the drug may tint the urine a brownish color.

The usual daily oral dosage of *nitrofurantoin* (CYANTIN, FURADANTIN, MACRODANTIN) for adults is 200 to 400 mg, divided for administration four times a day. The daily dosage for children is based on the calculation of 5 to 7 mg/kg of body weight, also divided for administration.

Nitrofurantoin sodium is administered intramuscularly or as a well-diluted intravenous infusion. The dosage that is given by the parenteral route to adults weighing 55 kg (120 lb) is 360 mg/day, usually divided for administration twice a day. The daily parenteral dosage for adults weighing less than 55 kg or children over 12 years of age is calculated on the basis of 7 mg/kg of body weight. Since the drug is irritating to tissues, intramuscular injections are employed infrequently.

Adverse effects of the drug include nausea, vomiting, and gastritis. Administration of the drug with food usually decreases the problems. Children frequently have skin rashes during therapy. Hemolytic anemia may appear in patients with *glucose-6-phosphate dehydrogenase* (G-6-PD) deficiency. Peripheral neuropathy has occurred in some patients, and some of the problems have included extensive involvement of the nerves, spinal cord, and striated muscles. The drug therapy is discontinued at the first evidence of numbness or tingling of the extremities to prevent progression of the neuropathy.

ANTIMYCOBACTERIAL DRUGS

The important mycobacteria are those pathogens causing tuberculosis or leprosy. The pathogens have thick lipoprotein cell walls that resist phagocytosis by the body's natural physiologic defense mechanisms, and the mycobacteria that survive within the macrophages can travel to widely disseminated tissue sites. The clusters of bacteria may remain dormant or may multiply slowly within the tissues where they reside.

The primary mycobacterial disease encountered in the populations of the world is caused by the organism *Mycobacterium tuberculosis,* and the presentation of drugs will initially focus on the drugs used for the control of tuberculosis. Control of the pathogen *Mycobacterium leprae* is a persistent problem in India, China, and Africa. The leprostatic drugs, which are used for the control of leprosy, may be employed in the Western hemisphere in this generation of worldwide travel that allows the global spread of pathogens. The presentation of the leprostatic drugs will follow the initial description of antitubercular drugs.

Isoniazid is the drug employed prophylactically for individuals who are exposed to but considered *uninfected* by the *Mycobacterium tuberculosis*. It is also used for the treatment of persons who have a positive reaction to tuberculin tests without positive sputum cultures, chest x-rays, or clinical evidence of infection. Prophylactic use is usually continued for a 12-month period for exposed, uninfected patients.

Isoniazid, ethambutol, rifampin, and *streptomycin sulfate* are the primary drugs employed in varying combinations for the treatment of *infected patients* or for *diseased patients.* The second-line drugs, *aminosalicylic acid, capreomycin, cycloserine, ethionamide, viomycin,* and *pyrazinamide,* are utilized when resistance to the primary drugs is indicated by lack of improvement in the patient's status and by positive sputum cultures. Resistance to the drugs develops readily, and the drugs are always employed in combinations for infected or diseased patient therapy to delay the emergence of resistant pathogens.

In selected situations therapy may be instituted with antitubercular drugs after sputum cultures are obtained (i.e., acutely ill positive tuberculin test reactors) because *Mycobacterium* cultures require a three-week incubation period. Combinations that commonly are employed for initial therapy are ethambutol, isoniazid, and rifampin; ethambutol, isoniazid, and streptomycin; and aminosalicyclic acid, isoniazid, and streptomycin. The initial group of drugs may be employed until resistance is evident, and at that time it is usual for at least two of the drugs to be replaced by others to which the organism is susceptible.

Therapy is often continued for 18 to 24 months, but the termination of therapy is defined as the presence of three consecutive negative sputum cultures. Persons with arrested tuberculosis are examined periodically because the organisms encapsulate in calcified tubercles in the lungs. Those tubercles can become active when the person's physical status or other conditions in the environment change (i.e., acute illness, immunosuppressive drug therapy).

Isoniazid

Action Mode. The drug interferes with the synthesis of the peptidoglycan structure of the *Mycobacterium* cell wall in reproducing pathogens. There is no evidence of the development of resistance to isoniazid when the drug is used as a single agent for prophylaxis, and that 12-month period of therapy seems to provide several years of protection against the disease.

Therapy Considerations. Children tolerate higher doses of isoniazid than do adults. The drug is most commonly administered orally (Table 16–8) and is well absorbed from the gastrointestinal tract. The circulating drug is widely distributed in body tissues and fluids. Peak plasma drug concentrations are reached in one to two hours. Drug concentrations comparable to those of the plasma are attained in the milk of nursing mothers and in the fetal circulation.

Isoniazid is metabolized in the liver by *acetylation* and *dehydrazination*. Individuals who are genetically *slow acetylators* of isoniazid may have serum drug concentrations that remain elevated and increase the incidence of adverse effects. Persons who are genetically *fast acetylators* more rapidly inactivate the drug, and their serum levels may be 50 percent lower than those found in slow isoniazid inactivators. Dosage adjustments are required to compensate for the differences in the serum drug concentrations.

The drug and its metabolites are excreted primarily in the urine by glomerular filtration, and approximately 70 percent of the drug is excreted within 24 hours. The presence of the drug and its metabolites in the urine may cause a false positive reaction with the cupric sulfate reagent Benedict's Qualitative Solution, but the effect on the less sensitive CLINITEST tablets is variable. Alternate reagents (i.e., TES-TAPE) should be used when testing for glycosuria.

Table 16–8.
Dosage Levels of Antitubercular Drugs

Drug	Route	Daily Dosage Adult	Child (mg/kg BW)	Number of Divided Doses
Aminosalicylic acid (PARASAL)	Oral	10–15 gm	—*	3–4
Capreomycin sulfate (CAPASTAT)	IM	1 gm	—*	1
Cycloserine (SEROMYCIN)	Oral	0.5–1 gm	10–20	3
Ethambutol hydrochloride (MYAMBUTOL)	Oral	15–25 mg/kg	—*	1
Ethionamide (TRECATOR-SC)	Oral	0.5–1 gm	—*	2–4
Isoniazid (HYZYD, INH, NICONYL, NYDAZID)	Oral IM	0.3 gm	10–30	1–2
Pyrazinoic acidamide	Oral	25–35 mg/kg	—*	3–4
Rifampin (RIFADIN, RIMACTANE)	Oral	0.6 gm	10–20	1
Streptomycin sulfate	IM	15–25 mg/kg	20	1–2
Viomycin sulfate (VIOCIN)	IM	2 gm	—*	2

* Dosage not established.

Adverse Effects. Some patients have a pyridoxine deficiency associated with the competition of the drug with pyridoxal phosphate for the enzyme *apotryptophanase*, which is required for the synthesis of the vitamin. Pyridoxine, or vitamin B_6, administration (i.e., 50 to 100 mg/day) often decreases the incidence and severity of the paresthesias of the extremities that are forerunners of more extensive neuropathies (i.e., hyperreflexia, vertigo, encephalopathy). Dietary counseling should also be planned because adequate nutrition can reduce the incidence of the problem.

Hepatotoxicity may appear during therapy with isoniazid, and the problems closely resemble those of viral hepatitis. The drug-related hepatic pathology, which usually occurs in the first three months of therapy, causes an elevation of the serum enzyme level (i.e., SGOT, SGPT) and bilirubinemia. The problems occur most frequently in slow acetylators and in persons who chronically ingest alcohol. They have not occurred in children. Adults who are receiving isoniazid are instructed to consult the professional personnel who are following their therapy when there is

any evidence of jaundice, yellowing of the sclera, dark-colored urine, clay-colored stools, excess fatigue, anorexia, or fever. Therapy is usually interrupted if symptoms of hepatitis or other allergic responses appear (i.e., skin eruptions, urticaria).

Gastrointestinal problems (i.e., nausea, vomiting, constipation, dryness of the mouth) may occur during therapy. Slow isoniazid acetylators may have a *lupus erythematosus-like syndrome* as a consequence of cumulative levels of the circulating drug. When slow acetylators are concurrently receiving phenytoin, their serum drug levels are monitored regularly because isoniazid inhibits hepatic metabolism of phenytoin. The increased levels of the anticonvulsant may cause toxic effects.

Ethambutol Hydrochloride

Action Mode. The drug rapidly enters the cytoplasm of reproducing mycobacteria. That action interferes with metabolic processes and the progression of pathogen multiplication. Ethambutol has a bacteriostatic effect on the bacteria.

Therapy Considerations. Ethambutol is absorbed readily after oral administration, and peak serum levels are attained within two to four hours. The serum drug level drops to one half the peak concentration within eight hours. The high concentration produced by the single dosage administration is considered essential to produce a level of drug that is bacteriostatic. The drug remains in the circulation and some of the drug enters the erythrocytes.

The drug is metabolized in the liver. One half of the drug is excreted in the urine within 24 hours after the oral dosage is administered. Up to 22 percent of the unchanged drug is excreted in the feces.

Adverse Effects. Optic nerve toxicity is the most common adverse effect of the drug, and the problems may include optic neuritis, decreased visual acuity, scotoma, and the loss of color discrimination. The toxic effects may appear within one to seven months after therapy is instituted. The problems may persist for several weeks after therapy is terminated. Regularly scheduled visual tests usually are planned during therapy. The patients should be told to promptly inform the professional personnel following their progress when vision problems arise. Those measures assist in early identification of the problems and prevention of their progression.

Peripheral neuritis may occur during therapy with ethambutol. Other adverse effects include gastrointestinal disturbances and allergic responses (i.e., fever, rash, pruritus, occasionally anaphylaxis).

Rifampin

Action Mode. The drug selectively inhibits the final step in the DNA-dependent synthesis of RNA in bacterial cells. That action provides a mycobactericidal effect by causing the production of nonfunctional cellular proteins. At dosage levels higher than those employed for control of *Mycobacterium,* the drug has a broad spectrum of activity against gram-negative organisms.

Therapy Considerations. Rifampin is administered orally as a single daily dose (Table 16–8). The dosage maximum for children over five years of age is 600 mg/day. The drug is well absorbed from the gastrointestinal tract, and peak serum drug levels usually are attained within 90 minutes. Approximately 75 to 90 percent of the circulating drug is bound to serum proteins. Highest tissues concentrations of the drug appear in the liver, lung, gallbladder, and kidneys. The drug diffuses readily into all body fluids. It is metabolized in the liver and the metabolite has antibacterial activity comparable to that of the parent drug. One half of the drug is excreted with the bile, and approximately 20 percent of the unchanged drug or its metabolite is excreted in the urine. Some of the drug is excreted in the milk of nursing mothers and it also appears in the glandular secretions. The drug and its metabolite impart a red-orange color to the feces, urine, and secretions (i.e., saliva, sweat, tears). Patients should be informed of the possible changes to prevent their anxiety when they observe the vivid discoloration.

Adverse Effects. The most common adverse effect is a "flulike syndrome" involving gastrointestinal disturbances (i.e., anorexia, nausea, vomiting, flatulence, abdominal cramping, diarrhea). Some evidence of central nervous system depression may also appear (i.e., drowsiness, fatigue, dizziness, mental confusion, inability to concentrate). Suprainfections (i.e., *Candida albicans*) and allergic reactions may occur (i.e., pruritus, urticaria, rashes, fever).

Interactions. Concurrent administration of aminosalicyclic acid may lower the serum levels of rifampin by interfering with its absorption. Scheduling 8-to-12-hour intervals between the administration of the drugs reduces the problem.

Rifampin induces the hepatic microsomal enzymes and that action may accelerate the elimination of digitalis derivatives, oral hypoglycemics, glucocorticoids, oral contraceptives, oral anticoagulants, or methadone. The dosage of those drugs may need adjustment to maintain their therapeutic effect.

Streptomycin Sulfate

The drug is an aminoglycoside antibiotic with a high potential for causing ototoxicity. The comprehensive presentation of the drug appears earlier in the chapter.

The use of intramuscular injections of streptomycin is a valuable adjunct in treatment of patients who require intensive therapy for tuberculosis (Table 16–8). The drug initially is administered in dosages of 20 mg/kg of body weight to adults. The initial plan of therapy may involve daily administration of the drug for a period of two to three weeks, and the intervals between injections may then be changed to two or three times a week.

Ambulatory patients frequently are able to receive the injections at the clinic or visiting nurse association office near their home at a time convenient to their daily living schedules. The transient headache that occasionally occurs after the injection can be lessened when the person sits quietly for a period of 15 to 30 minutes.

Aminosalicylic Acid

The drug has a bacteriostatic effect. The drug is absorbed by *Mycobacterium,* and there appears to be some binding action that interferes with the intracellular synthesis of proteins. The use of the drug with isoniazid increases and prolongs the serum levels of isoniazid thereby enhancing the antitubercular activity.

The drug formulations include *calcium aminosalicylate, potassium aminosalicylate,* and *sodium aminosalicylate.* The dosage ranges for each of the drugs is the same as for *aminosalicylic acid.* The drug formerly was employed in most primary treatment regimens, but the high incidence of gastrointestinal disturbances caused a high rate of noncompliance by the patients on long-term therapy.

The oral drug is rapidly absorbed from the intestinal tract, and the circulating drug is distributed in most body tissues and fluids. The drug is rapidly excreted, and 50 percent of the oral dose may appear in the urine within two hours. Metabolites produce a false positive reaction for glycosuria when Benedict's Qualitative Reagent is used for testing.

It is estimated that approximately 15 percent of the patients taking the drug have gastrointestinal disturbances. Allergic reactions occur in approximately 4 percent of the patients, and the problems include skin rashes, pruritus, and fever. There also may be changes in the blood cells (i.e., leukocytosis, eosinophilia). The most serious adverse effect is hepatotoxicity, which can be fatal. Drug therapy is terminated when there is evidence of fever without other causation because that is usually the first sign of liver tissue damage.

Capreomycin

The drug is an antibiotic that inhibits protein synthesis in reproducing *Mycobacterium.* The drug is employed as an alternate to streptomycin when bacterial resistance occurs if the cultures indicate pathogen susceptibility to capreomycin. Parenteral administration provides dependable elevated therapeutic serum levels of the drug in acutely ill patients. The intramuscular injections are painful, and there may be induration at the injection site. The potential for nephrotoxicity and ototoxicity, which involves both the auditory and vestibular branches of the eighth cranial nerve, limits usefulness of the drug for long-term therapy.

Cycloserine

The drug is an antibiotic that is available for oral use. It produces a bactericidal effect by interfering with the cell wall synthesis during the pathogen's reproductive cycle. Cycloserine produces peak blood levels within four to eight hours after administration, and the drug is widely distributed in body fluids. One half of the drug is eliminated within 12 hours after it is injected. Although the drug is less active than streptomycin, it is utilized as an alternate drug when bacterial resistance to that drug appears.

Central nervous system effects are the primary problems, but their incidence is relatively low at the dosage schedules employed for the control of tuberculosis (Table 16–8). The problems may include drowsiness, headache, mental confusion, psychotic reactions, or convulsions. The dosage usually is adjusted to maintain a blood concentration of 25 to 30 mcg/ml to prevent the adverse effects. Pyridoxine (i.e., 300 mg/day) may also be administered as a prophylactic measure.

Ethionamide

The drug is a bacteriostatic agent that is administered orally (Table 16–8). It is readily absorbed from the intestinal tract. The drug is slowly metabolized and the therapeutic serum drug concentrations are maintained for prolonged periods of time. At the maximum dosage level, adverse effects include gastrointestinal disturbances (i.e., anorexia, nausea, vomiting, metallic taste in the mouth, diarrhea). Administration of the drug with a snack or an antiemetic alleviates some of the problems. The appearance of a generalized skin rash necessitates termination of the drug therapy because it can progress to exfoliative dermatitis. Peripheral neuritis and mental depression can occur, and the drug is not utilized with other drugs that have the same neurotoxicity potential.

Viomycin

The drug is a semisynthetic antibiotic that is administered parenterally. It is utilized only selectively because it is less effective and potentially more neurotoxic than streptomycin or capreomycin. When cultures indicate that the organism is susceptible to viomycin, the drug may be administered at three-day intervals to decrease the emergence of resistance and the serious neurotoxicity.

Pyrazinamide

The drug is employed primarily for acutely ill patients who have been treated with other drugs and have *Mycobacterium* strains resistant to those drugs. It is always used in combination with other drugs. The drug causes a high incidence of hepatoxicity, which limits the duration of therapy. The liver pathology generally is reversible when therapy is terminated, but it has progressed to extensive destruction and fatalities. Liver function studies are evaluated during therapy, and any irregularities in the tests or physical evidence of jaundice, liver enlargement, or liver tenderness necessitate the termination of therapy.

Hyperuricemia also occurs frequently during therapy. The accumulation of uric acid may precipitate symptoms of gout in individuals predisposed to that problem. The drug can affect the blood-clotting mechanisms, and sideroblastic anemia has been reported.

Leprostatic Drugs

The drugs currently available for control of *Mycobacterium leprae* are the sulfones *dapsone* (AVLOSULFON) and *sodium sulfoxone* (DIASONE). The sulfones are employed for the treatment of *lepromatous leprosy* and *tuberculoid leprosy*. The characteristics of the lesions and of the *Mycobacterium* affect the progress of drug therapy.

Mycobacterium leprae produces a protective and nutritive substance that enhances its survival during the stages of reproduction. The characteristic lesions of lepromatous, or nodular, leprosy are ulcerations on the skin and mucous membranes containing large *Mycobacterium*-laden nodules, or granulomas. Tuberculoid, or anesthetic, leprosy involves macular skin lesions that are insensitive to stimuli within their borders. The lesions of tuberculoid leprosy can reappear after long periods of remission.

Action Mode. The sulfones have a competitive antimetabolite effect that interferes with the synthesis of folic acid by the pathogens. The absence of the *aminobenzoic acid* that is naturally synthesized by the microbes leads to the formation of nonfunctional proteins.

Therapy Considerations. The oral dosage of dapsone (25 to 100 mg/day) or sodium sulfoxone (330 to 660 mg/day) is administered as a single dose. The circulating drug enters the normal body tissues, with the exception of the ocular structures, and it enters the leprous tissues. The drug is metabolized in the liver, and the major metabolite has antibacterial activity. The primary excretion route is the urine, but small amounts of the drug appear in the sweat, saliva, tears, and milk of nursing mothers. The slow excretion rate of the drugs provides cumulative levels that enhance the therapeutic effect.

Therapy is continued for long periods of time (three to five years +), but the person periodically may be allowed to have short drug-free periods. The ulcerative lesions of the mucous membranes respond earliest to therapy, and there may be gradual improvement over the initial three to six months of therapy. Skin lesions respond very slowly to treatment; smears of the lesions remain positive for at least one and one-half years.

Adverse Effects. Anemia is a common problem in the early phase of therapy, and a sharp fall in the hemoglobin level (<10 gm/100 ml) or in the number of erythrocytes (<2.5 million per cubic millimeter) necessitates a reduction in the drug dosage. Concurrent improvement in the nutritional intake and the use of supplemental iron therapy usually produce an improvement in the person's health status. The drug dosage may be increased when the hematologic status improves. Leukopenia and methemoglobinemia may also occur, but the problems seldom necessitate the interruption of therapy.

An allergic reaction that is characteristic of the disease commonly occurs during therapy. The *erythema nodosum leprosum,* or "lepra" reaction, represents a response of the physiologic immune systems to the antigenic challenge of the substances released from the disintegrating *Mycobacterium.* The reaction exacerbates the lesions in the involved leprous tissues. When the reaction is severe, therapy may be interrupted to delay the progress of the allergic response and allow treatment of the allergy-related problems.

Allergic reactions that are specific to the sulfones are dermatologic reactions that include a generalized maculopapular rash or "fixed eruptions," which occur in approximately 2 percent of the patients within the first ten weeks of therapy. The reactions usually are related to the time when the dosage is increased from the initial level. The appearance of the generalized skin eruptions necessitates interruption of therapy to avoid the possibility of its progressing to exfoliative skin eruptions and the involvement of the epithelial tissues of the respiratory and gastrointestinal tract.

The nutritional status of the person is important during the disruptive infectious process, and the anorexia, nausea, or vomiting that occurs during therapy with the sulfones can interfere with eating. During the long period of therapy, the drugs cause few serious adverse effects. The periodic planned interruptions in therapy may be a factor in the low incidence of drug-related problems.

NURSING INTERVENTION

All pathogens are opportunists that are consistently available in the external and internal environment to cause infection when conditions in the host or the environment allow them to gain a foothold. The rapidity of their reproduction or their inability to resist the activity of physiologic processes for phagocytosis allows the emergence of an infectious process in the receptive host.

In the hospital environment a number of resistant strains of pathogens have emerged as a consequence of antibiotic therapy. There also are conditions in the environment and in the large number of receptive hosts that invite pathogen propagation.

Infection control investigators within the hospitals frequently have discovered the pathogen source of widespread infections in the cultures obtained from equipment utilized for seriously ill patients on the hospital units (i.e., inhalation therapy equipment, indwelling catheters). Regardless of the specific source of the pathogens, nosocomial infections can compromise the patient's recovery potential and inflate the costs of the illness by prolonging the period of hospitalization.

Prevention is always less costly than treatment, and the hygienic measures that are maintained by the patient and the professional personnel can decrease the exchange of pathogens in the hospital setting. The stringent procedures for the care of the insertion sites of catheters (i.e., intravenous, intra-arterial, bladder) are part of the preventive plan that has become standard practice in all hospital settings.

Disruption of the normal integrity of the tissues by wounds, burns, or infections can allow the entrance of pathogens. Drugs (i.e., glucocorticoids, antineoplastics) and other therapies that change the natural activity of the physiologic defense mechanisms (i.e., radiation therapy, tissue transplants) also predispose the person to infection.

Status Evaluation

Overt changes in the patient's status (i.e., purulent drainage from an incision, elevated body temperature) may forewarn of an infection, but in many instances the patient may provide the initial clues to physiologic changes that occur at inaccessible or internal body sites. Infections can evolve without causing overt evidence of their presence until they are well established.

Regularly planned examinations of body discharges and of the accessible tissues and body orifices allow identification of lesions, irritation, drainage, or inflammation at the common sites of infection (i.e., throat, lungs, bladder, skin). When changes are identified, sharing exact and vivid descriptions about the findings with the physician allows early treatment of the infection. Some patient protocols that have been established by health team members provide guidelines for events that require that cultures be obtained (i.e., blood cultures when temperature is >39° C (102.2° F). In all situations the material to be cultured must represent an adequate specimen for the planting of the culture and pathogen susceptibility, or sensitivity, test media. The laboratory procedures are expensive, and judgment should be exercised in the number of cultures obtained to minimize the cost to the patient.

A sudden high temperature elevation, chills, tachycardia, lowered level of consciousness, pallor, and hypotension are the early signs of a serious infection (i.e., bacteremia). It is usual, when those signs of infection appear, for the physician to examine the patient thoroughly. The physician usually prescribes cultures of the urine, sputum, feces, and wound drainage, and x-rays of the chest in an effort to determine the source of the problem. Because pathogens can enter the bloodstream from those tissues or from the insertion sites of catheters, tracheostomies, or drains, blood cultures may also be prescribed. The extent to which the physiologic defense mechanisms are mobilized is determined by obtaining and evaluating the leukocyte count and the differential distribution of the white blood cells. In acutely ill patients, drug therapy may be instituted immediately after the cultures are obtained.

Assessing Progress

An elevation of the body temperature is an indication of the high rate of physiologic activity associated with the invasion of pathogens. The high metabolic rate depletes the nutrient stores and disrupts the fluid and electrolyte balance. When the temperature is elevated, the superficial vasodilation that provides for dissipation of heat from the skin also increases the amount of fluid and sodium chloride that leaves the body. Nutrient, fluid, and sodium chloride replacement should be considered when offering meals or snacks to the patient. Antipyretics may be prescribed when the temperature consistently or sporadically is elevated above 38.5° C (101.3° F).

Observations of changes in the patient's status (i.e., lower temperature, wound healing) are vital in determining the effectiveness of the anti-infective drug therapy. Careful examination of body tissues for improvement in the basic infectious process provides an opportunity to identify the emergence of suprainfections (i.e., oral or vaginal *Candida* infections) that can occur during therapy with each of the anti-infective drugs. When the signs of infection remain stable without improvement, or when they worsen, the therapeutic plan is reevaluated by the health team. Pathogen susceptibility cultures may be repeated because the pathogen can become resistant to the drugs to which they initially showed susceptibility.

Drug Allergy Reactions

Allergic reactions may occur during therapy with any of the antimicrobial drugs, but they appear most commonly with antibiotic drug therapy. It is a routine aspect of the medical and nursing history-taking process to inquire about previous drug reactions. It is equally important to identify whether the person has frequent or recurrent reactions to foods, pollens, and other allergens. Individuals with those problems seem more frequently to have delayed allergic reactions during drug therapy (i.e., serum sickness, fever, skin rash, contact dermatitis). The person also may have become sensitized to a drug during its use topically or systemically without overt evidence of a reaction.

It is particularly important to observe the patient for an anaphylactic reaction when the first dose of a parenteral form of an antibiotic is being administered. Observing the patient for evidence of wheezing, dyspnea, or hypotension at five-minute intervals for a period of one-half hour assures immediate identification of the earliest evidence of the allergic response as the drug is disseminated throughout the body. Utilizing the half-hour time period to do nursing tasks within the patient's immediate environment allows frequent observation without inducing anxiety in the patient or family members. When an anaphylactic response occurs, treatment involves the administration of a bronchodilator, antihistamine, or vasoconstrictor and the use of resuscitative measures to maintain a patent airway and counteract shock.

Administration of a parenteral antibiotic to an ambulatory patient in the clinic or office should be followed by the same period of observation. The person should be asked to remain in the immediate area for a half-hour period after the drug is given. Although urticaria, angioedema, or the delayed allergic reactions may occur after the patient leaves the area, they are less serious problems than the life-threatening anaphylactic reaction. Symptomatic treatment (i.e., use of an antihistamine, topical application of an antipruritic lotion) usually alleviates the patient's discomfort.

Patients who have an allergic reaction to a drug should be advised to obtain from their local pharmacy a card, bracelet, or metal disc on a chain that is inscribed with a legend indicating the type of allergy. Identification of the problem is essential when the person is treated in a future emergency situation.

Counseling

Patients are very conscientious about taking their medications and following the instructions for control of the infection when symptoms are acute and disruptive to their living patterns. When the symptoms subside, that commitment may be decreased, and many patients terminate the therapy.

The problem of noncompliance is greatest when the persons are receiving anti-infective drugs for prophylaxis or for treatment over long periods of time. The most difficult aspect of the drug therapy plan for patients to comprehend is the necessity for continuance of therapy to its planned end point to avoid reemergence of the infection and the incidence of pathogen resistance to the drug. For example, persons receiving penicillin for a planned ten-day period for treatment of a *Streptococcus* infection in the nasopharyngeal tissues may discontinue taking the drug when the tissue inflammation no longer interferes with swallowing and the pain subsides. Although the immediate problems related to recurrence and resistant pathogens are primary concerns, future misuse of the drug also can cause pathogen resistance. It is usual for those same patients to utilize the remaining drug at a later time for self-treatment of infection.

The high rate of noncompliance with longterm therapy for control of tuberculosis in exposed or infected individuals has led to the practice of prescribing only a limited supply of the drugs (i.e., 30-day supply). That practice requires that the person visit the physician to obtain a prescription for the drugs. In some instances that practice has improved compliance, but the personal follow-up contact seems to be the only effective method for maintaining the patients' continual involvement in therapy.

Illness in any form interferes with routine or pleasurable patterns of living, and many individuals are impatient with those interruptions. It is essential to encourage the person who has an infection, or one who is recovering from a protracted period of infection, to rest and to modify his pace of activities until the body has an opportunity to repair tissue damage and to replenish reserve nutrient stores. Many patients find that any illness decreases their tolerance to full activity schedules for four or more weeks. Complete recovery without relapses of excess fatigue may be related to the time spent in allowing for the return of physiologic equilibrium.

Review Guides

1. Outline the factors that would be included when instructing the person in the following situations about the control of infection. Include in each outline the information about the drugs and their use, food and fluid intake, and the concurrent hygienic measures that are appropriate to each situation.
   A. The mother of a young child with nasopharyngitis who is to receive ampicillin suspension.
   B. An elderly woman with cystitis who is to take sulfisoxazole tablets.
   C. A man with tuberculosis who is to take isoniazid, ethambutol, and rifampin.
   D. A middle-aged woman with diverticulitis who is to take sufasalazine at home.

2. Formulate a nursing care plan for the following hospitalized patients who are receiving drugs for control of bacteremia.
   A. A patient with beta-hemolytic *Streptococcus* bacteremia that is being treated with penicillin intravenously.
   B. A patient with a tracheostomy who has a *Pseudomonas aeruginosa* bacteremia that is being treated with gentamicin sulfate and carbenicillin.
   C. A patient who had an intrapartum rupture of the uterus and *Bacteroides fragilis* bacteremia that is being treated with chloromycetin and gentamicin sulfate.

Additional Readings

Appel, Gerald B., and Neu, Harold C.: Nephrotoxicity of antimicrobial agents. *N. Engl. J. Med.,* **296:** part 1, pg. 663, March 24, 1977; part 2, pg. 722, March 31, 1977; part 3, pg. 784, April 7, 1977.

Assaad, D.; From, L.; Ricciatti, D.; and Shapiro, H.: Toxic epidermal necrolysis in Stevens-Johnson syndrome. *Can. Med. Assoc. J.,* **118:**154, January 21, 1978.

Avery, David, and Finn, Richard: Succinylcholine-prolonged apnea associated with clindamycin and abnormal liver function tests. *Dis. Nerv. Syst.,* **38:** 473, June, 1977.

Barlow, Peter B.: Treatment of tuberculosis. *Basics RD,* **5:**1, September, 1976.

Beletz, Elaine E., and Covo, Gabriela: The case of the hidden infections in the elderly. *Nursing 76,* **6:**14, August, 1976.

Brown, William J.: A classification of microorganisms frequently causing sepsis. *Heart Lung,* **5:**397, May–June, 1976.

Cunningham, F. Gary; Hauth, John C.; Strong, James D.; Herbert, William N. P.; Gilstrap, Larry C.; Wilson, Russell H.; and Kappus, Sheryl S.: Tetracycline or penicillin-ampicillin for pelvic inflammatory disease. *N. Engl. J. Med.,* **296:**1380, June 16, 1977.

Cushing, Ralph: Pulmonary infections. *Heart Lung,* **5:**611, July–August, 1976.

Dannenberg, Arthur M., Jr.: Macrophages in inflammation and infection. *N. Engl. J. Med.,* **293:** 489, September 4, 1975.

Derrick, C. Warren, and Dillon, Hugh C.: Erythromycin therapy for streptococcal pharyngitis. *Am. J. Dis. Child.,* **130:**175, February, 1976.

Ellard, G. A.: Variations between individuals and populations in the acetylation of isoniazid and its significance for the treatment of pulmonary tuberculosis. *Clin. Pharmacol. Ther.,* **19:**610, May, 1976.

Fisher, Evelyn J.: Antimicrobial therapy: some guidelines. *Heart Lung,* **5:**437, May–June, 1976.

Gardner, Pierce: Reasons for "antibiotic failures." *Hosp. Pract.,* **11:**41, February, 1976.

Kaufman, Richard E.; Johnson, Robert E.; Jaffe, Harold W.; Thornsberry, Clyde; Reynolds, Gladys H.; Wiesner, Paul J.; and The Cooperative Study Group: Gonorrhea therapy monitoring: treatment results. *N. Engl. J. Med.,* **294:**1, January 1, 1976.

Klein, Jerome O.: Shifts in microbial sensitivity: implications for pediatrics. *Hosp. Pract.,* **10:**81, May, 1975.

Lauter, Carl B.: Opportunistic infections. *Heart Lung,* **5:**601, July–August, 1976.

Lester, William: Chemotherapy for tuberculosis. *Postgrad. Med.,* **60:**112, September, 1976.

Linton, Adam L.: Diagnosis and treatment of infections of the urinary tract. *Heart Lung,* **5:**607, July–August, 1976.

Liu, Pinghui V.: Biology of *Pseudomonas aeruginosa. Hosp. Pract.,* **11:**138, January, 1976.

Luft, Friedrich C.: Antimicrobials in kidney and liver failure. *Am. Fam. Physician,* **14:**92, August, 1976.

Lumholtz, Bo; Siersbaek-Nielsen, Kaj; Skovsted, Liz; Kampmann, Jens; and Hansen, Jens Molholm: Sulfamethizole-induced inhibition of diphenylhydantoin, tolbutamide, and warfarin metabolism. *Clin. Pharmacol. Ther.,* **17:**731, June, 1975.

Mitchell, Richard W., and Robson, Hugh G.: Patients' compliance with follow-up treatment of gonococcal urethritis. *Can. Med. Assoc. J.,* **116:**48, January 8, 1977.

Moellering, Robert C., Jr., and Swartz, Morton N.: Drug therapy: the newer cephalosporins. *N. Engl. J. Med.,* **294:**24, January 1, 1976.

Nichols, Ronald Lee; Schumer, William; Nyhus, Lloyd M.; Bartlett, John G.; and Gorbach, Sherwood L.: Anaerobic infections. *Am. Fam. Physician,* **14:**100, October, 1976.

Pegram, Samuel, Jr., and Philip, James R.: Managing anaerobic infections. *Am. Fam. Physician,* **17:**186, March, 1978.

Peterson, Lois D., and Green, Juanita H.: Nurse-managed tuberculosis clinic. *Am. J. Nurs.* **77:**433, March, 1977.

Pollock, Allan A.; Berger, Stephen A.; Richmond, Alma S.; Simberkoff, Michael S.; and Rahal, James J.: Amikacin therapy for serious gram-negative infections. *J.A.M.A.,* **237:**562, February 7, 1977.

Rooney, John J., Jr.; Crocco, John A.; Kramer, Sybil; and Lyons, Harold A.: Further observations on tuberculin reactions in active tuberculosis. *Am. J. Med.,* **60:**577, April, 1976.

Rudoy, R. C., and Riley, Harris D., Jr.: Cephalexin: clinical and laboratory evaluation in infants and children. *Clin. Pediatr.,* **16:**639, July, 1977.

Shapera, Ronald M., and Matsen, John M.: Oxolinic

acid therapy for urinary tract infections in children. *Am. J. Dis. Child.,* **131:**34, January, 1977.

Smith, Arnold L.: Current concepts: antibiotics and invasive *H. influenzae. N. Engl. J. Med.,* **294:**1329, June 10, 1976.

Smith, Craig R.; Baughman, Kenneth L.; Edwards, Corwin Q.; Rogers, John F.; and Lietman, Paul S.: Controlled comparison of amikacin and gentamicin. *N. Engl. J. Med.,* **296:**349, February 17, 1977.

Stamey, Thomas A.; Condy, Mercy; and Mihara, Gladys: Nitrofurantoin and trimethoprim-sulfamethoxazole prophylaxis of urinary-tract infections. *N. Engl. J. Med.,* **296:**780, April 7, 1977.

Syphilis—recommended treatment schedules, 1976. *Am. Fam. Physician,* **14:**119, September, 1976.

Taylor, Carol M.: Pneumococcal pneumonia: your patient's second threat. *Nursing 76,* **6:**30, March, 1976.

Tobey, Lee E., and Covington, Tim R.: Antimicrobial drug interactions. *Am. J. Nurs.* **75:**1470, September, 1975.

Weg, John G.: Diagnostic standards of tuberculosis-revised. *J.A.M.A.,* **235:**1329, March 29, 1976.

Weinstein, Allan J.: Newer antibiotics: guidelines for use. *Postgrad. Med.,* **60:**75, October, 1976.

Weinstein, Allan J.; Gibbs, Ronald S.; and Gallagher, Mollie: Placental transfer of clindamycin and gentamicin in term pregnancy. *Am. J. Obstet. Gynecol.,* **124:**688, April 1, 1976.

17

Fungus Infection and Parasitic Infestation

The fungal infections and parasitic infestations that can be readily transmitted from one individual to another are persistent and somewhat neglected health problems. Public apathy about the problems probably is related to the seemingly innocuous status of organisms that infrequently create overt illness.

Physiologic Correlations

The physiologic processes that defend the body tissues against bacterial invasion also surge forth to prevent intrusion by fungus or parasites (i.e., protozoa, helminths, plasmodia). Some of those pathogens may gain a foothold and propagate in the superficial tissues or in the intestinal lumen. Unless the invaders cause tissue irritation at those sites, they generally remain protected from the body defense mechanisms and they are attacked only when they leave those havens. As long as the conditions of the environment that is selected by the pathogen are conducive to its growth and reproduction, its lifespan and that of its progeny may be limited only by the availability of nutrients from the host tissues.

Pathophysiologic Correlations

FUNGUS INFECTION

Infections by fungi may be primary infections or they may represent a suprainfection by organisms that naturally exist in the body. The sites of invasion and the growth characteristics affect plans for control of the organisms. The common therapeutic classifications of the fungal diseases include the *Candida infections, dermatophytic infections,* and *systemic fungal infections.*

Candida Infections

Candida albicans is the organism most commonly identified when patients have suprainfections in the oral cavity, intestinal tract, or vagina. The emergence of the fungus as a pathogen frequently is associated with the suppression of the normal flora by intensive antibiotic therapy. The fungal infection can also occur in individuals whose defense mechanisms are compromised by immunosuppressive drugs (i.e., antineoplastics, glucocorticoids).

Candida infections in the accessible body cavities (i.e., mouth, vagina) can be identified by their effects on the tissues. For example, the fungus in the oral cavity initially causes creamy-white or bluish-white patches that adhere to the mucous membranes. The patient who can drink liquids often complains that citrus fruit juices cause a burning sensation. Women who have a fungus infection of the vagina and vulva may complain of an increased discharge, burning, or pruritus. Cultures are necessary for the definitive diagnosis, but the characteristic appearance of the lesions allows immediate institution of therapy for relief of the discomfort.

Dermatophytic Infections

The infections can be caused by several species of *Epidermophyton, Trichophyton,* or *Microsporum.* Tinea capitis, tinea corporis, and tinea pedis are the most common fungal infections on the superficial tissues of the body. The fungi proliferate beneath the thin layers of the superficial tissues, and their presence is detectable by the opaque scaling or unevenness of tissues on the scalp, skin, or nails. The organisms grow and propagate rapidly in a warm, moist environment, and their abundant numbers may cause widespread irritation and desquamation of tissues in pressure areas. For example, tinea pedis, or "athlete's foot," can rapidly become irritated, itching, burning, and desquamated when continual wearing of sneakers causes persistent sweating of the feet in hot weather.

Systemic Fungal Infections

Fungi that become widely disseminated in the internal body tissues can cause the uncommon but important mycotic diseases *blastomycosis, coccidioidomycosis, cryptococcosis, histoplasmosis,* and *sporotrichosis.* The organisms become sequestered in body tissues and their eradication may require months or years of treatment. For example, blastomycosis may involve the skin, lungs, and bones; coccidioidomycosis, the lungs, skin, subcutaneous tissues, conjunctiva, and bones; cryptococcosis, the brain, skin, and lungs; histoplasmosis, the lungs, lymphatics, spleen, liver, heart, bone, and skin; and sporotrichosis, the lungs, mouth, conjunctiva, bones, joints, and muscles.

Dermal reaction tests may be done to determine whether the person has been exposed to fungi. Antibodies that are produced at the time of the exposure cause a positive test when the fungus tissue extract is injected into the intradermal tissues. Culturing of an infected tissue exudate is required to confirm the diagnosis. Although preliminary identification of the cultured organism may be available slightly earlier, final reports of the fungus growth and identification of the causative organism usually require a four-week incubation period.

PROTOZOAL INFESTATIONS

The most common protozoal infestation is caused by *Trichomonas vaginalis*. The presence of the flagellate in the vagina or in the urethra of the male causes a persistent irritation and a white, frothy discharge. The persistent infection is readily transmitted between sexual partners and the organism may invade the extravaginal or extraurethral tissues, glands, or ducts. The organism can be identified by microscopic examination of fresh smears made from vaginal tissue scrapings or from the prostatic fluid obtained from the male.

Intestinal Amebiasis

Entamoeba histolytica is the protozoa that infests the human intestine, and the disease is called amebiasis. The amebic cysts enter the body through the mouth with food or other items (Fig. 17–1). The cysts are dissolved in the small intestine and that process releases the vegetative ameba, or *trophozoite*.

Amebae digest a small segment of tissue to form a cavity in the intestinal wall where they reproduce and colonize. The availability of food residue in the intestine and proteins from the intestinal wall facilitates their growth. Their periodic reproduction of quadrinucleated cysts and the excretion of those cysts with the feces maintain the ameba transmission route between humans. The cysts in the stools provide the evidence of amebiasis that is essential for specific therapy for eradication of the parasite. Amebae sometimes remain as harmless parasites within the intestinal lumen, and the asymptomatic per-

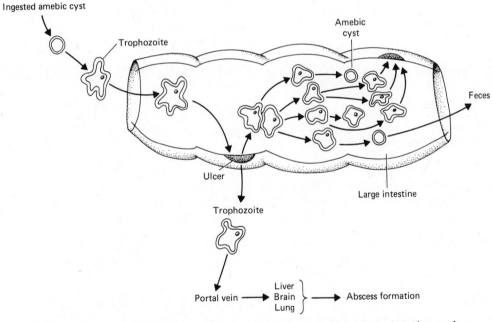

Fig. 17–1. The wall of the amebic cyst is digested by enzymes in the intestine, and that action liberates the trophozoite. The digestion of proteins in the intestinal wall by the ameba causes ulceration. Reproduction of trophozoites increases the numbers of intestinal parasites. Some of the amebae penetrate the intestinal wall and travel to other organs. The cysts, which are formed periodically, are excreted with the feces.

son's intestine may be a reservoir for the formation of cysts that are excreted with the feces.

Amebiasis is a chronic health problem that periodically causes intestinal disturbances, weight loss, and generalized muscle aching. Extensive irritation of the colon can cause debilitating amebic dysentery. The propulsive movements of the intestinal wall cause bleeding, and there may be perforation at the sites of the deepest ulcerations.

Extraintestinal Amebiasis

Trophozoites may penetrate the intestinal wall and travel through the portal venous circulation to hepatic sites. Their erosion of hepatic tissues causes ulceration and abscess formation. The activity of the amebae gradually disrupts liver function. Symptoms of hepatitis may provide the earliest evidence of their presence. The parasites may also invade pulmonary or brain tissues but the liver is the most common site of extraintestinal amebiasis.

HELMINTH INFESTATION

Intestinal Helminthiasis

Pinworms, hookworms, and tapeworms are the helminths most frequently found in the human intestine. The parasites propagate in the intestine. Their movement from those tissues is blocked by the immunoglobin G, complement, and eosinophil activity that is stimulated by the presence of the foreign protein outside of the intestinal lumen.

Pinworms. There are approximately 20 million cases of pinworms in the United States each year. *Enterobius vermicularis,* or pinworm, infestation often is annoying but it is relatively innocous.

The eggs are readily transmitted from one child to another during their many sharing activities (i.e., gum, food, toys). The eggs hatch in the duodenum and the larvae travel to the large intestine where they become sexually mature worms within 35 days. The female worm emerges from the colon during the night to lay eggs in the anal skin folds. That activity causes anal irritation, and the restlessness and sleep disturbance of the child are often the first indication that there is a worm infestation.

The worms that emerge from the anal area may enter the urethra and migrate to the bladder of females. The *Escherichia coli* that the worm carries into the bladder can cause cystitis.

The emerging worms can be seen at night with a flashlight that is directed at the anus when the child is restless. A transparent strip of cellophane tape can be utilized to collect the eggs, which are readily identified under a microscope.

Hookworms. *Necator americanus* and *Ancylostoma duodenale* infestations occur after the larvae enter the skin. They cause a severe pruritic eruption at the cutaneous site of entry (i.e., soles of the feet). The larvae enter the circulation and travel to the lungs. They migrate across the pulmonary capillary bed and travel through the lungs to the tracheobronchial structures. When they enter the esophagus, they migrate through the digestive tract to the jejunum.

The parasites feed on the blood they obtain by biting into the tissues. The blood loss becomes significant as the worms multiply and the person with the worm infestation gradually becomes anemic. The public health regulation that shoes be worn in stores is directed at decreasing the transmission of hookworms.

Tapeworms. Tapeworm infestations are caused by *Diphyllobothrium latum,* or fish tapeworm; *Hymenolepis nana,* or dwarf tapeworm; *Taenia saginata,* or beef tapeworm; and *Taenia solium,* or pork tapeworm. The head, or *scolex,* of the worms has hooks or suckers that allow the worm to attach to the wall of the intestine. Although the attachment site on the intestinal wall may become inflamed or infected, there may be no evidence of the infestation until the food ingested by the worm reduces the nutrient absorption from the intestine of the host.

The free larvae (cysticerci) of *Taenia solium* may travel to extraintestinal sites, and their invasion and propagation can disrupt the function of the invaded organ.

Extraintestinal Helminthiasis

Infestations by flukes and their larvae can disrupt the function of the tissues that are invaded by the parasites. *Clonorchis sinensis,* or liver flukes, propagate in the intestine and invade the biliary structures. They feed on the blood from the wall of the structures where they attach. When they increase in numbers, they can obstruct the bile ducts. *Schistosoma haematobium* and *S. mansoni,* or blood flukes, and *Paragonimus westermani* and *P. kellicotti,* or lung flukes, produce larvae that are difficult to eradicate from the tissues.

PLASMODIA INFESTATION

Plasmodium vivax is the organism that most frequently causes *benign tertian malaria.* More rarely, *P. ovale* causes a milder tertian malaria. *P. vivax* reproduction occurs in the red blood cells and exoerythrocyte tissues. *P. falciparum* causes *pernicious malignant tertian malaria.* The reproduction cycle of *P. falciparum* occurs in the erythrocytes. *P. malariae* causes a quartian malaria that may be latent for many years.

Malaria is a worldwide health problem that causes illness and death in a large segment of the world population. Persons who travel to areas where the disease is prevalent are given drugs to provide *causal prophylaxis.* The term is employed to describe the plan for the drug to intercede at primary tissue sites to eradicate the organism before it begins its reproduction cycle.

Plasmodium Life-Cycle

The infected female *anopheles* mosquito deposits the *Plasmodium sporozoite* when she bites an individual. That sporozoite travels to the liver where it begins the *trophozoite-schizont-* *merozoite* reproduction cycle that later is repeated in the red blood cells (Fig. 17–2). The *trophozoites* are large, solid multinucleated cells. The division of their nuclei leads to the production of several nucleated structures, or *schizonts,* within the walls of the trophozoites. When the schizonts are released at the time of the trophozoite rupture, they have developed to asexual *merozoites* that enter the red blood cells to repeat the reproduction cycle. Their proliferation in the blood cells causes the cells to rupture and the merozoites enter other erythrocytes. Schizonts periodically produce sexual *gametocytes* that may be withdrawn with blood when a female *anopheles* mosquito bites the infected person. The unbridled reproduction continues until cellular semi-immunity develops in the untreated host.

Benign Tertian Malaria

The benign tertian malaria that is caused by *P. vivax* is characterized by symptoms that occur at regular 48-hour intervals. The cyclic occurrence of chills, fever, headache, muscle aching, and gastrointestinal disturbances is associated with the release of metabolic and erythrocyte products during the period of merozoite release from the red blood cells and exoerythrocyte tissues.

Pernicious Malignant Tertian Malaria

The pernicious malignant tertian malaria caused by *P. falciparum* is characterized by an acute hemolytic state and the release of copious erythrocyte products that form emboli and occlude small blood vessels. The rapid destruction of red blood cells causes anemia, and a shock state may occur within hours. Phagocytes ingest some of the hemoglobin pigments that are released from the ruptured erythrocytes. The pigments that enter the blood cause jaundice, hemoglobinemia, and hemoglobinuria. Excess pigments in the urine cause a reddish black discoloration ("blackwater" fever). Acute renal failure occurs as a consequence of the deposition of the pigments in the tubules. Pernicious malignant tertian

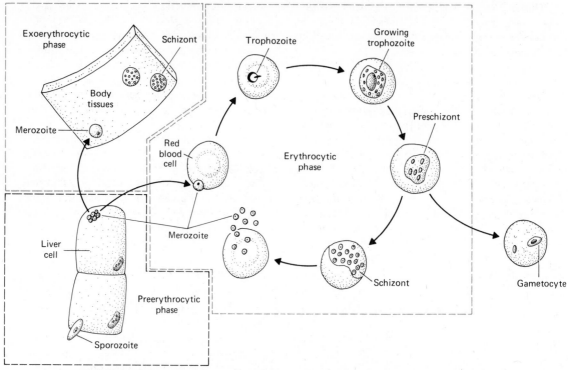

Fig. 17–2. The reproductive cycle of the malarial plasmodium *P. falciparum* takes place in the red blood cells. The cycle of *P. vivax* involves an erythrocyte and an exoerythrocyte phase. The development of merozoites in the cells causes their rupture, and the plasmodia enter other blood cells. Gametocytes that are released by the schizonts provide the reproductive cells that are removed when a mosquito bites the infected person.

malaria is a medical emergency that requires antimalarial therapy, heparinization to decrease clot formation, and the immediate treatment of shock, renal failure, and anemia.

Antifungal Drugs

The drugs that are employed for the control of widely disseminated fungal infections are administered parenterally. Infections in the gastrointestinal tract or external tissues can be treated with drugs that are administered orally or topically to the tissues that are infected by fungi. The oral systemically absorbed antifungal drugs are sometimes administered concurrently with topical agents to facilitate the eradication of the fungi.

DRUGS USED FOR SYSTEMIC INFECTIONS

The drugs that are employed for the control of the systemic mycotic infections are *amphoteri-*

cin B and *flucytosine*. The drugs are utilized for the eradication of the serious and persistent infections caused by fungi.

Amphotericin B (FUNGIZONE)

The drug is a fungistatic antibiotic that is clinically effective in the control of infections caused by *Aspergillus fumigatus, Blastomyces dermatitidis, Coccidioides immitis, Cryptococcus neoformans, Histoplasma capsulatum, Mucor mucedo, Paracoccidioides brasiliensis, Rhodotorula,* and *Sporothrix schenckii.* It is also used for the control of systemic infections caused by *Candida albicans, C. guilliermondi,* and *C. tropicalis.*

Action Mode. The drug binds to the sterols of the fungal cell membrane and that action produces a detergent-like effect that weakens the membrane. The increased permeability of the cell membrane allows leaking of the potassium and other intracellular constituents. The concurrent action of the drug on sterol-containing membranes of normal body cells (i.e., erythrocytes, renal cells) contributes to some of the adverse effects that occur during therapy with the drug.

Therapy Considerations. Amphotericin B is administered intravenously for the treatment of systemic fungal infections. The initial daily dosage of the drug is based on the calculation of 250 mcg/kg of body weight and that dose is infused over a six-hour period. The daily dosage is gradually increased to a maximum level that is calculated on the basis of 1 mg/kg of body weight. The use of a large vein and a scalp-vein needle for the infusion decreases the incidence of pain, phlebitis, or thrombophlebitis that is caused by the irritating effects of the drug.

The drug solution deteriorates rapidly when it is exposed to light. The bottle of solution and the tubing that is used for the infusion are covered with brown paper, aluminum foil, or another opaque material to protect the drug solution from exposure to light.

The patient usually is hospitalized during the initial treatment period. During the many months that are required for eradication of the fungus infection, the person may receive the intravenous infusion daily, or on alternate days, in an ambulatory care facility.

Approximately 10 percent of the circulating drug is bound to plasma proteins. Minimal quantities of the drug cross the blood-brain barrier, and the drug is administered intrathecally when the fungus infection involves the meninges. The cerebrospinal fluid circulation of the drug provides a therapeutic effect on the infected central nervous system tissues. The drug is taken up by the arachnoid villi. Some of the drug is thought to be retained in the extracellular fluids of the brain, which serve as a reservoir for the drug.

The elimination half-life of the drug is 18 to 24 hours. Approximately 40 percent of a single dose of the drug is excreted in the urine over a seven-day period.

Adverse Effects. There is a high incidence of adverse effects during intravenous therapy with amphotericin B. Almost 50 percent of the patients have headache, shaking chills, and body temperatures up to 40.5° C (104.9° F). The temperature elevation usually occurs within one to two hours after the intravenous infusion is started and it subsides about four hours after the infusion is completed. The elevations gradually become less pronounced during subsequent daily intravenous therapy. The administration of antipyretics and the use of an automatic hypothermia blanket usually are planned to control the problems and allow continuation of therapy.

Malaise, muscle and joint pain, weight loss, and gastrointestinal disturbances (i.e., nausea, vomiting, anorexia, abdominal cramping, epigastric pain, dyspepsia) are also common problems during therapy with amphotericin B. Symptomatic therapy usually is planned (i.e., antiemetics, analgesics), and alternate-day therapy sometimes is employed to reduce the incidence of the problems. Anaphylactic reactions rarely occur during therapy with the antibiotic.

Nephrotoxicity is often a dose-limiting factor. Approximately 75 percent of the patients who receive the drug have a gradual decrease in renal function. The lysis of the steroid-containing renal tubular cells and the direct vasoconstricting action of the drug are primary factors in the gradual disruption of kidney function. Hypokalemia and the output of a dilute urine with a low specific gravity precede the retention of nitrogenous products, which indicates that there is decreased tubule function. The blood urea nitrogen (BUN) and serum creatinine levels are evaluated daily during the time the dosage is being increased and weekly throughout the entire course of therapy to allow early identification of renal tubule dysfunction. When the BUN is higher than 40 mg/100 ml or the serum creatinine level exceeds 3 mg/100 ml, the drug dosage may be reduced or therapy may be interrupted to allow time for the return of renal function.

Most of the patients who receive the drug have muscle weakness that is associated with hypokalemia. The use of potassium supplements or the addition of potassium-rich foods to the diet may avert the problem. Intravenous administration of potassium chloride may be necessary when the patient is nauseated. The serum magnesium levels occasionally may be low during therapy. The serum potassium and magnesium levels are evaluated at least once a week during the entire course of treatment.

The reversible normocytic, normochromic anemia that appears during therapy is related to the action of the drug on the sterols in the cell membrane of developing red blood cells. Intrathecal administration of the drug can cause headache, nausea, vomiting, urine retention, transient paresis, paresthesias, pain in the back, legs, or abdomen, and vision changes.

Flucytosine (ANCOBON)

The drug is employed for the control of fungal infections that are caused by *Cryptococcus neoformans, Candida albicans,* and *C. tropicalis.* Other organisms that have shown sensitivity to the drug include strains of *Aspergillus, Clado-* *sporium, Phialophora, Torulopsis,* and *Sporothrix.*

Action Mode. The drug enters the fungal cell where it is deaminated to the antimetabolite *fluorouracil.* That antimetabolite interferes with fungal protein synthesis by competing with uracil during the metabolism of pyrimidines.

Therapy Considerations. The dosage of the oral capsules for adults and children weighing more than 50 kg (110 lb) is calculated on the basis of 50 to 150 mg/kg of body weight per day, divided for administration at six-hour intervals. The dosage for children who weigh less than 50 kg is calculated on the basis of 1.5 to 4.5 gm/M^2 body surface area per day.

The oral drug is absorbed well from the gastrointestinal tract and peak serum drug levels are attained within six hours after a single dose of the drug is taken. The peak serum drug levels are attained within two hours when the drug has been taken regularly for a period of four days. The drug is distributed widely in body tissues and fluids. It enters the ocular fluids. The concentrations in the cerebrospinal fluid are 60 to 100 percent of the serum drug concentration. Approximately 50 percent of the circulating drug is bound to serum proteins. The elimination half-life of the drug is about three hours. Approximately 90 percent of the unchanged drug is excreted in the urine, and the urinary concentrations of the drug may be 10 to 100 times those of the serum.

Adverse Effects. The toxic effects of the drug on rapidly proliferating gastrointestinal tissues and bone marrow are the same as those that occur when fluoracil is employed for antineoplastic drug therapy. The toxic effects on the tissues of the gastrointestinal tract produce nausea, vomiting, anorexia, diarrhea, and gaseous distention of the intestines. Bone marrow hypoplasia that is produced by the drug causes anemia, leukopenia, pancytopenia, and thrombocytopenia. Drug therapy may be interrupted to allow tissue repair when diarrhea or leukopenia occurs.

Other adverse effects that may appear during therapy with flucytosine include confusion, hallucinations, headaches, sedation, vertigo, and liver enlargement. The seriousness of the adverse effects is the rationale for the frequent-interval evaluation of hematologic values and liver enzyme studies (i.e., SGOT, SGPT) during therapy with the drug.

DRUGS USED FOR LOCALIZED INFECTIONS

Griseofulvin is administered orally for the control of fungus infections of superficial tissues (i.e., skin, hair, nails). *Nystatin* is administered orally for the control of fungus infections in the oral cavity or in the gastrointestinal tract. Several drugs are employed topically for the control of fungus infections of the skin or the mucous membranes of the vagina or anal areas.

Griseofulvin

The drug is a fungistatic antibiotic employed for the control of mycotic infections caused by *Epidermophyton, Microsporum,* or *Trichophyton* (i.e., tinea barbae, tinea capitis, tinea corporis, tinea cruris, tinea pedis, and tinea unguium).

Action Mode. The drug disrupts the mitotic spindle structure during the reproduction of the cell. That action arrests the cell division in the metaphase. Griseofulvin is deposited in keratin cells and fungi are unable to invade, grow, or reproduce in the drug-containing cells.

Therapy Considerations. Microsize griseofulvin (FULVICIN-U/F, GRISACTIN, GRISOWEN) is available as capsules, as tablets, or as an oral suspension. The usual adult dosage is 0.5 to 1 gm/day. The daily pediatric dosage is based on the calculation of 10 to 12.5 mg/kg of body weight.

The drug is also available as *ultramicrosize griseofulvin* (GRIS-PEG). The adult dosage of ultramicrosize griseofulvin is 250 to 500 mg/day. The daily pediatric dosage is calculated on the basis of 5 mg/kg of body weight.

The course of therapy is continued until cultures indicate the absence of fungi and new keratinized tissue has replaced the infected tissue. The eradication of tinea capitis may require four to six weeks of therapy; tinea corporis, two to four weeks; tinea pedis, four to eight weeks; and tinea unguium, more than three to four months to eradicate the fungus from the fingernails and more than six months to eradicate it from the toenails.

Ultramicrosize griseofulvin is absorbed almost completely from the duodenum, but only 25 to 70 percent of the microsize griseofulvin is absorbed. Peak serum levels of the drug are attained within four to eight hours after the drug is taken. There is an indication that the intake of a high-fat meal at the time that the microsize griseofulvin is taken can increase the intestinal absorption rate of the drug.

The absorbed drug is concentrated in the skin, hair, nails, liver, fat, and skeletal muscles. It can be found in the stratum corneum soon after it is taken. Within two days after therapy is terminated, there is no detectable drug in the skin. The concentrations of the drug are higher in the outer horny layers than in the deeper layers of the skin. That reverse concentration of the drug, which is delivered to the skin by the internal circulation, is thought to be related to the dissolution of the drug in perspiration and the subsequent deposition of the drug on the horny layers when the perspiration evaporates.

The drug is metabolized primarily in the liver. The elimination half-life of the drug is 9 to 21 hours. The inactive metabolites of the drug are excreted in the urine and in perspiration.

Adverse Effects. Headache, which may be severe, frequently occurs in the initial days of therapy but tends to occur less frequently when therapy is continued. Other adverse effects include excessive thirst and gastrointestinal disturbances (i.e., epigastric discomfort, nausea, vomiting, flatulence, diarrhea). Allergic reactions that may occur during the period of therapy are skin rashes, urticaria, and photosensitivity reactions. Large doses of the drug occasionally cause mental confusion and psychotic symptoms. Periodic evaluations of blood values are planned during therapy because there have been reports of leukopenia.

Drug Interactions. Concurrent use of alcohol can cause tachycardia and flushing associated with the vasodilation effects of each drug. The barbiturates induce the hepatic microcomal enzymes, and that action accelerates the metabolism of griseofulvin when the drugs are used concurrently. The introduction of griseofulvin into the drug therapy plan of a patient who is receiving warfarin may decrease the person's prothrombin times.

Nystatin (MYCOSTATIN, NILSTAT)

The drug is an antifungal antibiotic. It is employed for the control of infections in the oral cavity or intestinal tract that are caused by *Candida albicans*.

Action Mode. The drug binds with the sterols in the fungal cell membrane. That action causes a detergent-like effect that increases the permeability of the membrane and allows leaking of the intracellular content.

Therapy Considerations. The drug is available as tablets and as a suspension. It is also available in capsules and suspensions in combination with tetracyclines.

Nystatin is administered orally for the treatment of intestinal infections in dosages that range from 1.5 to 3 million units/day. That dosage is divided for administration three times per day. Infants with severe infections in the diaper area may be given 400,000 units/day, divided for administration four times per day. Concurrent topical application of nystatin cream or ointment may be planned to hasten the control of the fungal infection.

The daily dosage of the oral suspension for adults or children who have a fungal infection in the oral cavity is 1.6 to 2.4 million units, and the daily dosage for infants is 0.8 million units/day. The daily dosage is divided for administration four times per day. At the time of each treatment, the dosage is divided, and one half the dose is placed in each side of the mouth where it is retained for several minutes before it is swallowed. The treatments are continued for at least 48 hours after the cultures of the tissues are negative.

The oral formulations are absorbed in minimal amounts from the intestinal tract. Nystatin is not absorbed from the intact skin or mucous membranes.

Adverse Effects. The low absorption rate of the drug limits its adverse effects. Mild and transient nausea, vomiting, and diarrhea occasionally occur. Allergic reactions rarely appear during therapy with nystatin.

Topical Antifungal Drugs

Amphotericin B. The drug is available as a 3 percent cream, lotion, or ointment for topical application in the control of cutaneous or mucocutaneous infections that are caused by *Candida albicans*. The topical formulation is applied to the affected areas two to four times per day. Whenever possible, the affected areas are kept dry and exposed to maintain an environment that is unfavorable to the growth of the fungi.

Hygienic measures (i.e., cleansing of the affected area, hand washing) are an important aspect of the therapy. Those measures are also essential to prevent reinfection by *Candida* from the intestinal tract after the initial infection is eradicated. The treatment may be continued for one to four weeks before the infection is cleared from cutaneous sites, and it may take several months for eradication of the infection from the nails.

The lotion, ointment, or cream may cause erythema, pruritus, or a burning sensation at the site of its application. The topical preparations may discolor the skin and fabrics. The stains that are made by the cream or ointment on fabrics may be removed by using cleaning fluid, and those made by the lotion may be removed by washing the fabric with warm water and soap.

Nystatin. The drug is available as creams, ointment, powder, or as vaginal suppositories for the treatment of infections caused by *Candida albicans.* The creams, ointments, and otic suspension contain nystatin in combination with corticosteroids or antibacterial agents. The cream or the ointment is used for the treatment of dry areas that are infected and the powder is used for moist or wet areas.

The vaginal suppositories are inserted high in the vagina one or two times per day for the control of vulvovaginal infections. The treatment is continued during menstruation. Use of the suppositories for three to six weeks prior to delivery may prevent transmission of the maternal vaginal infection to the infant during its passage through the birth canal.

Other Antifungal Drugs. Vulvovaginal *Candida* infections may be treated with *candicidin*

(CANDEPTIN) cream ointment, or vaginal tablets or capsules, *clotrimazole* (GYNE-LOTRIMIN) vaginal tablets, or *miconazole nitrate* (MONISTAT 7) vaginal cream. Instructions about the use of the drugs should include hygienic measures and the necessity for consistent treatment until the infection is controlled. Approximately 7.5 percent of the patients have vulvovaginal itching, burning, or irritation in the first week of therapy.

The dermatophytes may be treated by the topical application of clotrimazole (LOTRIMIN) cream or solution, *haloprogin* (HALOTEX) cream or solution, *miconazole nitrate* (MICATIN) cream, or *tolnaftate* (TINACTIN) cream, powder, or solution. Many over-the-counter preparations also are used by persons who have fungal infections. Complete eradication of the fungi from the infected tissues requires prolonged and consistent therapy. The end point of the treatment is the desquamation of infected tissue and the growth of new noninfected keratinized tissue. When patients understand that tissue change as being the therapy end point, they may continue the treatment. Many persons stop using the drug when the discomfort is relieved.

Antiparasitic Drugs

The drugs employed for the control of parasites include the *antiprotozoal drugs,* which are used for the control of ameba or *trichomonal* infestations; the *antihelminth drugs,* which are used for the control of worm infestations; the *antiplasmodial drugs,* which are used for the control of malaria; and the *scabicides* and *pediculicides.*

ANTIPROTOZOAL DRUGS

Amebiasis is a persistent health problem throughout the world. Approximately 10 percent of the American population have ameba infestations. Amebiasis occurs when the amebic cyst is ingested with foods or from other articles that are put into the mouth.

The drugs that are employed for the control of ameba infestations in the intestine are *diiodo-*

hydroxyquin, carbazone, and *paramomycin.* The antibiotics *tetracycline, chlortetracycline,* and *oxytetracycline* sometimes are used to decrease the bacterial flora of the intestine thereby decreasing the food supply of the ameba.

The drugs employed for the treatment of intestinal and extraintestinal amebiasis are *metronidazole* and *emetine. Metronidazole* and the trichomonicidal drug *furazolidone* are employed for the treatment of infestations of the genital tract by the protozoa *Trichomonas vaginalis.*

Diiodohydroxyquin (DIODOQUIN, MOEBIQUIN, YODOXIN)

The drug is an iodine-containing preparation (64 percent iodine) that is a direct-acting amebicide. It is effective in the elimination of trophozoites from the intestine, and that action leads to the elimination of amebic cysts. The exact mode of its action on the plasmodia is unknown.

Therapy Considerations. The drug is administered orally and insignificant amounts of the dose are absorbed from the gastrointestinal tract. The usual daily dosage for adults and children over nine years of age is 1.89 to 1.95 gm, divided for administration three times per day after meals. The dosage for children nine years of age or younger is based on the calculation of 35 to 40 mg/kg/day, divided for administration two to three times per day after meals. The drug is usually given for a three-week period, and that course of therapy may be repeated after a two-to-three-week drug-free interval when cysts are present in the feces.

The drug is used for the treatment of asymptomatic carriers and has been employed for the mass treatment or prophylaxis of persons in countries where amebiasis is prevalent. The total daily dosage may be taken at one time when the drug is used prophylactically.

Adverse Effects. Symptoms of iodism occasionally may occur (i.e., acne, rash, sore throat, rhinitis, headache, chills, fever). The problems occur most frequently in persons who have iodine intolerance. Diarrhea, constipation, transitory abdominal cramps, anal pruritus, lethargy, or an increased sense of warmth occasionally occurs during therapy.

Carbarsone

The drug is an organic arsenical that contains 28 percent arsenic. It is effective in the control of trophozoites in the intestinal lumen and in the wall ulcerations. The mode of action has not been identified.

Therapy Considerations. Carbarsone is administered orally or as a retention enema solution. The daily oral dosage for adults is 500 to 750 mg, divided for administration two to three times per day. The oral dosage for children is calculated on the basis of 75 mg/kg of body weight for the total treatment course of ten days. The daily dosage is divided for administration three times per day. The initial ten-day course of treatment may be repeated after a 10-to-14-day drug-free period when cysts are found in the feces. The person usually is advised to maintain a light diet and to modify activity during the course of treatment. The oral drug is readily absorbed from the gastrointestinal tract but is excreted slowly in the urine.

The retention enema is utilized when deep ulcerative lesions persist in the lower colon. A solution of 500 ml of 2 percent sodium bicarbonate is given as a cleansing enema, and the drug solution of 2 gm carbasone in 200 ml of 2 percent sodium bicarbonate is then given as a retention enema. The enema is given on alternate evenings until five doses have been administered.

Adverse Effects. The drugs can produce serious adverse effects that include vomiting, increased diarrhea, pulmonary congestion, neuritis, pruritus, rash, hepatitis, splenomegaly, and albuminuria. Therapy is terminated when those adverse effects appear. There also have been reports of fatal exfoliative dermatitis and hepatic necrosis. The drug is used infrequently because of the toxic effects that occur during therapy.

Paromomycin (HUMATIN)

The drug is an antibiotic employed for its direct amebicidal action in the intestinal tract. The drug is poorly absorbed from the gastrointestinal tract and almost 100 percent of the drug is excreted in the feces.

Therapy Considerations. The drug is administered orally three times a day with meals. The daily dosage for children and adults who have intestinal amebiasis is based on the calculation of 25 to 35 mg/kg of body weight. Treatment is usually continued for a period of five to ten days.

Adverse Effects. The most common adverse effects of the drug are nausea, abdominal cramps, and diarrhea. When a high dosage is required for the treatment of resistant infestations, the drug may cause severe diarrhea and abdominal cramps. A few patients have heartburn, vomiting, headache, skin rash, or anal pruritus. The drug-induced suppression of the normal intestinal flora may produce a suprainfection with *Candida albicans,* which can become the dominant intestinal organism.

Metronidazole (FLAGYL)

The drug is employed primarily for the treatment of infestations that are caused by *Entamoeba histolytica* and *Trichomonas vaginalis.* It is a direct amebicide that is active in the control of ameba trophozoites in the intestinal lumen, intestinal wall, and extraintestinal sites. Metronidazole also is active in the vaginal secretions and semen, and that activity provides a trichomonicidal effect when the drug is taken by the sexual partners. The mode of action has not been identified.

Therapy Considerations. The usual daily adult dosage of the oral tablets for the treatment of acute intestinal amebiasis is 2.25 gm and the dosage for the treatment of amebic liver abscess is 1.5 to 2.25 gm/day. The daily oral dosage is divided for administration three times per day for a period of five to ten days.

The daily dosage for children with acute intestinal amebiasis or amebic liver abscess is based on the calculation of 35 to 50 mg/kg of body weight. That dosage is divided for administration three times per day for ten days.

The oral dosage for women who have a trichomonal infestation of the urogenital tract is 750 mg/day for a seven-day period. The total daily dosage is divided for use three times per day. The same dosage is taken by the sexual partner during the same time period.

The initial course of oral drug therapy may be repeated after a drug-free period of four to six weeks when the infestation is refractory to treat-

ment. The female may have vaginal itching, burning, or dryness and urethral discomfort while taking the oral drug.

The oral drug is well absorbed from the small intestine. Effective serum drug concentrations are attained within one to three hours after the drug is ingested orally and those levels persist for 12 hours. Approximately 30 to 40 percent of the drug is metabolized in the liver. The drug crosses the placental barrier.

The metabolites and the unchanged drug are excreted in the urine. The metabolites sometimes produce a dark or reddish-brown discoloration of the urine. Some of the drug appears in glandular secretions and the drug concentration in the milk of nursing mothers is similar to that of their serum concentration.

Metronidazole initially was the drug of choice for the control of ameba and *Trichomonas* infestations. There is increasing evidence of the emergence of organisms that are resistant to the effects of the drug and that may limit its use for some patients. It has also caused carcinogenicity in animal studies, and the labels carry the warning message to alert patients to the potential problem in humans.

Adverse Effects. The most common adverse effects are gastrointestinal disturbances (i.e., anorexia, nausea, vomiting, epigastric distress, abdominal cramps, diarrhea, constipation). The person may complain of a metallic, sharp, and unpleasant taste and dryness of the mouth during therapy with the drug. A furry tongue, glossitis, stomatitis, dizziness, vertigo, or ataxia may occur occasionally. Rashes, urticaria, or suprainfections with fungi also may occur during therapy. Mild leukopenia has been reported during therapy with metronidazole.

Persons should be cautioned against drinking alcoholic beverages during the time that they are taking the drug because the ingestion of alcohol may produce abdominal distress, nausea, vomiting, or headache. Those symptoms and the altered taste of the alcohol that occurs are similar to the effects of disulfiram (ANTABUSE), which is utilized by alcoholics as a deterrent to drinking.

Emetine Hydrochloride

The drug is a direct amebicide that is employed for the treatment of amebic dysentery, amebic hepatitis, and amebic abscesses of the liver or other organs that are invaded by the protozoa. It is used in combination with other drugs (i.e., diiodohydroxyquin) that destroy the amebic cysts because it is ineffective in penetrating the cysts.

Action Mode. Emetine causes degeneration of the nucleus of the ameba and reticulation of the ameba cytoplasm. The high concentrations of the drug that are attained in the liver tissues facilitate the eradication of the ameba at those sites.

Therapy Considerations. Emetine hydrochloride is administered by deep subcutaneous or intramuscular injection for a period of four to six days for the treatment of acute amebiasis. Regional myositis with aching, stiffness, tenderness, and weakness often occurs as a local reaction to the injections. The maximum dosage level for adults is 60 mg/day. The maximum dosage for children over eight years of age is 20 mg/day and that for children younger than eight years of age is 10 mg/day. The four-to-six-day course of treatment may be repeated after a one-month period when the infestation persists.

Larger quantities of the drug and a longer course of therapy are required for the treatment of hepatic amebic infestations. Adults may receive 60 mg/day for a period of nine days. That course of treatment may be repeated after a drug-free period of one week. The second course of therapy is usually six days in length.

The drug is slowly absorbed from the subcutaneous injection site. It is slowly excreted in the urine and traces of the drug may be found in the urine 40 to 60 days after therapy is terminated.

Adverse Effects. The slow excretion rate of the drug causes its accumulation, and there is a higher incidence of adverse effects during repeat courses of therapy. Up to 75 percent of the patients who receive the drug have adverse effects. The drug produces cellular degeneration in the hepatic, cardiac, intestinal, renal, and skeletal muscle tissues. Therapy is terminated when toxic effects appear.

The most serious and frequent adverse effects are cardiovascular problems that may include hypotension, arrhythmias, precordial pain, dyspnea, tachycardia, and cardiac dilation. Congestive heart failure occasionally occurs. The patients are confined to bed during the treatment and for several days after the course of treatment to reduce the incidence of adverse effects and to allow frequent monitoring of the cardiovascular status (i.e., blood pressure, heart rate, electrocardiographic changes). Other adverse effects that may occur during or following the course of therapy include nausea, vomiting, diarrhea, vertigo, dizziness, severe skeletal muscle weakness, and eczematous, urticarial, or purpural areas on the skin surfaces.

Furazolidone (FUROXONE)

The drug is available as vaginal suppositories and as a powder insufflate for the treatment of vaginal infestations by *Trichomonas vaginalis*. The formulations also contain the antifungal agent *nifuroxine* (TRICOFURON).

The therapy involves concurrent use of the suppositories and the powder. The suppositories are inserted into the vagina at night and in the morning for a one-week period. The vaginal powder is used two times per week after the genitalia and vagina are cleansed and dried thoroughly. After the initial one-week period of therapy, the suppositories may be used before retiring every night including the time of menstruation. The end point of therapy is the time when the plasmodia are eradicated from the genital areas.

ANTIHELMINTH DRUGS

The drugs that are available for the control of helminth infestations are *mebendazole, gentian violet, piperazine, diethylcarbamazine citrate, pyrantel pamoate, pyrvinium pamoate, quinicrine hydrochloride,* and *thiabendazole.* When unusual worm infestations are identified, specific drugs for their control are obtained from the Center for Disease Control in Atlanta, Georgia. The formulary of the Parasitic Disease Drug Service at the Center lists the drugs that are approved by the Food and Drug Administration for use on an investigational basis.

Mebendazole (VERMOX)

The drug is employed for the control of infestations of the intestine by trichuriasis (whipworm), enterobiasis (pinworm), ascariasis (roundworm), or *Ancylostoma duodenale* and *Necator americanus* (hookworms). It produces egg reductions and cure rates in 90 percent of the persons who are treated for pinworm, roundworm, or hookworm infestations. When the drug is used for the eradication of whipworms, it produces a reduction in eggs in 90 percent and cure rate of 70 percent of the persons who are treated. Eradication of the whipworms and eggs in heavily infested persons occurs after two to three courses of treatment.

Action Mode. Mebendazole acts primarily by irreversibly inhibiting the uptake of carbohydrates and other nutrients by the helminths. That action slowly causes degenerative changes and nutritional death of the parasites. It may take up to three days to clear the intestine of the parasites.

Therapy Considerations. The drug is available as chewable tablets. The treatment of enterobiasis requires a single dosage of 100 mg for adults or children over two years of age. A dosage of 100 mg two times per day (i.e., morning and evening) is used for three consecutive days for adults or children over two years of age who have infestations with trichuriasis, ascariasis, or hookworms or when there is a mixed infestation of the helminths. When examination of the feces shows that ova remain in the intestine, a second course of therapy may be utilized after a three-to-four-week drug-free period.

A very small amount of the orally administered dose is absorbed from the intestine. Most of the unchanged drug and its metabolites are excreted in the urine within 72 hours.

Hygienic measures are an important aspect of the eradication of worm infestations. To prevent autoinfestation, the person should be advised to wash the hands thoroughly after toileting. The hand washing must include cleaning under the fingernails to assure the removal of worm eggs from those protected sites. The transmission of the worms from one individual to another can be reduced by the thorough washing of all foods that are not cooked before being eaten.

Adverse Effects. Diarrhea occasionally occurs during the course of therapy with mebendazole. When there is a massive worm infestation, the person may have a transient episode of propulsive diarrhea that expels large numbers of immobilized worms.

Gentian Violet

The drug paralyzes parasites by acting on their neuromuscular systems. Although it is effective in the control of pinworms, threadworms, and liver flukes, the gastrointestinal disturbances that frequently occur during therapy have led to the preferential use of newer drugs that cause fewer adverse effects.

Therapy Considerations. The daily dosage of the enteric-coated drug tablets for adults and children over 16 years of age is 150 mg, divided for administration three times per day before or after meals for a period of eight to ten days for the control of pinworm infestations; 16 to 18 days for threadworms; and 30 days for the control of liver flukes. The daily dosage for children 15 to 16 years of age is 250 mg; for children 12 to 14 years of age it is 200 mg; for children 9 to 11 years of age it is 150 mg; and for children six to eight years of age it is 100 mg. The daily dosage for children less than six years of age is calculated on the basis of 9.6 mg for each year of age to a maximum dosage of 90 mg. The dosage is divided for administration two to three times per day before or after meals, and the course of therapy, like that for adults, depends on the parasite infestation that is being treated.

Adverse Effects. Biting into the tablets can produce irritation and a deep purple stain on the oral tissues or fabrics that come into contact with the drug. The drug is available as a solution for administration to young children. Gastrointestinal disturbances that occur during therapy include mild nausea and abdominal pain, vomiting, and diarrhea.

Piperazine (ANTEPAR, MULTIFUGE, PIPERAVAL)

The drug is employed primarily for the control of infestations with pinworms or roundworms (*Ascaris lumbricoides*). A two-day course of treatment usually eliminates the infestation.

Action Mode. Piperazine paralyzes the musculature of the parasite, and the live but inactivated worms are expelled in the feces. The drug produces a curare-like effect by interfering with muscular receptor response to acetylcholine stimulation. It is thought to produce hyperpolarity of the muscle by altering the permeability of the cell membrane to the ions required for the maintenance of the resting potential.

Therapy Considerations. The drug is taken orally as a single daily dose for two consecutive days for the treatment of roundworms. The adult daily dosage is 3.5 gm. The daily dosage for children is based on the calculation of 75 mg/kg of body weight.

The drug is taken as a single daily dose for seven consecutive days for the treatment of pinworms. The daily oral dosage for adults or children is based on the calculation of 65 mg/kg of body weight to a maximum daily dosage of 2.5 gm. When examination of the feces reveals the presence of ova after the initial period of therapy, the course of therapy may be repeated after a one-week drug-free period.

Piperazine is absorbed from the gastrointestinal tract at a variable rate, and the unchanged drug is excreted in the urine. The drug is available as *piperazine citrate* or as *piperazine phosphate* tablets or syrup. The presence of food in the stomach or intestine does not affect the action of the drug.

Adverse Effects. The drug rarely produces adverse effects. Nausea, vomiting, diarrhea, or headache may occur in a few persons during therapy. The toxic effects that can occur with accidental overdose include neuromuscular problems (i.e., tremor, incoordination, generalized muscular weakness, vertigo, blurred vision), convulsions, and lapses of memory.

Diethylcarbamazine Citrate

The drug is employed primarily for the treatment of persons with bancroftian filariasis, Malayan filariasis, dipetalonemiasis, or loiasis. Diethylcarbamazine does not reverse the lymphangitis, which causes elephantiasis or hydrocele, but it may prevent further lymphatic involvement.

Action Mode. The specific action mode of the drug has not been defined. It is considered to sensitize the parasite's cuticle, which allows the phagocytic destruction of the helminth by the host's defense mechanisms. The absence of microfilariae during treatment with the drug suggests that the adult parasites are destroyed or sterilized.

Therapy Considerations. A lower initial dosage is usually employed to decrease the incidence of the allergic reactions that occur when large numbers of dying worms or their degradation products are released into the circulation. The initial daily dosage for adults and children is 2 mg/kg of body weight on the first day. The dosage may be based on the calculation of 4 mg/kg on the second day and of 6 mg/kg of body weight on each succeeding day throughout the three to four weeks of treatment required for filariasis, dipetalonemiasis, or loiasis. The daily dosage is divided for administration three times per day immediately after meals.

The drug is readily absorbed from the gastrointestinal tract. The circulating drug is distributed to all except the adipose tissues in the body. Approximately 95 percent of the oral dose is excreted as the metabolites in the urine within 30 hours.

Adverse Effects. Headache, malaise, weakness, and lassitude are the most frequent adverse effects. Other effects, which are usually mild and of short duration, include arthralgia, myalgia, nausea, vomiting, anorexia, skin rash, and dizziness. Allergic reactions to the proteins that are released by the dying worms are mild in bancroftian filariasis, more intense in Malayan filariasis, severe in loiasis, and very severe in onchocerciasis. Within a few hours after the initial dose of the drug is given, the symptoms appear (i.e., fever, sweating, headache, tachycardia, cough, tachypnea, nausea, vomiting, syncope, hypotension, rash, pruritus, urticaria, angioedema, lymphangitis). An elevation of the leukocyte and eosinophil counts provides evidence of the activity of the body's defense mechanisms in response to the protein release.

Pyrantel Pamoate (ANTIMINTH)

The drug frequently is employed for the treatment of persons who have infestations with roundworms or pinworms. The drug is highly effective in the control of those helminth infestations.

Action Mode. Pyrantel produces a selective and transient blockade of the neuromuscular transmission system of the animal. The depolarization of the muscles of the helminths causes a curare-like paralysis that allows their expulsion by the normal peristaltic activity of the host intestine.

Therapy Considerations. The drug is available as an oral suspension that is used in a single dose for the eradication of pinworm infestations. The drug is poorly absorbed from the gastrointestinal tract. The absorbed drug is rapidly metabolized and excreted in the urine.

The single dose for adults or children with pinworms is calculated on the basis of 11 mg/kg of body weight to a maximum total dose of 1 gm. The oral suspension may be administered with milk or fruit juice. The course of therapy may be repeated after a one-month drug-free period when the helminths remain in the intestine.

Adverse Effects. The most common adverse effects are gastrointestinal disturbances (i.e., nausea, vomiting, abdominal cramps, anorexia). Headache, dizziness, drowsiness, insomnia, or skin rash occasionally appears during therapy. There may also be a transient elevation of the serum glutamic oxalacetic transaminase levels (SGOT), which indicates irritation of the hepatic tissues. The mild adverse effects of the drug do not persist and seldom require symptomatic treatment.

Pyrivinium Pamoate (POVAN)

The drug is employed for the treatment of persons with infestations of pinworms. It is one of the most frequently used drugs for the control of pinworm infestations in children.

Action Mode. The drug is a cyanine dye that interferes with the absorption of the host's intestinal carbohydrate supplies by the helminths. That action leads to the nutritional death of the animal.

Therapy Considerations. A single dose of 5 mg/kg of body weight is taken by children or adults with pinworm infestations. That dosage is repeated after a period of two weeks to eliminate worms that have developed from ova.

Pyrivinium is a highly polar cyanine dye, and minimal amounts of the drug are absorbed from the gastrointestinal tract. The oral suspension may stain the clothing or other fabrics bright red if it is spilled. The tablets are swallowed without biting or chewing them to avoid the same red staining of the oral mucosa. Persons who take the oral suspension or tablets should be told that the stools will be bright red because of the presence of the drug.

Adverse Effects. Nausea, vomiting, or abdominal cramps may occur with large doses of the drug. There have been allergic reactions and a rare occurrence of photosensitivity.

Quinacrine Hydrochloride (ATABRINE)

The drug is an acridine dye that is employed as an alternate agent for the control of infestation with *Taenia saginata* (beef tapeworm) or *Diphyllobothrium lata* (fish tapeworm). Its use has been limited by the incidence of adverse effects that occur during antihelminth therapy.

The oral drug is readily absorbed from the intestine. It is distributed widely in body tissues and accumulates in the tissues when the drug continues to be taken. It is slowly liberated from those sites. The drug may be found in the urine for more than two months after therapy is terminated.

Therapy Considerations. The drug is taken orally after the pretreatment preparation provides a nearly empty gastrointestinal tract. A bland, semisolid, nonfat diet is eaten during the day before the drug is taken, and the person fasts after supper. A saline cathartic (i.e., magnesium sulfate) is given the evening before the antihelminth drug is to be taken. A cleansing enema may also be given before the treatment is started. Evacuation of the feces from the intestine reduces the amount of fecal material that must be examined for the scolex of the tapeworm after the drug is administered. The treatment is ineffective when the scolex is retained in the intestine because reproduction may be resumed by the animal.

The oral drug is given to the fasting adult or child over 14 years of age in the morning. Sodium bicarbonate (500 to 600 mg) may be given with each dose of quinacrine to decrease the incidence of nausea and vomiting. The total dosage of 800 mg may be divided for ingestion in four to eight doses that are taken at ten-minute intervals. The dividing of the dosage decreases the incidence of vomiting. The total dosage for children 11 to 14 years of age is 600 mg, and for those five to ten years of age it is 400 mg. Children may be given 300 mg of sodium bicarbonate with each of the three to four doses, which are given at ten-minute intervals.

A saline cathartic is given one to two hours after the drug is taken. The worm segments that are excreted are stained yellow by the drug, which facilitates identification of the scolex.

Adverse Effects. The large dosages of quinacrine that are required for the elimination of tapeworm infestations can cause a transient and benign toxic psychosis that may persist for two to four weeks. Headache, mild gastrointestinal disturbances, and dermatitis may also occur. Much of the drug is absorbed by the skin, and the acridine dye may cause a temporary yellowish coloration of the skin. The drug can precipitate a severe attack of psoriasis in persons with a history of psoriasis.

Thiabendazole (MINTEZOL)

The drug is employed primarily for the treatment of persons with infestations by *Strongyloides stercolaris* and the larvae of *Ancylostoma braziliense,* which cause "creeping eruption," or cutaneous larva migrans. Although the drug is known to inhibit some enzyme systems in the helminths, its exact mode of action is unknown.

Therapy Considerations. The drug is available as an oral suspension that is administered after meals. The dosage for adults and children who have enterobiasis infestations is based on the calculation of 50 mg/kg of body weight to a maximum dosage of 3 gm. That dosage is divided for administration in two doses on a single day of therapy. The same dosage is given seven days after the first treatment period. The dosage of thiabendazole for children weighing less than 15 kg has not been established.

The daily oral drug dosage for adults or children with cutaneous larva migrans is based on the same dosage calculation, but the drug is given for two successive days. A second course of therapy is used when the infestation persists after the initial two-day period of therapy. The drug is rapidly absorbed from the intestinal tract. Most of the drug is excreted in the urine within 24 hours.

Adverse Effects. The most frequent adverse effects are nausea, vomiting, anorexia, and dizziness. Less frequent effects include diarrhea, epigastric distress, abdominal cramping, headache, flushing, chills, drowsiness, and body odor. Fever, angioedema, pruritus, and rash also occur during therapy. Transient hepatic or bone marrow involvement is manifested as jaundice or leukopenia and may be dose related.

ANTIPLASMODIAL DRUGS

The incidence of malaria is related to the proliferation rate of the mosquito carriers that maintain the life-cycle of the plasmodia. Their rate of reproduction has increased with the recent limitations on broadcast spraying for pest control. In many countries the mosquitoes have developed resistance to insecticides. The plasmodia have developed resistance to some of the drugs that formerly were effective therapeutic agents.

Plasmodium Vulnerability to Drugs

The antimalarial drugs are employed to control the reproduction of the *Plasmodium* during its erythrocyte or exoerythrocyte cycle in man. Travelers to countries where the disease is endemic may receive the antimalarial drugs to provide *causal prophylaxis* or *suppressive prophylaxis* to reduce the risk of acquiring malaria. *Causal prophylaxis* is the term employed to describe the effects of the antimalarial drug that intercedes at primary tissue sites to prevent the invasion of the sporozoites or the initial merozoite invasion of the erythrocytes. *Suppressive prophylaxis* is provided by drugs that interfere early in the asexual red blood cell cycle for reproduction (Fig. 17–3).

The antimalarial drugs are also employed for the treatment of persons who have been exposed to the disease. They provide *suppressive cure* by their action during each erythrocyte reproduction cycle. Their use over a prolonged period of time progressively eradicates the plasmodia. *Clinical cure* describes the effects of the drugs that are used for the relief of symptoms when the person has an exacerbation of the disease. *Radical cure* is the term employed to describe the complete elimination of all plasmodia from the erythrocytes and from exoerythrocyte tissues.

The erythrocyte phase of malaria may be controlled by the synthetic antimalarial drugs that are known as the *4-aminoquinolines* and by *quinine*. By controlling the erythrocyte production cycle of *P. falciparum, P. vivax,* and *P. malariae,* the drugs provide suppressive prophylaxis and clinical cure of malaria. They provide radical cure of *P. falciparum,* but the absence of exoerythrocyte activity limits their use for the radical cure of *P. vivax* and *P. malariae* infections. The drugs also have a gamecyticidal action that prevents the transmission of the sexual forms of the malaria *Plasmodium* (except *P. falciparum*) by the mosquito that draws blood from an infected person.

Primaquine phosphate acts on the plasmodia at exoerythrocyte tissues, and that action provides causal prophylaxis and radical cure of *P. vivax* when the drug is used in high dosage. It provides protection against propagation of the *P. falciparum* sporozoites and gametocytes.

Pyrimethamine provides causal prophylaxis against *P. falciparum* and also provides slight causal prophylaxis against infestations caused by *P. vivax.* It provides suppressive prophylaxis against both *P. falciparum* and *P. vivax* and suppressive cure of malaria caused by *P. vivax.* The drug renders the gametocytes noninfective.

4-Aminoquinolines

The similarity in the chemical, pharmacologic, therapeutic, and adverse effects of the drugs al-

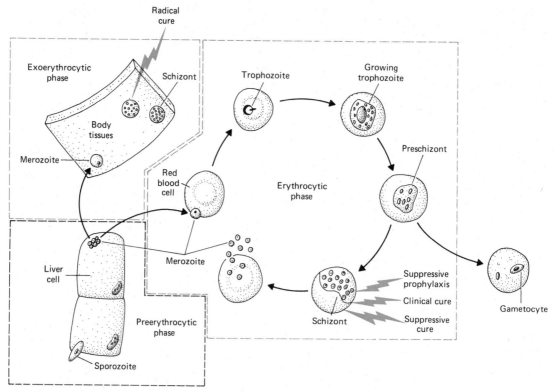

Fig. 17–3. The treatment of malaria is based on the vulnerability of the *Plasmodium* during the erythrocyte or exoerythrocyte phases of its life-cycle in man.

lows their discussion as a class, or group, of anti-malarial drugs. The drugs include *amodiaquine, chloroquine,* and *hydroxychloroquine.*

Action Mode. The drugs provide an anti-malarial effect by their interaction with *deoxyribonucleic acid* (DNA) during the plasmodial erythrocyte cycle. The drugs inhibit DNA polymerase and also affect the polymerase of *ribonucleic acid* (RNA). That action interferes with the reproduction of the plasmodium.

Therapy Considerations. When the drugs are administered for the treatment of acute malaria, their rapid action provides an afebrile state within 24 to 48 hours and the peripheral blood smears usually are negative within 48 to 72 hours. The drugs generally are taken orally with meals to decrease gastrointestinal irritation.

The 4-aminoquinolines frequently are employed to provide suppressive prophylaxis. The traveler to a country where the disease is endemic is protected when the drug is taken at weekly intervals for two weeks prior to entering the area, during the period of time that is spent in the area, and for eight weeks after leaving the area. Because regular use of the drug is important for prophylaxis, the traveler is advised to take the drug on a particular day of the week. That plan reduces the incidence of dosage omission during the period of exposure to the *Plasmodium.*

The drugs are absorbed rapidly and almost completely from the gastrointestinal tract within 30 to 60 minutes. The maximum plasma drug concentrations are attained within one to two hours after the drugs are ingested. The drugs are widely distributed in body tissues. Their high affinity for nucleoproteins provides tissue drug concentrations in the erythrocytes, brain, liver, spleen, kidney, and lungs that exceed those of the plasma. The drugs also accumulate in the eye by selectively binding to the melanin pigments.

The drugs are partially metabolized in the liver, and some of the metabolites possess antimalarial activity. The unchanged drug and the metabolites are slowly excreted in the urine. The urinary excretion rate is increased by acidification of the urine and is decreased by alkalinization of the urine.

Adverse Effects. The antimalarial dosage of the drugs may produce mild adverse effects. The transient gastrointestinal disturbances include nausea, vomiting, epigastric distress, anorexia, abdominal cramps, and diarrhea. Headache and pruritus may also occur during therapy.

Reversible ocular changes that may occur include sensitivity, edema, and opaque deposits in the cornea. The problems may appear a few weeks after therapy is started or may occur after therapy with the drugs has been continued for months.

Serious retinopathy occasionally appears when the drugs are utilized at high dosage for prolonged periods of therapy. Retention of the drug in the tissues of the retina allows the progression of the pathology when the drug therapy is terminated and may cause permanent damage to the retina. The problem initially is evident as an increased granularity and edema of the retinal tissues that readily is identified by an ophthalmologic examination. The initial lesion is a patchy depigmentation of the retina that is surrounded by a concentric area of pigmentation. Visual field defects (i.e., scotomata) are associated with the lesions. Areas of pigmentation or decoloration also occasionally appear on the skin, hair, and eyebrows. Drug therapy is discontinued when the ocular changes occur and the person is observed for the progression of the problems.

Amodiaquine Hydrochloride (CAMOQUIN). The dosage of the oral drug that is used to provide suppressive prophylaxis for adults and children over 15 years of age is 400 to 600 mg/week. Children from 5 to 15 years of age are given 400 mg/week; children two to five years of age are given 200 mg/week; and children under two years of age are given 100 mg/week.

The adult dosage for the treatment of acute attacks of malaria is given over a three-day period. The dosage is 600 mg initially. A 300-mg dose is given six hours later and that dose is repeated in 24 to 48 hours. The daily dosage for children during the three-day course of therapy is calculated on the basis of 10 mg/kg of body weight, divided for administration in three doses, which are given at 12-hour intervals.

Chloroquine (ARLEN, ROQUINE). The drug is available as *chloroquine phosphate* tablets. The tablets are also available in combination with *hydroxychloroquine sulfate, quinacrine hydrochloride,* or *primaquine phosphate. Chloroquine hydrochloride* is the injectable form of the drug.

The initial dose for the treatment of adults with acute attacks of malaria is 600 mg. A 300-mg dosage is given six hours after the initial dose and that dosage is given at 24- and 48-hour intervals after the second dose. The initial dosage for children is calculated on the basis of 10 mg/kg of body weight. A dosage based on 15 mg/kg of body weight is given six hours later and that dose is repeated 24 and 48 hours after the second dose.

The adult dosage for intramuscular injection is 200 to 250 mg, and that dosage may be repeated at six-hour intervals to a maximum 24-hour dosage of 900 mg. Adults may also receive the drug (400 mg) as an intravenous infusion. Children may receive an intramuscular dosage that is based on the calculation of 5 mg/kg of body weight, and that dosage may be repeated at six-hour intervals to a maximum total daily dosage equivalent to 10 mg/kg of body weight.

The adult dosage for suppressive prophylaxis

is 300 mg/week. The dosage for children is based on the calculation of 5 mg/kg of body weight (maximum 300 mg) and that dosage is given one time per week.

Hydroxychloroquine Sulfate (PLAQUENIL). The initial dosage for the treatment of adults with acute attacks of malaria is 620 mg, and a dose of 310 mg is given six hours after the initial dose. On the second and third days of the course of treatment the dosage is 310 mg/day. The initial dosage for children is based on the calculation of 10 mg/kg of body weight. The dose that is given six hours after that initial dose and the daily dosage for the next two days is based on the calculation of 5 mg/kg of body weight (maximum 310 mg).

The adult dosage for suppressive prophylaxis of malaria is 310 mg/week. The weekly dosage for children is calculated on the basis of 5 mg/kg of body weight.

Quinine

The drug is an alternate agent that is used when the plasmodia are resistant to the newer and less toxic synthetic agents. Quinine, an alkaloid that is extracted from the bark of the cinchona tree, has a long history of use in countries where malaria is endemic. At the present time it is employed primarily for the treatment of severe attacks of relapsing malaria caused by *P. falciparum* that is chloroquine resistant.

The oral dosage of *quinine sulfate* for adults with malaria is 325 mg at six-hour intervals. The course of therapy is 7 to 14 days. The dosage for children is based on the calculation of 10 mg/kg of body weight and that dose is given three times per day for a period of seven days. Patients should be informed that the drug may produce a brown to black discoloration of the urine.

Primaquine Phosphate

The drug is important for its action at exoerythrocyte tissues. It produces a radical cure of *P. vivax*. It is also used with an antimalarial drug that is effective in the suppression of the erythrocyte stage of malaria, to provide causal prophylaxis, or to prevent relapses of benign tertian malaria. It may be used for its gametocyticidal effect when patients are recovering from infestations by *P. falciparum.*

Therapy Considerations. The oral tablets may be given to adults to provide radical cure and suppressive prophylaxis or to prevent relapses of *P. vivax* malaria at a dosage of 15 mg/day for a period of 14 days after the person leaves the area where the disease is endemic. Primaquine phosphate is used concurrently with or following the course of chloroquine therapy. Children may receive a dosage calculated on the basis of 1.75 mg/4.5 kg of body weight per day for a period of 14 days. When the drug is taken daily for 14 days, it provides a radical cure of *P. vivax.*

Adverse Effects. The most common adverse effects are abdominal cramps, epigastric distress, nausea, headache, visual disturbances, and pruritus. The gastrointestinal problems may be alleviated by taking the drug with meals or with an antacid. Food also masks the bitter taste of the drug.

The most serious adverse effect is the hemolytic anemia that occurs in individuals with a *glucose-6-phosphate dehydrogenase* (G-6-PD) deficiency. The schedule for taking the drug may be modified to weekly intervals when the ethnic origin of the individual indicates the possibility that the enzyme deficiency is present (i.e., African, Mediterranean, Oriental countries of origin). Methemoglobinemia commonly occurs during therapy with primaquine phosphate but seldom necessitates interruption of the antimalarial drug therapy. Quinacrine potentiates the toxicity of primaquine.

Pyrimethamine (DARAPRIM)

The drug is used primarily in combination with a sulfonamide for the treatment of plasmodia infestations that are resistant to the action of chloroquine. The drugs are slow acting and another antimalarial agent (i.e., quinine) may be employed to provide a prompt effect.

Action Mode. The drug is a folic acid antagonist. It interferes with the activity of the enzyme *dihydrofolic acid reductase,* which is essential for the plasmodia to synthesize *tetrahydrofolic acid* (Fig. 17–4). When the drug is employed in combination with a sulfonamide, the inhibition of aminobenzoic acid utilization that is effected by that drug provides a dual block to the plasmodial synthesis of its essential nucleic acids.

Therapy Considerations. The oral dosage for suppressive prophylaxis of malaria for adults and children over ten years of age is 25 mg/week. Children who are five to eight years of age may receive 12.5 mg/week; children one to four years of age may receive 6.25 to 12.5 mg/week; and infants may receive 6.25 mg/week. The drug is taken on the same day of the week during the two-week period before entering the country where the disease is endemic, during the period of

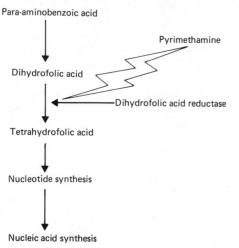

Para-aminobenzoic acid

Pyrimethamine

Dihydrofolic acid

Dihydrofolic acid reductase

Tetrahydrofolic acid

Nucleotide synthesis

Nucleic acid synthesis

Fig. 17–4. Pyrimethamine inhibits the synthesis of folic acid in plasmodia by blocking the enzymatic conversion of dihydrofolic acid to tetrahydrofolic acid.

exposure, and for eight weeks after leaving that country.

Adverse Effects. The antimalarial drug dosage seldom causes adverse effects. Accidental ingestion of large doses of the drug by children can produce convulsions, megaloblastic anemia, leukopenia, thrombocytopenia, and atrophic glossitis.

SCABICIDES AND PEDICULICIDES

The mites that cause scabies and the lice that cause pediculosis readily are transmitted from one person to another. Although there are drugs that can readily eradicate the infestations, the problems remain prevalent in a large segment of the population.

The treatment of scabies requires application of the drug solution, lotion, or ointment to the entire skin surface below the chin line. That treatment plan assures that the females, which live in burrows in the skin, come in contact with the drug. It is essential that the interdigital webs of the hands, the palms, soles of the feet, axillae, buttocks, nipples, and inner aspects of the thigh are treated because those are the primary sites of the infestations. To prevent reinfestation with the eggs or mites, all contact materials (i.e., bedding and clothing) must be thoroughly laundered and fresh clothing is worn after the treatment.

Head lice are transmitted primarily by children who readily share their combs, brushes, or hats with others. The tiny, whitish eggs, or nits, are readily identifiable when the hair is examined closely. The females lay their eggs on the hair follicles, and those nits are held in place by the gelatinous substance that they secrete. They can be differentiated from flakes of dandruff by the crunching sound that occurs when they are crushed between the fingernails. When there is a heavy infestation, the nits are also found on the eyebrows and the eyelashes.

The drugs most frequently employed for the control of pediculosis are *gamma benzene hexachloride* and *copper oleate.* Gamma benzene hexachloride and crotamitin are the drugs most frequently used for the control of scabies.

Gamma Benzene Hexachloride (GAMENE, KWELL)

The drug is the primary agent for the treatment of pediculosis. It is applied topically to the infested areas as a 1 percent cream, lotion, or shampoo. After application of the drug to the scalp and hair, a brush may be used to distribute it evenly and a towel may be wrapped around the head for one hour. One treatment usually eradicates the lice and their eggs.

The drug is irritating to the tissues and care should be taken to avoid its contact with the mucous membranes and eyes. The treated area must remain unwashed for a period of 24 hours after the treatment. Shampooing the hair after that period of time is important to prevent absorption of the drug from the scalp. The treatment may be repeated after one week if the infestation persists after the initial drug application. Three treatments are the maximum used because the drug can irritate the tissues and drug absorption from the scalp can cause convulsions.

Copper Oleate (CUPREX)

The drug is used as a pediculicide. The solution (15 to 30 ml) is gently rubbed into the scalp by parting the hair and applying the solution in a pattern that assures even application of the solution. After 15 minutes, the hair is washed with soap and water. The dead lice and nits may be removed with a "head lice" fine comb after the shampoo. One other treatment may be used within a 48-hour period when the infestations persist after the first application of the drug.

Crotamiton (EURAX)

The drug is used as a scabicide. The ointment or lotion is massaged into all of the skin surface below the chin line. The treatment is repeated 24 hours after the initial application of the drug. The skin may be washed 48 to 72 hours after the last application.

NURSING INTERVENTION

Systemic mycotic infections, extraintestinal amebiasis, and *P. falciparum* malaria are serious health problems. During the acute phase of the illness, the primary emphasis is on eradicating the causative organism from the tissues and maintaining the physiologic equilibrium of the patient. The nursing intervention appropriate for maintaining the health status of persons with those illnesses is similar to that employed when patients have widely disseminated bacterial infections.

Counseling is an important aspect of nursing intervention when persons have a fungus infection that can be readily transmitted from one part of the body to another or a parasitic infestation that can be readily transmitted from one person to another. The eradication of many of those infections is dependent on the person's persistent compliance with the therapeutic plan and the concurrent use of hygienic measures to prevent autoinfestation or the infestation of others by the parasites or their eggs and larvae.

When drug therapy is planned for the treatment of carriers who are asymptomatic or for contacts who unavoidably come in contact with the parasites, their compliance may be improved if they understand the rationale for the treatment and the predictable end points of therapy. For example, sexual partners may more consistently take the prescribed medication for the eradication of an infestation with *Trichomonas vaginalis* when they understand the transmission potential of the parasite and the probability that the uncomfortable genital infection can be eradicated by a seven-day course of drug taking by both persons.

The characteristic mode of transmission of invading parasites provides the basic guidelines for discussing the hygienic measures appropriate in the individual situation. Specific measures should be discussed with all infested persons. For example, some families have recurring problems with pinworm infestations and each member of the group may receive the antithelminth drug for eradication of the infestations. The concurrent use of hygienic measures to halt the transmission of the eggs is an essential aspect of the plan for eradication of the parasitic infestations.

Counseling about hygienic measures should focus on the hazard of transmitting the eggs from the anal area after toileting or scratching. The measures that limit egg sharing include washing uncooked foods before eating them, wearing snug-fitting cotton underpants to avoid anal contact when scratching during the night, cutting the fingernails, and thorough hand washing on arising in the morning and after toileting. An explicit description of the use of an orangewood stick or the tip of a fingernail file to assure that the eggs are removed from the protected sites under the nails is an essential part of the hand-washing instructions. The foregoing measures are so essential to the eradication of the pinworm infestation that some physicians prescribe washing the anal area early in the morning and applying an antibiotic ointment to the area or the use of an antibiotic ointment on the fingertips and under the fingernails concurrent with the use of an oral antithelminth drug.

It is also important that the underwear and bedding be handled carefully to prevent the dissemination of eggs in the environment. Laundering the clothing and bedding and thorough cleaning of the toilet at the time of treatment may also prevent reinfestation. There may be additional measures that would be suggested when the preliminary assessment reveals that the individual's living conditions and health practices can increase the potential for transmission of the parasites.

The same specificity as is demonstrated in the foregoing example is important when discussing hygienic measures that should be employed for the control of most of the parasitic infestations and nonsystemic fungal infections. The person's use of hygienic measures is more consistent when the guidelines that are suggested include examples of the measures that are necessary to prevent the transmission of the organisms. When prolonged therapy is required, the compliance rate is higher when there are a small number of clearly identified instructions for the person to follow than when the person implements numerous measures in an overzealous attempt to shorten the period of therapy. The latter often leads to cessation of the treatment after the initial discomfort is relieved.

Review Guides

1. For each of the drugs listed below describe
   a. The common helminth infestations for which the drug is used
   b. Factors that would be included when instructing the person who is to take the drug (i.e., measures to provide maximum effect of the drug, common adverse effects, predictable outcomes of the treatment, hygienic measures to be implemented)

   mebendazole   *pyrivinium pamoate*
   piperazine   *quinacrine hydrochloride*
   pyrantel pamoate   *thiabenazole*

2. Outline a nursing care plan for the patient who is receiving emetine and diiodohydroxyquin for the control of amebiasis.

3. Outline the factors that should be included in the instruction of persons who are to take primaquine and hydroxychloroquin for suppressive prophylaxis when traveling to a country where *P. vivax* malaria is prevalent.

4. Formulate a nursing care plan for the patient who is receiving amphotericin B by intravenous infusion.

5. Describe the factors that would be included when explaining the rationale for the treatment and instructing the person about the use of nystatin

(oral and topical) and griseofulvin (oral and topical).

6. List two precautions that should be taken when using gamma benzene hexachloride for the control of pediculosis and list three hygienic measures that should be implemented to prevent reinfestation.

Additional Readings

Adeckman, Michael, and Tuthill, Timothy M.: Pulmonary filtrates and eosinophils associated with drug reactions and parasitic infections. *Postgrad. Med.*, **60:**143, September, 1976.

Aisner, Joseph; Schimpff, Stephen C.; Sutherland, John C.; Young, Viola; and Wiernik, Peter H.: Torulopsis glabrata infections in patients with cancer. *Am. J. Med.*, **61:**23, July, 1976.

Balfour, Henry H., Jr., and Burke, Barbara A.: Viral and mycoplasmal pneumonias. *Postgrad. Med.*, **58:**48, December, 1976.

Blumenthal, Daniel S.: Current concepts: intestinal nematodes in the United States. *N. Engl. J. Med.*, **297:**1437, December 29, 1977.

Botero, David: Clinical trial methodology in intestinal parasitic diseases. *Clin. Pharmacol. Ther.*, **19:**630, May, 1976.

Burke, Joseph A.: Giardiasis in children. *Am. J. Dis. Child.*, **129:**1304, November, 1975.

Codish, Stephen D., and Tobias, Jeffrey S.: Managing systemic mycoses in the compromised host. *J.A.M.A.*, **235:**2132, May 10, 1976.

Cvitkovich, D.; Burch, K. H.: Quinn, E. L.; Madhavan, T.; Cox, F.; and Fisher, E.: Uncommon causes of infection related to a rural environment. *Clin. Med.*, **83:**13, February, 1976.

Dvorak, James A., and Miller, Louis H.: Invasion of erythrocytes by malaria merozoites. *Science,* **187:**748, February 28, 1975.

Dykers, John R., Jr.: Single-dose metronidazole for trichomoniasis: patient and consort. *N. Engl. J. Med.*, **293:**23, July 3, 1975.

Egorin, Merrill J.; Trump, Donald L.; and Wainwright, Charles W.: Quinacrine ochronosis and rheumatoid arthritis. *J.A.M.A.*, **236:**385, July 26, 1976.

Gauder, John P.: Cryptococcal cellulitis. *J.A.M.A.*, **237:**672, February 14, 1977.

Hazelrigg, Donald E.: Scraping for scabies. *Am. Fam. Physician,* **17:**129, January, 1978.

Jacobs, Paul H.: Fungal infections of the skin. *Primary Care,* **2:**39, March, 1975.

Kean, B. H.: The treatment of amebiasis. *J.A.M.A.,* **235:**501, February 2, 1976.

Kean, B. H., and Reilly, Phillip C., Jr.: Malaria—the mime. *Am. J. Med.,* **61:**159, August, 1976.

Krogstad, Donald J.; Spencer, Harrison, C., Jr.; and Healy, George R.: Current concepts in parasitology: amebiasis. *N. Engl. J. Med.,* **298:**262, February 2, 1978.

Kumar, U. Nanda; Varkey, Basil; and Landis, Francis B.: Allergic bronchopulmonary aspergillosis: an increasing clinical problem. *Postgrad. Med.,* **58:**141, November, 1975.

Mahmood, Khalid: Granulomatous oophoritis due to Schistosoma mansoni. *Am. J. Obstet. Gynecol.,* **123:**919, December 15, 1975.

Markell, Edward K.: Diagnosis of the more common parasitic diseases. *Primary Care,* **5:**57, March, 1978.

Medoff, Gerald, and Kobayaski, George S.: Amphotericin B: old drug, new therapy. *J.A.M.A.,* **232:**619, May 12, 1975.

Milliken, Larry E.: Superficial and cutaneous fungal infections: diagnosis and treatment. *Postgrad. Med.,* **60:**52, July, 1976.

Murray, Henry W.; Fialk, Mark A.; and Roberts, Richard B.: Candida arthritis: a manifestation of disseminated candidiasis. *Am. J. Med.,* **60:**587, April, 1976.

Orkin, Milton, and Maibach, Howard I.: Current concepts in parasitology: this scabies pandemic. *N. Engl. J. Med.,* **298:**496, March 2, 1978.

Prince, Daniel S., and Hardin, Joe G.: Hydroxychloroquine-induced vertigo. *J.A.M.A.,* **233:**984, September 1, 1975.

Quinn, E. L.; Burch, K. H.; Cox, F.; Fisher, E.; Madhaven, T.; Haas, E. J.; and Del Busto, R.: Pseudomonas infections. *Am. Fam. Physician,* **14:**84, November, 1976.

Restrepo, Angela; Robledo, Mario; Giraldo, Roberto; Hernández, Humberto; Sierra, Fernando; Gutiérrez, Fernando; Londoño, Fernaldo; López, Roberto; and Calle, Gonzalo. The gamut of paracoccidioidomycosis. *Am. J. Med.,* **61:**33, July, 1976.

Spencer, F. J.: The scourge of shigellosis. *Clin. Med.,* **83:**20, February, 1976.

Stevens, David A.; Levine, H. B.; and Deresinski, Stanley C. Miconazole in coccidioidomycosis. 11. Therapeutic and pharmacologic studies on man. *Am. J. Med.,* **60:**191, February, 1976.

Trenholme, Gordon M.; Williams, Roger L.; Riechmann, Karl H.; Frischer, Henri; and Carson, Paul E.: Quinine disposition during malaria and during induced fever. *Clin. Pharmacol. Ther.,* **19:** 459, April, 1976.

Tudor, Richard B.: Pediatrics: ridding children of common worm infections. *Postgrad. Med.,* **58:**115, December, 1975.

Wadlington, William B.; Faber, Robert; and O'Neill, James A., Jr.: Recent experience with hepatic amebiasis. *Clin. Pediatr.,* **14:**163, February, 1975.

Webster, Leslie T., Jr.; Butterworth, Anthony E.; Mahmoud, Adel A. F.; Magola, Eric N.; and Warren, Kenneth S.: Suppression of delayed hypersensitivity in schistosome-infected patients by niridazole. *N. Engl. J. Med.,* **292:**1144, May 29, 1975.

Young, Edward J.: Human brucellosis. *Clin. Med.,* **83:**9, May, 1976.

18

Immune and Allergic Responses

The immune responses protect the body tissues from the effects of trauma or toxins and from invasion by bacteria, fungi, viruses, and protozoa. The same immune responses can contribute to the incidence of allergic reactions and autoimmune disorders. There is considerable evidence that they also contribute to some of the chronic diseases (i.e., multiple sclerosis, Parkinson's disease). The chronic diseases are thought to occur as immune responses to the progeny or residual products of viruses that have remained dormant in the body for long periods of time after the initial virus exposure.

Physiologic Correlations

The development of adaptive or acquired immunity is a normal physiologic process that begins in utero and continues throughout the lifetime of an individual. The two types of immunity are *cellular immunity* and *humoral immunity*. The lymphocytes that provide cellular immunity and the antibodies that provide humoral immunity both originate from the stem cells of the hematopoietic tissues of the liver and spleen.

CELLULAR IMMUNITY

The preprocessing of cells for the cellular immune system begins in the human fetus during the eighth week of gestation. Stem cells from the fetal liver and spleen travel to the *thymus gland* where the cells divide to form the *T cells,* or *T lymphocytes,* which are the cellular immune bodies. The T cells are named for the gland that produces them. During the process of lymphocyte synthesis in the thymus, the massive challenge by normal circulating body proteins destroys those lymphocytes responding to them. The T cells that are released into the circulation are T lymphocytes that are sensitized only to nonself-antigens or foreign proteins, polysaccharides, or mucopolysaccharides. The sensitized cells are capable of engulfing and destroying specific bacteria, viruses, or toxins. When those antigenic substances contact a sensitized lymphocyte in the lymphoid tissues or other body tissues, the challenge leads to the rapid proliferation of the clones of sensitized T lymphocytes (Fig. 18–1).

Cellular immunity provides protection against slow-growing bacteria (i.e., *Mycobacterium tu-berculosis*), cancer cells, fungus, or virus. It also participates in the rejection response to transplanted tissues and organs and is involved in the autoimmune responses. The T lymphocytes have a *direct action* and an *indirect action* that destroy foreign or antigenic substances.

Direct Action

The sensitized T lymphocytes can destroy antigens by directly binding with them. During the bonding the lymphocyte swells and releases a cytotoxic substance (i.e., lysosomal enzyme) that destroys the antigen. The indirect action of the sensitized T lymphocytes, which mobilizes other phagocytes of the normal physiologic immune processes, reinforces the direct activity of the lymphocytes.

Indirect Action

The indirect response occurs as the lymphocytes combine with the antigens and release a *transfer factor* that endows other nonsensitized lymphocytes in the area with the ability to

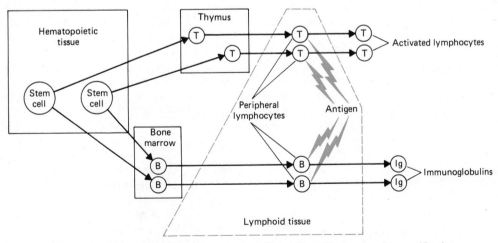

Fig. 18–1. Stem cells from the liver and spleen diversify in the thymus gland to form the T lymphocytes of the cellular immunity system. Stem cells also diversify in the bone marrow to form the B lymphocytes of the humoral immunity system. An antigen challenge leads to the proliferation and release of the immune bodies that are sensitized to that allergen.

destroy the antigen in a manner comparable to that of the sensitized T cell. In addition to that inactivation process, the sensitized lymphocytes emit a *chemotactic factor* that attracts granulocytes and macrophages to the site of the antigen challenge. The arrival of the neutrophils and macrophages magnifies the phagocytic activity in the area of the antigen-antibody reaction. The release of lysosomal enzymes during the processes of phagocytosis causes a local inflammatory response in tissues adjacent to the area.

HUMORAL IMMUNITY

The primary difference between the T lymphocytes of cellular immunity and the B lymphocytes that produce the antibodies of the humoral immunity system is the lifespan of the two types of *immunologically competent cells*. The thymus-derived lymphocytes provide immune responses over a time span that ranges from ten years to a lifetime, but B lymphocytes have a span of activity of a few months or years.

Immunoglobulin Synthesis

The synthesis pathway for the B lymphocytes that later will synthesize immunologically active antibodies, or immunoglobulins, begins with the stem cells in the fetal liver and spleen (Fig. 18–1). The preprocessing of the stem cells is thought to occur in selected sites in the bone marrow. Although the specific marrow production site in humans has not been defined, the site of the lymphocyte precursors has been identified as the *bursa of Fabricius* in birds. The designation of the human lymphocytes as *B lymphocytes* reflects that avian site of origin.

The *B lymphocytes* travel to the lymphoid tissues where they remain as dormant clones of cells. When an antigen enters the lymphoid tissues, the immunoglobulins on the membranes of the B lymphocytes that are specific for its configuration interact with the antigen. The interaction converts the B lymphocytes into plasma cells, which form the immunoglobulin antibodies required for inactivation of the antigen.

The initial fetal synthesis of immunoglobulins from B lymphocytes begins between the tenth and eleventh weeks of gestation. During that time period, immunoglobulin M is synthesized and other antibodies are synthesized during the later weeks of gestation. The maternal-fetal transfer of immunoglobulin G, which occurs at about the thirty-eighth day of gestation, provides passive immunity to the newborn infant. The transfer precedes the fetal synthesis of that immunoglobulin, which normally begins during the twelfth week of gestation.

Immunoglobulin Structure

Each immunoglobulin molecule has one pair of *light polypeptide chains* and an equal number of paired *heavy polypeptide chains*. The light chains are designated as either *kappa* or *lambda* types. The pairs of heavy chains may be one of five types, and the characteristic polypeptides determine the particular immunoglobulin class. They may have *alpha, delta, epsilon, gamma,* or *mu* chains, and their name designates the heavy chains of their structure: *immunoglobulin A* (IgA); *immunoglobulin D* (IgD); *immunoglobulin E* (IgE); *immunoglobulin G* (IgG); or *immunoglobulin M* (IgM). The immunoglobulin receptor sites have mirror images of the configuration of the antigen's structure for which they have specificity and they can rapidly form a tight union with the specific antigens.

Immunoglobulin Function

IgA is present in the vasculature (40 percent), saliva, and intestinal and respiratory secretions. It neutralizes viruses and provides protection against infections on the body surfaces that are exposed to the environment.

IgD comprises 0.2 percent of the immunoglobulins. Its functions have not been clearly defined.

IgE comprises only 0.5 percent of the immunoglobulins but is prevalent during allergic reactions. It mediates the vascular responses of those reactions. It governs the responses of the immediate type of hypersensitivity reactions and provides skin-sensitizing antibody.

IgG comprises 75 percent of the immunoglobulins. It neutralizes viruses and toxins and destroys bacteria.

IgM is found primarily in the vasculature (80 percent). It provides protection against gram-negative bacteria and neutralizes viruses.

Complement Activation

The destruction of antigens by IgG and IgM is facilitated by their ability to activate the complement system of enzymes. After the immunoglobulins combine with the antigen, the complement attaches to the surface of the antigen. The enzymes increase the antigen's susceptibility to phagocytosis. They also cause the agglutination of the antigens and the coagulation of tissue proteins that interfere with the movement of the antigens. Those actions concentrate the antigens for more effective interaction.

Complement also provides the chemotaxis that attracts neutrophils and macrophages to the antigen-antibody action site where they participate with the complement in the lysis and phagocytosis of antigens. The antigen-antibody complement interaction processes produce an inflammatory reaction in the tissues adjacent to that activity.

Pathophysiologic Correlations

ALLERGIC REACTIONS

Immunoglobulin E acts through the *anaphylactic system* to prevent the movement of allergens and to reduce their destructive effects on body tissues. IgE attaches to the tissue-bound mast cells and to the circulating basophils, which are functionally similar to the mast cells. The attachment of IgE to the mast cells and basophils causes those cells to secrete histamine and serotonin.

Effects on Tissues

Mast cells are most prominent in the tissues that are frequently exposed to environmental allergens. IgE is also found primarily in the lymphoid tissues at those sites that are commonly assaulted by allergens (i.e., skin, respiratory and gastrointestinal tract tissues).

Their union with IgE causes the swelling and rupture of the mast cells and basophils. That process releases additional histamine into the tissues surrounding the allergen. The action of histamine at the vascular histamine (H_1) receptors causes local vasodilation and an increased porosity of the capillaries at the interaction site. The tissues become hyperemic and swelling occurs as a consequence of the movement of fluid and plasma proteins from the capillaries into the tissues. The concurrent release of bradykinins from the cells further increases the vascular permeability and causes an irritation of the nerve endings that adds to the pain and discomfort experienced during an allergic response. The concurrent release of *eosinophil chemotactic factor* of anaphylaxis (ECF-A) provides additional phagocytic activity by those cells that arrive at the interaction site. The release of the *slow-reacting substance of anaphylaxis* (SRS-A) from the mast cells intensifies and prolongs the constriction of the smooth muscles of the bronchi when the interaction occurs at those respiratory tract sites.

Immediate Allergic Reactions

The anaphylactic system causes widespread allergen-antibody reactions as a consequence of the dissemination of the allergen to diverse body tissues. The initial exposure to the allergen may be uneventful or there may be a minor reaction. During that exposure the IgE that contacts the allergen retains a memory pattern for the formation of antibodies that are specific for the allergen. Reexposure to the same allergen causes a rapid proliferation of the allergen-specific immunoglobulins and there is an immediate antibody response at the tissue sites where the challenge occurs.

The types of allergic responses that occur immediately on reexposure include *anaphylaxis, urticaria,* and *angioedema.* Drugs are the most common allergens producing the reexposure response, but the reactions can occur when the person is reexposed to a variety of proteins, polysaccharides, or mucopolysaccharides.

Inherited Allergic Traits

The immediate allergic reactions can also occur in persons who have genetically inherited traits that cause the formation of sensitized immunoglobulins, or *reagins.* The preformed immunoglobulins (IgE) cause an allergic reaction when they are initially exposed to the allergenic substances to which they are sensitized. The allergic response tends to occur in a particular target organ where the sensitized immunoglobulins are most abundant, and the responses vary according to the tissue site involved in the allergen-reagin interaction. For example, the interaction in the nasal passages usually involves the release of large quantities of histamine and the mucosa is hyperemic and swollen. Excess fluid leaks from the tissues and there are copious secretions and localized tissue irritation. When the allergen-reagin interaction occurs in the bronchial structures, there is a higher level of slow-reacting substance of anaphylaxis and less histamine secretion at the interaction site. The constriction of the bronchial structures that is caused by the slow-reacting substance is the basis of the acute respiratory distress that occurs during an asthmatic attack.

Delayed-Reaction Allergies

Lymphocyte Response. The cellular immune system also responds to the challenge of allergens (i.e., chemicals, drugs, cosmetics, poison ivy toxin). The initial exposure to the allergen causes the formation of sensitized T lymphocytes with specificity for the particular substance. Reexposure, or rechallenge, causes an allergen-lymphocyte interaction that produces hyperemia, swelling, and irritation at the sites of the interaction within 12 to 48 hours after that exposure.

Immunoglobulin Response. The allergic reactions can also occur within a period of seven to ten days after the exposure to the allergen. That period correlates with the time that is required for the immunoglobulins that come in contact with the allergen to proliferate. The reaction occurs when the numbers of sensitized immunoglobulins are sufficient to produce overt evidence of the allergen-antibody interaction at tissue sites. For example, *serum sickness, Arthus reaction, rash,* or *fever* may occur from seven to ten days after the administration of a single dosage of a drug that causes the synthesis of sensitized immunoglobulins.

AUTOIMMUNITY

The autoimmune responses are associated with failure of the immune systems to differentiate between self and nonself. The T lymphocytes may produce an immune reaction when the proteins of the cornea or of the thyroid (thyroglobulins) are released by inflammation, infection, or trauma. Those proteins remain sequestered in their natural locations during the fetal processing of proteins in the thymus gland, and their release at a later time allows the lymphocytes that are sensitized to antigens with similar configurations to attack and destroy them. The antigen-lymphocyte interaction can cause destruction in the tissues of origin (i.e., corneal opacity, degenerative thyroiditis).

Body tissues can be destroyed in the antigen-antibody responses to bacterial toxins and other antigens. For example, the interaction that is associated with the toxins of streptococcal infections can cause destruction of the toxins and of the collagen tissues that are the site of their liberation during the infection (i.e., cardiac, renal, or joint tissues).

Autoimmunity is also thought to occur as a consequence of viral invasion that alters the antigenicity of body tissues. Some of those responses appear to be associated with the combining of tissue products with proteins, bacteria, or viruses that are antigenic substances. That union can cause the antigen-antibody interactions that destroy tissues. For example, the paralysis of muscles that is characteristic of myasthenia gravis or the diffuse destruction of tissues that is associated with lupus erythematosus is thought to occur consequent to alterations in the antigenicity of tissue proteins.

TISSUE REJECTION

Cellular immunity and humoral immunity independently can provide protection against antigens. When there is a massive challenge by foreign protein (i.e., tissue or organ implants), both types of immunity may respond to the challenge. Sensitized T lymphocytes proliferate rapidly and are sufficient in numbers to cause initial evidence of a rejection response within a period of 48 hours after the protein challenge occurs. The humoral immunity response also participates in the rejection response after sensitized immunoglobulins have been reproduced. Those antibodies provide a second wave or intensification of the rejection reaction approximately four days after the initial massive protein challenge.

The intensity of the response of the immune systems has delayed the progress of organ transplantation. Tissue matching, or *histocompatibility* testing, is done prior to organ implantation to assure that the protein tissue from the donor is compatible with the "self" proteins of the recipient. When organs are implanted, it is necessary to utilize drugs (i.e., antilymphocyte serum, glucocorticoids, antineoplastic drugs) to destroy the T lymphocytes and the immunoglobulins that predictably will respond to the protein challenge.

STRESS-INDUCED GLUCOCORTICOID RELEASE

The adrenal gland secretes corticosteroids each day. The regular diurnal release of the hormones is highest between 2 A.M. and 8 A.M. and minimal between 4 P.M. and midnight in individuals who maintain a daytime schedule of activities. The hormonal release is physiologically adjusted to occur prior to the usual activity periods in persons who have different work and sleep patterns. Physiologic adjustments can also provide up to a tenfold increase in the release of corticosteroids during periods of maximal stress.

Physiologic stress (i.e., extensive surgery, severe infection, or trauma) provides the stimulus for the release of corticotropin-releasing hormone (CRH) from the hypothalamus. The hormone travels through the hypothalamus-pituitary blood system to the anterior pituitary gland where it stimulates the release of *adrenocorticotropic hormone* (ACTH). That hormone stimulates the release of *glucocorticoid* and *mineralocorticoid* from the adrenal cortex (Fig. 18–2). The glucocorticoid that is released into the bloodstream travels to the liver and other body tissues where it causes the catabolism of labile proteins, fats, and glycogen. That activity provides increased amounts of glucose that are released into the bloodstream.

The concurrent activity of mineralocorticoids and of the antidiuretic hormone from the posterior pituitary gland becomes significant when the periods of stress are intense, prolonged, or repetitive. Under those circumstances, the elevated blood levels of mineralocorticoids contribute to the increased renal tubule reabsorption of sodium ions and the excretion of potassium ions. The associated activity of antidiuretic hormone increases the reabsorption of water from the distal renal tubules.

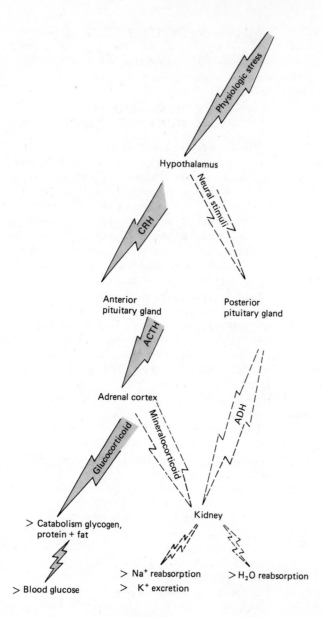

Fig. 18–2. Physiologic stress provides the stimulus for the release of corticotropin-releasing hormone (CRH) from the hypothalamus. Adrenocorticotropic hormone (ACTH) stimulates the release of adrenal glucocorticoid and the subsequent catabolism of glycogen, protein, and fat stores that provide elevated blood glucose levels. During long periods of stress, mineralocorticoid and antidiuretic hormone (ADH) action at renal tubule receptors increases sodium and water reabsorption and potassium excretion.

Glucocorticoids

DRUG THERAPY

The glucocorticoids are employed for replacement of the physiologic hormones when there is decreased function of the adrenal gland (i.e., Addison's disease), but they are more commonly utilized to suppress inflammatory, allergic, or immune responses. The drugs are also employed with antineoplastic drugs for the treatment of hematologic and malignant diseases (i.e., leukemia, lymphoma). The therapeutic effects and the adverse effects of the drugs generally represent extensions of the physiologic functions of the natural endogenous hormone.

Action Mode

The glucocorticoids affect most physiologic processes. They are the carbohydrate-regulating hormones of the adrenal cortex. Their effect on electrolyte (i.e., sodium and potassium) and water regulation is considerably less than that of the mineralocorticoids.

The glucocorticoids suppress the immune response by their effect on the lymphatic system. They produce lymphopenia, depress antibody production, and reduce the size of enlarged lymph nodes. They reduce the inflammation that is associated with the immune response by decreasing the number of circulating eosinophils and stabilizing the membranes of the lysosomes that release enzymes into the tissues. The decreased response of the immune systems to antigen or allergen challenges reduces the adverse effects on body tissues that are associated with the allergic reactions, tissue implants, or autoimmune disease.

Therapy Considerations

The oral formulations of the glucocorticoids are absorbed readily from the intestinal tract and are rapidly distributed in the body tissues. The drugs cross the placental barrier. The liver is the primary site of their accumulation and is the principal site of metabolism. The drugs are rapidly eliminated by glomerular filtration and tubule secretion.

The onset of action occurs approximately two to eight hours after the drug is taken orally, and the drug provides an anti-inflammatory effect for 24 hours after the last dose of the drug is taken. The soluble parenteral forms provide peak concentrations within a few minutes after the intravenous or intramuscular injection of the drug.

Topical application of the drugs to the skin or eyes or local application of the drug by inhalation or as retention enemas is more effective for some lesions and circumvents the adverse effects of systemic drug therapy. Some of the drug may be absorbed when it is applied topically under occlusive dressings. Long-term use of glucocorticoid creams, lotions, or solutions on intertriginous areas or under occlusive dressings may cause a thinning and striation of the skin associated with the drug-induced rupture of the subcutaneous collagen fibers.

The intra-articular, sublesional, or intralesional injection of glucocorticoid formulations is also used to provide an anti-inflammatory effect without clinically significant systemic distribution of the drug. The anti-inflammatory effect on the tissues may persist for one to two weeks after the injection. In many instances, the drug injection and a period of limited joint movement may completely alleviate the problem (i.e., bursitis). The person must be cautioned against exercising the extremity until the inflammation of the tissues has subsided.

Adverse Effects

Inflammation. The anti-inflammatory effect of the glucocorticoids is a positive outcome of their use, but it can also allow the uninhibited proliferation of invading virus, bacteria, or fungi. In the absence of the usual signs of the natural physiologic responses to pathogen invasion (i.e., elevated temperature, tissue inflammation), serious infections may become established. The problem is referred to as the "masking" effect of the glucocorticoids.

The concurrent inhibition of fibroblastic activity and collagen tissue breakdown that are caused by the drugs can activate *Mycobacterium tuberculosis* by liberating the dormant organisms from the depots in pulmonary tissues. A tuberculin test is usually performed before institution of long-term therapy. The test results may show a false negative result when the test antigen is injected after the drugs have suppressed the immune response. Prophylactic therapy is planned for persons who have a positive test reaction.

Suppression of Corticotropin Secretion. The hypothalamic-pituitary-adrenal interaction that leads to the natural endogenous release of glucocorticoids is a negative feedback mechanism. The administration of the hormones significantly suppresses the activity of that natural interactive mechanism, and some adrenal cortical tissue atrophy occurs when the glucocorticoids are administered for more than one week. The drugs may be used on an alternate-day schedule during long-term therapy to reduce the suppression of corticotropin secretion and adrenocortical atrophy.

The hazard of adrenocortical insufficiency is also reduced by gradual reduction in the drug dosage at the termination of therapy. After prolonged periods of therapy, decrements in the dosage may be made at weekly intervals. The daily dosage may be given as a single dose in the morning with breakfast to provide the glucocorticoid during the daytime hours. That plan allows the adrenocorticotropic hormone to reestablish the natural early-morning (2 A.M. to 8 A.M.) pattern for endogenous glucocorticoid release. Withdrawal of the drug after shorter periods of therapy (i.e., one to two weeks) is often accomplished by making 50 percent decrements in the total daily dosage while maintaining the previously scheduled intervals for taking the drug.

The person is observed for evidence of weakness, hypotension, nausea, or anorexia during the withdrawal process, and the dosage may be increased when there is evidence of adrenal insufficiency. Throughout the period of therapy with glucocorticoids those same symptoms indicate the presence of a physiologic stress syndrome that necessitates an increase in drug dosage.

Gastritis and Peptic Ulcers. The drugs frequently cause gastritis and sometimes cause peptic ulcers by decreasing the protective mucus barrier of the stomach and interfering with tissue repair. In some patients the drugs also increase the production of gastric acid and pepsinogen.

The problems occur when the drugs are administered parenterally or orally, and they are unrelated to local gastric tissue irritation by the drug.

Antacids usually are administered when the patient is receiving glucocorticoids. The pain, eructation, or food intolerance that usually forewarns of peptic ulcers is associated with inflammation of the gastric mucosa, and that local tissue response is usually absent during glucocorticoid therapy. Guaiac testing of the stools, gastric aspirate, and vomitus allows early identification of gastric bleeding. Antacids are usually administered during the time the patient is receiving glucocorticoids.

Diabetogenic Effect. The catabolism of proteins, fats, and glycogen that is caused by the glucocorticoids increases the blood glucose level, and latent diabetes may become clinically apparent. During the initial period of therapy, blood and urine glucose levels are evaluated regularly to allow early detection of excess glucose content.

Dietary regulation may reduce the blood glucose level. Persistently elevated blood glucose levels may necessitate the use of antidiabetic drugs. When the glucocorticoids are administered to individuals who receive insulin or hypoglycemic agents for the control of diabetes, an increase in the dosage of those drugs may be required to control the blood glucose levels.

Protein and Lipid Catabolism. Long-term therapy with glucocorticoids may cause muscle wasting and porosity of the bones by drug-induced mobilization of proteins from those structures. The fragility of the bones and the decrease in muscle strength can contribute to bone fractures when there is minimal trauma. The development of the long bones may be retarded when the drugs are given to children. Some protection against extensive tissue protein catabolism can be provided by increasing the protein content of the diet because the drugs more readily utilize labile proteins than those of the muscles and bones.

The catabolism and redistribution of lipids in

the body tissues cause their deposition in the subcutaneous tissues of the face, abdomen, and suprascapular areas. The collection of lipids in the mandibular area is the easiest to recognize because the face has a rounded appearance that is called "moonface." The redistribution of lipids may also accelerate atherosclerosis.

Edema and Hypokalemia. The natural glucocorticoids *cortisone* and *hydrocortisone, prednisolone* and *prednisone* also have mineralocorticoid activity. The drugs are useful for hormone replacement for patients with adrenal insufficiency.

The mineralocorticoid action at the renal distal tubules increases the reabsorption of sodium ions and the excretion of potassium ions. The electrolyte imbalances and the edema and muscle weakness that are associated with the imbalances may be prevented by restriction of the dietary sodium content. When patients have significant edema, the therapeutic agent may be changed to one of the synthetic glucocorticoids, which are designed to provide minimal mineralocorticoid activity and maximal glucocorticoid activity.

Central Nervous System Effects. The large doses of glucocorticoids required for the suppression of some of the severe inflammatory responses can cause behavioral and personality changes. The problems may include euphoria, insomnia, nervousness, irritability, or psychotic episodes. A reduction in dosage may alleviate the symptoms, but control of the disease process often necessitates continuation of the glucocorticoid therapy.

Other Adverse Effects. Acne, hirsutism, menstrual disorders, weight gain, headache, hypertension, hyperhidrosis and flushing, vertigo, and asthenia may occur during therapy with the drugs. There have been reports of *pseudotumor cerebri*, or benign intracranial hypertension, in children. The problem occurs most frequently during the withdrawal of the drugs. Following prolonged therapy, children may also have posterior subcapsular cataract formation. The systemic use of glucocorticoids for children is usually restricted to the control of life-threatening inflammatory processes when the benefits outweigh the risks of the adverse effects of the drugs.

Preparations Available

Betamethasone. The drug is available as a syrup and tablets for oral use (Table 18–1). *Betamethasone sodium phosphate and betamethasone acetate* are repository suspensions employed for intramuscular or localized injections (6 to 12 mg every three to seven days). The effects appear within two to three hours after injection of the drug. When the drug is injected into the joints or other tissues, the effects persist for three to seven weeks. The drug is also available as a topical preparation.

Cortisone Acetate. The drug is available as tablets for oral use and as a suspension for intramuscular injection (Table 18–1). The absorption of the drug from the muscle occurs over a period of 24 to 48 hours. The mineralocorticoid activity of the drug may cause sodium retention and hypokalemia.

Dexamethasone. The drug is available as tablets and as a liquid for oral use (Table 18–1). *Dexamethasone sodium phosphate* is available as solutions for intramuscular or intravenous injection. It is available with lidocaine for intrasynovial or intra-articular injection. It is also available as an inhalant. Three inhalations provide the 250-mcg adult dosage that usually is used three or four times per day to a maximum of 12 inhalations per day. Children may be given two inhalations, or 168 mcg, three or four times per day to a maximum of eight inhalations per day. Excessive use of the drug (i.e. > 12 inhalations per day) causes the absorption of significant amounts of the drug. Dexamethasone is also available as a cream, ointment, and gel for topical use.

Fluprednisolone. The drug is available as tablets for oral use (Table 18–1). The low sodium-retaining activity of the drug makes it necessary for the patient with adrenocortical in-

Table 18–1.
Glucocorticoids Employed for the Control of Inflammation

Drug	Route	Daily Dosage	
		Adult Dosage (mg)	Number of Divided Doses
Betamethasone (CELESTONE)	Oral	0.6–7.2	1
	IM	0.5–9	2
Cortisone (CORTONE)	Oral	12.5–400	1–4
	IM	100–300	3
Dexamethasone (DECADRON, DERONIL, DEXAMETH, HEXADROL)	Oral	0.5–10	1
	IM/IV	2–24	2–4
Fluprednisolone (ALPHADROL)	Oral	2.5–30	1–2
Hydrocortisone (CORTEF, CORTRIL, HYDROCORTONE)	Oral	20–240	1–2
	IM/IV	12.5–250	2
Meprednisone (BETAPAR)	Oral	8–60	1–4
Methylprednisolone (MEDROL)	Oral	4–48	1–2
	IM/IV	10–40	1
Paramethasone acetate (HALDRONE)	Oral	2–24	1
Prednisolone (DELTA-CORTEF, METICORTELONE)	Oral	5–60	1–2
	IM		
Prednisone (DELTA-DOME, PARACORT)	Oral	4–60	1
Triamcinolone (ARISTOCORT, KENACORT)	Oral	5–60	1

sufficiency (i.e., Addison's disease) to receive a mineralocorticoid for adrenal hormone replacement therapy.

Hydrocortisone. The drug is available as tablets and as a suspension for oral use (Table 18–1). The solution for intravenous injection may be infused (100 mg) slowly over a two-to-three-hour period for the control of acute adrenal insufficiency. The drug may also be given by intramuscular injection (100 to 250 mg) in emergency situations. It is absorbed from the muscle site over a four-to-eight-hour period. *Hydrocortisone acetate* is the insoluble solution that is utilized for intra-articular injection. The drug is also available as an ointment, cream, lotion, gel, and spray for topical application and as a retention enema (CORTENEMA).

Meprednisone. The drug is available in tablets for oral use (Table 18–1). It is employed primarily for the control of inflammatory responses and has no mineralocorticoid activity.

Methylprednisolone. The drug is available as tablets and extended-release tablets for oral use (Table 18–1). It is also available as an ointment, cream, or aerosol for topical use. *Methylprednisolone acetate* is used for intramuscular injections and is slowly absorbed over a period of five to seven days. When it is injected into the intrasynovial or soft tissues, the effects appear within 12 to 24 hours and persist for approximately one week. *Methylprednisolone sodium succinate* provides a prompt effect when it is administered by intramuscular injection.

Paramethasone Acetate. The drug is available as tablets for oral use (Table 18–1). It provides an anti-inflammatory effect within 30 minutes after it is taken orally.

Prednisolone. The drug is available in tablets for oral use (Table 18–1). It is available as the acetate or terbutate in solutions for intramuscular, intravenous, intra-articular, or intrabursal injection. The drug is also available as a cream or an aerosol solution and as a solution or ointment for ophthalmic use. The intravenous solution is injected over a one-minute period (25 to 50 mg) in acute situations, and the drug injection provides an anti-inflammatory effect within one hour. It may also be given two times per day in an infusion that provides 100 mg of the drug. The mineralocorticoid activity of the drug is approximately one quarter to one half that of cortisone or hydrocortisone.

Prednisone. The drug is available as tablets for oral use (Table 18–1). The mineralocorticoid activity of the drug is approximately one quarter to one half that of cortisone and hydrocortisone.

Triamcinolone. The drug is available as tablets for oral use (Table 18–1) and as an ointment, cream, lotion, gel, foam, and spray for topical use. It is also available as *triamcinolone acetonide* or *triamcinolone diacetate* suspensions that provide repository parenteral drug for therapy. The slow release of the drug (i.e., 40 to 80 mg) from the intramuscular tissues occurs over a period of time ranging from four to seven days.

Beclomethasone Dipropionate (VANCERIL). The drug is a relatively new formulation that is available as an aerosol spray. It is employed for the treatment of persons with severe asthma. It provides specific topical tracheobronchial anti-inflammatory activity with low systemic toxicity. Persons whose glucocorticoid therapy is changed from systemic use of the drug to aerosol administration should be observed for evidence of steroid withdrawal symptoms (i.e., joint and muscular pain, lassitude, depression) during the transition period. The therapy plan usually involves two inhalations (100 mcg) of the drug two to four times per day. The maximum therapy for adults is 20 inhalations per day.

Adrenocorticotropic Hormone

DRUG THERAPY

The pituitary gland is considered to be the master gland for hormonal production, and decreased function of the vital organ necessitates replacement of the hormones that it naturally produces. Adrenocorticotropic hormone (ACTH), or corticotropin, may be employed to replace the hormone when there is hypopituitarism, but it is used more commonly to increase the endogenous release of glucocorticoids from the adrenal cortex. ACTH is also used for diagnostic testing of adrenocortical function.

Action Mode

ACTH stimulates the adrenal gland to secrete its entire spectrum of cortical hormones. During therapy with the drug there is an increase in the circulating levels of glucocorticoid, mineralocorticoid, and androgen. The stimulus to glucocorticoid production provides the increased anti-inflammatory activity that periodically is useful in some of the chronic disease states (i.e., asthma, myasthenia gravis, multiple sclerosis, rheumatoid arthritis).

Therapy Considerations

Corticotropin (ACTHAR) is a protein extract from the anterior pituitary gland of animals that is administered parenterally. The rapid tissue utilization of the drug necessitates its administration at six-hour intervals to maintain the desired adrenocortical production of glucocorticoids.

During the initial period of therapy for hospitalized patients, it may be administered as an infusion over a period of eight hours and that provides a therapeutic effect for a 24-hour period. The dosage is adjusted to the anti-inflammatory effect that is provided by the drug. There is considerable individual variation in the adrenocortical sensitivity to the stimulation by the hormone. The initial daily dosage range is 40 to 80 units. The dosage may be increased gradually to the daily dosage maximum of 200 units. The total daily dosage is divided for administration four times per day when the drug is administered by subcutaneous or intramuscular injection. The dosage is lowered for prolonged therapy because more than 40 units/day can produce uncontrollable adverse effects.

The drug is available as *repository corticotropin* (ACTH GEL, CORTICOTROPIN GEL, CORTROPHIN GEL, HP ACTHAR GEL) and as *corticotropin-zinc hydroxide* (CORTROPHIN-ZINC). The slow absorption of the repository drug from the muscle (18 to 24 hours) allows it to be given as a single daily intramuscular injection.

The drug dosage is gradually reduced at the termination of therapy. During the readjustment period, the patient is observed for evidence of adrenal insufficiency (i.e., muscle weakness, lassitude, fatigue, hypotension), and the drug dosage may be increased if these symptoms appear.

Adverse Effects

The consistently higher circulating blood levels of the glucocorticoids that are provided by the use of ACTH may cause the same adverse effects as those that occur with administration of the adrenocortical hormone. ACTH-induced overstimulation of the adrenals may cause weight loss with a negative nitrogen balance, hyperglycemia, edema and hypertension that are associated with sodium and water retention, "moonface," hirsutism, abdominal striae, and osteoporosis.

Hypokalemia is usually averted by the addition of potassium-rich foods to the diet to provide at least a 5-gm potassium intake per day. In the absence of that supplementation, there may be muscle weakness, exhaustion, fatigue, or paresthesias during therapy with ACTH.

Hypoprothrombinemia occurs during ACTH therapy in some patients. The drug seldom causes psychotic episodes, but the high dosage that is required for intensive therapy may precipitate behavioral changes. Hallucinations, delusions of reference, exaggerated euphoria, pronounced insomnia, agitated depression, or a decreased ability to concentrate may occur during therapy. Patients intermittently are aware of their behavioral problems and they usually can relate them to the effects of the drug. A reduction in dosage usually modifies the problem.

Antihistamines

DRUG THERAPY

The antihistamines frequently are employed to alleviate the discomfort of erythema, pruritus, and edema that are associated with allergic reactions. Many antihistamine preparations are available as over-the-counter (OTC) products for topical or internal use, and they commonly are employed for the control of skin rashes (i.e., poison ivy reaction) or the initial coryza that is associated with the invasion by the cold virus.

Action Mode

The antihistamines compete with histamine for the H_1 receptor sites on the smooth muscle of the blood vessels, gastrointestinal tract, uterus, and bronchial muscle. They are effective in preventing the histamine-induced vasodilation and capillary porosity. That action decreases the erythema and swelling and the production of secretions at sites of allergen-antibody or allergen-lymphocyte interaction. The effects of the drugs are greatest when they are used early in the allergic response because they intercede before histamine stimulates the receptors. At the time of administration, the drugs interfere with histamine activity, but the histamine-induced responses that occur prior to the time of drug administration are unaffected by the drugs.

Therapy Considerations

The antihistamines are absorbed rapidly after oral or parenteral administration. The onset of action occurs within 15 to 30 minutes after oral administration and the duration of action is approximately three to six hours or longer. The drugs are rapidly converted to inactive metabolites that are excreted in the urine.

Preparations Available

The antihistamines that are employed for the control of allergic responses are classified by their structural commonalities. The classes include *ethanolamine derivatives, ethylenediamine derivatives, phenothiazine derivatives, propylamine derivatives,* and *miscellaneous antihistamines.* The adverse effects that commonly occur during therapy with the drugs within the structural groupings should be considered when discussing the drug therapy plan with the patient.

Ethanolamine Derivatives

The group of drugs includes *carbinoxamine, diphenhydramine, diphenylpyraline,* and *doxylamine* (Table 18–2). The drugs produce a higher frequency of anticholinergic effects than other antihistamines. The problems include dryness of the mouth, blurring of vision, constipation, dysuria, impotence, vertigo, tinnitus, sweating, tachycardia, personality changes, headache, faintness, and paresthesias.

Central nervous system depressant effects occur in approximately 50 percent of the patients taking the drugs. The problems include drowsiness, dizziness, lassitude, disturbed coordination, and muscular weakness. The sedative effects may be beneficial for persons whose rest and sleep have been disturbed by the allergic response. Tolerance to the sedative effects gradually occurs when therapy is continued. During the initial days of therapy the person should be cautioned against performing tasks that could jeopardize safety when dizziness or drowsiness occurs.

Carbinoxamine Maleate. The drug is available as tablets, extended-release tablets, elixir, and syrup for oral administration. The daily dosage of the drug for children older than six years of age ranges from 12 to 16 mg, divided for administration three or four times per day. The daily dosage for children younger than six years of age is 6 to 16 mg, divided for administration three to four times per day.

The extended-release formulation is a layered tablet that contains 8 to 12 mg of the drug. It is usually taken at 8-to-12-hour intervals.

Diphenhydramine Hydrochloride. The drug is available as an elixir, capsules, and enteric-coated tablets for oral administration. It is available in solutions for intramuscular or intravenous injection. The drug is found in many solutions, creams, and lotions in combination with other drugs. Antihistamines can cause allergic reactions, and their use topically is usually limited to short periods of treatment of acute allergic skin reactions. The lotion or cream containing diphenhydramine hydrochloride with calamine (CALADRYL) is frequently employed for that purpose.

The oral dosage for children over 12 years of age is based on the adult dosage. The daily oral and intravenous dosage for children younger than 12 years of age is based on the calculation of 5 mg/kg of body weight, divided for administration three or four times per day. The intramuscular dosage for children under 12 years of age is 12.5 to 25 mg. The drug should be injected into a large muscle mass to avoid tissue irritation.

Diphenylpyraline Hydrochloride. The drug is available as tablets and extended-release tablets

Table 18–2.
Antihistamines That Are Employed for the Control of Allergic Reactions

Drug	Daily Dosage (Adult)			Occurrence of Adverse Effects (Frequency)
	Route	Range (mg)	Number of Divided Doses	
Ethanolamine derivatives				
Carbinoxamine (CLISTIN)	Oral	12–32	3–4	*High:* Anticholinergic effects, central nervous system depression
Diphenhydramine (BENADRYL)	Oral	75–200	3–4	
	IM			
	IV	40–400	4	*Low:* Gastrointestinal disturbances
Diphenylpyraline (DIAFEN, HISPRIL)	Oral	6–12	3–6	
Doxylamine succinate (DECAPRYN)	Oral	50–150	4–6	
Ethylenediamine derivatives				
Methapyrilene (HISTADYL)	Oral	100–300	4–5	*High:* Gastrointestinal disturbances (mild)
	SC/IM	80–240	4–6	
	IV	40–160	3–4	
Tripelennamine (PYRIBENZAMINE)	Oral	100–600	2–4	*Moderate:* Central nervous system depression (drowsiness)
	IM/IV	25–50	2	
Phenothiazine derivatives				
Methdilazine (TACARYL)	Oral	14.4–32	2–4	*Moderate:* Central nervous system depression or stimulation
Trimeprazine (TEMARIL)	Oral	10–20	3–4	
Propylamine derivatives				
Brompheniramine (DIMETANE)	Oral	12–32	3–4	*Moderate:* Central nervous system depression or stimulation
	SC			
	IM			
	IV	10–40	2–4	
Chlorpheniramine (CHLOR-TRIMETON, HISTACHLOR, PHENETRON)	Oral	6–16	3–4	
	SC			
	IM			
	IV	10–40	1–4	
Dexbrompheniramine (DISOMER)	Oral	12–24	2–3	
Dexchlorpheniramine (POLARMINE)	Oral	6–8	3–4	
Triprolidine (ACTIDIL)	Oral	5–7.5	2–3	
Miscellaneous				
Cyproheptadine (PERIACTIN)	Oral	4–32	3–4	*High:* Drowsiness
				Low: Dryness of the mouth, dizziness
Dimethindene (FORHISTAL)	Oral	1–6	1–3	*High:* Drowsiness
				Moderate: Dizziness, headache, gastrointestinal disturbances

for oral administration. Children over 12 years of age may be given a dosage that is based on the adult dosage range. The daily dosage for children 6 to 12 years of age is 4 to 8 mg, divided for administration two to four times per day. The daily dosage for children under six years of age is 1 to 2 mg. The higher dosage (2 mg) may be divided for administration two times per day.

Doxylamine Succinate. The drug is available as tablets and syrup for oral administration. The daily dosage for children older than 12 years of age is 50 to 150 mg, divided for administration four to six times per day. The daily dosage for children under 12 years of age is 15 to 37.5 mg, divided for administration four to six times per day.

Ethylenediamine Derivatives

The ethylenediamine derivatives include *methapyrilene* and *tripelennamine* (Table 18–2). The drugs cause a high frequency of mild gastrointestinal disturbances, which may include epigastric distress, anorexia, nausea, vomiting, diarrhea, or constipation. The drugs may be administered with meals, with a snack, or with milk to decrease the gastric irritation that causes the problems. The incidence of central nervous system depression is much lower than that occurring with the ethanolamine derivatives.

Methapyrilene Hydrochloride. The drug is available in capsules, tablets, and a syrup for oral administration. It is available as solutions for subcutaneous or intramuscular injection. It is also available as solutions for nasal use, ointment for ophthalmic use, and topical ointment. It is an ingredient of some of the nonprescription drugs that are used for the treatment of insomnia (i.e., DORMIN, NYTOL).

The oral daily dosage for children and infants is calculated on the basis of 3.5 to 8 mg/kg of body weight, divided for administration four to six times per day. The single parenteral dosage for children and infants is based on the calculation of 400 mcg/kg of body weight.

Tripelennamine. The drug is available as *tripelennamine citrate* elixir for oral administration. *Tripelennamine hydrochloride* is available as tablets and extended-release tablets for oral administration. It is also available in solutions in nasal spray bottles and as cream and ointment for topical use.

The daily oral dosage for children is calculated on the basis of 5 mg/kg of body weight, divided for administration four to six times per day. Children may be given 100 to 150 mg of the extended-release formulation daily, divided for administration two to three times per day. The dosage of tripelennamine citrate usually is one and one-half times the dosage of the hydrochloride. For example, infants may be given 10 to 20 mg of the hydrochloride or 15 to 30 mg of the citrate. The dosage on the labels of the preparations is given as the equivalent of the hydrochloride salt.

Phenothiazine Derivatives

The phenothiazine derivatives that are employed for the control of allergic responses include *methdilazine* and *trimeprazine* (Table 18–2). The drugs produce a moderate frequency of central nervous system depression or stimulation.

Methdilazine Hydrochloride. The drug is available as a syrup or as tablets for oral use. *Methdilazine* is available as chewable tablets. The tablets form the hydrochloride when they enter the stomach. Rapid chewing and swallowing of the tablets are necessary to avoid the slight local anesthetic effect of the drug on the oral mucosa.

The dosage for children over three years of age is based on the adult dosage. Younger children may receive 8 mg/day, divided for administration two times per day. Infants may be given 4 mg/day, divided for administration two times per day.

Trimeprazine Tartrate. The drug is available as tablets, as a syrup, and as extended-release capsules. The dosage for children over 12 years of age is based on the dosage for adults. Children from 3 to 12 years of age may receive 3.5 to 7.5 mg/day, divided for administration three times per day. Children from six months to three years of age may be given 1.25 to 3.75 mg/day, divided for administration three or four times per day. Prolonged therapy (i.e., four to ten weeks) can cause the adverse effects that commonly occur when the phenothiazines are used for long-term therapy (i.e., cholestatic jaundice, extrapyramidal reactions, blood dyscrasias).

Propylamine Derivatives

The propylamine derivatives are the most active of the antihistamine drugs. The group includes *brompheniramine, chlorpheniramine, dexbrompheniramine, dexchlorpheniramine,* and *triprolidine* (Table 18–2). The drugs produce a moderate frequency of central nervous system depression or stimulation. Parenteral administration of the drugs can cause a local reaction, jitteriness, sweating, pallor, transient hypotension, and syncope. The drugs can also produce allergic, or hypersensitivity, reactions, which may include skin rash, urticaria, hypotension, or thrombocytopenia.

Brompheniramine Maleate. The drug is available as an elixir, tablets, and extended-release tablets for oral administration. It is also available as solutions for subcutaneous, intramuscular, or intravenous injection. The daily oral dosage for children over six years of age is 12 to 16 mg, divided for administration three to four times per day. The daily oral dosage for children under six years of age is based on the calculation of 440 to 500 mcg/kg of body weight, divided for administration three to four times per day. The parenteral dosage for children over 12 years of age is 0.5 mg/kg/24 hr, divided into three to four doses.

Chlorpheniramine Maleate. The drug is available as tablets, capsules, extended-release tablets, and syrup for oral administration. It is also available in solutions for subcutaneous, intramuscular, or intravenous injection. Chlorpheniramine maleate, gluconate, or tannate is also an ingredi-

ent in many preparations used for the control of allergic reactions in the respiratory tract.

The daily oral dosage for children over 12 years of age is calculated on the basis of the adult dosage. The daily oral dosage for children 6 to 12 years of age is 6 to 8 mg. The daily dosage for children two to six years of age is 3 to 4 mg. The childrens' dosage is divided for administration three to four times per day. The extended-release formulation may be prescribed for children over six years of age, and the dosage is 8 to 16 mg/day. The dosage is usually divided for administration once during the day and at bedtime.

Dexbrompheniramine Maleate. The drug is available as tablets, as extended-release tablets, and as a syrup for oral administration. The daily dosage for children over six years of age is 3 to 8 mg. The daily oral dosage for children three to six years of age is 3 mg. The daily dosage for children under three years of age is calculated on the basis of 220 mcg/kg of body weight. The daily dosage for children is divided for administration three times per day.

Dexchlorpheniramine Maleate. The drug is available as tablets, as extended-release tablets, and as a syrup for oral administration. The daily oral dosage for children over 12 years of age is based on the adult dosage. The daily dosage for children younger than 12 years is 1.5 to 5 mg (one half the adult dosage) and for infants it is one quarter of the adult dosage. The daily dosage is divided for administration to children or infants three or four times per day. The extended-release formulation may be used to provide the daily dosage for adults.

Triprolidine Hydrochloride. The drug is available as tablets and syrup for oral administration. The daily dosage for children over two years of age is 2.5 to 3.75 mg and for infants it is 1.25 to 1.87 mg. The dosage for children and infants is divided for administration two or three times per day.

Miscellaneous Antihistamines

The drugs included in the miscellaneous grouping include *cyproheptadine* and *dimethindene* (Table 18–2). The drugs have the same therapeutic uses and actions as other antihistamines but they have varying chemical structures.

Cyproheptadine Hydrochloride. The drug is available as tablets and syrup for oral administration. The usual daily dosage for children 7 to 14 years of age is 8 to 12 mg and for children two to six years of age it is 4 to 6 mg. That dosage may be divided for administration two to three times per day. In addition to transient drowsiness, dryness of the mouth, and dizziness, jitteriness, nausea, and skin rash may occur during therapy with the drug.

Dimethindene Maleate. The drug is available as tablets and extended-release tablets for oral administration. The daily dosage for children over six years is the same as the adult dosage (1 to 6 mg/day). The daily dosage for children under six years of age is 0.5 to 1.5 mg, divided for administration one to three times per day. The extended-release tablets may be given to adults and children over six years of age.

The adverse effects that may occur during therapy include drowsiness, dizziness, headache, dryness of the mouth, nausea, diarrhea, and urinary urgency. There may also be evidence of central nervous system stimulation (i.e., insomnia, hyperirritability, excitation). A reduction in the dosage usually modifies the problems.

Interactions

Monoamine oxidase inhibitors and alpha-sympathomimetic amines prolong or intensify the anticholinergic effects of the antihistamines. There also may be additive sedative effects when the antihistamines are given concurrently with other central nervous system depressants.

Immunizing Agents

DIAGNOSTIC ANTIGEN CHALLENGE TESTS

Intradermal injections of antigens are employed to determine the presence of sensitized immunoglobulins or lymphocytes when it is desirable to ascertain whether there has been exposure to disease-producing organisms or allergy-producing drugs. Agents are available for testing a person's prior exposure to the uncommon fungal invaders (i.e., *Coccidioides immitis, Histoplasma capsulatum*), viruses, parasites, *Mycobacterium*, or penicillin (Table 18–3).

The agents are sterile diluted preparations that are injected into the intradermal tissues of the upper arm or the flexor surface of the forearm. A positive test reaction is usually seen as redness, induration, or edema in a circumscribed area around the injection site. A positive diagnostic antigen challenge test result indicates an exposure-induced production of immune bodies that are sensitized to the antigenic substance. The exposure may have occurred without producing overt manifestations of the disease that generally is caused by the organism.

A positive test reaction to *coccidioidin, histoplasmin,* or *tuberculin* indicates that the exposure to the organisms has produced some immunologically competent cells. The person's clinical status and other tests are evaluated before therapy is instituted. For example, a positive reaction to *purified protein derivative of tuberculin* (PPD) may be followed by chest x-rays and sputum analyses. Those diagnostic tests are required to determine whether the disease is active or dormant. Positive x-ray findings and sputum cultures indicate the need for drug therapy for the treatment of tuberculosis.

A positive test result after the intradermal injection of *diphtheria toxin* or *mumps skin test antigen* is an indication that the immunologically competent cells are available to protect the indi-

Table 18–3.
Agents Employed for Diagnostic Antigen Challenge Tests

Dermal Test Agent	Antigen Source	Exposure Tested	Reaction Onset Time
Coccidioidin	*Coccidioides immitis* (10 strains)	Coccidioidomycosis	24–48 hr
Diphtheria toxin, Diagnostic Diphtheria toxin, Inactivated diagnostic	*Corynebacterium diphtheriae*	Diphtheria	48–72 hr
Histoplasmin	*Histoplasma capsulatum*	Histoplasmosis	24–48 hr (up to 3 days)
Mumps skin test antigen	Jeryl Lynn B strain of mumps virus	Mumps (epidemic parotitis)	24–36 hr
Tuberculin, Old	*Mycobacterium tuberculosis*	Tuberculosis	48–72 hr
Tuberculin, Purified protein derivative (PPD)			
Penicilloyl-polylysine (PPL)	Penicilloic acid	Penicillin	15 min

vidual who is exposed to those diseases. When the test result is negative, vaccination may be planned to provide immunity for the unprotected person.

A positive reaction to *penicilloyl-polysine* (PPL) indicates the presence of antibodies that could cause an anaphylactic response during a rechallenge with the drug. It is usual for an alternate drug to be employed for the control of an infection when the penicillin antigen test result is positive.

SERUM THERAPY

Passive immunity can be provided for the unprotected person who is exposed to a disease-producing organism by the injection of serum from humans or animals who have immunologically competent cells that are specific for the antigen causing the disease. Injection of the serum provides sensitized antibodies that immediately become available to destroy the invading antigens and they provide that protection for approximately three weeks. The serum products that are commonly employed include antitoxins, antivenins, and immunoglobulins:

Antitoxins and Antivenins
  Antirabies serum (equine)
  Botulism antitoxin, bivalent
  Crotaline antivenin, polyvalent
  Diphtheria antitoxin
  Lactrodectus mactans antivenin
  Micrurus fulvis antivenin
  Gas gangrene antitoxin, pentavalent
  Tetanus antitoxin

Immunoglobulins
  Hepatitis B immune globulin (human)
  Immune serum globulin (human)
  Mumps immune globulin (human)
  Pertussis immune human serum
  Rabies immune globulin (human)
  Rh_o (D) immune globulin (human)
  Tetanus immune globulin (human)

Antitoxins and Antivenins

The serum products are the antibodies that are obtained from horse or bovine sources. A state of hyperimmunity is attained in the animal by periodic injection of preparations of venom, viruses, or toxin-producing bacteria. The serum antibody level, or *titer,* is gradually elevated by progressive increases in the strength of the antigenic substance.

Each of the serum products has specificity for a particular antigen or proteins with similar structures. For example, *Lactrodectus mactans antivenin* is produced by the injection of black widow spider venom into the animal, and the antibodies are sensitized to that venom. *Polyvalent crotaline antivenin* has a broader spectrum of specificity because the antigens that are used to stimulate antibody production include Eastern and Western diamondback, Central and South American rattlesnake, and fer-de-lance venom. The antivenin can be employed to provide passive immunity for the individual who is bitten by any one of the species of snakes whose venom is used as the antigen, or venom, stimulus for antibody production in the animal. The antivenin is administered parenterally and some of the serum may be injected around the site of the snakebite to neutralize the venom at the entry site.

Serum Sickness

The original preparations of horse serums, which were used to provide passive immunity, caused a high incidence of allergic reactions. The preparations that are currently in use have been purified to remove most of the allergy-inducing proteins.

Sensitivity testing usually is planned before the administration of horse serum. The injection of 0.05 ml of the diluted serum (1:20) into the intradermal tissues or its instillation into the conjunctival sac produces redness within 5 to 20 minutes when the individual has antibodies that are sensitized to the serum from prior exposure to it. Bovine serum may be employed for treatment of the person who is sensitized to horse serum. When it is necessary to utilize the horse serum for sensitized persons, it is diluted and administered in small quantities (i.e., 0.05 to 0.5 ml) at 30-minute intervals while the individual is under close obser-

vation. Epinephrine hydrochloride and resuscitative equipment should be on hand because an anaphylactic reaction can occur during the period of horse serum administration.

Serum sickness can occur when sensitized immune cells are produced from seven to ten days after the serum is injected. The allergic response includes urticaria, edema, and swelling of the joints. The symptoms usually are relieved by the use of calamine lotion and the application of cold packs to the affected areas. The urticaria also responds well to antihistamine therapy but high dosages may be required.

Immunoglobulins

The immunoglobulins are obtained from human sources. *Immune serum globulin* is obtained by the collection and pooling of placental extracts from widely separated geographic areas. That process increases the spectrum of sensitized immunoglobulins that are in the solution. The globulin solution provides passive immunity against hepatitis, rubella, rubeola, and poliomyelitis.

Hepatitis, mumps, pertussis, rabies, and *tetanus immunoglobulins* provide immediate protection against the antigens for which they have specificity and that protection persists for a period of two to three weeks. The duration of immunity to the specific antigens is usually adequate to provide protection when close association with an infected individual cannot be avoided.

Rh₀ (D) immune globulin, unlike the other immunoglobulins, is administered to suppress antibody formation. It is employed to protect the Rh-negative mother from antibodies that can be produced after delivery of an Rh-positive baby. The placental products that are released during separation of the fetus can stimulate the formation of Rh-positive antibodies in the mother. At the time of subsequent pregnancies those antibodies would cause *erythroblastosis fetalis* or the abortion of an Rh-positive fetus. The umbilical cord blood is analyzed after delivery of the baby. Rh₀ (D) is administered intramuscularly to the mother within 72 hours after the delivery when the tests show that the newborn is Rh positive.

IMMUNIZATION

Active immunity against bacterial toxins, rickettsiae, or viruses may be provided by administration of live or attenuated organisms or their toxins (Table 18–4). Administration of the antigenic substances causes the endogenous production of sensitized T lymphocytes or immunoglobulins that can reproduce and destroy the antigens when an exposure occurs. The antigenic substance produces a subclinical disease that provides the memory pattern for the exposure-induced production of immune bodies.

Some of the immunizing agents are available as combined solutions. That combination of agents makes it possible to complete the immunity-building plan, which requires the use of three doses of each agent, without the trauma of numerous injections. *Diphtheria toxoid, pertussis vaccine, attenuated polymyelitis vaccine,* and *tetanus toxoid* are the agents available as a combined inoculating solution for injection.

Some of the immunizing agents are available as alum-precipitated, aluminum hydroxide–adsorbed, or aluminum phosphate–adsorbed preparations. The additives, or adjuvants, provide a tissue depot of the immunizing agent that is slowly absorbed from the injection site (i.e., diphtheria toxoid, pertussis vaccine, tetanus toxoid). The delayed rate of absorption provides higher immune body titers by maintaining the antigenic challenge over a prolonged period of time.

The adjuvants are irritating to the tissues, and a small air bubble is left in the syringe when the solution is prepared for administration. The injection of the air after the solution is injected completely clears the drug from the syringe and needle. The procedure prevents tissue contact with droplets of the solution when the needle is withdrawn.

Several of the immunizing agents are prepared by using chicken eggs as the growth media, and it is important to ascertain whether the individual has a known sensitivity to egg products before the immunizing agent is administered. Many individuals are sensitized to chicken or fowl products. Those persons may have an allergic reaction to the vaccines that are prepared in eggs (i.e., mono-

Table 18–4.
Agents Employed to Stimulate Endogenous Immune Body Production

Inoculant	Immunization Plan		Immunity Duration
	Indication	Doses Required	
BCG vaccine, attenuated (bacillus Calmette Guérin strain of *Mycobacterium tuberculosis*)	Preexposure (post negative dermal reaction testing)	1 injection	4 yr +
Cholera vaccine, inactivated (*Vibrio cholerae*)	Preexposure	3 injections at 1-wk intervals	3–6 mo
Diphtheria toxoid (*Corynebacterium diphtheriae* toxin)	Age 6–8 wk or preexposure	3 injections at 4-wk intervals	5 yr +
Influenza vaccine, bivalent, inactivated* (type A_2 Japan; type A_2 Taiwan; type B_2 Massachusetts) Monovalent, inactivated* (type A Asian strain) Polyvalent, inactivated* (type A PR; type A_1 Ann Arbor;	Preexposure	2 injections at 2-mo intervals	1 yr +

Table 18–4

| Inoculant | Immunization Plan | | Immunity Duration |
	Indication	Doses Required	
type A₂ Japan; type A₂ Taiwan; type B₂ Massachusetts)			
Measles virus vaccine, live, attenuated*† (Edmonston, Schwarz, or Enders strains)	Age 12 mo or preexposure	1 injection	4 yr +
Meningococcal polysaccharide vaccine, Group C (*Neisseria meningitidis* strain C 11)	Preexposure and postexposure	1 injection	Unknown
Mumps virus vaccine inactivated*	Preexposure	2 injections at 4-wk intervals	6–12 mo
Live, attenuated* (Jeryl Lynn B strain)	Age 12 mo or preexposure	1 injection	2 yr +
Pertussis vaccine, inactivated (*Bordetella pertussis*)	Age 6 mo or preexposure	3 injections at 1-mo intervals	1–4 yr
Plague vaccine, inactivated (*Pasteurella pestis*)	Preexposure	2 injections at 1-wk intervals	4–6 mo
Pneumococcal vaccine, polyvalent	Preexposure	1 injection	4 yr +
Poliomyelitis vaccine Attenuated (type 1 Brunhilde; type 2 Lansing; type 3 Leon)	Age 6–12 wk or preexposure	3 injections at 1-mo intervals	4 yr +
Live, oral, monovalent (types 1, 2, 3 Sabin strains)	Age 6–24 wk or preexposure	1 drink of each type at 6-wk intervals	4 yr +
Live, oral, trivalent (types 1, 2, 3 Sabin strains)	Age 10–12 mo or preexposure	1 drink 6 mo after monovalent series	4 yr +
Rabies vaccine, inactivated*‡	Preexposure and postexposure	2 injections at 1-mo intervals	6 mo
Rocky Mountain spotted fever vaccine, inactivated* (*Rickettsia rickettsii*)	Preexposure	3 injections at 1-wk intervals	1 yr
Rubella virus vaccine, live*† (Cendehill HPV-77 strains)	Age 12 mo or preexposure	1 injection	4 yr +
Smallpox vaccine, attenuated* (vaccinia virus)	Age 15–18 mo or preexposure	1 injection	3 yr +
Tetanus toxoid (*Clostridium tetani* toxin)	Age 6–8 wk or preexposure	3 injections at 4-wk intervals	5 yr +
Typhoid vaccine, inactivated (*Salmonella typhi*)	Preexposure	3 injections at 1–4-wk intervals	1 yr
Typhoid and paratyphoid vaccine, inactivated (*Salmonella typhi, S, paratyphi, S, schott-mülleri*)	Preexposure	3 injections at 1-wk intervals	1 yr
Typhus vaccine, inactivated* (*Rickettsia prowazewki*)	Preexposure	2 injections at 1-wk intervals	6 mo
Yellow fever vaccine, attenuated*	Preexposure	1 injection	6 yr

* Product may be from chick or fowl media.
† Product may be from canine media.
‡ Product may be from rabbit brain media.

valent, bivalent, or polyvalent influenza vaccine, measles virus vaccine, mumps virus vaccine, rabies vaccine, Rocky Mountain spotted fever vaccine, rubella virus vaccine, smallpox vaccine, typhus vaccine, yellow fever vaccine). The allergic individuals may receive vaccines that are obtained from canine or rabbit sources. *Measles virus vaccine* and *rubella virus vaccine* are obtained from canines, and those products can be used as alternate immunizing agents. *Rabies vaccine* may be prepared by using the brains of rabbits, and it

provides an alternate immunizing solution for individuals who are allergic to the products that are prepared in eggs.

Some of the biologic products contain small amounts of antibiotics. Although the additive seldom causes an allergic response, it could precipitate a reaction in highly sensitized individuals. Antibiotics are used in the preparation of *measles virus vaccine, live attenuated mumps vaccine, poliomyelitis vaccines, rubella virus vaccine,* and *smallpox vaccine.*

Antiviral Drugs

The primary method for control of invasion by disease-producing virus is immunization. The only antiviral drug presently available for systemic use for the control of viral infection is *amantadine hydrochloride.*

DRUG THERAPY

The drug is a synthetic antiviral agent. It is employed for the treatment of Parkinson's disease and drug-induced extrapyramidal reactions (pseudoparkinsonism) and for the prevention or treatment of influenza caused by strains of influenza A and C viruses and the Sendai strain of parainfluenza virus. The mechanism of its action in the control of symptoms of parkinsonism is unclear. It is thought to increase the levels of dopamine at the basal ganglia by blocking the uptake of the neurotransmitter by the presynaptic neurons.

The drug is frequently employed to prevent an influenza virus infection in acutely ill patients or other persons to whom the disease poses a threat to life. Prophylactic use of the drug for those persons who are unavoidably exposed to the disease may decrease the incidence of viral infection or the severity of the influenza.

Action Mode

Amantadine hydrochloride (SYMMETREL) is thought to control the reproduction of virus by

preventing the uncoating of the viral particle that is required for its replication. It also prevents the entrance of the virus into the host cells. Because the drug intercedes between the viruses and the cells, it is more effective when it is administered prophylactically or at the time of the initial exposure to the pathogen.

Therapy Considerations

The drug is administered orally. The usual daily dosage for adults and for children over nine years of age is 200 mg, which may be given as a single dose to adults or may be divided for administration two times per day. Children under nine years of age may receive a daily dosage of the drug calculated on the basis of 4.4 to 8.8 mg/kg of body weight to a maximum of 150 mg/day. That dosage may be divided for administration two to three times per day. The minimum course of therapy is ten days, and it may be extended to 90 days when continued exposure to the influenza virus is unavoidable.

The oral drug is absorbed well from the gastrointestinal tract. Peak serum drug levels are attained within one hour after the drug is ingested. The average plasma half-life of the drug is 24 hours. The unchanged drug is excreted in the urine. It is excreted more rapidly when the urine pH is lowered by acidifying agents. The drug is excreted in the milk of nursing mothers.

Adverse Effects

The central nervous system and psychic effects of the drug may appear within a few hours or days after therapy is instituted. The problems vary in their severity and range from nervousness, irritability, fatigue, anxiety, insomnia, inability to concentrate, confusion, forgetfulness, and detachment to mental depression and psychosis. The problems occur less frequently and are less severe when the drug is administered in divided doses two times per day. Planning the time for taking the afternoon dosage at least six hours before retiring usually decreases the insomnia that occurs during therapy with the drug.

Allergic reactions include skin rash, dermatitis, and photosensitivity. Other adverse effects that may occur during use of the drug are related to its anticholinergic activity (i.e., dryness of the mouth, blurred vision, constipation, urine retention).

NURSING INTERVENTION

Allergy History Taking

Medical histories in the patient's clinical record generally include a statement about the allergies that are described by the patient during an interview. When there is an indication of a previous allergic reaction to a drug, that information is indicated prominently by a bold label on the cover of the patient's clinical record and it also may be written in the "doctor's order sheet." That practice is intended to reduce the risk that the patient will receive any drug known to produce an allergic reaction.

Lymphocytes and antibodies are sensitized to particular substances, but that specificity or "commitment" can include allergens with similar chemical structures. For example, individuals who have an allergic reaction during therapy with the natural penicillins usually are sensitized to the semisynthetic penicillins and they sometimes may react to the cephalosporins, which have a similar chemical structure.

The possibility that an allergic reaction can occur with products having similar structures makes it essential to explore the question of allergies carefully when taking the nursing history. Many individuals avoid exposure to those substances that have caused skin reactions, coryza, shortness of breath, or gastrointestinal problems. Their statements may not include those problems unless the inquiry by the nurse is specific and directive. The provocative questioning can assist the person to recall that there was a skin reaction to a particular cosmetic, shave cream, deodorant, or hair dye. The single incident loses significance for the individual when the change to another product solves the problem. Similar questioning about chemicals, dust, pollens, and foods may elicit information about respiratory and gastrointestinal allergies.

Each allergen that is identified by the patient may not be significant to the plan of therapy, but the frequent occurrence of allergic responses to topical or systemic drugs in patients with allergies to other chemicals makes it important to identify the base-line allergic status before therapy is instituted. An essential aspect of the discussion of causative factors is the description of the intensity and characteristics of the allergic response. The composite description is included in the clinical record, and it is discussed with the physician to assure its consideration when drugs are prescribed for treatment of the current health problem.

Counseling

Glucocorticoid Therapy. The glucocorticoids are frequently administered to hospitalized patients and are also frequently prescribed for use by ambulatory patients. Short-term therapy with the drugs is often aproblematic. The patient who is to maintain a long-term drug therapy program may receive the maximum benefit from the drugs and encounter fewer adverse effects when there is an initial period of instruction and regularly scheduled contacts for evaluation of progress and problems.

The person who is to take glucocorticoids for a prolonged period of time at home must be aware of the necessity for maintaining the uninterrupted schedule for taking the drugs. When there is an intercurrent illness that causes persistent nausea and vomiting, it is important that the person contact the physician. In addition to the necessity for making arrangements for parenteral administration of the usual drug dosage, an additional quantity of the drug may be required during the period of physiologic stress caused by the illness.

The person is examined at the time of each scheduled visit to the clinic or office. During the interim time periods self-examination or assessments by family members are important for the identification of infectious processes that can occur during therapy with the glucocorticoids. The fungi are opportunist organisms that can cause serious diseases (i.e., candidiasis, pneumocystic pneumonia, cryptococcosis, aspergillosis, sporotrichosis). Hygienic practices (i.e., hand washing, meticulous mouth care) and avoidance of unnecessary contact with persons who have infections are primary measures that can be employed to prevent infection. A minor elevation in the body temperature, cough, malaise, excess fatigue, and changes in the characteristics of body secretions (i.e., thick, opaque saliva) or the urine (i.e., odiferous, concentrated despite adequate hydration) can be described to the person as examples of body changes that are indicators of an infectious process.

The catabolism of proteins slows the healing of wounds and also increases the fragility of bones. In addition to encouraging the person to increase the daily intake of protein, it is important to suggest precautionary measures that can be used to prevent falls. For example, small amounts of water on the kitchen floor, scatter rugs, highly waxed floors, or low footstools may cause slipping or tripping. The suggested hazards usually alert the patient to accident-causing situations in the home that can be remedied.

Accidents in the home are common problems and occur most frequently when the individual is unsteady or unstable when ambulating. The discussion of accident prevention should be geared to the reality of the situation.

The porosity of bones is associated with muscle wasting. The person who has a well-developed musculature probably requires only a reminder that obvious hazards should be avoided. The more fragile elderly person will benefit by discussion of potential hazards as well as use of protective devices (i.e., handrails on stairs, adhesive strips in the bathtub) to prevent falls.

Antihistamine Therapy. Antihistamines are usually employed for short-term treatment of acute allergic reactions. Persons using the drugs should be cautioned against shortening the scheduled time intervals prescribed for use of the drug in an attempt to accelerate the course of therapy. The antihistamines can cause allergic contact dermatitis, and the intensive use of the drugs can provide the irritation that is required to sensitize the lymphocytes. The individual should be informed that the use of the drug is to be discontinued when a rash appears or when there is an extension of the inflammation. When an allergic reaction to an antihistamine occurs, there will be a similar response with future use of the drug. The person should be told to read the labels of over-the-counter preparations to prevent exposure to the allergy-producing drug when purchasing a product for the subsequent treatment of a similar health problem.

The drowsiness that commonly occurs when the patient is taking antihistamines can be a hazard when the individual performs tasks requiring mental alertness and a short reaction time. The person should be advised to schedule the times for taking the drugs when such activities are minimal. The person should also be made aware that other central nervous system depressants (i.e., alcohol) will increase the drowsiness produced by the drugs.

Review Guides

1. Outline a plan for assessing the adverse effects of dexamethasone when the patient is receiving the drug for the prevention of cerebral edema after brain surgery.
2. Describe the factors about the drug that would be explained to the ambulatory patient who is to take cortisone for the treatment of rheumatoid arthritis.
3. Outline a plan for assessing the therapeutic effects of the drug when prednisone is being given to a patient with asthma.
4. Explain the rationale for rest of the extremity after a patient has an injection of prednisolone terbutate into the bursa of the right arm.
5. Formulate a plan for nursing care of a patient who is receiving an intravenous infusion of adrenocorticotropic hormone (ACTH) over an eight-hour period each day. Describe in the plan the explanations that would be given to the patient about the effects and adverse effects of the drug.
6. The patient has giant hives over most of the body that appeared after an intravenous dosage of penicillin was given. Outline the factors that would be included in the explanation of the cause of the hives and the expected effect of the antihistamine that has been prescribed for control of the allergic reaction.
7. Describe the rationale for administration of amantadine hydrochloride to the patients on a cardiac surgical unit when there is an epidemic of influenza.
8. Explain the factors that influence the decision to administer Rh_o (D) immune globulin to a mother after her baby is born.

Additional Readings

Beaven, Michael A.: Histamine. *N. Engl. J. Med.,* **294:** part 1, p. 30, January 1, 1976; part 2, p. 320, February 5, 1976.

Bodey, Gerald P.; Hersh, Evan M.; Valdivieso, Manuel; Feld, Ronald; and Rodriquez, Victorio: Effects of cytotoxic and immunosuppressive agents on the immune system. *Postgrad. Med.,* **58:**67, December, 1975.

Bowman, Herbert S.: Effectiveness of prophylactic Rh immunosuppression after transfusion with D-positive blood. *Am. J. Obstet. Gynecol.,* **124:**80, January 1, 1976.

Bridgewater, Sharon C.; Voignier, Ruth R.; and Smith, C. Steven: Allergies in children. *Am. J. Nurs.,* **78:** 614, April, 1978.

Byyny, Richard L.: Drug therapy: withdrawal from glucocorticoid therapy. *N. Engl. J. Med.,* **295:**30, July 1, 1976.

Campbell, Allan M.: How viruses insert their DNA into the DNA of the host cell. *Sci. Am.,* **235:**114, December, 1976.

Carty, Rita M.: Some facts about allergy. *Pediatr. Nurs.,* **3:**7, March/April, 1977.

Donley, Diana: Nursing the patient who is immunosuppressed. *Am. J. Nurs.,* **76:**1619, October, 1976.

Elders, M. Joycelyn; Wingfield, Barbara S.; McNatt, M. Loretta; Clarke, James S.; and Hughes, Edwin R.: Glucocorticoid therapy in children. *Am. J. Dis. Child.,* **129:**1393, December, 1975.

Freda, Vincent J.; Pollack, William; and Gorman, John G.: Rh disease: how near the end? *Hosp. Pract.,* **13:**61, June, 1978.

Glasser, Ronald J.: How the body works against itself . . . . autoimmune disease. *Nursing 77,* **7:** 38, September, 1977.

Gould, Lawrence; Reddy, C. V. Ramana; Swamy, Narayana; Chau, Windell; and Dorismond, Jean-Claude: Hemodynamic effects of steroids in cardiac disease. *Am. Heart J.,* **92:**133, August, 1976.

Gutterman, Jordon U.; Mavligit, Giora M.; and Hersh, Evan M.: Chemoimmunotherapy of human solid tumors. *Med. Clin. North Am.,* **60:**441, May, 1976.

Halberg, Franz: Implications of biologic rhythms for clinical practice. *Hosp. Pract.,* **12:**139, January, 1977.

Johnson, Herbert H., Jr.: Itching. *Primary Care,* **2:**593, December, 1975.

Kerigan, A. T.; Pugsley, S. O.; Cockcroft, D. W.; and Hargreave, F. E.: Substitution of inhaled beclomethasone dipropionate for ingested prednisone in steroid-dependent asthmatics. *Can. Med. Assoc. J.,* **116:**867, April 23, 1977.

Kobrzycki, Paula: Renal transplant complications. *Am. J. Nurs.,* **77:**641, April, 1977.

Light, Wilma C., and Reisman, Robert E.: Stinging insect allergy: changing concepts. *Postgrad. Med.,* **59:**153, April, 1976.

Loeb, John N.: Corticosteroids and growth. *N. Engl. J. Med.,* **295:**547, September 2, 1976.

McCalla, June L.: Immunotherapy: concepts and nursing implications. *Nurs. Clin. North Am.,* **11:** 59, March, 1976.

Marks, Meyer B.: Recognizing the allergic person. *Am. Fam. Physician,* **16:**72, July, 1977.

Migeon, Claude J.: Diagnosis and management of congenital adrenal hyperplasia. *Hosp. Pract.,* **12:** 75, March, 1977.

Moss, Edward M.: The child with atopic dermatitis. *Primary Care,* **2:**615, December, 1975.

Newton, David W.; Nichols, Arlene O.; and Newton, Marian: Corticosteroids. *Nursing 77,* **7:**26, June, 1977.

Norman, Philip S.: The clinical significance of IgF *Hosp. Pract.,* **10:**41, August, 1975.

Nysather, John O.; Katz, Arnold E.; and Lenth, Janet L.: The immune system: its development and functions. *Am. J. Nurs.,* **76:**1614, October, 1976.

O'Loughlin, John M.: Infections in the immunosuppressed patient. *Med. Clin. North Am.,* **59:**495, March, 1975.

O'Malley, Bert W., and Schrader, William T.: The receptors of steroid hormones. *Sci. Am.,* **234:**32, February, 1976.

Ostler, H. Bruce; Thygeson, Phillips; Okumoto, Masao; and Wendell, Joan: Opportunist ocular infections. *Am. Fam. Physician,* **17:**134, April, 1978.

Parker, Charles W.: Drug therapy: drug allergy. *N. Engl. J. Med.,* **292:** p. 511, March 6, 1975; p. 732, April 3, 1975; p. 957, May 1, 1975.

Rhodes, Mitchell L., and Smith, Jan B.: The lung in autoimmune collagen vascular disease (A-CVD). *Heart Lung,* **6:**653, July–August, 1977.

Richards, Frank F.; Konigsberg, W. H.; Rosenstein, R. W.; and Varga, Janos M.: On the specificity of antibodies. *Science,* **187:**130, January 17, 1975.

Rose, Leslie I., and Saccar, Connie: Choosing corticosteroid preparations. *Am. Fam. Physician,* **17:** 198, March, 1978.

Rudolph, Robert I., and Leyden, James J.: Dermatologic therapy with immunosuppressive agents. *Postgrad. Med.,* **58:**103, August, 1975.

Schatz, Michael; Patterson, Roy; Zeitz, Stanley; O'Rourke, John; and Melam, Howard: Corticosteroid therapy for the pregnant asthmatic patient. *J.A.M.A.,* **233:**804, August 18, 1975.

Smolensky, M. H., and Reinberg, A.: The chronotherapy of corticosteroids: practical application of chronobiologic findings to nursing. *Nurs. Clin. North Am.,* **11:**609, December, 1976.

Sparks, Frank C.: Hazards and complications of BCG immunotherapy. *Med. Clin. North Am.,* **60:**499, May, 1976.

Speer, Frederic: Food allergy: the 10 common offenders. *Am. Fam. Physician,* **13:**106, February, 1976.

Streeten, David H. P., and Phil, D.: Corticosteroid therapy. I. Pharmacological properties and principles of corticosteroid use. *J.A.M.A.,* **232:**944, June 2, 1975;

———: Corticosteroid therapy. II. Complications and therapeutic indications. *J.A.M.A.,* **232:**1046, June 9, 1975.

Warrenfeltz, Annette, and Graham, William P., III: Avulsion injuries in patients receiving corticosteroids. *Am. Fam. Physician,* **11:**74, June, 1975.

Weigle, William O.: Immunologic tolerance and immunopathy. *Hosp. Pract.,* **12:**71, June, 1977.

Wells, James H.: Understanding atopic syndromes. *Postgrad. Med.,* **58:**67, October, 1975.

West, Sheila; Brandon, Brenda; Stolley, Paul; and Rumrill, Richard: A review of antihistamines and the common cold. *Pediatrics,* **56:**100, July, 1975.

Wolf, A. Ford: Hypersensitivity states. *Hosp. Med.,* **11:**56, November, 1976.

Zepp, E. A.; Thomas, J. A.; and Knotts, G. R.: Some pharmacologic aspects of the antihistamines. A survey of current clinical applications. *Clin. Pediatr.,* **14:**1119, December, 1975.

19

Sex Hormone Deficiency and Fertility Control

CHAPTER OUTLINE

Reproduction is a natural biologic process that assures propagation of the species. Technologic advances in the past decade have produced oral agents and intrauterine devices that provide the female with relatively safe and effective alternatives to the finality of sterilization for the control of reproduction. The wide acceptance of the conception control measures seems to be related to the element of personal choice involved in their elective use for family planning. Current drug research is directed at the development of agents that can be employed by the male for the same reversible control of conception.

Physiologic Correlations

Reproduction requires synchronized hormonal activity for its fruition. Although the gonads are the centers of the reproduction processes, the production of ova in the female or spermatozoa in the male is dependent on the hypothalamic releasing factors that control the secretion of hormones from storage sites in the anterior lobe of the pituitary gland. The neuromessengers from the hypothalamus that induce hormone secretion from the pituitary gland are *follicle-stimulating hormone releasing factor*, which induces the secretion of *follicle-stimulating hormone* (FSH),

401

and *luteinizing hormone releasing factor,* which induces the *secretion of luteinizing hormone* (LH). The gonadotropic hormones stimulate the release of steroid hormones from the gonads

(Fig. 19–1). Those hormones act on highly specific receptors of the reproductive organs to convert inactive cells to an active state.

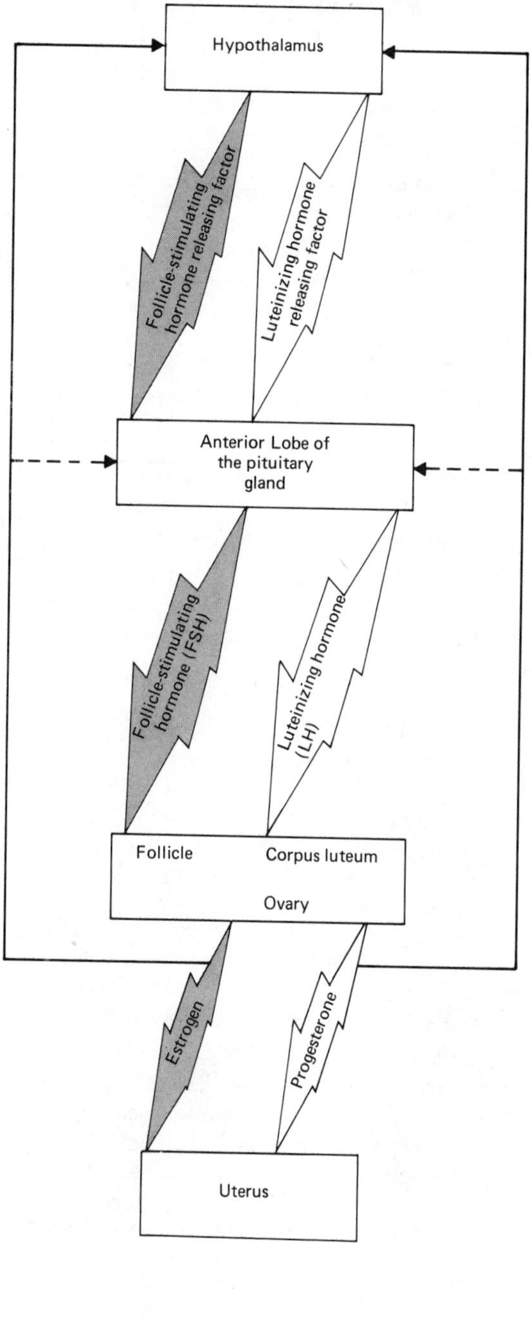

FEMALE SEXUAL CYCLE

Each of the gonadotropic hormones has a specialized function in the female and they work in unison to maintain the sexual cycle. The process of ovarian egg development begins in utero, and at birth the female infant's ovaries are estimated to have approximately one-half million primary follicles that contain oogonia, or germ cells. Spontaneous degeneration of the follicles during the following decade decreases their number appreciably, and only about 0.8 percent of the original number of follicles is estimated to be viable during the reproductive years.

The sexual cycle during the reproductive years of the woman generally is repeated at 28-day intervals, but the cyclic pattern may be 20 to 45 days in length. During each cycle the hormonal activity produces maturation of an ovum and prepares the uterine lining to harbor a fertilized egg.

Ovum Maturation

The female sex cycle is initiated by the activity of FSH, which starts the development of the primary ovarian graafian follicles a few days before menstruation signals the completion of the previous sex cycle. The maturing follicles produce estrogen and that hormone brings the immature egg to maturity. Within ten days, the follicle reaches maturity. LH is required for the final ovulation process, which releases the mature egg from the follicle on the fourteenth day of the female sexual cycle, or midcycle. The gonadal hor-

Fig. 19–1. The hypothalamic-releasing factor stimulates the pituitary release of FSH, which is required to activate estrogen-induced maturation of the follicles and the ova. Subsequent release of LH stimulates the release of progesterone from the corpus luteum. The synchronized activity of estrogen and progesterone produces the proliferative and secretory phases of endometrial development.

mone feedback at the time of ovulation suppresses the pituitary release of FSH, and the decline in blood levels of the gonadotropic hormone prevents supplementary ovulations.

Corpus Luteum Function

The ruptured and empty follicle becomes a secretory structure, or corpus luteum, which produces progesterone under the stimulus of LH. Prolactin, a third gonadotropic hormone produced by the pituitary gland, is also thought to contribute to the activity of the corpus luteum during its fourteen-day lifespan. The luteal cells reduce progesterone production about ten days after ovulation in each nonfertile cycle. Four to five days later the endometrium begins to break down and menstruation occurs. In the absence of pregnancy, the decline in blood steroid concentrations during the latter luteal phase stimulates hypothalamic-induced pituitary release of FSH and LH. During menstruation when the uterine lining is being shed, a subsequent fertilization cycle begins.

Endometrium Preparation

Before ovulation, the ovarian graafian follicles secrete increasing amounts of estrogenic steroids, primarily estradiol, that stimulate the proliferation of the endometrium and increase its vascularization. A final increase in the levels of estrogen in the bloodstream induces the hypothalamic midcycle release of LH, which precipitates ovulation within 24 hours. The change from estrogen to progesterone predominance is essential for the final preparation of the uterine lining for ovum implantation. The progesterone-induced endometrial development provides a thick lining that is moist with secretions.

HORMONE EFFECTS ON FEMALE SEXUAL CHARACTERISTICS

The primary action of estrogen is development of the organs of reproduction. At the time of puberty the gonadotropic hormones markedly increase the levels of estrogen, and there is a consequent rapid development of the fallopian tubes, uterus, and vagina.

Estrogen-induced proliferation of the uterine lining, replacement of the fragile cervical and vaginal epithelium with a stratified, trauma-resistant epithelium (cornification), and increased production of secretions are the primary changes that ready the organs for reproduction. There is a concurrent development of the secretory glands, enlargement of the external genitalia, and deposition of fat in the mons pubis and the labia majora.

The estrogens produce breast development by an increase in the deposition of fat, development of the stromal tissues, and growth of the ductile system of the mature female breasts. Progesterone activity is also required for the proliferation and enlargement of the alveoli of the breasts. The increased progesterone activity induces swelling of the breasts that is thought to be a consequence of the production of secretions in the alveoli and lobules and the accumulation of fluid in the subcutaneous tissues.

Estrogen-induced deposition of fat in the subcutaneous tissues gradually produces the contour of the adult female body. The larger amounts of fat in the buttocks and thighs produce the roundness that is characteristic of the female figure. A concurrent increase in the elasticity and vascularization of the skin produces softer, warmer tissues.

At the time of puberty, the activity of estrogens causes a rapid acceleration of linear bone growth, and the female is taller than most males of the same age. The osteoblastic activity, which provides that rapid growth spurt, also accelerates the closure of the epiphyses of the long bones. That process halts the linear growth of females earlier than that of males in the same age group. The osteoblastic activity also changes the contour of the pelvic bones to a broader structure with an ovoid outlet that can accommodate the passage of the mature fetus at birth.

The cyclic production of hormones continues throughout the reproductive years of women. Prior to the time of natural menopause, there is a gradual reduction in follicle activity, and the production of hormones declines. The sexual cycles become more irregular and finally cease at menopause.

MALE SEXUAL DEVELOPMENT

The placental release of chorionic gonadotropin produces a small quantity of testosterone, and that hormone provides the stimulus for the development of the testes. The subsequent release of testosterone from the fetal testes stimulates the production of spermatogonia, or germ cells.

There are approximately one to two thousand spermatogonia in the testes of the male fetus at the end of the second month of intrauterine life. Testosterone activity also produces the development of the penis, scrotum, prostate gland, seminal vesicles, and genital ducts and causes the descent of the testes into the scrotum during the last two months of gestation.

A large quantity of testosterone is released at the time of puberty, and the levels remain relatively high until the male climacteric when the hormone levels very gradually decline. The activity of testosterone at puberty produces enlargement of the penis, scrotum, and testes and a rapid development of the secondary male sexual characteristics.

Throughout the lifespan of the male there is a relatively consistent division of the spermatogonia, or spermatogenesis, in the seminiferous tubules. The process involves the transformation of the spermatogonium into motile spermatozoa with 23 chromosomes, or the haploid number, that are required for the fertilization of an ovum. Sperm production is dependent on the activity of luteinizing hormone, which stimulates the Leydig cells to produce the high local concentration of testosterone required to maintain spermatogenesis in the tubules. FSH binds to the cells of the seminiferous tubules to stimulate the proliferation of spermatogonia.

The spermatozoa travel from the seminiferous tubules to the long tubular structure of the epididymis where they become independently motile and less immature. Of the hundreds of millions of spermatazoa that are ejaculated during sexual intercourse, only a few hundred survive the journey to the upper segment of the fallopian tubes and only one sperm penetrates the viscous envelope that surrounds the egg.

The activity of the male hormone is more generalized than that of the female hormones. The testosterone that attaches to cellular receptors is converted in the cells to *dihydrotestosterone,* which activates the cellular processes. The adrenal glands of both the male and female secrete five or more androgens, but the quantities that enter the bloodstream are insufficient to provide significant masculinizing effects.

Testosterone accelerates the growth of body hair and provides the typical male distribution of hair over the pubic area, face, and chest. The hormone also produces baldness in males who have that genetically inherited trait. Testosterone-induced hypertrophy of the laryngeal mucosa and enlargement of the larynx produce the deeper voice of the adult male.

Testosterone increases the anabolism of protein, and there is a rapid development of the musculature. The protein building also increases the thickness of the skin and subcutaneous tissues. An increase of the protein matrix of the bones and the rapid deposition of calcium salts increase the thickness and length of the bones, and there is an acceleration of linear growth in the adolescent male.

REPRODUCTION

After its union with the sperm, the fertilized ovum travels through the undulating open end of the fallopian tube to the uterus. At approximately the nineteenth to twentieth day of the female sexual cycle, the cluster of cells, or blastocyst, is unattached and it is encircled by a single row of nourishing cells. The outer cells gradually nestle into the endometrium and begin to form the placenta.

The blastocyst produces copious amounts of gonadotropic molecules, or chorionic gonadotropin (CG), which provides the stimulus for continued release of progesterone from the corpus luteum. At the fifth week of gestation, when the lifespan of the corpus luteum is ended, the placenta provides the progesterone required for maintenance of the endometrial lining of the uterus.

LABOR INDUCTION

At the termination of the period of gestation, the clonic contractions of the uterus herald the onset of labor. The contractions, which are intensified by the voluntary abdominal muscular contractions of the mother, move the fetus forward through the predilated cervix and the birth canal.

The neural impulses that are transmitted to the hypothalamus by the dilated cervix provide the impetus for the transmission of neuromessengers that stimulate the secretion of oxytocin from the posterior pituitary gland. Oxytocin-induced uterine contractions facilitate evacuation of the placenta. The direct pressure on the capillaries and arterioles that is provided by the post-delivery contractions also decreases the endometrial bleeding after separation of the placenta.

LACTATION

The decrease in the levels of estrogen and progesterone that occurs after evacuation of the placenta reduces the amount of *prolactin inhibitory factor* that is released from the hypothalamus. The subsequent release of prolactin from the anterior pituitary gland stimulates the mammary glands to synthesize large quantities of fat, lactose, and casein, which are required for the production of milk.

The suckling of the infant provides the neural impulses that stimulate the hypothalamic-pituitary neuromessengers. The subsequent secretion of oxytocin from the anterior pituitary gland intensifies uterine contractions. Oxytocin also causes contraction of the myoepithelial cells that surround the alveoli of the breast, and that action expresses the alveolar milk into the ducts.

Drug Therapy

Hormone therapy is employed primarily to provide the male or female hormones when their endogenous production is deficient. The female hormones are used to inhibit or enhance conception and they are widely employed in obstetrics to induce labor, increase uterine contractions post-delivery, or to inhibit milk production. The hormones are employed selectively to change the hormone dominance in the treatment of patients with carcinoma of the reproductive organs. The use of hormones as antineoplastic agents is discussed in detail in Chapter 15.

Estrogen Therapy

The exogenous administration of estrogens provides all of the responses that are produced by the endogenous hormone. Estrogens are used for the treatment of females with a deficiency of the hormone as a consequence of underdeveloped ovaries (hypogonadism) or hypopituitarism. The administration of estrogen completes the maturation of poorly developed fallopian tubes, uterus, vagina, labia, and mammary glands. The hormones produce the changes in the reproductive organs that are common to the postpuberty female: proliferation of the endometrium and increased uterine tone; increased height of the cervical mucosal cells and increased secretions; and thickening and cornification of the vaginal mucosa. The hormones also provide the elasticity of the skin, deposition of fat in the breasts, buttocks, and thighs, and linear bone growth that are the natural secondary sexual characteristics in the female. The estrogen may be given for 14 days and progestogen may be given for the following 14 days for the establishment of the female sexual cycle. The treatment course usually is continued for three to six months. The termination of drug therapy is planned to allow evaluation of the status of the drug-free sexual cycle in the female.

The administration of estrogens to women during the pre- or postmenopausal period decreases the incidence of "hot flashes," sweats, chills, paresthesias, muscle cramps, myalgia, and arthralgia that are associated with the reduction of estrogen activity. The maintenance of estrogen levels also delays the elevation of blood cholesterol and phospholipid levels that occurs in postmenopausal women.

The administration of estrogens immediately after delivery maintains the hypothalamic release of *prolactin inhibitory factor,* and the production of breast milk is suppressed. Estrogen-progestogen combinations are employed to maintain menstrual periods in persons with undeveloped or nonfunctioning ovaries and are also used for ovulation control in the prevention of conception.

Therapy Considerations

The natural unconjugated estrogens are administered parenterally because they are inactivated in the gastrointestinal tract and the liver (estradiol, estrone). Conjugated estrogens, some synthetic derivatives of the natural estrogens, and the nonsteroidal estrogens are administered orally.

Most of the orally administered estrogens are rapidly absorbed and metabolized. The crystalline estrogen aqueous suspensions and the oil solutions are given by intramuscular injection; the immediate absorption of some of the depot drug provides prompt estrogenic activity and the slow absorption of the remainder from the depot site provides hormonal activity that continues for several days. The drug content of topical preparations is readily absorbed through the skin and mucous membranes, and the absorbed hormone produces systemic effects.

Estrogens are widely distributed in the body and high concentrations are found in most of the fatty tissues. The circulating hormones are 50 to 80 percent bound to red blood cells and other plasma proteins. The drugs cross the placental barrier.

The primary site of estrogen metabolism is the liver, but other tissues also metabolize the hormones (i.e., kidneys, gonads, muscles). The unchanged hormones and their metabolites are excreted primarily in the urine. Small amounts also enter the feces with the bile.

Preparations Available

Chlorotrianisene (TACE). The drug is a nonsteroidal estrogenic compound. Its estrogenic activity is dependent on liver metabolism, which produces a compound with higher hormonal activity than that of the weak parent drug. The drug is stored in adipose tissues, and its slow release from those tissues delays the onset of action and prolongs the duration of action.

The oral dosage of the drug is 12 to 25 mg daily for 21 days when it is employed for the treatment of women with estrogen deficiency. The oral dosage that is used in the postpartum period to prevent lactation and breast engorgement is 12 mg four times per day for seven days or 50 mg every six hours for six doses.

Conjugated Estrogenic Substances (GENESIS, PREMARIN). The drug contains the mixed conjugated forms of the naturally occurring estrogens *sodium estrone sulfate* and *sodium equilin sulfate.* The usual oral dosage for suppression of lactation is 1.25 mg for five days or 3.75 mg for five doses. The drug is administered every four hours when either of those dosage schedules is used.

Female hypogonadism is treated with a daily dosage of 2.5 to 7.5 mg/day. The drug is given in divided doses each day for a period of 20 days that is followed by a ten-day drug-free period, and the course of therapy is repeated until bleeding occurs. The usual dosage for the treatment of women with an estrogen deficiency related to menopause, surgical castration, or primary ovarian failure is 1.25 mg/day. The drug is administered in three-week cycles that are followed by a one-week drug-free period.

A dosage of 0.3 to 1.25 mg/day may be employed for treatment of women with senile vaginitis, pruritus vulvae, or kraurosis vulvae. The vaginal cream may be used for treatment of those vaginal disorders. It is used in an amount (2 to 4 gm) that supplies 1.25 to 2.5 mg of conjugated estrogens per day.

Dienestrol. The drug is a synthetic, nonsteroidal estrogen. The usual oral dosage for the treatment of patients with estrogen deficiency is 0.1 to 1.5 mg/day. The oral dosage used to prevent lactation and breast engorgement is 1.5 mg for three days and 0.5 for the following week.

Dienestrol is also used as a vaginal cream or foam in the treatment of vaginal disorders (i.e., atrophic vaginitis). The usual initial dosage of the cream is 0.5 to 1 mg/day for one to two weeks. The cream may be used at one half the initial dosage for an additional period of one to two weeks. The maintenance dosage is 0.5 mg one to three times per week.

Diethylstilbestrol (DES). The drug is a synthetic compound. It is the most active of the nonsteroidal estrogens. Use of the drug is contraindicated during pregnancy because cervical adenocarcinoma has been identified years later in the female offspring of women who received the drug while pregnant.

Diethylstilbestrol is administered orally. It is also available as a suppository for intravaginal use. *Diethylstilbestrol diphosphate* is administered orally. It is administered intravenously when it is used for the treatment of prostatic cancer. The usual oral dosage for treatment of women with estrogen deficiency is 0.1 to 0.5 mg/day. During prolonged therapy a cyclic treatment plan may be used. For example, the patient may receive three-week courses of drug treatment with a one-week drug-free period between each treatment course.

Diethylstilbestrol may be used both orally and intravaginally in the treatment of vaginal disorders. The vaginal suppositories (0.1 to 1 mg diethylstilbestrol) may be used daily, and the oral drug is taken concurrently at a dosage of 0.1 to 0.5 mg/day for 10 to 14 days on the cyclic plan of therapy. The oral dosage of diethylstilbestrol that is used for the suppression of lactation and breast engorgement is 5 mg one to three times per day until a total dosage of 30 mg has been given.

Diethylstilbestrol is the only estrogen that has been approved by the FDA for use as a postcoital contraceptive. The use of the drug is considered to be an emergency measure to prevent conception in victims of rape or incest and in select situations where the person's physical or mental health would be jeopardized by pregnancy. The drug is highly effective when it is taken within 24 to 72 hours after coitus. The dosage is 25 mg two times per day for five consecutive days. The woman should be informed that the drug must be taken in spite of the nausea that commonly occurs to prevent conception.

Esterified Estrogens (AMNESTROGEN, EVEX). The drug is a preparation of mixed natural estrone sulfate and sodium equilin sulfate. The proportion of estrone is higher and the proportion of equilin is lower than that of the conjugated estrogens. The dosages employed for therapy and the clinical uses of the drug are essentially the same as those of conjugated estrogens.

Estrogenic Substances (URETRIN, MENAGEN). The drug is a preparation of mixed natural estrogens. The dosage employed for suppression of lactation is 4 to 6 mg/day for six days. Women with an estrogen deficiency are given a dosage of 1 to 2 mg daily on a 20-day cyclic pattern that allows a ten-day drug-free period between each course of therapy.

Estradiol. The drug is a steroidal estrogen available in forms for oral use and for subcutaneous or intramuscular injection. It is the most active of the naturally occurring estrogens.

Estradiol (ESTRACE) initially is given by intramuscular injection at a dosage of 1 to 1.5 mg one to three times per week for the treatment of estrogen deficiency. The usual maintenance dosage is 0.5 to 1 mg/week. After two to three weeks of treatment, the dosage gradually is reduced. In the treatment of amenorrhea associated with hypogonadism the drug may be given by intramuscular injection at a dosage of 1 to 1.5 mg/week for two to three weeks. Progesterone usually is given during the following 14 days to complete the 28-day sexual cycle. The course of therapy usually continues for three to six months.

Ethinyl estradiol (ESTINYL, FEMINONE) is administered orally at a dosage of 20 to 50 mcg/day for treatment of estrogen deficiency for 21 days of planned 28-day cycles. The dosage usually employed for treatment of hypogonadism is 50 to 150 mcg/day for 14 days, and progesterone is administered for the following 14 days. Therapy is continued for three to six months. The dosage of ethinyl estradiol for the suppression of lactation is 50 mcg to 1 mg/day for three days. The dosage is then gradually reduced to 0.1 mg, and therapy is terminated after seven days.

Estradiol cypionate in oil (CYPIONATE, DEPO-ESTRADIOL) is a cottonseed oil solution that is administered by intramuscular injection for the treatment of patients with an estrogen deficiency at an initial dosage of 1 to 5 mg. That dosage may be given at weekly intervals during the following two to three weeks. The drug is given intramuscularly at a dosage of 5 to 10 mg in the treatment of patients with kraurosis vulvae. The injection may be repeated in two to three weeks.

Estradiol valerate in oil (DELESTROGEN, DURA-GEN, DURATRAD, ESTATE, ESTRAVAL, SPAN-EST, VALERGEN) is administered by intramuscular injection. The usual initial dosage is 5 to 20 mg for the treatment of estrogen deficiency. That dose provides two to three weeks of estrogenic effect. Two to three weeks later a dose of 5 to 20 mg may be given in combination with a progestin. A single dose of 10 to 25 mg is given at the termination of the first stage of labor to provide suppression of lactation in mothers who do not plan to breast-feed their infants.

Estrone (ESTROVAG, THEELIN). The drug is a steroidal estrogen. It is given intramuscularly at a dosage of 0.1 to 0.5 mg two to three times per week in the treatment of women with estrogen deficiency. Atropic vaginitis may be treated with the nightly use of a 0.2-mg vaginal suppository.

Piperazine estrone sulfate (OGEN) is the preparation usually used when estrone is given orally. The dosage is 3.75 mg every four hours for 20 hours after delivery to control the functional bleeding. Atropic vaginitis may be treated with a dosage of 0.625 to 2.5 mg/day. The oral dosage for treatment of women with estrogen deficiency is 2.5 mg/day for three to four weeks with a five-to-seven-day drug-free period following each treatment period. When the deficiency is associated with hypogonadism, the dosage is 1.25 to 3.75 mg/day for 21 days with a ten-day drug-free period in each treatment cycle. A dosage of 3.75 mg every four hours for five doses is used for suppression of lactation in the postpartum patient.

Adverse Effects

Nausea is the most common adverse effect during the initial days of therapy with the estrogens. The nausea usually disappears when therapy is continued. The estrogens may also produce other gastrointestinal effects (i.e., thirst, vomiting, anorexia, abdominal cramps, diarrhea). Headache, vertigo, scotomata, insomnia, lassitude, anxiety, paresthesias, or breast engorgement and tenderness may also occur during therapy with the hormones. There have also been reports of purpura, hypersensitivity reactions, edema, leg cramps, porphyria cutanea tarda, and chloasma. Prolonged therapy may produce hypercalcemia. Cyclic plans are usually used for prolonged periods of therapy with estrogens to avoid the endometrial hyperplasia and uterine bleeding that occur with continued administration of the hormone. Intravaginal application of the estrogens produces increased mucus secretion, and there may be a vaginal discharge. Anterior pituitary function may be inhibited by prolonged administration of the estrogens. Administration of the drug to adolescent females may cause premature epiphyseal closure in the long bones after the initial stimulation of linear bone growth.

Thromboembolic episodes have been associated with the estrogens that are used in oral contraceptives, and there is a potential risk of thrombosis during prolonged use of estrogens. Fluid retention and electrolyte imbalances may occur with prolonged use of the drugs.

Progestins

The drugs produce all of the responses that occur as a consequence of progesterone activity in the female. The drugs produce secretory changes and withdrawal bleeding in the endothelium that previously has been developed by the action of estrogen and they relax the uterine smooth muscle. The hormones also stimulate the development of mammary alveolar tissue and the production of secretions in the alveoli and lobules.

The hormones are used for the treatment of functional uterine bleeding associated with a hyperplastic nonsecretory endometrium, for the prevention of spontaneous abortion, and for the treatment of amenorrhea or infertility related to inadequacy of corpus luteum function. The drugs are also used in combination with estrogens for suppression of ovulation in the control of conception.

Therapy Considerations

Therapeutic plans for the control of functional uterine bleeding and amenorrhea involve the use of the progestins during the fifth through the twenty-fifth days (three weeks) of a female sexual cycle. Larger dosages of the progestins may be used during the sixteenth to the twenty-first days of the first cycle and repeated during the same period of three consecutive sexual cycles. The effects of the progestin are dependent on the endometrial proliferation produced by endogenous estrogen. In the absence of endogenous estrogen, that hormone is administered before the course of treatment with progestin.

Therapeutic plans for the control of infertility involve the use of the progestins immediately after ovulation and prior to conception. Therapy may be interrupted at the predicted time of menstruation, or alternate-day therapy may be planned after the tenth day of treatment to allow the onset of menstruation in the nonpregnant female. Although withdrawal of the drug usually produces shedding of the uterine lining, or menstruation, promptly in women who are not pregnant, there may be a three-week period before that event occurs.

Cyclic therapy with progestins, similar to that previously described, may also be employed for the treatment of infertility. The progestins may also be used to maintain the endometrial lining in women with a history of habitual abortion. The drug is usually given through the thirty-eighth week of gestation and is withdrawn when fetal viability is evident.

Preparations Available

Dydrogesterone (DUPHASTON, GYNOREST). The drug, a derivative of progesterone, is administered orally. In the treatment of functional uterine bleeding, the drug is given at a dosage of 10 to 20 mg/day for five to seven days. A dose of 10 mg is given daily from the twentieth to the twenty-fifth days of each cycle. Females with primary or secondary amenorrhea may be given 10 to 20 mg/day in divided doses from the fifteenth to twenty-fifth days of the sexual cycle, and those with functional amenorrhea may receive 10 mg/day for five consecutive days of each cycle. Infertility may be treated with 10 mg/day from the fifth to the twenty-fifth days of the cycle. The drug may also be given for treatment of dysmenorrhea at a dosage of 10 to 20 mg/day from the fifth to the twenty-fifth days of three to six consecutive cycles. Therapy then is interrupted to see if the normal cyclic menstrual pattern has returned.

Hydroxyprogesterone Caproate in Oil (DELA-LUTIN). The drug is a progesterone derivative with a duration of action of 7 to 14 days. The usual dosage for intramuscular injection in the treatment of amenorrhea is 375 mg 12 days before the predicted time of menstruation. When menstruation occurs, therapy is withheld for two to three cycles to assess whether the cycle continues without therapy.

Medroxyprogesterone Acetate (PROVERA). The drug is a synthetic progestin that usually is administered orally. The oral dosage used for the treatment of amenorrhea or functional uterine bleeding is 5 to 10 mg/day for five to ten days. The therapy is started on the estimated sixteenth or twenty-first day of the cycle. The drug may be given for prevention of abortion in an oral dosage of 10 to 30 mg/day until fetal viability is evident. An oral dosage of 10 mg/day may be given during the first trimester; 20 mg/day during the second trimester; and 40 mg/day in the third trimester to women with a history of habitual abortion. The women may also receive the drug by intramuscular injection at a dosage of 50 mg during the first trimester. The dosage then may be 100 mg every two weeks until the end of the eighth month of gestation.

Norethindrone (NORLUTIN, NORETHISTERONE). The drug is a synthetic progestin that is administered orally. It has androgenic activity, and the dosage levels are reduced when it is used for the treatment of patients with threatened abortion. Short-term use or dosage reduction prevents the hazard of masculinization of the female fetus. The oral drug also is available as *norethindrone acetate* (NORLUTATE), which is used at one half the dosage of norethindrone.

The dosage of norethindrone is 2.5 to 10 mg/day for the treatment of amenorrhea, or functional uterine bleeding. Therapy is started on the fifth day and stopped on the twenty-fifth day of the cycle. The dosage for the treatment of women who have a history of habitual abortion is 10 mg/day, and for threatened abortion it is 40 mg/day for five days with a reduction to 10 mg/day after the initial period of therapy. Endometriosis is treated with a dosage of 10 mg/day for a period of two weeks, and the dosage then is increased in increments of 5 mg every two weeks to a maintenance dosage of 20 to 30 mg/day. Therapy may be continued for six to nine months unless breakthrough bleeding necessitates interruption of therapy.

Progesterone (GESTEROL, LIPO-LUTIN, PROGE-LAN). The drug is available as an aqueous and as an oil solution. It is similar to the natural hormone that is secreted from the corpus luteum. It is administered by intramuscular injection at a dosage of 5 to 10 mg/day for six to eight doses for the control of functional uterine bleeding or the management of amenorrhea. In women who receive the drug for the treatment of amenorrhea, withdrawal bleeding may occur 48 to 72 hours after the last injection, and the normal cycles follow. The dosage for treatment of women with a history of habitual abortion is 2 to 20 mg one to three times per week and for threatened abortion it is 5 to 50 mg/day.

Adverse Effects

Short-term use of the progestins may produce spotting and irregular bleeding, nausea, or lethargy. Adverse effects are numerous during prolonged therapy with high dosages of the drugs. Decreased glucose tolerance, fluid retention, or electrolyte imbalances that are caused by the progestins can precipitate or aggravate chronic health problems (i.e., epilepsy, migraine, asthma). There have been reports of gastrointestinal disturbances, edema, headache, dizziness, amenorrhea, congestion of the breasts, and decreased libido. Jaundice has also occurred during prolonged therapy with the progestins. The drugs may produce some estrogenic and androgenic effects.

Androgens

DRUG THERAPY

The hormones provide the same responses as those produced by the male endogenous hormone *testosterone,* which is the principal androgen. Administration of the drugs produces development of the accessory sex organs (testes, prostate gland, penis), improves the functional capacity of those organs (i.e., spermatogenesis, libido, potency), and promotes the development of secondary sex characteristics. The androgens commonly employed for treatment of prepubertal or postpubertal males with hypogonadism are *testosterone, methyltestosterone,* and *fluoxymesterone.* The androgen *danazol* is employed primarily to change the hormone dominance of women who have mild to moderate endometriosis. The androgens are also employed in combination with an estrogen to suppress postpartum lactation. The use of androgens for the treatment of metastatic mammary carcinoma in postmenopausal women is discussed in detail in Chapter 15. The antineoplastic dosages of androgens are two to three times the dosages used for treatment of androgen deficiency.

Preparations Available

Testosterones. The preparations are the natural synthetic steroid that is similar to the endogenous male hormone. *Testosterone* (NEOHOMBREOL F) is the aqueous short-acting preparation that is administered at a dosage of 25 to 50 mg two to five times per week for the treatment of males with androgen deficiency. Testosterone pellets (ORETON), which have a three-to-four-month duration of action, may be implanted in the subcutaneous tissues to provide a dose of 150 to 450 mg in the treatment of males with hypogonadism. *Testosterone propionate* (ORETON PROPIONATE) is administered as buccal tablets at a dosage of 5 to 20 mg/day. The drug solution in sesame oil also is administered as an intramuscular injection at a dosage of 25 mg two to five times per week. The tablets may be used in the immediate postpartum period at a dosage of 25 to 50 mg/day for three to four days for suppression of lactation. *Testosterone enanthate* (DELATESTRYL) or *testosterone cypionate* (DEPO-TESTOSTERONE) usually is administered at a dosage of 200 to 400 mg every four weeks in the treatment of males with a deficiency of androgen. The drugs also are employed for the treatment of oligospermia at a dosage of 100 to 200 mg every four to six weeks.

Methyltestosterone. The drug is available as oral tablets (METANDREN, NEO-HOMBREOL M, ORETON METHYL), which usually are employed at a dosage of 10 to 50 mg/day for the treatment of hypogonadism. It is also available as buccal tablets, which are used at a dosage of 5 to 20 mg/day. The dosage of the oral drug that is employed for suppression of lactation is 80 mg/day, and that of the buccal tablets is 40 mg/day in divided doses for two days during the early postpartum period. The buccal tablets provide twice the bioavailable drug as the tablets that are taken orally.

Fluoxymesterone. The drug is available as oral tablets (HALOTESTIN, ORA-TESTRYL, ULTANDREN), which usually are employed at a dosage of 2 to 10 mg/day for treatment of males with hypogonadism. The drug is also available in combination with ethinyl estradiol (HALODRIN), and the tablets are used for suppression of lactation.

Danazol. *Danazol* (DANOCRINE) is a synthetic androgen and a derivative of testosterone ethisterone that is employed as an alternate drug for the treatment of women who have mild to moderate endometriosis that is unresponsive to therapy with female hormones. Endometriosis usually recurs within 60 to 90 days when treatment with danazol is terminated. The drug is used orally at a dosage of 400 mg two times per day for a period of three to six months. Therapy may be extended to nine months when continued treatment is needed. The drug decreases estrogen and progesterone activity by suppressing the pituitary release of the gonadotropins FSH and LH. The subsequent suppression of ovarian function produces atrophy and involution of endometrial tissues at uterine and ectopic sites. The drug-induced suppression of ovulation produces amenorrhea within six to eight weeks after therapy is initiated.

Anabolic Androgens. The anabolic steroids (Table 19–1) are synthetic agents with primary anabolic activity and minor androgenic activity. They are employed primarily for their protein-building effects when patients have severe muscle wasting or extensive tissue destruction (i.e., osteoporosis, burns, decubiti). Some of the steroids (i.e., dromostranolone propionate) are also used for the treatment of postmenopausal, or surgically castrated, women with advanced breast carcinoma. In approximately 20 percent of those women, there is a temporary recalcification of the bone metastases and regression of soft tissue lesions during therapy. The anabolic androgens also may be used to minimize the nitrogen losses associated with corticosteroid therapy and to stimulate erythropoiesis in treatment of patients with refractory anemia (i.e., aplastic anemia). The drugs are employed at higher dosages when they are used for their effect on red blood cell production. For example, the dosage of oxmetholone is 5 to 15 mg/day when it is given for its protein-building effects on body tissues. The dosage is 50 to 100 mg/day when it is used for the stimulation of the renal and extrarenal production of erythropoietin and the hormonal stimulation of bone marrow that accelerate red blood cell production. The use of the drugs at high dosage increases the incidence of adverse effects, and drug-free periods of two to three weeks may be planned at three-to-six-month intervals when the person is to receive the drugs for long periods of time.

Adverse Effects

The administration of androgens to children initially accelerates maturation of bone. The bone growth may be followed by closure of the epiphyses of the long bones and a consequent cessation of linear growth that decreases the adult height maximum of the male. Periodic x-ray evaluations of the status of bone matura-

Table 19–1.
Dosage Range of Anabolic Steroids

Drug	Route	Usual Adult Dosage*	Usual Child Dosage*
Ethylestrenol (MAXIBOLIN)	Oral	4–8 mg/day	1–3 mg/day
Methandriol (STENEDIOL)	IM	10–40 mg/day	5–10 mg/day
Methandrostenolone (DIANABOL)	Oral	2.5–5 mg/day	0.02–0.03 mg/kg/day
Nandrolone decanoate (DECA-DURABOLIN)	IM	50–100 mg/3–4 wk	25–50 mg/3–4 wk
Nandrolone phenpropionate (DURABOLIN)	IM	25–50 mg/wk	12.5–25 mg/2–4 wk
Oxandrolone (ANAVAR)	Oral	5–10 mg/day	0.25 mg/kg/day
Oxmetholone (ADROYD)	Oral	7.5–15 mg/day	2.5–5 mg/4–6 wk
Stanozolol (WINSTROL)	Oral	6 mg/day	2–6 mg/day

* Efficacy is evaluated after at least three months of therapy.

tion are planned at six-month intervals during androgen therapy in children to follow the progression of skeletal development.

The androgens produce virilizing effects in males with adequate endogenous androgen production. When the drugs are given to male children prepuberty, development of the accessory sex organs and male characteristics is accelerated. The child may have pubic hair, enlargement of the penis, and frequent erections. The appearance of abnormal, painful, continued erections (priapism) necessitates the interruption of therapy to decrease the high endogenous levels of androgens.

The androgens produce masculinization in females, and there may be hirsutism and enlargement of the clitoris that generally are reversible,

flushing of the skin, acne, oily skin, alopecia, increased libido, irregularities of menstruation, and deepening of the voice, which usually is irreversible. Hypercalcemia may appear in women who receive the drug at high dosage for treatment of advanced breast cancer.

Hepatic dysfunction has occurred in persons receiving methyltestosterone or fluoxymesterone, and it has also occurred during therapy with the anabolic androgens oxandrolone, oxymetholone, and stanozolol. The jaundice that results from intrahepatic cholestasis is reversible when therapy is terminated. Edema, which is associated with the sodium and water retention effects of the androgens, is most common in elderly persons and individuals with cardiac or renal dysfunction.

Growth Hormone

Somatotropin (ASELLACRIN) is employed for treatment of persons with growth failure caused by a deficiency of endogenous growth hormone. The agent is the purified extract of human pituitary glands.

Action Mode

Like the endogenous hormone, the drug stimulates the hepatic synthesis of *somatomedins* in a manner similar to the action of endogenous growth hormone. The *somatomedins* produce the anabolic activity in body tissues (i.e., bone, skin, muscle, collagen, visceral organs). The drugs are used primarily to stimulate normal linear bone growth, before epiphyseal closure, in children with a deficiency of the hormone.

Somatomedins enhance the intracellular transport of amino acids, and the synthesis of nucleic acids and proteins. The drug-induced stimulation of skeletal bone development increases intestinal absorption of calcium from the intestine and reabsorption of phosphorus in the renal tubules. The somatomedins also increase hemoglobin synthesis and induce lymphocytosis and erythropoiesis in the bone marrow.

Somatomedins produce gluconeogenesis and

increase hepatic glycogen production. The blood glucose levels are maintained by the inhibition of intracellular glucose metabolism and decreased activity of insulin that are caused by somatotropin. The lipolytic effect of the hormone mobilizes free fatty acids and glycerol from the fat stores of body tissues.

Therapy Considerations

The drug initially is administered intramuscularly at a dosage of 2 IU three times a week with a minimum of 48 hours between doses. The injection sites should be alternated to prevent the discomfort, pain, and swelling caused by the drug. Administration of the hormone is expected to produce a more than 2.5-cm increase in growth during a six-month period. Therapy is terminated when the normal linear growth for an adult is attained, there is epiphyseal closure, or the drug therapy fails to promote growth.

Adverse Effects

In a small number of patients (5 percent), somatotropin-neutralizing antibody titers become elevated to neutralizing levels during the first three to six months of therapy. When the response to therapy declines, antibody titers are evaluated and therapy is interrupted until the levels fall. The somatotropin antibodies are also thought to produce the infrequent allergic reactions that occur during therapy. About 30 to 40 percent of persons receiving the drug show antibodies to somatotropin, but their titers are not normally at neutralizing levels.

Interactions

Concurrent administration of thyroid hormones and androgens may accelerate epiphyseal closure. The use of glucocorticoids during therapy with somatotropin produces a synergistic effect that increases the blood glucose levels and decreases the sensitivity to insulin. The glucocorticoids also reduce the growth-stimulating effects of somatotropin.

Gonadotropic Hormones

DRUG THERAPY

The gonadotropic hormones *chorionic gonadotropin* and *menotropins* are employed for the treatment of deficient gonadal function. Chorionic gonadotropin is an extract from the urine of pregnant women, and menotropins is a purified preparation of the hormones FSH and LH, which is extracted from the urine of postmenopausal women. *Clomiphene citrate* is a nonsteroidal agent employed to stimulate ovulation in anovulatory women.

Chorionic Gonadotropin

Therapy Considerations.   The drug is available as ANDROID-HCG, ANTUITRIN-S, A.P.L., CHOREX, FOLLUTEIN, GONADEX, LIBIGEN, PREGNYL, and STEMUTROLIN for injection. The natural endogenous hormone, which is produced by the placenta during pregnancy, stimulates development of the gonads in the fetus. The drug is employed for the treatment of adult males with deficient endogenous androgen production due to hypopituitarism. The hormone stimulates the development of the Leydig cells of the testes and increases their production of androgen. It also stimulates maturation of the seminiferous tubule cells.

Administration of the drug to postpubertal females with functioning ovaries produces ovulation in the follicles that previously have matured under the influence of estrogen activity. Chorionic gonadotropin is also used in conjunction with menotropins to induce ovulation in anovulatory women who desire pregnancy.

The drug is administered by intramuscular injection. The usual initial dosage for the treatment of cryptorchidism is 4000 USP units three times per week for a period of three weeks. The dosage then is 5000 U every two days for four doses, followed by 100 to 1000 U over a six-week period, and a final course of 500 to 1000 U three times per week for four to six weeks. The therapy should produce the desired descent of the testes into the scrotum. Hypogonadism usually is treated with a dosage of 500 to 1000 USP units three times per week. The usual dosage for the treatment of corpus luteum deficiency and induction of ovulation is a single dose of 5000 to 10,000 USP units on the day after the last dose of the menotropins pretreatment was given. Drug administration is started on the fifteenth day of the female sexual cycle, and the course of therapy may be repeated during the same time period for three to four subsequent cycles.

Adverse Effects.   Fluid retention occasionally may occur as a consequence of increased androgen activity in males. Sexual precocity is a potential problem in prepubertal males who are treated with the drug.

Menotropins

The drug is used for the treatment of anovulatory females who desire pregnancy. Prior to use of the drug, the reproductive organs are examined to detect anatomic problems or primary ovarian failure. The fertility status of the sexual partner is also evaluated before therapy is started.

Therapy Considerations. Menotropins is administered by intramuscular injection at an initial dosage that contains 75 IU of follicle-stimulating hormone and 75 IU of luteinizing hormone. That dosage is given daily for 9 to 12 days. The end point of therapy is the occurrence of follicle maturation. The estrogen-induced changes in the vaginal cells and cervical mucosa and the increased quantity of cervical secretions are observable estrogen effects that are associated with follicle maturation. The urinary excretion of estrogen is a reliable objective indicator of the maturation process. A single dose of chorionic gonadotropin (10,000 USP units) is administered one day after the last dose of menotropins is given. Daily sexual intercourse is essential on each consecutive day from the time the last dose of menotropins is given to the time that ovulation occurs. The effects of progesterone, which appear at the time of ovulation, are a slight elevation in the basal body temperature and secretory and cellular changes in the vagina and cervix, which are evident during vaginal examination. When pregnancy does not follow ovulation, the course of treatment is repeated at the same dosage levels. The dosage of menotropins may be two times the initial level during two subsequent courses of therapy.

Adverse Effects. The most frequent adverse effect of the treatment plan is mild to moderate ovarian enlargement, with an associated distention of the abdomen or pain, which may persist for two to three weeks. Chorionic gonadotropin is not administered, and sexual intercourse is restricted to avoid rupture of ovarian cysts when there is an enlargement of the ovaries during the period of menotropins therapy.

There have been a few reports of a hyperstimulation syndrome within two weeks after therapy. The syndrome, which develops over three to four days, involves sudden ovarian enlargement and ascites or pleural effusion. The movement of intravascular fluid into the abdomen can produce hemoconcentration. Women who are taking the drug are examined every two days for evidence of excess ovarian stimulation during the treatment period and for two weeks after each course of therapy is completed.

Multiple pregnancies have occurred in approximately 20 percent of the patients who conceived as a result of menotropins-chorionic gonadotropin therapy. Nausea, vomiting, and diarrhea can also occur during the period of treatment.

Clomiphene Citrate

The specific action mode of clomiphene citrate in inducing ovulation is unclear. It stimulates the release of the gonadotropins FSH and LH from the pituitary gland, and that action produces the maturation of the ovarian follicle and ovulation and development of the corpus luteum.

Therapy Considerations. The drug is administered orally in a dosage of 50 mg daily for five days during the initial course of treatment. Ovulation is usually established after the first course of therapy with clomiphene citrate, and subsequent courses of therapy are started on the fifth day of each sex cycle. The drug may be given at a dosage of 100 mg/day for five days to women who fail to ovulate within 30 days after the first course of drug therapy. Most women ovulate after three courses of therapy.

Adverse Effects. Ovarian enlargement, cyst formation, and vasomotor symptoms (i.e., hot flashes) are the most common side effects of the drug. Therapy is interrupted when there is ovarian enlargement, and it may be reinstituted after the ovaries return to their pretreatment size.

During therapy with clomiphene citrate there may be abdominal distention or pain. Ocular toxicity associated with the action of the drug on the retina may produce transient blurring of vision, diplopia, scotomata, or photophobia. The drug may also produce nausea, vomiting, increased volume of urine and frequency of urination, heavier menses, weight gain associated with increased appetite, and dermatologic reactions (i.e., reversible hair loss, urticaria, skin rash, allergic dermatitis). Breast tenderness, increased nervous tension, headache, restlessness, insomnia, dizziness, lightheadedness, depression, and fatigue also may occur during the period of therapy. Multiple pregnancies frequently occur when the woman conceives during a clomiphene citrate treatment cycle.

Oral Contraceptives

DRUG THERAPY

The contraceptives are estrogen-progestins that are used in combination tablets to suppress gonadotropin secretion from the pituitary gland. The estrogen component of the combination tablet suppresses the secretion of FSH, and the progestin inhibits the midcycle, or preovulatory, release of LH when the tablets are taken during 20 to 21 days of the sexual cycle. A placebo tablet, which is similar in appearance to the drug-containing tablets, is taken on the remaining seven days of the cycle. The inhibition of ovulation alters the endometrium and cervical mucus in a manner that creates an unfavorable environment for the final maturation of the sperm, which usually occurs in an estrogen-prepared vaginal-uterine passage.

The contraceptives provide a shortened period of endometrial proliferation that is followed by a phase of limited endometrial secretory activity. Thinning of the endometrium may occur after several cycles, and the menstrual flow is reduced by the decreased thickness of the endometrial lining of the uterus. When therapy is terminated, the pituitary release of gonatropic hormones resumes and the hormones stimulate ovarian function. Ovulation usually occurs within three cycles. The endometrium may require up to three months to attain the normal proliferative and secretory activity of the sexual cycle.

The action of the estrogen component of the drugs on hepatic tissues may produce metabolic changes that primarily are manifested as alterations in carbohydrate and lipid metabolism. The drugs suppress lactation when they are taken in the immediate postpartum period. When the contraceptives are taken by nursing mothers, the hormones appear in the breast milk.

Preparations Available

The estrogen of the contraceptives is *ethinyl estradiol* or *mestranol* and the progestin is *ethynodiol diacetate, norethindrone acetate, norethynodrel,* or *norgestrel.* The preparations include

  Ethinyl estradiol and ethynodiol diacetate (DEMULEN)
  Ethinyl estradiol and norethindrone acetate (NORLESTRIN)
  Ethinyl estradiol and norgestrel (OVRAL)
  Mestranol and ethynodiol diacetate (OVULEN)
  Mestranol and norethindrone (ORTHO-NOVUM, NORINYL)
  Mestranol and norethynodrel (ENOVID, ENOVID-E)

The primary difference between the various preparations is the ratio of estrogen to progestin. Most of the preparations are provided in a 21-day dispenser and a 28-day dispenser that provides seven placebo tablets. The 28-day packet is considered to decrease omission of the drug by establishing a regular and continuous daily schedule for taking the contraceptive. The woman is advised to take the tablets regularly after the evening meal or at bedtime to minimize nausea. When the 21-day packet is used, the drug is taken from the fifth to the twenty-fifth day of the cycle, and there is a seven-day period before the drug schedule is resumed. The woman is advised to employ, or have her sexual partner employ, contraceptive measures during the first week of the initial period of therapy. Similar precautions are necessary for a period of seven days when two days of scheduled drug use are missed because there is a possibility that ovulation has occurred. The two missed doses necessitate taking two tablets daily for the next two days and resumption of the regular schedule after that period of time. When only one dose is missed, the tablet is taken as soon as the omission is remembered. The woman should be advised to stop taking the contraceptive when three doses are missed. Therapy is started seven days after the last dose was taken and alternate contraceptive measures should be used until the drug has been taken for seven days. The possibility of ovulation and breakthrough uterine bleeding increases with each missed dose. The drug therapy is continued when spotting occurs, but the schedule is interrupted when there is menstrual-type breakthrough bleeding. A new regimen is started on the fifth day after the onset of the bleeding.

Adverse Effects

Nausea is the most common adverse effect. Other gastrointestinal disturbances include vomiting, abdominal cramps, bloating, diarrhea, or constipation. The drugs may produce an increase or a decrease in appetite and weight, and edema may be present. Chloasma, or melasma, frequently occurs in women who had that dermatologic reaction during a previous pregnancy and occasionally occurs in other women during therapy. The irregular brown macules appear on the face, and they may remain after the drug therapy is terminated. Acne may be severe during the initial days of therapy, but the drug-induced decrease in the production of sebum generally produces an improvement in acne. A few women develop acne during contraceptive therapy. Other dermatologic reactions include rash, urticaria, erythema multiforme, erythema nodosum, hemorrhagic eruption, and pruritus. There have been a few reports of hirsutism and alopecia.

Tenderness and enlargement of the breasts and the production of secretions also may occur. Women are advised of the necessity for an annual gynecologic examination for evaluation of tissue changes (i.e., breast neoplasms, cervical erosion, cervical secretions), and a Papanicolaou smear is done to identify neoplastic changes as a routine part of that examination.

Hypertension has been associated with the use of oral contraceptives. Although the elevations usually are minor, some women have persistently high blood pressure. Those women are advised to use alternate contraceptive measures. The hypertension is reversible when therapy is terminated. The blood pressure elevation is considered to be related to stimulation of the renin-angiotensin system by the estrogen of the contraceptives.

Thrombophlebitis has occurred in a small number of women taking the drugs (i.e., thrombophlebitis, pulmonary embolism, cerebral thrombosis). The estrogen component of the drug enhances platelet aggregation, which may be the source of the problem. The woman is advised to inform the physician if there is severe headache, blurred vision, pain in the legs or chest, or a cough that is unrelated to a cold.

Mental depression, fatigue, nervousness, aggressiveness, anxiety, and irritability may occur. Depression occurs most frequently in women who have a history of premenstrual depression.

The drugs change the pH of the vaginal tract from acidic to alkaline, and there is an increased incidence of *Candida* infections. The contraceptive therapy may also produce cholestatic jaundice within two weeks to two months after therapy is started. The cholestasis produces malaise, anorexia, and pruritus.

There is considerable evidence that the risk of heart disease and stroke is twice as high in women who take the contraceptives as compared with other females. The risk is considered to be ten times as high when the women who take the drugs are over 35 years of age and smoke more than 15 cigarettes per day.

Many of the adverse effects of the oral contraceptives represent an imbalance between the estrogen:progestin ratio and the person's hormonal status. The factors that indicate an imbalance include:

Estrogen excess: nausea, migraine headache, breast tenderness, edema, hypertension, cervical mucorrhea, polyposis, and chloasma (melasma).

Estrogen deficiency: hypomenorrhea, increased spotting, and early or midcycle breakthrough bleeding.

Progestin excess: increased appetite and weight gain, tiredness and fatigue, hypomenorrhea, monilial vaginitis, hair loss or hirsutism, acne and oily skin, breast regression, and depression.

Progestin deficiency: amenorrhea and late breakthrough bleeding.

Oxytocics

DRUG THERAPY

The oxytocic drugs provide the uterine contractions that eject or evacuate the uterine contents. *Dinoprost tromethamine* is used to evacuate the products of conception and induce abortion. *Oxytocin, ergonovine maleate,* and *methylergonovine maleate* are used to provide uterine contractions that evacuate the placenta after the delivery of the fetus.

Dinoprost Tromethamine

The drug (PROSTINE F₂ ALPHA) is a derivative of the naturally occurring compound *prostaglandin F₂ alpha*. It has been approved for use in clinical trials by the FDA for intra-amniotic instillation to terminate pregnancy during the second trimester. When the drug-induced abortion is incomplete, instrumental or suction currettage may be required to complete the abortion.

Action Mode. Dinoprost tromethamine acts on the myometrium to produce uterine contractions. The drug also produces stimulation of the smooth muscle of the gastrointestinal tract. Large doses of the drug can cause bronchoconstriction and alterations in the blood pressure and heart rate.

Therapy Considerations. The drug is introduced into the amniotic fluid through a transabdominal intrauterine catheter. Abortion occurs within 20 hours after the instillation of 40 mg of the drug in approximately 50 percent of the patients. An additional instillation of 10 to 40 mg

may be given 24 hours later to women who do not abort after the initial instillation of the drug. The drug initially is introduced slowly at a maximum rate of 1 mg/minute until an initial 5-mg test dose has been given. The woman is observed closely for signs of drug sensitivity (i.e., vomiting, pain, bronchoconstriction) during the initial period of the instillation. The catheter is left in place to allow subsequent administration of the drug.

The drug is widely distributed in fetal tissues, and the highest concentrations are found in the fetal liver. The drug slowly diffuses into the maternal bloodstream after it is administered into the intra-amniotic fluid. It is rapidly metabolized in the maternal lungs and liver. The metabolites are completely excreted in the urine within 24 hours. Small amounts (5 percent) are excreted in the feces.

Adverse Effects. Approximately 50 percent of the patients who receive the drug have transient vomiting. About 25 percent of the women have nausea, abdominal cramps, or uterine pain. Diarrhea occurs infrequently. The gastrointestinal disturbances occur as a consequence of the drug-induced stimulation of the smooth muscle of the gastrointestinal tract. Lactation, which follows successful termination of the pregnancy, may last for several days. There have been occasional reports of unspecified pain, bradycardia, headache, flushing, dizziness, dyspnea, posterior cervical perforations, chills, endometritis, diaphoresis, coughing, wheezing, major motor seizures, paresthesias, hypertension, breast tenderness, urine retention, and uterine rupture.

Oxytocin

The drug (PITOCIN, SYNTOCINON) is a synthetic preparation that has the same activity as the endogenous hormone, which is released from the posterior pituitary gland. It is used to induce labor, to stimulate contractions in the postpartum uterus, and to control uterine bleeding after delivery.

Action Mode. Oxytocin acts directly on the uterine smooth muscle to produce clonic contractions. It concurrently stimulates the myoepithelial cells in the mammary gland and that action increases the flow of breast milk in the postpartum woman.

Therapy Considerations. The drug has a rapid onset of action. The buccal tablets provide uterine contractions within 30 minutes, and that activity persists for 30 to 60 minutes. Intramuscular injection of 0.25 to 0.5 unit of the drug provides uterine contractions in three to seven minutes, and they persist for 30 to 60 minutes. Intravenous injection is a safer and more reliable method of administration. It provides contractions within one minute but the duration of action is shorter than that occurring with the other routes of administration.

Oxytocin is used for the induction of labor only when medical problems (i.e., preeclampsia near term, maternal diabetes, ruptured membranes) threaten the life or health of the mother or fetus. Although the drug formerly was used for the elective induction of labor, the F.D.A. recently recommended these limitations on its use as a means of avoiding the adverse effects that can cause serious problems for the mother or fetus. The revised labeling of the drug and dosage information represent the new recommendations.

The drug is given as a dilute solution by intravenous infusion to induce labor at term. The drip rate is controlled to initially deliver 1 to 2 milliunits of oxytocin per minute. The dilation of the cervix, progression of uterine contractions, and status of the fetus are monitored regularly during the induction process. When labor is not induced by administration of the drug at the initial dosage level, the infusion rate is gradually increased in increments of 1 to 2 milliunits per minute until the mother's contraction pattern resembles that of normal labor.

Oxytocin is given by intramuscular injection at a total dosage of 3 to 10 units to produce uterine contractions postdelivery. It may also be used as a dilute intravenous injection that provides 0.5 to 2 units of the drug for the control of uterine hemorrhage in the postpartum patient.

Adverse Effects. Dilution of the intravenously administered drug is a necessary precaution to prevent the hypertension, tachycardia, and electrocardiographic changes that are associated with injection of concentrated solutions. Fetal cardiac arrhythmias (i.e., bradycardia, tachycardia) can occur during buccal administration of oxytocin. There have been a few reports of anxiety, dyspnea, precordial pain, cardiovascular spasm, edema, cyanosis, or redness of the skin during administration of the drug. Rupture of the uterus and fetal asphyxia may result from tetanic contractions when the drug is administered in excessive dosage or prematurely.

Ergonovine Maleate

Action Mode. The drug (ERGOTRATE) produces direct stimulation of the smooth muscle of the uterus, which increases the tone, rate, and amplitude of rhythmic contractions. It is used primarily for the prevention and control of uterine hemorrhage and to hasten involution of the uterus in the postpartum period.

Therapy Considerations. The drug is given at an oral or sublingual dosage of 200 to 400 mcg two to four times daily for 48 hours. The regular, firm uterine contractions constrict the uterine vessels and prevent bleeding or hemorrhage after separation of the placenta. The drug also may be given at a dosage of 200 mcg by intramuscular or intravenous injection to control postpartum hemorrhage. Hypertension or bradycardia occasionally is associated with use of ergonovine maleate. Parenteral administration is limited to emergency situations because there is a high incidence of adverse effects.

Methylergonovine Maleate

Therapy Considerations. The drug (METHERGINE) is a synthetic homolog of ergonovine and has a similar effect on the uterine smooth muscle. It produces stronger and more prolonged contractions than does ergonovine. Intravenous injection of the drug produces uterine contractions within 30 to 60 seconds. The contractions occur within two to five minutes after an intramuscular injection and within three to five minutes after oral administration. It is given by intramuscular or intravenous injection at a dosage of 200 mcg immediately after the delivery of the anterior shoulder in the second stage of labor or after the delivery of the placenta. The dosage may be given every two to four hours when uterine atony or hemorrhage persists. The oral dosage for subinvolution of the uterus during the postpartum period is 200 mcg three to four times per day.

Adverse Effects. The drug may produce headache, dizziness, and abdominal cramps. Hypertension and bradycardia occur less frequently with use of methylergonovine than with ergonovine maleate.

NURSING INTERVENTION

Nurses frequently have an opportunity, during day-to-day interactions with patients, to counsel them about sexual problems. Despite the widespread dissemination of information about sex issues (i.e., abortion, family planning, sexual identity, sexual preference) many persons have misconceptions about those and other aspects of human sexuality. For example, surgically castrated women frequently perceive themselves as being unable to participate actively in sexual intercourse. They also envision a loss of their female characteristics and a rapid onset of the aging process. Those persons benefit from the nurse's sharing of information about the anatomic integrity of the vaginal canal and the continued low-level production of estrogens from endogenous tissues.

The adrenal glands provide the precursors for the synthesis of estrone in the adipose tissues of the body. Although there is a lower circulating level of the hormone and estrone is less potent than the estradiol produced by the ovaries, the estrogen level is adequate to maintain the secondary sex characteristics. The changes in skin texture and hair distribution occur gradually rather than, as it often is perceived by the woman with a total hysterectomy, as a sudden physical change to a geriatric status.

Nurses frequently find it necessary to use provocative questioning to obtain essential information about the individual's perceptions and concerns. Many females seem highly sophisticated when the problems of sexual function are discussed. The ready availability of information concerning sex provides a general frame of reference and produces a pseudosophistication that can be misleading when obtaining information from the person. There is a difference between the person's ability to use appropriate terminology in the discussion of anatomy or reproduction control and the understanding of personal health problems or practices.

The reticence of health professionals to discuss sex-related matters is evident in the absence of relevant data in the clinical record of females who are being treated for nongynecologic problems. There is seldom a reference to the female's menstrual cycle or directives for the resumption of the use of oral contraceptive therapy predischarge from the hospital.

The predictable time of menstruation and problems that regularly occur during the sex cycle can have implications for care of the patient. For example, the menstrual process is preceded by a two-to-three-day period when the female functions physically and mentally at less than peak efficiency. Knowledge of that predictable period of time makes it possible to arrange major procedures at times other than those when the person is less capable of coping with the physical or emotional stress of the procedures. The nurse can optimize the health care of patients by identifying problems or concerns and assisting the person in their management.

The sharing of accurate information about hormone activity with patients is particularly important at the present time because the benefit-to-risk ratio is being considered carefully in each situation where the female hormones can be employed for therapy. Non-hormonal measures are being used for the control of many problems that previously were almost categorically treated with hormone therapy. For example, there is a trend toward dependence on the natural endogenous processes to decrease lactation. Women who are familiar with the relatively trouble-free suppression of lactation provided by the use of hormones may benefit from the nurse's sharing of information about the natural endogenous hormonal control of lactation. The use of a supportive bra or binder decreases the movement of the engorged breasts, and the application of ice packs also may ameliorate the discomfort of lactation in the nonnursing postpartum patient. The production of breast milk ceases, and breast engorgement gradually subsides in the absence of nipple stimulation by the suckling infant.

The potential for misconceptions about the hazards of hormone therapy is high when the drugs are employed for therapy. Most women are aware of the widely publicized relationship between endometrial cancer in the female offspring of women who received estrogens during pregnancy; the incidence of thrombophlebitis, hypertension, or prolonged anovulatory periods at the termination of therapy in females taking oral contraceptives; and the occurrence of endometrial hyperplasia in women taking estrogens for the control of premenopausal symptoms. In addition, the Food and Drug Administration requires that each person who receives a preparation containing an estrogen be given a printed description of the known hazards of the hormones. The person's awareness of those estrogen-related problems can induce fear of hormone therapy and lead to noncompliance with the therapy plan.

The person who is to take an estrogen-containing preparation should be informed of the protective measures that are being employed to assure safe use of the drug. For example, many of the current dosage recommendations are lower than those formerly employed, and there are planned drug-free periods, or cyclic patterns, that interrupt the drug therapy on a regular basis during the prolonged use of the estrogens. At the present time, the judicious use of the drugs, or the decision not to use the hormones, is based on the individual requirements of the person.

Review Guides

1. Describe the natural endogenous source of chorionic gonadotropin and its contribution to the development of sexual function and characteristics.

2. Outline the problems that the person should be told to discuss immediately with the physician during therapy with chorionic gonadotropic hormone and menotropins.

3. List the factors that would be included when counseling the person about the use of clomiphene citrate.

4. Describe the differences in the assessments that would be planned when estrogens are being given to a young female child and a premenopausal woman.

5. List the expected outcomes of therapy when a testosterone preparation is being given to a young male child and a 30-year-old adult male.
6. Outline the factors that would be included when explaining the effects of hormone therapy to the person who is receiving the drugs for suppression of lactation.
7. Describe the actions of the drug and the precautions to be observed when the person is receiving oxytocin for the induction of labor.
8. Outline the factors that indicate there is a problem in the matching of the hormone content of an oral contraceptive with the hormone status of the individual.

Additional Readings

Balin, Howard: Oral contraceptives. *Am. Fam. Physician*, **13:**109, January, 1976.

Barberia, Juan M.; Abu-Fadil, Salim; Kletzky, Oscar A.; Nakamura, Robert M.; and Mishell, David A., Jr.: Serum prolactin patterns in early human gestation. *Am. J. Obstet. Gynecol.*, **121:**1107, April 15, 1975.

Beck, Paul, and Lilling, Max I.: Induction of labor with intravenous prostaglandin. *Am. J. Obstet. Gynecol.*, **125:**648, July 1, 1976.

Billiar, R. B.; Jassani, M.; and Little, B.: Estrogen and the metabolism of progesterone in vivo. *Am. J. Obstet. Gynecol.*, **121:**877, April 1, 1975.

Bridgewater, Sharon C.; Voignier, Ruth R.; and Smith, C. Steven: Allergies in children. *Am. J. Nurs.*, **78:**614, April, 1978.

Buckman, Marie T., and Peake, Glenn T.: Prolaction in clinical practice. *J.A.M.A.*, **236:**871, August 16, 1976.

Chan, Lawrence, and O'Malley, Bert W.: Mechanism of action of the sex steroid hormones. *N. Engl. J. Med.*, **294:** part 1, p. 1322, June 10, 1976; part 2, p. 1372, June 17, 1976; part 3, p. 1430, June 24, 1976.

Chung, Hyo Jin: Arresting premature labor. *Am. J. Nurs.*, **76:**810, May, 1976.

Cowart, Marie, and Newton, David W.: Oral contraceptives: how best to explain their effects to patients. *Nursing 76*, **6:**44, June, 1976.

Csapo, A. I.: Effects of progesterone, prostaglandin F_{2a} and its analogue ICI 81008 on the excitability and threshold of the uterus. *Am. J. Obstet. Gynecol.*, **124:**367, February 15, 1976.

Dickey, Richard P.: Menstrual problems of the adolescent. *Postgrad. Med.*, **60:**183, October, 1976.

Ehara, Y.; Yen, S. S. C.; and Siler, T. M.: Serum prolactin levels during puberty. *Am. J. Obstet. Gynecol.*, **121:**995, April, 1, 1975.

Evans, James, and Townsend, Lance: The induction of ovulation. *Am. J. Obstet. Gynecol.*, **125:**321, June 1, 1976.

Evrard, John R.; Buxton, Bertram H. Jr.; and Erickson, Donna: Amenorrhea following oral contraception. *Am. J. Obstet. Gynecol.*, **124:**88, January 1, 1976.

Field, Peggy Anne, and Funke, Jeanette: The premenstrual syndrome: current findings, treatment and implications for nurses. *JOGN Nurs.*, **5:**23, September/October, 1976.

Frantz, Andrew G.: Physiology in medicine: prolactin. *N. Engl. J. Med.*, **298:**201, January 26, 1978.

Freeman, William S.: When patients "can't" take the pill. *Am. Fam. Physician*, **17:**143, January, 1978.

Goldzieher, Joseph W.; de la Peña, Armando; Chenault, C. Brandon; and Wontersz, T. B.: Comparative studies of the ethynl estrogens used in oral contraceptives. II. Anti-ovulatory potency. *Am. J. Obstet. Gynecol.*, **122:**619, July 1, 1975.

Graber, Edward A., and Barber, Hugh R. K.: The case for and against estrogen therapy. *Am. J. Nurs.*, **75:**1766, October, 1975.

Gwens, James R.; Andersin, Richard N.; Wiser, Winifred L.; Umstot, Edward S.; and Fish, Stewart A.: The effectiveness of two oral contraceptives in suppressing plasma androstenedione, testosterone, LH, and FSH, and in stimulating plasma testosterone-binding capacity in hirsute women. *Am. J. Obstet. Gynecol.*, **124:**333, February 15, 1976.

Horenstein, Simon: Oral contraceptives, stroke, and related phenomena. *Current Concepts Cerebrovasc. Dis. (Stroke)*, **X:** part I, p. 25, September–October, 1975; part II, p. 29, November–December, 1975.

Jewelewicz, Raphael: Management of infertility resulting from anovulation. *Am. J. Obstet. Gynecol.*, **122:**909, August 15, 1975.

Johnson, Wayne L.; Harbert, Guy M.; and Marting,

Chester B.: Pharmacologic control of uterine contactility. *Am. J. Obstet. Gynecol.,* **123:**364, October 15, 1975.

Jones, D. E. Darnell, and Halbert, David R.: Oral contraceptives: clinical problems and choices. *Am. Fam. Physician,* **12:**115, October, 1975.

Kerr, M. Dorothea, and Vaughan, Cynthia: Psychohormonal treatment during the menopause. *Am. Fam. Physician,* **11:**99, February, 1975.

Langer, Alvin; Devanesan, Mona; Pelosi, Marco A.; Apuzzio, Joseph J.; and Frattarola, Michael: Choice of an oral contraceptive. *Am. J. Obstet. Gynecol.,* **126:**153, September 15, 1976.

McEwen, Bruce S.: Interactions between hormones and nerve tissue. *Sci. Am.,* **235:**48, July, 1976.

Maloney, Joanne M.: Titrating with intravenous oxytocins. *JOGN Nurs.,* **4:**42, May–June, 1975.

May, W. Joseph: Current status of estrogen replacement therapy. *Am. Fam. Physician,* **16:**108, December, 1977.

Mills, Lewis C.: Drug-induced impotence. *Am. Fam. Physician,* **12:**104, August, 1975.

Oski, Frank I.: Oxytocin and neonatal hyperbilirubinemia. *Am. J. Dis. Child.,* **129:**1139, October, 1975.

Proudfit, Carol M.: Estrogens and menopause. *J.A.M.A.,* **236:**939, August 23, 1976.

Reichlin, Seymour: Regulation of the hypophysiotropic secretions of the brain. *Arch. Intern. Med.,* **135:**1350, October, 1975.

Reiter, Edward O., and Root, Allen W.: Hormonal changes of adolescence. *Med. Clin. North Am.,* **59:**1289, November, 1975.

Segal, Sheldon J.: The physiology of human reproduction. *Sci. Am.,* **231:**53, September, 1974.

Seki, Katsuyoshi; Seki, Metsunori; Okumura, Toshiko; and Huang, Ke-En: Effect of clomiphene citrate on serum prolactin in infertile women with ovarian dsyfunction. *Am. J. Obstet. Gynecol.,* **124:**125, January 15, 1976.

Shearin, Robert B.: Contraception for adolescents. *Am. Fam. Physician,* **13:**117, March, 1976.

Swerdloff, Ronald S.: Physiological control of puberty. *Med. Clin. North Am.,* **63:**351, March, 1978.

Tichy, Anna M., and Malasanos, Lois J.: The physiological role of hormones in puberty. *Am. J. Maternal Child Nurs.,* **1:**384, November–December, 1976.

Tyson, John E.: Mechanisms of puerperal lactation. *Med. Clin. North Am.,* **61:**153, January, 1977.

Umbeck, Kathleen, and Diamond, Frayda: An oxytocin challenge test protocol. *JOGN Nurs.,* **6:**29, January–February, 1977.

Weitzman, Elliot D.: Biologic rhythms and hormone secretion patterns. *Hosp. Pract.,* **11:**79, August, 1976.

Whitley, Nancy: Uterine contractile physiology: applications in nursing care and patient teaching. *JOGN Nurs.,* **4:**54, September–October, 1975.

Yen, Samuel S. C.: Estrogen and menopause. *Am. Fam. Physician,* **16:**87, July, 1977.

Ziel, Harry K., and Finkle, William D.: Association of estrone with the development of endometrial carcinoma. *Am. J. Obstet. Gynecol.,* **124:**735, April 1, 1976.

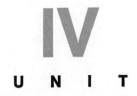

U N I T

Drugs Used to Maintain Gas Exchange and Removal of Toxicants and Wastes

20

Bronchial Constriction, Cough, Excess Mucus

The common cold is a recurrent health problem that plagues the population. In addition to the use of a variety of home remedies, it is estimated that Americans spend 700 million dollars each year for medications to treat colds. Realistically, those remedies may provide symptomatic relief, but, whether treated or untreated, the common cold generally persists for a period of five to seven days. Allergic rhinitis, which presents similar symptoms, is an antigenic reaction frequently confused with the common cold.

Asthma, which is the most common cause of bronchial constriction, is a health problem of approximately six million people in the country. Their respiratory status is dependent on the use of bronchodilators to maintain a patent airway during the recurrent episodes of bronchial constriction caused by the syndrome.

Physiologic Correlations

Travel Pathway of Inspired Air

The extensive and highly vascularized structure of the nasal passages provides for the warming and moistening of inspired air. The fine hairlike projections that line the mucous membranes, and the mucus secretions, ensnare the dust and other large particles that enter with the air on inspiration.

Intermittent mouth breathing significantly reduces the exposure of the inspired air to the protective surfaces of the nasal passages. Air that circulates over the smooth surfaces of the oral passages rapidly causes drying of those structures.

The ciliated columnar epithelium of the oropharyngeal and tracheobronchial structures provides for the warming, moistening, and filtering of inspired air that enters from the nasopharynx or the mouth. The air that reaches the lungs enters the alveoli and is available to perfuse the blood at the alveolar-capillary membranes.

Oxygen Utilization

Increased metabolic work, which occurs during periods of strenuous exercise or activity, raises the oxygen requirements of body tissues, and the gas is rapidly extracted from the circulating blood. The blood that returns to the pulmonary capillary beds has a low oxygen content, and the rate of oxygen diffusion across the alveolar-capillary membrane is increased by that deficit.

Carbon Dioxide Production

An increased metabolic rate increases the production of carbon dioxide, and the blood level of carbonic acid (H_2CO_3) is elevated. That increase in hydrogen ions and carbon dioxide in the blood stimulates the respiratory control centers in the medulla, and the efferent neural impulses from those centers increase the rate and volume of respirations. The blood levels of carbonic acid are lowered by the rapid diffusion of carbon dioxide across the capillary-alveolar membrane. The carbon dioxide is eliminated during expiration.

Sympathetic Nerve Stimulation

The sympathetic nerve division of the autonomic nervous system provides the adjustments that maintain physiologic equilibrium during periods of physical activity. The sympathetic nerve–induced cardioacceleration provides an increased circulation rate for the distribution of oxygen to active tissues, and the concurrent bronchodilation increases the ventilatory capacity.

The physiologic adjustments are provided by the action of the endogenous catecholamines *norepinephrine* and *epinephrine*. Those neurotransmitters stimulate the sympathetic, or adrenergic, receptors in the cardiac and bronchial tissues.

Beta-Adrenergic Receptors. The adrenergic receptors of the heart are described as beta$_1$ receptors and those of the bronchial tissues as beta$_2$ receptors. The differentiation of the beta receptors is related to their responses to stimulation by drugs.

Endogenous norepinephrine is the neurotransmitter that maintains the adjustments in the heart rate during periods of moderate activity. Exogenous norepinephrine has a weaker effect than epinephrine on the cardiac beta$_1$ receptors.

The administration of epinephrine, or the release of that hormone from the adrenal medulla during periods of strenuous activity, stimulates the beta$_1$ receptors in the cardiac tissues, and the heart rate and the strength of contractions are markedly increased. The concurrent stimulation of beta$_2$ receptors in the bronchial tissues produces bronchial dilation.

Pathophysiologic Correlations

THE COMMON COLD

A variety of viruses cause the common cold in adults and children. *Rhinoviruses* (60 types), *Coxsackie* viruses (29 types), and *ECHO* viruses (31 types) are the offending organisms in the symptom complex known as the common cold. The catarrhal infection of the nose and throat is associated with local discomfort due to congestion, excess mucus secretion, general malaise, and fatigue. Viral invasion of the lungs or superimposed bacterial infection may produce coughing, fever, and general malaise. Gastrointestinal disturbances may also contribute to the general discomfort of the pulmonary infection.

The tissue responses occur when antibodies in-

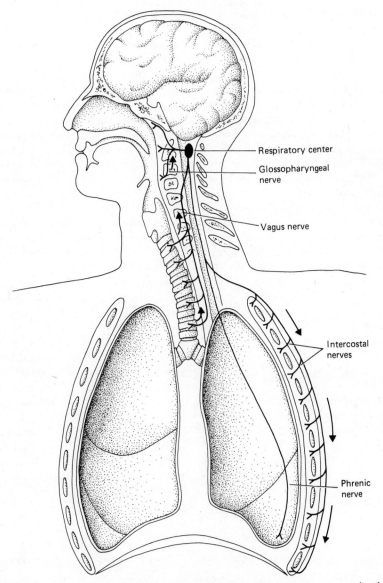

Fig. 20–1.   Afferent nerve endings in the tracheobronchial structures transmit stimuli to the medullary respiratory control centers. Efferent impulses to the muscles of respiration produce the explosive cough that is required to expel mucus or irritating substances.

teract with the viral antigen at local tissue sites. That union causes the mast cells, which are present in the tissues, to swell and rupture. The release of histamine from the disintegrating mast cells produces capillary dilation and an increased porosity of the capillaries. The hyperemic tissues become swollen when fluid and proteins slowly leak out of the capillaries. That sequence of events produces the initial swelling and congestion of the respiratory passages that herald the onset of a cold. When the tissues become overdistended with fluid, it begins to leak into the upper respiratory passages.

The local irritation, swelling, and fluid production stimulate the cough-sensitive nerve endings in the oropharynx, trachea, and main bronchus. The sensory branches of the vagus nerve transmit the stimuli to the respiratory center in the medulla. The efferent impulses to the muscles of respiration produce the contraction required for coughing (Fig. 20–1). The cough is a physiologic protective mechanism that maintains a patent airway for the passage of respiratory gases.

ASTHMA

The symptom complex characteristic of asthma generally represents an allergic response in the bronchial tissues. Approximately one third of the persons with asthma have no demonstrable allergic component during their asthmatic attacks, but the airway obstruction is comparable to that of the allergy-induced response.

The tissue response occurs when immunoglobu-lin E (IgE) and complement interact with the allergen at bronchial tissue sites. That interaction causes the release of histamine and *slow-reacting substance of anaphylaxis* (SRS-A) from the mast cells. The release of the slow-reacting substance is the more important factor in asthma because it produces and maintains the constriction of the smooth muscles of the bronchi. That problem is compounded by histamine-induced edema of the walls of the small bronchioles. Obstruction of the bronchiole lumen by inspissated mucus, spasm, and localized edema contributes to the marked reduction in the individual's maximum respiratory capacity.

Expansion of the lungs on inspiration partially opens the bronchioles, and air passes into the alveoli. On expiration the lung tissues compress and close the bronchioles and the alveoli. The increased bronchiolar resistance presents a barrier to the movement of air from the alveoli. The expiratory time is prolonged, and there is an increase in the functional residual capacity and the residual volume of air in the lungs.

Dyspnea, which is associated with the increased work of breathing, is characteristic of an acute asthma attack. The person uses all of the accessory muscles (i.e., abdominal, cervical, dorsal, pectoral) in an effort to expel the entrapped alveolar air. The heart rate is rapid and the respirations are rapid and shallow. The person usually sits in an upright or slightly chest-forward position, perspires profusely, and has an obvious look of fear or panic.

Bronchodilators

An acute asthma attack is a medical emergency. The primary focus is to provide an open airway. An adrenergic drug (i.e., epinephrine) usually is administered initially, and a theophylline drug may also be administered to maintain the open airway.

Various formulations of those agents are also used regularly as prophylactic agents, or they may be employed at the onset of an attack to prevent progression of the bronchiolar constriction.

ADRENERGIC DRUGS

The adrenergic, or sympathomimetic, drugs are employed for their bronchodilating action in treatment of the acute bronchoconstriction that occurs in asthma or other allergic states (i.e., drug-induced anaphylaxis). They are also used for symptomatic treatment of the mild bronchospasm that occurs with bronchial asthma or chronic obstructive lung disease (COLD). *Terbutaline sulfate* and *epinephrine hydrochloride* are the drugs most frequently employed for treatment of acute bronchoconstriction. Other adrenergic drugs used for their bronchodilating action are *ephedrine sulfate, ethylnorepinephrine hydrochloride, isoproterenol hydrochloride, metaproterenol sulfate, methoxyphenamine hydrochloride,* and *protokylol hydrochloride.*

Action Mode

The drugs stimulate the beta$_2$-adrenergic receptors in the bronchial tissues. They produce relaxation of the bronchial smooth muscle by stimulating the activity of the enzyme *adenyl cyclase* at the receptors. The enzyme increases the production of *cyclic adenosine 3′,5′-monophosphate* (cAMP), and that hormonal messenger produces the physiologic response. Each of the drugs, with the exception of terbutaline and metaproterenol, also stimulates the beta$_1$ receptors of the heart and that action causes an increase in the cardiac rate.

Epinephrine and ephedrine act on both alpha- and beta-adrenergic receptors in most of the tissues that are innervated by the sympathetic nervous system. Like other adrenergic agents, their beta-adrenergic effects are produced by stimulating the activity of the enzyme *adenyl cyclase.* The alpha-adrenergic effects are produced by inhibiting the activity of the enzyme. Parenteral doses of epinephrine primarily provide beta-adrenergic stimulation that produces bronchial smooth muscle relaxation, cardioacceleration, and dilation of the skeletal muscle vasculature.

Isoetharine Hydrochloride (BRONKOSOL)

The drug is diluted (0.25 to 1 ml in three parts saline sol.) for delivery as an aerosol to patients using a respirator or oxygen. *Isoetharine mesylate* (BRONKOMETER) is an oral nebulized drug which delivers a metered dose of 340 mg. Isoetharine is used at four-hour intervals. More frequent use can produce adverse adrenergic effects.

Terbutaline Sulfate

The drug action on beta$_2$-adrenergic receptors provides relaxation of the bronchial smooth muscles. It has little activity at the cardiac beta$_1$ receptors. Its action on the beta$_2$ receptors of the vasculature and the uterus relaxes the smooth muscles of the peripheral vasculature and the uterus. The peripheral dilation may reflexly cause a slight increase in the cardiac rate.

Therapy Considerations. Terbutaline sulfate is administered orally or by subcutaneous injection into the lateral deltoid area. The adult oral dose of the drug (Table 20–1) is usually administered three times a day at six-hour intervals during the waking hours to a maximum daily dosage of 15 mg. The daily dosage for children 12 to 15 years of age is 7.5 mg, divided for administration three times per day.

The adult subcutaneous dosage (0.25 mg) may be readministered after a 15-to-30-minute interval when bronchoconstriction persists. The maximum dosage for a four-hour period is 0.5 mg. The dosage for children under 12 years of age is investigational in the United States.

The drug is well absorbed from the subcutaneous tissues. Approximately 33 to 50 percent of the drug is absorbed from the gastrointestinal tract. The dosage represents an adjustment that compensates for the relatively low absorption and provides therapeutic serum drug concentrations. Following oral use of the drug, the onset of action appears within 30 minutes. There is significant improvement in the person's respiratory status within one to two hours. The peak effect is evident in two to three hours, and the duration of that effect is four to eight hours.

The onset of action of the drug occurs within 15 to 30 minutes after subcutaneous administration. The peak effect occurs within 30 to 60 minutes, and that effect lasts for one and one-half to four hours.

Terbutaline is metabolized in the liver. The unchanged drug (60 percent) and the metabolites (37 percent) are excreted in the urine within 72

Table 20–1.

Adrenergic Drugs Employed for a Bronchodilating Action

Drug	Route	Usual Adult Single Dosage (mg)	Usual Child Single Dosage
Ephedrine sulfate	Oral	25–50	See text
Epinephrine (SUS-PHRINE)	SC	0.5–1.5	0.01 mg/kg BW
Epinephrine hydrochloride (ADRENALIN CHLORIDE, VAPONEFRIN)	SC	0.2–1	0.01 mg/kg BW
Ethylnorepinephrine hydrochloride (BRONKEPHRINE)	SC IM	0.66–2	0.2–1 mg
Isoproterenol hydrochloride (ISUPREL)	SL	10–15	5–10 mg
Metaproterenol sulfate (ALUPENT, METAPREL)	Oral	20	See text
Methoxyphenamine hydrochloride (ORTHOXINE)	Oral	50–100	25–50 mg
Protokylol hydrochloride (VENTAIRE)	Oral	2–4	1–2 mg
Terbutaline sulfate (BRICANYL, BRETHINE)	Oral SC	2.5–5 0.25	3.5–5 mcg/kg BW*

* Dosage is investigational.

to 96 hours. Approximately, 3 percent of the drug enters the intestinal tract with the bile and is eliminated with the feces.

Adverse Effects. The most frequent adverse effects are tachycardia and transient episodes of palpitation, nervousness, tremor, and dizziness. There have also been reports of nausea, vomiting, headache, anxiety, restlessness, lethargy, drowsiness, tinnitus, and diaphoresis. The cardiovascular effects may be additive when other sympathomimetic drugs are administered concurrently.

Epinephrine

Therapy Considerations. The drug is most frequently administered as *epinephrine hydrochloride* for the treatment of acute bronchoconstriction. The adult subcutaneous dosage (Table 20–1) may be repeated in two hours when bronchoconstriction persists. The dosage for children may be repeated in four hours.

The drug is well absorbed from the subcutaneous tissues, and its absorption can be accelerated by massaging the site of the injection. Bronchodilation is produced within five to ten minutes after subcutaneous injection of the drug, and a maximal effect occurs in 20 minutes.

Epinephrine (SUS-PHRINE) provides a concentrated drug suspension (1:200) and is used when prolonged action is desired. The initial subcutaneous dosage for adults is 0.5 mg and that for children is 0.25 mg. The low initial dosage of the drug is planned to provide an opportunity to assess the effects of the drug on the respiratory and cardiovascular status of the patient. The drug may be given after a time interval of four hours when bronchoconstriction persists. The maximum dosage for adults is 1.5 mg and that for children is 0.75 mg.

The drug is also available as *epinephrine bitartrate* (MEDIHALER-EPI). The premeasured dose of epinephrine base that is provided with each inhalation of the mist is 0.2 mg. The inhaler is used by the person when the drug is required for control of bronchoconstriction, and the inhalant produces bronchodilation within one minute. Only minimal amounts of the drug are absorbed from the tissues of the respiratory tract. Rebound bronchospasm sometimes occurs when the effect of the inhaled drug is terminated. Dryness of the oropharyngeal membranes, which occurs during the inhalation of the drug, may be reduced by rinsing the mouth with water after the treatment.

Adverse Effects. The most frequent adverse effects are cardiac arrhythmias (i.e., premature ventricular contractions, palpitations, sinus tachycardia). Anxiety, tremors, tenseness, excitability, or insomnia may also occur. Other adverse effects include nausea, headache, pallor, bronchial edema, and inflammation.

Interactions. The cardiac beta-adrenergic effects can be antagonized by beta-adrenergic-blocking drugs (i.e., propranolol).The tricyclic antidepressants, monoamine oxidase inhibitors, some antihistamines, and sodium levothyroxine can potentiate the tachycardia induced by epinephrine.

Ephedrine Sulfate

The action, therapeutic uses, and adverse effects of the drug generally are similar to those of epinephrine. Ephedrine, unlike epinephrine, may deplete the presynaptic sympathetic neurons of their stores of norepinephrine by releasing it from the granule storage sites. That action gradually leads to tolerance of the cardiac and pressor effects of the drug.

Therapy Considerations. The drug is usually administered orally (Table 20–1). The dosage for adults may be repeated at three- or four-hour intervals. The oral dosage for children 6 to 12 years of age is 6.25 to 12.5 mg every four to six hours. The daily dosage for younger children is based on the calculation of 0.3 to 0.5 mg/kg of body weight, divided for administration four to six times per day.

The orally administered dosage is rapidly absorbed. The bronchodilating effect is evident within 15 to 60 minutes after the drug is ingested, and that effect persists for two to four hours. The cardioacceleration and the vasopressor effects of the drug may persist for four hours after the drug is administered at the therapeutic dosage level. The absorbed drug crosses the placenta and appears in the milk of nursing mothers. The drug is metabolized in the liver and excreted in the urine.

Adverse Effects. The orally administered drug may produce pronounced central nervous system activity (i.e., nervousness, anxiety, apprehension, fear, tension, agitation, excitement, restlessness, weakness, irritability, talkativeness, insomnia). Tolerance to the bronchodilating effects generally occurs, and the person may increase the dosage in an attempt to obtain the bronchodilator effects. The increased dosage can produce a reversible psychotic episode (i.e., paranoid psychosis, visual or auditory hallucinations).

Ethylnorepinephrine Hydrochloride

The beta adrenergic action of the drug produces bronchodilation, cardiac stimulation, and peripheral vasodilation. Although the effects, therapy considerations, and adverse effects are similar to those of isoproterenol, it less frequently is employed for treatment of acute bronchoconstriction.

Isoproterenol

The primary effects of the therapeutic dose of the drug are bronchodilation, cardiac stimulation, and peripheral vasodilation. Tolterance to the bronchodilating and cardiac effects may develop with frequent or prolonged use of the drug. In addition to the actions that are common to other adrenergic drugs, isoproterenol inhibits the release of histamine and the slow-reacting substance of anaphylaxis (SRS-A) at the sites of allergen-antibody interactions.

Therapy Considerations. *Isoproterenol hydrochloride* is used sublingually three or four times per day by adults and children for the relief of bronchospasm (Table 20–1). The maximum dosage for adults is 60 mg/day and that for children is 30 mg/day. The drug is commonly used at bedtime to decrease the moderate bronchoconstriction that causes noisy, wheezing respirations during the night.

Isoproterenol hydrochloride may occasionally be administered as an intravenous infusion at the rate of 0.08 to 1.7 mcg/kg of body weight per minute for the treatment of *status asthmaticus*.

The infusion rate is monitored carefully because higher dosage produces serious adverse effects. The intravenously administered drug produces an almost immediate bronchodilating action.

Isoproterenol sulfate (MEDIHALER-ISO) is available in an easy-to-use hand-held propellant nebulizer, which delivers 0.075 mg of isoproterenol per inhalation. The usual dose is one to two deep inhalations, and that dosage is repeated one or two times at five-to-ten-minute intervals when it is required for the relief of bronchoconstriction. That course of treatment can be repeated at four-to-six-hour intervals.

The drug is also available for use in a hand-held bulb nebulizer, which delivers approximately 125 mcg of the drug with each release. The person is instructed to take one to two deep inhalations of the solution, and that course of treatment is repeated at two-to-five-minute intervals to a maximum of six inhalations per hour when it is required.

The patient should be given instructions about the proper use of the nebulizer to assure that they obtain the maximum drug effect. Inappropriate use of the equipment can lead to swallowing of the drug.

Adverse Effects. The oral inhalant is rapidly absorbed from the tissues of the respiratory tract, and the drug may produce adverse effects similar to those of the absorbed sublingual drug. The most frequent adverse effects are cardiac irritability (i.e., palpitations, ventricular tachycardia, or fibrillation) and central nervous system stimulation (i.e., nervousness, excitability, insomnia, tremor). Concurrent administration of beta-adrenergic-blocking agents (i.e., propranolol) may cause a decrease in the bronchodilation, cardioacceleration, and vasodilation effects of isoproterenol.

Metaproterenol Sulfate

The drug has a more prolonged action and a lower incidence of the severe cardiac effects that occur with isoproterenol. It also has the advantage of being an effective bronchodilator when used orally. Metaproterenol produces relaxation of the smooth muscles of the bronchi and the peripheral vasculature at therapeutic doses.

Therapy Considerations. The oral dosage for adults is administered three to four times per day. The same dosage may be given to children over nine years of age (Table 20–1). The dosage for children six to nine years of age is 10 mg, and that dosage may be taken three to four times per day.

The drug is well absorbed from the gastrointestinal tract. Approximately 40 percent of the dose is metabolized in the first passage through the liver, and the dosage represents an adjustment to provide the desired therapeutic effect. The onset of the bronchodilator effect occurs within 15 minutes and the peak effect occurs within four hours. The duration of effect is somewhat shorter after long-term use of the drug.

Metaproterenol sulfate is available as an oral inhalant, which delivers 0.65 mg of the drug per inhalation. Adults and children are instructed to take two to three deep inhalations at four-hour intervals when the drug is required to relieve bronchoconstriction. The total daily dosage maximum is 12 inhalations. The drug produces a bronchodilating effect within one minute after it is inhaled.

Adverse Effects. The most frequent adverse effects are tachycardia, palpitation, hypertension, tremor, nervousness, headache, dizziness, nausea, vomiting, and a bad taste in the mouth. Propranolol and metaproterenol are mutually antagonistic when they are employed concurrently.

Methoxyphenamine Hydrochloride

The drug, like ephedrine, depletes the norepinephrine stores in the presynaptic sympathetic nerve endings. That action can produce tolerance to the vasopressor effects of the drug.

Therapy Considerations. The drug is taken orally three to four times per day by adults or children (Table 20–1). The bronchodilation effect occurs within 30 to 60 minutes after the drug is ingested, and the effect lasts for three to four hours.

Adverse Effects. The most frequent adverse effect is dryness of the oral mucosa and mild anorexia or nausea. The drug occasionally produces a slight increase in the blood pressure and the pulse rate, cardiac palpitation, anxiety, nervousness, wakefulness, lightheadedness, dizziness, and flushing. Concurrent use of other sympathomimetic drugs may produce additive effects. Propranolol and methoxyphenamine hydrochloride are mutually antagonistic.

Protokylol Hydrochloride

The drug is similar to isoproterenol in chemical structure and pharmacologic action. It has the advantage of providing bronchodilation when it is taken orally.

Therapy Considerations. The oral dosage is taken by adults four times per day. Children may receive the drug three to four times per day (Table 20–1).

The drug is well absorbed from the gastrointestinal tract. The onset of the bronchodilator action occurs in 30 to 90 minutes, and that effect lasts for three to four hours. The drug is metabolized in the liver at a slower rate than that of isoproterenol. The metabolites are excreted in the urine.

Adverse Effects. The most frequent adverse effects are tachycardia and palpitation. The drug occasionally produces central nervous stimulation (i.e., tremulousness, tenseness, insomnia, dizziness, vertigo).

THEOPHYLLINE DRUGS

The synthetic drugs that are included in the group are salts or derivatives of theophylline, and their action is dependent on their theophylline content. Caffeine is also structurally classed as a theophylline derivative, and that natural theophylline is found in tea.

Aminophylline is the theophylline most commonly employed for control of asthma. The group of drugs also includes *dyphylline, oxtriphylline, theophylline anhydrous, theophylline monoethanolamine,* and *theophylline sodium glycinate.*

Action Mode

The theophyllines have identical pharmacologic actions. They competitively inhibit the enzyme *phosphodiesterase,* which is the enzyme that degrades cyclic 3′,5′-adenosine monophosphate (cAMP). That action increases the quantity of intracellular cAMP that is available to mediate bronchodilation or inhibit the release of bronchoconstricting agents. A concurrent intracellular translocation of calcium ions also is considered to enhance the effects of theophylline. The drug also relieves bronchoconstriction or bronchospasm by a direct relaxant effect on the smooth muscles of the bronchi. Theophylline directly dilates the coronary, pulmonary, renal, and general systemic arteries and veins. Those actions decrease the peripheral vascular resistance and the venous pressure. At therapeutic dosage levels, theophylline constricts the cerebral vasculature, and it stimulates all levels of the central nervous system. The drug affects many physiologic processes. It has a low therapeutic index, and its use is maintained strictly within the limits of safe dosage to avert serious adverse effects.

Therapy Considerations

The theophyllines are available in formulations for oral or rectal use and for intramuscular or intravenous injection. The oral theophyllines are readily absorbed from the gastrointestinal tract. The presence of food in the digestive tract may delay absorption but does not reduce the total absorption percentage of the drug. The drug is slowly and incompletely absorbed from the intramuscular sites of injection. Rectal suppositories are absorbed slowly and erratically, but theophylline is well absorbed when it is given as a retention enema.

Serum theophylline concentrations of 10 to 20 mcg/ml provide a therapeutic bronchodilator response. The lower level of the range usually provides the bronchodilation required for the relief of mild bronchoconstriction. Adverse effects appear when the serum drug concentrations are elevated above the 20 mcg/ml level.

Intravenous administration of the theophyllines produces the rapid onset of action that is required during an acute episode of bronchoconstriction. Oral administration of the liquid capsules, or uncoated tablets, produces a peak plasma drug concentration within one to two hours. Enteric-coated tablets provide a peak serum drug concentration in five hours. The rectal suppositories produce peak serum drug concentrations in three to five hours, and the theophylline retention enemas provide peak concentrations within one to two hours.

The circulating drug is rapidly distributed throughout the body tissues and the extracellular fluids. Theophylline crosses the placental barrier. The drug is approximately 56 percent bound to plasma proteins. The rate of plasma binding is lower (36 percent) in premature infants. The plasma half-life is about five hours in adults and three and one-half hours in children. The concentration of the drug in saliva is generally 60 percent of the serum drug concentration. The drug is metabolized in the liver, and the unchanged drug (<10 percent) and its metabolites are excreted in the urine. Theophylline is secreted in the milk of nursing mothers, and the concentration of the drug may be 70 percent of the serum concentration.

Adverse Effects

The most frequent adverse effects are central nervous system stimulation (i.e., headache, irritability, restlessness, nervousness, insomnia, dizziness, convulsions) and gastrointestinal disturbances (i.e., nausea, vomiting, epigastric pain, abdominal cramps, anorexia). The central nervous system stimulation is usually more severe in children than in adults, and therapy is terminated when dosage reduction does not alleviate the problems. Gastric irritation is reduced when the oral drugs are administered with food, milk, or a snack.

Cardiovascular effects are usually mild and transient (i.e., palpitations, tachycardia). The drug may also produce transient urinary frequency, dehydration, or twitching of the fingers and hands. There have been some reports of allergic reactions (i.e., urticaria, pruritus, angioedema).

Interactions

Theophylline accelerates the excretion of lithium carbonate, and that interaction may decrease its therapeutic effect. The drug may also have a synergistic toxic effect with sympathomimetics that increases the potential for cardiac arrhythmias. The erythromycins and troleandomycin can decrease the hepatic clearance of theophylline and thereby produce elevated serum concentrations of the bronchodilator.

Toxicity

Serum drug concentrations above 20 mcg/ml increase the incidence and severity of adverse effects. The toxic drug levels characteristically produce agitated maniacal behavior, frequent vomiting, extreme thirst, slight fever, tinnitus, palpitation, and arrhythmias. Other distinguishing effects that occur with toxic serum drug levels are delirium, muscle twitching, severe dehydration, albuminuria, "coffee ground" vomitus, hyperthermia, and profuse diaphoresis. Seizures may occur before there is other evidence of toxicity. The treatment of toxicity involves gastric lavage, when the overdose occurred by the oral route, and symptomatic therapy.

Preparations Available

Aminophylline. The drug is available in forms for administration orally or rectally, and it is the only theophylline salt that is available for intravenous injection (Table 20–2). The intravenous injection is given slowly at a rate of 20 to 40 mg/

Table 20–2.

Theophylline Drugs Employed for Bronchodilating Action

Drug	Route	Usual Adult Single Dosage (mg)	Usual Child Daily Dosage
Aminophylline (theophylline	Oral	200–300	20 mg/kg ÷ 4
ethylenediamine)	IM	500	—
	IV	300–450	15 mg/kg ÷ 3
	Rectal	255–387	12 mg/kg ÷ 3
Dyphylline (AIRET, DILOR,	Oral	200–800	14–26 mg/kg ÷ 3–4
LYFYLLIN, NEOTHYLLINE)	IM	250–500	—
Oxtriphylline (CHOLEDYL)	Oral	200	15 mg/kg ÷ 4*
Theophylline anhydrous	Oral	100–200	10 mg/kg ÷ 4
(AEROLATE, AQUALIN, ELIXOPHYLLIN,			—
SLOPHYLLIN, THEOBID)	Rectal	250–500	10–12 mg/kg ÷ 4
Theophylline monoethanolamine			
(FLEET THEOPHYLLINE)	Rectal	312–625	—
Theophylline sodium			
glycinate (GLYNAZAN)	Oral	330–660	See text

* Children 2 to 12 yr of age.

minute to adults and is administered over a 10-to-30-minute period to children. Rapid intravenous injection of the drug produces dizziness, faintness, lightheadedness, palpitations, syncope, precordial pain, flushing, marked bradycardia, premature ventricular contractions, severe hypotension, and cardiac arrest.

In the treatment of adults with acute bronchoconstriction, an initial loading dose based on the calculation of 6 mg/kg of body weight may be given intravenously over a 20-to-30-minute period. That dosage usually is followed by a maintenance infusion of 0.9 mg/kg/hour to attain a serum level of approximately 10 mcg/ml. The initial intravenous loading dose for children with acute bronchospasm is based on the calculation of 4.4 to 7.2 mg/kg, given over a 15-to-30-minute period. That dose is followed by a maintenance infusion of 0.88 to 1.32 mg/kg/hour.

The usual adult oral dosage of 3.5 mg/kg of body weight is administered at six-hour intervals. The dosage maximum is 5 mg/kg every six hours unless serum levels can be monitored. The rectal suppositories may be administered at eight-hour intervals. Frequent use of the suppositories causes irritation of the rectal mucosa.

Dyphylline. The drug is the only theophylline that is administered intramuscularly because aminophylline, which also is available for intramuscular use, is irritating to the tissues (Table 20–2). The injections are usually repeated several times per day when bronchial constriction interferes with the patient's breathing.

The oral drug is administered to adults, children, or infants three or four times a day. The dosage for infants is calculated on the basis of 4.4 to 6.6 mg/kg of body weight per day.

Oxtriphylline. The drug is administered orally to adults and children (Table 20–2). The dosage usually is taken four times per day with meals and at bedtime.

Theophylline Anhydrous. The oral dosage for adults and children (Table 20–2) is administered at six-hour intervals. The rectal dosage is also given to adults or children at six-hour intervals.

Theophylline Monoethanolamine. The drug is available in a disposable container for administration to adults as a rectal enema (Table 20–2). It is the least irritating of the theophyllines that are given rectally. The enemas may be administered at 12-hour intervals when the drug is required for relief of bronchial constriction.

Theophylline Sodium Glycinate. The oral tablets may be given to adults at six-to-eight-hour intervals after meals (Table 20–2). Children over 12 years of age may receive 220 to 330 mg; children 6 to 12 years receive 100 to 200 mg; children three to six years receive 110 to 165 mg; children one to three years, 55 to 110 mg. The drug is given to children at six-to-eight-hour intervals after meals.

Antiasthmatic Drugs

CROMOLYN SODIUM

Cromolyn sodium is the only drug currently approved for prophylactic use as an antiasthmatic agent. It is employed as an adjunct to the overall therapeutic plan for the management of severe, recurrent bronchial asthma. The drug is prophylactic in nature and usually is effective when the person's pulmonary function tests show that there is a reversible bronchodilator component to the airway obstruction. The drug is not effective when an asthmatic attack has started.

Action Mode

Cromolyn sodium prevents the release of histamine and the slow-reacting substance of anaphylaxis (SRS-A) by inhibiting the degranulation of sensitized mast cells. That local action in the mucosa of the tracheobronchial structures decreases the erythema, edema, and bronchiole constriction associated with the allergic response. There is some indication that the drug also provides some hyposensitization after long-term use by preventing the release of the enzyme *phospholipase A,* which aids in the release of chemical mediators from nonsensitized mast cells.

Therapy Considerations

Cromolyn sodium (AARANE, INTAL) is available as 20-mg capsules that are loaded into the inhaler (SPINHALER). Patients who are to use the inhaler require detailed instructions to assure that they obtain the maximum effect of the drug. The patient is instructed to exhale as completely as possible before placing the mouthpiece of the inhaler between the lips. The head is tilted backward to hyperextend the neck and provide a straight-line pathway for the inhalant to travel toward the pulmonary passages. That position decreases the tendency to swallow on inhalation. After a rapid deep inhalation of the drug, the inhaler is removed from the mouth and the patient holds the breath for a few seconds before exhaling. That procedure is followed until all of the powder contained in the capsule has been inhaled. The moisture of exhaled air wets the powder, and it is necessary to remind the patient to remove the inhaler immediately after each inhalation. Adults and children over five years of age repeat the treatments four times per day at regularly spaced intervals.

The use of the drug has decreased the corticosteroid dosage required for the control of symptoms in patients with asthma. The response to therapy is evident within two to four weeks. Some patients fail to respond to cromolyn therapy, but the reason for those therapeutic failures is unclear.

The amount of drug that reaches the lung tissues is dependent on the correct use of the inhaler, the degree of bronchoconstriction, and the amount of secretions in the tracheobronchial structures. Approximately 5 to 10 percent of the inhaled drug dose reaches the lungs. The drug is absorbed from the lung tissues and enters the systemic circulation. More than 90 percent of the drug is usually swallowed. The highly polarized and lipid-insoluble drug is poorly absorbed from the gastrointestinal tract and is excreted in the feces.

The elimination half-life of the absorbed drug is approximately 81 minutes. The unchanged drug is rapidly excreted in the urine. It also enters the intestine with the bile and is excreted with the feces.

Adverse Effects

Irritation of the oropharyngeal tissues, cough, and bronchospasm frequently are associated with inhalation of the dry powder or with the lactose vehicle used in the drug preparation. Prior inhalation of a bronchodilator may be planned to control the patient's cough and bronchospasm when the problems interfere with the treatments.

There have been reports of nausea or cutaneous reactions (i.e., urticaria, rash, erythema). If therapy is to be terminated, the dosage is reduced gradually because asthma symptoms may recur when dosage reduction is rapid.

Corticosteroid Aerosols

BECLOMETHASONE DIPROPIONATE

Topical corticosteroid therapy is a relatively new approach to the prevention of the allergic responses that produce the symptoms of asthma. *Beclomethasone dipropionate* (VANCERIL) recently was released by the Food and Drug Administration for treatment of chronic asthma. Individuals who are dependent on steroids for the control of asthma usually benefit from the aerosol drug, and the use of systemic glucocorticoids can gradually be terminated. The changeover to the topical steroid is planned concurrently with a progressive reduction in the systemic steroid dosage. Gradual dosage reduction over a prolonged period of time prevents the occurrence of acute adrenal insufficiency or nonpulmonary allergic problems (i.e., eczema, rhinitis).

The usual adult dosage is two inhalations, providing 50 mcg of the drug with each inhalation, three to four times per day. The maximum adult daily dosage is 20 inhalations. The usual dosage for children more than six years of age is one to two inhalations three to four times per day to a maximum of ten inhalations daily.

The low effective dosage of the aerosol drug produces few systemic adverse effects. The most common problem is *Candida albicans* infection in the mouth or oropharynx, which usually is preceded by hoarseness. The infection occurs in approximately 5 to 15 percent of the patients who use the aerosol drug. A reduction in dosage to 100 to 200 mcg/day and use of amphotericin lozenges usually clear the fungus infection from the tissues. Prolonged use of systemic corticosteroids produces skin atrophy, and there is a hazard of local atrophic changes in the respiratory passages with the topical use of the corticosteroid.

Cough Suppressants

DRUG THERAPY

The drugs employed for suppression of nonproductive cough include *antihistaminic, local anesthetic, centrally acting cough suppressants,* or antitussives. The cough suppressants are used when irritation of the nerve endings in the tracheobronchial structures is causing persistent coughing that is exhausting for the individual. Auscultation of the lungs is planned prior to the use of the suppressants to rule out the presence of secretions in those structures as a cause of the cough.

Antihistamine Cough Suppressants

The antihistamines are employed for control of spasmodic bronchial cough that occurs as a consequence of an allergic response in the tracheobronchial structures (Fig 20–2). Their concurrent selective central nervous system depression enhances the depression of the cough reflex. The drugs also have an anticholinergic action that may cause dryness of the mucosa and thickening of the bronchial secretions. The antihistamines employed for cough suppression include *diphenhydramine hydrochloride* and *tripelennamine citrate*.

Diphenhydramine Hydrochloride (BENADRYL). The adult oral dosage of the drug is 12.5 to 50 mg, and that dosage is administered up to six times a day to a maximum of 150 mg/24 hours. Children may receive an oral dosage calculated on the basis of 5 mg/kg of body weight daily, divided for administration four to six times a day. The maximum daily dosage for children 6 to 12 years of age is 75 mg, and for children two to four years of age it is 37.5 mg.

Tripelennamine Citrate (PYRIBENZAMINE). The drug is available as a syrup or as an elixir. The dosage for either preparation is 5 to 10 ml (37.5 to 75 mg) for adults. The dosage for children is 2.5 to 5 ml (18.75 to 37.5 mg). The drug may be used at four-to-six-hour intervals.

Local Anesthetic Cough Suppressants

The drugs suppress cough by their action at the afferent endings of the vagus nerve. That action suppresses the transmission of efferent impulses from the respiratory center that precipitate cough (Fig. 20–2). Benzonatate is the only local anesthetic cough suppressant currently in use.

Benzonatate (TESSALON). The oral dosage for adults and children over ten years of age is 100 to 200 mg, and the dose may be given three times per day. The dosage for children under ten years of age usually is 50 mg three or four times per day. The oral drug produces a cough suppressant effect within 15 to 20 minutes that last for three to eight hours. The person should be cautioned not to chew the oral capsules because the drug will produce a local anesthetic effect on the oral mucosa.

Centrally Acting Cough Suppressants

The drugs suppress the cough reflex by their direct effect on the respiratory center in the me-

dulla (Fig. 20–2). The cough suppressants have a drying effect on the respiratory tract mucosa that increases the viscosity of secretions. The centrally acting cough suppressants include *chlophedianol hydrochloride, codeine, dextromethorphan hydrobromide, hydrocodone bitartrate, levopropoxyphene napsylate,* and *noscapine.* The drugs are often ingredients in cough preparations. *Codeine* and *hydrocodone* are narcotics and are subject to the controls of the Federal Controlled Substances Act of 1970.

Adverse Effects. The drugs infrequently produce adverse effects at therapeutic dosage levels. Nausea, vomiting, dizziness, sedation, palpitation, pruritus, and constipation may occur with repeated use of the drugs. An overdose of the antitussive narcotics can produce toxic effects, which may include exhilaration, excitement, nightmares, convulsions, delirium, hypotension, miosis, bradycardia or tachycardia, flushed facies, tinnitus, lassitude, muscle weakness, or cardiopulmonary failure.

Chlophedianol Hydrochloride (ULO). The oral dosage of the drug for adults and for children over 12 years of age is 25 mg, and that dose is given three to four times per day. Children 6 to 12 years of age may be given 12.5 mg three to four times per day. At high dosage the drug produces dryness of the mouth, visual disturbances, and vertigo.

Codeine. Codeine, *codeine sulfate,* and *codeine phosphate* are administered orally for cough suppression. *Codeine resin* is used as an ingredient of cough preparations. The usual dosage is 8 to 20 mg four to six times per day to a maximum of 120 mg/24 hours. The dosage for children is based on the calculation of 1.0 to 1.5 mg/kg of body weight per day, divided for administration in six doses. The maximum total 24-hour dosage for children 6 to 12 years of age is 60 mg and for younger children it is 30 mg.

The drug is well absorbed from the gastrointestinal tract. The peak antitussive effect occurs within one to two hours, and that effect may persist for four hours. The drug is secreted in the

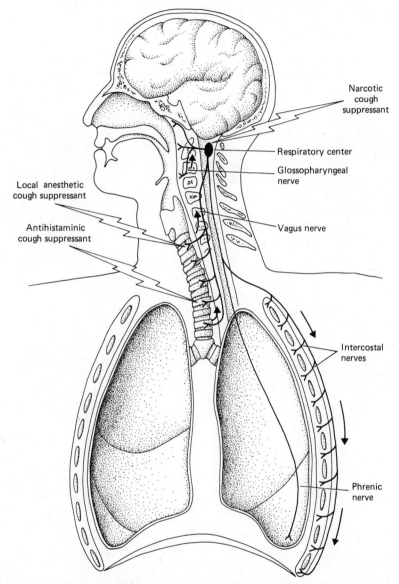

Narcotic
cough
suppressant

Respiratory center

Glossopharyngeal
nerve

Local anesthetic
cough suppressant

Antihistaminic
cough suppressant

Vagus nerve

Intercostal
nerves

Phrenic
nerve

Fig. 20–2. Cough suppressants act by depressing the afferent nerve responses to stimuli or by depressing neural transmission in the medulla respiratory control centers.

milk of nursing mothers. The metabolites of the drug are excreted in the urine.

Dextromethorphan Hydrobromide (METHO-RATE, ROMILAR). The oral dosage for adults is 10 to 20 mg one to four times per day. Children over four years of age are given 5 to 10 mg and children under four years of age are given 2.5 to 5 mg one to four times per day. The drug is well absorbed from the intestinal tract and provides an antitussive effect within 15 to 30 minutes after it is ingested. The duration of that effect is approximately three to six hours.

Hydrocodone Bitartrate (DICODID). The drug is a narcotic that is administered orally. *Hydrocodone resin* is used as an ingredient in many cough preparations. The usual adult dosage of hydrocodone bitartrate is 5 to 10 mg three to four times per day. Children may be given a dosage based on the calculation of 600 mcg/kg of body weight per day, divided for administration in three or four doses. The maximum single dose for children over 12 years of age is 10 mg; for children 2 to 12 years of age it is 5 mg; and for children younger than two years of age it is 1.25 mg. The antitussive action of the drug is evident within 30 minutes, and that effect lasts for four to six hours.

Levopropoxyphene Napsylate (NOVRAD). The oral antitussive dosage for adults is 100 mg every four hours to a maximum of 600 mg/day. The dosage for children who weigh 23 to 45 kg (50 to 100 lb) is 50 mg (maximum 150 to 200 mg/day), and for children or infants weighing less than 23 kg it is 25 mg (maximum 75 mg/day). The dosage is given to children every four hours as required for the control of coughing.

Noscapine (TUSSCAPINE). The oral adult dosage is 15 to 30 mg three to four times per day. Children over one year of age may be given a dosage of 7.5 to 15 mg three or four times per day.

Expectorants and Mucolytics

DRUG THERAPY

The drugs are utilized as oral preparations, which act systemically to facilitate the removal of secretions or as aerosols that act topically to liquefy secretions. Thick secretions cling tenaciously to the cilia of the upper respiratory passages and are difficult for the person to remove by coughing. The drugs are useful adjunctive agents in an overall plan for tissue hydration and topical moistening of secretions. The drugs facilitate the removal of secretions by coughing or by suctioning when it is required.

Expectorants

The preparations that provide thinner mucus secretions include *ammonium chloride, guaifenesin, terpin hydrate,* and the iodide-containing drugs *calcium iodide, diluted hydriodic acid, iodinated glycerol,* and *potassium iodide.* The orally administered drugs are considered to act reflexly to provide a thinning of secretions by their irritating effect on the gastric mucosa. The gastric irritation stimulates vagus nerve activity. There is a consequent reflex vagus nerve–mediated stimulation of the bronchial mucous glands that increases the production of mucus.

Ammonium Chloride. The drug is often used in combination with other expectorants and cough mixtures. The usual oral adult dosage is 250 to 500 mg every two to four hours. Ammonium chloride is available as a syrup and as a tablet that is taken with a full glass of fluid. The drug produces few adverse effects at the dosage levels that are required for an expectorant effect. There may be gastric disturbances (i.e., anorexia, nausea, vomiting) and a slight diuretic effect.

Guaifenesin (ROBITUSSIN). The adult oral dosage of the drug syrup is 100 to 200 mg every two to four hours. The dosage for children is 50 to 100 mg three to four times per day. The drug is employed for the control of productive and nonproductive cough. Persons taking the syrup usually complain about the bitter aromatic taste. Adverse effects rarely occur when the drug is used at the recommended dosage levels. Nausea and drowsiness occur occasionally.

Terpin Hydrate. The elixir contains alcohol, 42.5 percent, and that is thought to contribute to its effectiveness as an expectorant. The dosage of the elixir is 5 to 10 ml. It is employed more frequently with codeine than alone. The alcohol content precludes its use for alcoholics who are on an abstinence program.

Calcium Iodide (CALCIDIN). The oral adult expectorant dosage is 150 mg every hour or 300 to 600 mg every two to four hours. The drug is taken with a half glass of hot water. Like other iodides, the drug is selectively excreted and concentrated in the lungs, and that is thought to contribute to the therapeutic effects. Prolonged administration of iodide-containing expectorants can lead to iodism, hypothyroidism, and goiter. Iodism is manifested as inflammation of the respiratory tract tissues, skin eruptions, and accumulation of fluid in the nasal passages, lungs, and eyelids.

Hydroidic Acid Syrup. The oral dosage of the drug syrup is 65 to 70 mg (5 ml) two to three times per day after meals. The drug is administered well diluted. Hydriodic acid syrup is given in 5-to-10-ml doses with a full glass of water. Drinking the solution through a straw avoids injury to the teeth by the concentrated acid syrup.

Iodinated Glycerol (ORGANIDIN). The oral expectorant dosage for adults is 30 to 60 mg four times per day. Children may receive up to 15 to 30 mg/day. The drug is taken with liquids.

Potassium Iodide. The solution of potassium iodide is standardized to contain 1 gm of potassium iodide per milliliter, and it frequently is referred to as saturated solution of *potassium iodide* (SSKI). The dosage is 300 to 600 mg three to four times per day. After the expectorant effect is obtained, the dosage intervals usually are extended. Patients find the drug solution distasteful even when it is partially masked by mixing it with milk. The solution or the tablets are taken with fluid to reduce gastric irritation.

Mucolytics

The mucolytic agents *acetylcysteine, tyloxapol,* and *trypsin* are topical agents employed for their liquefying effect on the mucus secretions in tracheobronchial and pulmonary tissues. They are used as adjuncts in the treatment of persons with acute or chronic bronchopulmonary disorders (i.e., bronchitis, emphysema, cystic fibrosis). Acute bronchospasm has occurred in some patients with asthma who used the drug inhalants.

Acetylcysteine (MUCOMYST, RESPAIRE). The drug acts by breaking up the mucoprotein linkages and reducing the viscosity of secretions. It is more active in an alkaline pH (i.e., 7 to 9). The drug may be used in a nebulizer or may be instilled directly into a tracheostomy opening. Acetylcysteine (2 to 20 ml of 10 percent solution or 1 to 10 ml of 20 percent solution) may be put in the nebulizer of respiratory equipment (i.e., face mask, intermittent positive breathing equipment) every two to six hours.

Tyloxapol (ALEVAIRE). The drug has a detergent effect that lowers the surface tension and reduces the viscosity of thick, tenacious secretions. It is administered through a nebulizer that is attached to a pressurized air or oxygen source. The solution is used at full strength (0.125 percent with 5 percent sodium bicarbonate and 5 percent glycerin), and 500 ml is adequate to supply the nebulized drug for a period of 12 to 24 hours of continuous administration. It is also used in a small nebulizer or respiratory assistor equipment for intervals of 30 to 90 minutes three or four times per day.

Trypsin (TRYPTAR). The drug is an enzyme mucolytic that is obtained from beef pancreas. The drug dosage of 125,000 to 250,000 units is dissolved in 6 ml of sterile water or saline and used as an aerosol inhalant one time per day. Use of the aerosol may produce dyspnea, chills, fever, and a histamine-like response in some patients. Anaphylaxis has been reported during therapy with trypsin.

Nasal Decongestants

DRUG THERAPY

The sympathomimetic drugs employed for relief of nasal congestion include the orally administered drug *pseudoephedrine hydrochloride* and several drugs that are applied topically.

Pseudoephedrine Hydrochloride (D-FEDA, NOVAFED, SUDAFED)

The oral drug frequently is employed as a nasal decongestant. The alpha adrenergic action of the drug provides vasoconstriction that shrinks the swollen mucosa and reduces the hyperemia, edema, and congestion. That action promotes the drainage of the sinuses and the eustachian tubes. The drug also has beta adrenergic action that produces bronchodilation.

The adult dosage is 60 mg three to four times per day and that same dosage plan is used for children over 12 years of age. The dosage for children younger than 12 years of age is based on the calculation of 4 mg/kg of body weight, divided for administration four times per day.

Topical Nasal Decongestants

The topically applied drugs *ephedrine sulfate, epinephrine hydrochloride, methylhexanelamine* (FORTHANE), *naphazoline hydrochloride* (PRIVINE), *oxymetazoline hydrochloride* (AFRIN), *phenylephrine hydrochloride* (NEOSYNEPHRINE), *prophylhexedrine* (BENZEDREX, DRISTAN), *tetrahydrozoline hydrochloride* (TYZINE), *tuaminoheptane sulfate* (TUAMINE), and *xylometazoline hydrochloride* (OTRIVIN, SINE-OFF).

The drugs are considered to stimulate the alpha-adrenergic receptors of the sympathetic nervous system. *Propylhexedrine* indirectly stimulates the alpha-adrenergic receptors, and the other topical nasal decongestants have a direct action on those receptors.

Intranasal use of the solutions produces constriction of the dilated arterioles and reduces the hyperemia and congestion that are blocking the nostrils, sinuses, and eustachian ostia. Topical use of the drugs usually provides a decongestant effect within five to ten minutes that persists for five to six hours. The drugs seldom cause systemic effects. There infrequently may be systemic sympathomimetic effects (i.e., blood pressure elevation, nervousness, nausea, dizziness, headache, insomnia, palpitation, tachycardia, or arrhythmias). The local effects of the drugs include sneezing and burning, stinging, and dryness of the nasal mucosa. Overuse of the drugs can produce rebound congestion (i.e., chronic redness, swelling, and rhinitis).

Children often resist taking nosedrops because they cause irritation of the throat and a gagging sensation. Those problems can be averted and the effects of the drug on the nasal mucosa can be maximized by having the child lie on the bed in a supine position with the head over the edge of the bed. In that position, the nosedrops that are administered run downward over the nasal septum and the turbinates to the roof of the pharynx rather than over the floor of the nasal cavity and down into the throat. After the solution is instilled, turning to a prone position with the head over the edge of the bed allows distribution of the drug over the nasal turbinates.

NURSING INTERVENTION

The common cold is a health problem that frequently is encountered in the hospital or in the community. There often are opportunities for the nurse to provide health teaching focused on preventive measures and the appropriate use of drugs for control of the symptoms of a cold.

The problem of bronchial constriction is also encountered frequently and can constitute a distressing or life-threatening event for the patient. The following guidelines provide an outline of the nursing intervention that can assist the person who requires the consistent use of a bronchodilator to maintain the plan of therapy.

Guidelines for Nursing Intervention

I. Establish base lines for assessing the effect of the bronchodilator drug on pulmonary function.
  A. Obtain the patient's statement of the problem and the functional limits caused by the problem.
  B. Obtain information about the psychosocial factors affecting resolution of the problem (i.e., health history, health care practices, compliance with prescribed therapies, previous problems with drugs).
  C. Examine the patient for signs of obstruction of the respiratory tract.
    1. Observe the rate, depth, and characteristics of the breathing patterns.
      a. Use of accessory muscles of respiration (i.e., stridor, sternal retractions, flaring nostrils, mouth breathing).
      b. Equality of the inspiratory-expiratory time.
      c. Mobility of the chest cage, anteroposterior chest diameter (barrel chest).
      d. Equality of the chest movements bilaterally.
      e. Mobility of the diaphragm during respiratory cycles.
      f. Elevation of the abdomen on inspiration.
    2. Auscultate the patient's chest for breath sounds (i.e., dullness, rales).
    3. Listen to the effects of the respiratory problem on speech patterns (i.e., shortened sentences, telegraphic speech).
    4. Assess the patient's tolerance and reactions to activity (i.e., fatigue, elevated pulse and respiration rates, coughing).
    5. Observe the effectiveness of coughing.
      a. Chest expansion and ventilation of the upper and lower lobes of the lung.
      b. Sensitivity of the cough reflex.
      c. Ability to expectorate or swallow the secretions raised.
      d. Amount, characteristics, and consistency of secretions.
  D. Examine the patient for signs of decreased gas exchange.
    1. Decreased oxygen exchange (hypoxia).
      a. Elevated pulse rate (tachycardia).
      b. Restlessness, excitement, irritability, headache.
      c. Slowing of mental processes (i.e., depression, decreased mental acuity, apathy, slowness of thought, emotional disturbances, stupor, loss of memory, defective judgment, fatigue).
    2. Decreased carbon dioxide exchange (hypercapnia).
      a. Headache.
      b. Muscle twitching.
      c. Tremulousness.
      d. Convulsions, coma.
  E. Examine the clinical records for relevant data. These include
    1. Pulmonary function studies (i.e., vital capacity, tidal volume).
    2. Blood gas values (i.e., venous or arterial pO_2 and pCO_2 levels, pH).
    3. White blood count (including eosinophils), hematocrit, and hemoglobin values.
II. Plan measures to maximize the bronchodilator drug effect and maintain gas exchange.

A. Explain to the patient the effect of the bronchodilator, ventilatory assistors (i.e., oxygen, compressed air, IPPB), and tissue hydration (i.e., fluid intake) on respiration and secretion mobilization.

B. Schedule administration of the bronchodilator drug to allow easier breathing during the required activities and maximum benefit from concurrent therapies.

C. Implement a plan for maximum lung expansion (i.e., positioning) and removal of retained secretions (i.e., mobilization, breathing exercises, coughing, IPPB) that allows spaced activities and rest periods.

D. Include the patient in health team planning for implementation of the prescribed restrictions.

E. Monitor the breathing patterns and secretion mobilization.

F. Reassess the patient's physiologic status to define the effectiveness of the bronchodilator drug and the adverse effects of the drug.

III. Prepare the patient and a family member to assess the progress of the bronchodilator drug regimen.

A. Teach the patient how to assess the changes in ventilatory status. These include
1. Decreased tolerance to activity.
2. Fatigue, dizziness.

B. Review with the patient, and a family member, the plan for use of the bronchodilator, breathing exercises, and nebulized medications.
1. Plan with the patient for implementation of the specific drug therapy plan within the usual daily schedule of activities.
2. Provide specific written instructions for the patient to use at home.

C. Explain to the patient the factors that change the respiratory status and the requirements for the bronchodilator drug. These include
1. Exposure to cold air.
2. Air pollutants.
3. Respiratory tract infections.
4. Emotional stressors or fatigue.

D. Describe to the patient the problems that require physician contact. These include
1. Feeling of suffocation or an increased work of breathing that is unrelieved by the bronchodilator.
2. Major adverse effects of the particular bronchodilator.

E. Describe to the patient the measures that can be employed to support the drug action. These include
1. Elevation of the head of the bed and use of pillows.
2. Modification of breathing patterns (i.e., pursed lips with exhalation, use of abdominal muscles to mobilize the diaphragm).

F. Reassess the patient's readiness to maintain the drug therapy plan at home.

Review Guides

1. Describe the measures that would be appropriate when monitoring the patient's status to determine the effects and adverse effects of the drugs when the patient is receiving (a) terbutaline sulfate, (b) aminophylline, (c) epinephrine

2. Outline the observations that would be appropriate before administering (a) diphenhydramine hydrochloride, (b) benzonatate citrate, (c) hydrocodone bitartrate

3. Define the factors that would be included when instructing the parent about the use of dextromethorphan hydrobromide cough preparation and xylometazoline hydrochloride nosedrops to a child who is six years old.

4. Identify the time sequence that would be indicated when planning the routine morning care (i.e., bed bath, bedding change) of a patient who has received an aminophylline suppository at 9 A.M.

5. List two nursing problems that naturally would be the focus of activities when the person is receiving guaifenesin to facilitate the removal of thick, tenacious secretions.

Additional Readings

American Academy of Pediatrics Committee on Drugs: Adverse reactions to iodide therapy of asthma and other pulmonary diseases. *Pediatrics,* **57:**272, February, 1976.

Aranda, Jacob V.; Sitar, Daniel S.; Parsons, William D.; Loughnan, Peter M.; and Neims, Allen H.: Pharmacokinetic aspects of theophylline in premature infants. *N. Engl. J. Med.,* **295:**413, August 19, 1976.

Ballin, John C.: Evaluation of a new aerosolized steroid for asthma therapy. *J.A.M.A.,* **236:**2891, December 20, 1976.

Berger, Albert J.; Mitchell, Robert A.; and Sveringhaus, John W.: Regulation of respiration. *N. Engl. J. Med.,* **297:** part 1, p. 92, July 14, 1977; part 2, p. 138, July 21, 1977; part 3, p. 194, July 28, 1977.

Bergner, Renée K., and Bergner, Arthur: Rational asthma therapy for the outpatient. *J.A.M.A.,* **235:**288, January 19, 1976.

Bondarevsky, Ernesto; Shapiro, Menachem S.; Schey, George; Shahor, Josua; and Bruderman, Israel: Beclomethasone diproprionate use in chronic asthma patients. **236:**1969, October 25, 1976.

Brandon, Milan L.: Long-term metoproterenol therapy in asthmatic children. *J.A.M.A.,* **235:**736, February 16, 1976.

Codd, John, and Grohar, Mary Ellen: Postoperative pulmonary complications. *Nurs. Clin. North Am.,* **10:**5, March, 1975.

Dolovich, Jerry; Hargreave, Frederick E.; and Wilson, William M.: Control of asthma in children. *Primary Care,* **2:**19, March, 1975.

Ellis, Elliott F.: Pharmacologic therapy of asthma. *Postgrad. Med.,* **59:**127, April, 1976.

Eney, R. Donald, and Goldstein, Eugene O.: Compliance of chronic asthmatics with oral administration of theophylline as measured by serum and salivary levels. *Pediatrics,* **57:**513, April, 1976.

Farr, Richards: Asthma in adults: the ambulatory patient. *Hosp. Pract.,* **13:**113, April, 1978.

Flod, Natalie E.; Franz, Michael L.; and Galant, Stanley P.: Recent advances in bronchial asthma. *Am. J. Dis. Child.,* **130:**890, August, 1976.

Ghory, Joseph E.: The ABCs of educating the patient with chronic bronchial asthma. *Clin. Pediatr.,* **16:**879, October, 1977.

Gold, Warren M.: Asthma. *Basics RD,* **4:**1, January, 1976.

Goodman, Daniel H., and Wert, Alvin D.: Approaches to asthma management. *Am. Fam. Physician,* **11:**74, March, 1975.

Hyde, John S.; Yamshon, Daniel; Isenberg, Paul D.; and Schur, Samuel: Metaproterenol in children with chronic asthma. *Clin. Pharmacol. Ther.,* **20:**207, August, 1976.

Johnson, Marion: Outcome criteria to evaluate postoperative respiratory status. *Am. J. Nurs.,* **75:**1474, September, 1975.

Lecks, Harold I.: Appraisals of cromolyn sodium and corticosteroids in the treatment of the asthmatic child. *Clin. Pediatr.,* **16:**861, October, 1977.

Lilienfield, Laurence S.; Rose, John C.; and Princiotto, Joseph V.: Antitussive activity of diphenhydramine in chronic cough. *Clin. Pharmacol. Ther.,* **19:**421, April, 1976.

Marks, Meyer B.: Therapeutic effectiveness of cromolyn sodium with 38 severely asthmatic children under five years of age. *Clin. Pediatr.,* **15:**169, February, 1976.

Newhouse, M.; Sanchis, J.; and Bienenstock, J.: Lung defense mechanisms. Part 1. *N. Engl. J. Med.,* **295:**990, October 28, 1976.

Nicholson, David P.: A problem in clinical research: asthma and cromolyn sodium. *Heart Lung,* **5:**71, January–February, 1976.

Parry, William H.; Martorano, Frank; and Cotton, Ernest K.: Management of life-threatening asthma with intravenous isoproterenol infusions. *Am. J. Dis. Child.,* **130:**39, January, 1976.

Piafsky, Kenneth M., and Ogilvie, Richard I.: Drug therapy: dosage of theophylline in bronchial asthma. *N. Engl. J. Med.,* **292:**1218, June 5, 1975.

Plummer, Alan L.: Choosing a drug regimen for obstructive pulmonary disease. 2. Agents other than bronchodilators. *Postgrad. Med.,* **63**:113, May, 1978.

Richerson, Hal B.: Asthma in adults. II: The patient in status asthmaticus. *Hosp. Pract.,* **13**:109, May, 1978.

Robertson, K. Joy, and Guzzetta, Cathleen E.: Arterial blood-gas interpretations in the respiratory intensive-care unit. *Heart Lung,* **5**:256, March–April, 1976.

Ryo, Ung Yun; Kang, Bann; and Townley, Robert G.: Cromolyn sodium in patients with bronchial asthma. *J.A.M.A.,* **236**:927, August 23, 1976.

Sheffer, Albert L.; Rocklin, Ross E.; and Goetzl, Edward J.: Immunologic components of hypersensitivity to reactions to cromolyn sodium. *N. Engl. J. Med.,* **293**:1220, December 11, 1975.

Simons, F. Estelle R.; Pierson, William E.; and Bierman, C. Warren: Current status of the use of theophyllines in children. *Pediatrics,* **55**:735, May, 1975.

Sokol, William N., and Beall, Gildon N.: Asthma. *Hosp. Med.,* **13**:10, May, 1977.

Speir, William A.: Outpatient management of chronic bronchitis and emphysema. *Geriatrics,* **31**:77, September, 1976.

Talamo, Richard C.: Managing the adolescent asthmatic. *Med. Clin. North Am.,* **59**:1489, November, 1975.

Tinkelman, David G., and Avner, Sanford E.: Ephedrine therapy in asthmatic children. *J.A.M.A.,* **237**:553, February 7, 1977.

Walsh, Elizabeth Hawkins, and Pettrone, Ciel R.: Pediatric allergy and asthma. *Pediatr. Nurs.,* **3**:12, March–April, 1977.

Weinbirger, Miles W.; Matthay, Richard A.; Ginchansky, Elliot J.; Chidsey, Charles A.; and Petty, Thomas L.: Intravenous aminophylline dosage. *J.A.M.A.,* **235**:2110, May 10, 1976.

Weisberg, Stephen C., and Kaiser, Harold B.: New drugs in the treatment of asthma. *Postgrad. Med.,* **60**:133, September, 1976.

Wilson, Archie F.: Drug treatment of acute asthma. *J.A.M.A.,* **237**:1141, March 14, 1977.

Yurchak, Anthony M., and Jusko, William J.: Theophylline secretion into breast milk. *Pediatrics,* **57**:518, April, 1976.

Zaske, Darwin E.; Miller, Kenneth W.; Strem, Edward L.; Austrian, Sol; and Johnson, Paul B.: Oral aminophylline therapy. *J.A.M.A.,* **237**:1453, April 4, 1977.

21

Metabolic Waste and Toxicant Retention

The accidental ingestion of drugs by children is a major health problem. The use of "child-proof" caps on drug bottles has markedly decreased the high incidence of aspirin and iron tablet ingestion, but the problems are not entirely eliminated.

Progress has also been made in the prevention of lead poisoning and the identification and treatment of children who have ingested the heavy metal. Public awareness of that health hazard has accelerated the action programs for stripping the lead paint from the woodwork of homes where there are young children. Public service messages on television frequently provide instructions for persons who plan to remove paint from the wood in their homes. The advice about proper clothing, use of masks, and safe disposal of the debris is directed at preventing the ingestion, inhalation, or absorption of lead during the paint-stripping process.

POISON CONTROL

A national network of government-subsidized poison control centers can be contacted at any hour of the day or night for information about ingested substances. The centers maintain a computer bank of data about the potentially poisonous ingredients of commercial products that may be used in the home. The centers have a statewide toll-free telephone number that can be called by residents of suburban or rural areas, or the number of the closest center can be obtained by calling directory assistance. The staff provide instructions about appropriate emergency measures and the observations that should be made. They also advise contact with a physician for further instructions after the emergency measures are implemented.

During National Poison Control Week, community pharmacies distribute pamphlets that provide information about preventive measures that can be used in the home. They also give a 30-ml vial of the emetic *ipecac syrup*, with instructions for its use in an emergency situation, to the parents of young children in the community. During contact with parents of young children, the nurse also has an opportunity to advise them about poison prevention and to encourage them to record the telephone number of the poison control center and the local pharmacy with their listing of other readily accessible emergency numbers (i.e., police, fire department, physician).

Many agents can be employed to bind poisons in the gastrointestinal tract and prevent their absorption. Those agents are listed in the poison treatment charts that are widely distributed by the National Poison Center Network.

The drugs that are discussed in this chapter are the *adsorbents* and *emetics,* which are employed to prevent the absorption of orally ingested poisons; the heavy metal *antagonists,* which are used to remove poisons from body tissues; the *alcohol deterrent,* which provides a hypersensitivity that reduces the person's desire to ingest alcohol; the *potassium-removing resin,* which is employed to reduce hyperkalemia; the *drugs controlling hyperuricemia,* which are utilized to reduce the serum and tissue levels of urates; the *drugs that reduce blood ammonia levels;* and the *biliary stone dissolution agent.* The drugs have relatively specific applications in the control of particular toxicants. In this chapter the pathophysiologic correlations and the guides for nursing intervention are included with discussions of the drug therapy.

Adsorbents

Activated charcoal (CHARACOCAPS, CHARCOAID, CHARCODOTE, CHARCOTABS) is a fine black powder that is an effective nonspecific adsorbent of many drugs and chemicals. It is not used when the oral poison is a corrosive agent, cyanide, iron, mineral acid, or organic solvent. A dosage that is calculated to be five to ten times the estimated weight of the ingested poison, or a single 30- to 50-gm dose of the powder, is mixed with tap water until it is the consistency of thick soup. Larger doses are required when there is food in the stomach. The oral drug may be mixed with concentrated

fruit juice or chocolate powder to increase its palatability. The soupy mixture may also be introduced into the stomach through a nasogastric tube after gastric lavage.

The drug remains in the gastrointestinal tract and the time of excretion can be identified by the black coloration of the feces. Activated charcoal is most effective when it is administered within 30 minutes of the poison ingestion. Its action is enhanced by evacuation of the stomach and upper intestine by emesis before it is given.

Emetics

DRUG THERAPY

Ipecac syrup and *apomorphine* are the drugs employed to induce vomiting after the person has ingested an oral overdose of selected poisons. The drugs provide useful alternatives to gastric lavage in conscious persons. They are not used when the ingested poison is a convulsant, caustic, corrosive, or volatile oil.

The emesis that follows the use of the drugs removes the residual poison from the stomach and upper intestine and that action prevents its absorption. Although the emetic action of ipecac syrup is slower than that of apomorphine, the oral route for administration of ipecac syrup usually makes it possible for the treatment to be done in the home. For example, the parent who is instructed by the physician or the poison control center personnel can administer the drug to the child and plan appropriate observations for toxic effects of the absorbed drug. Ipecac syrup produces no central nervous system depression, and the child can resume the normal activities in the home after the emetic event.

Ipecac Syrup

Ipecac syrup is available cost free at community pharmacies for use at the time that an emetic is indicated for poison ingestion. Ipecac syrup produces emesis by irritating the gastric mucosa and by stimulating the chemoreceptor emetic trigger zone in the medulla. The gastric irritation produces parasympathetic nerve impulses, which stimulate the vomiting center in the medulla, and there is a concurrent stimulation of the center by impulses from the chemoreceptor trigger zone.

Therapy Considerations.   The dual vomiting center stimulation provided by the action of ipecac produces forceful vomiting in 80 to 99 percent of the persons taking the drug and 90 percent vomit within 30 minutes. The dosage for adults and children older than one year of age is 15 to 30 ml, and for children younger than one year of age it is 5 to 10 ml. The person should drink at least 200 to 300 ml of milk with the drug. Evaporated milk has adsorbent properties and is the ideal liquid to take with the drug. Water may increase the absorption of the poison.

Physical activity enhances the action of the drug, and the person should be encouraged to move around until the emetic event occurs. When vomiting is delayed for 20 minutes, the dosage of the drug is repeated. Activated charcoal usually is given to adsorb the ipecac syrup and the ingested poison when vomiting does not occur within 30 minutes after the second dose of the drug. Gastric lavage may also be planned for removal of the residual drugs.

Apomorphine Hydrochloride

The drug is a semisynthetic alkaloidal salt without analgesic activity that is derived from mor-phine. It is usually administered subcutaneously to induce vomiting in the emergency treatment of persons who have ingested oral poisons that are not caustics or central nervous system depressants. Apomorphine induces vomiting by directly stimulating the chemoreceptor emetic trigger zone of the medulla.

Therapy Considerations.   The drug is administered as a single subcutaneous injection to children or adults at a dosage of 70 to 100 mcg/kg of body weight. It is occasionally administered intravenously at a dosage of 10 mcg/kg of body weight. The concurrent administration of 240 ml of milk to adults and 120 ml to young children facilitates emesis. Larger amounts of fluid are contraindicated because they can accelerate the absorption of poisons from the gastrointestinal tract. Emesis tends to occur earlier when the person remains physically active.

Emesis usually occurs within five minutes after the drug is administered. Approximately 90 percent of the persons taking the drug vomit within 15 minutes. When emesis does not occur after a 15-minute period, other measures are employed to decrease the absorption of the poison (i.e., gastric lavage). The central nervous system action of apomorphine produces a combination of excitation and sedative effects that appear within a few minutes after the drug is injected, and those effects persist for approximately two hours.

Adverse Effects.   The most frequent adverse effect is protracted vomiting. The action of the drug on the medullary control centers may produce respiratory depression, and it occasionally produces circulatory depression. Narcotic antagonists (i.e., naloxone hydrochloride) are usually effective in controlling the vomiting and decreasing the respiratory and central nervous system depression. The other adverse effects that occasionally appear are mild nausea, salivation, syncope, perspiration, weakness, and pallor. There have been reports of central nervous system stimulation manifested as euphoria, restlessness, tremor, tachycardia, or hyperpnea.

Heavy Metal Antagonists

DRUG THERAPY

The drugs are employed to remove heavy metals from sequestered sites in body tissues in individuals acutely or chronically exposed to toxicants (i.e., iron, lead, calcium, copper). The heavy metal antagonists include *deferoxamine, edetate calcium disodium, edetate disodium, penicillamine,* and *dimercaprol.* The circulating drugs remove the poison by binding, or chelating, the toxicant. The soluble metal-drug molecules, or chelates, are excreted in the urine. The chelates are nephrotoxic, and fluid intake should be at a minimal level of 2 to 3 liters/day to assure their excretion. The heavy metal antagonists are most effective when they are administered soon after the poisoning for the treatment of acute toxicity.

Deferoxamine Mesylate (DESFERAL)

The drug has a high affinity for iron and is primarily effective in chelating loosely bound stored iron. It removes iron from ferritin, hemosiderin, and transferrin but does not affect the iron content of hemoglobin or cytochromes. The drug acts by finding ferric ions, and the resulting *ferrioxamine* molecule, which is formed in the plasma and in many tissues, is a stable water-soluble complex that is readily excreted by the kidneys.

Therapy Considerations. Deferoxamine mesylate is usually administered intramuscularly. The injection sites are alternated to decrease the pain and induration caused by the injection. The drug may also be administered by slow intravenous infusion in the treatment of cardiovascular collapse associated with acute iron intoxication. The usual dosage for adults and children is 1 gm when it is administered by either route. A second 500-mg dose is given in four hours, and that dosage is repeated after a four-hour interval has elapsed. When the clinical response of the patient indicates the need for continued administration, subsequent doses of 500 mg are given every 4 to 12 hours. The maximum dosage for a 24-hour period is 6 gm. Iron is poorly mobilized in children younger than three years of age who have a small iron overload, and the drug is administered only when a test dose of deferoxamine mesylate produces urinary excretion of more than 1 mg of iron in 24 hours.

The drug is administered intramuscularly at a dosage of 500 mg to 1 gm daily to adults and children with chronic iron overload as a consequence of multiple transfusions (i.e., thalassemia, chronic anemia). The drug may also be administered by slow infusion at a dosage of 2 gm at a separate venous site each time the person receives a transfusion with a unit of blood.

Deferoxamine and the ferrioxamine molecules are excreted primarily in the urine. The ferrioxamine imparts a reddish color to the urine. The maximal excretion of iron occurs during the initial period of therapy when the more accessible metal is chelated.

The ingestion of toxic quantities of iron tablets may produce vomiting, diarrhea, tarry stools, and hematemesis, and the absorbed iron can cause a fast and weak pulse, lethargy, hypotension, and coma. In untreated patients, signs of peripheral circulatory collapse appear one-half to one hour after the ingestion of a toxic dose. The early symptoms disappear in four to six hours, and the patient usually improves rapidly and remains asymptomatic for 6 to 24 hours. A second crisis occurs in the next 12 to 48 hours, and there may be cyanosis, pulmonary edema, circulatory collapse, convulsions, coma, and death.

The immediate treatment of acute iron intoxication includes administration of milk, induction of emesis, or gastric lavage with 5 percent sodium bicarbonate solution. Deferoxamine is administered when symptoms are severe (i.e., convulsions, coma, shock). The ferrioxamine molecules can be removed by dialysis when necessary.

The potentially lethal dose is 300 mg of elemental iron per kilogram of body weight. Those persons who recover may have gastrointestinal disturbances one to two months later. The problems are caused by necrotic alterations of the gastric and intestinal mucosa that occur at the sites of iron tablet disintegration at the time of the initial iron ingestion. Antacids usually are prescribed after the initial period of therapy to reduce the severity of the gastrointestinal ulcerations.

Adverse Effects. Deferoxamine mesylate is relatively nontoxic when it is used for the treatment of acute iron intoxication. Rapid intravenous infusion of the drug can produce generalized erythema, urticaria, hypotension, and shock that are thought to be related to the histamine-liberating action of the drug. Prolonged treatment of persons with iron storage diseases can cause allergic reactions (i.e., rash, pruritus, cutaneous wheal formation, anaphylaxis). Blurred vision, abdominal discomfort, diarrhea, leg cramps, tachycardia, and fever have also been reported.

Edetate Calcium Disodium (CALCIUM DISODIUM VERSENATE)

The drug, which usually is referred to as calcium EDTA, is used primarily for chelation of lead in persons with chronic lead poisoning. It also chelates zinc, and to a lesser extent it binds cadmium, manganese, iron, copper, chromium, nickel, vanadium, and radiation or nuclear fission products (plutonium, thorium, uranium, and yttrium).

The calcium of the molecule is displaced by the divalent and trivalent metals to form stable soluble complexes that are excreted in the urine. Saturation of the molecule with calcium prevents the sharp reduction in serum and tissue calcium that occurs with edetate disodium.

Therapy Considerations. The drug is usually given by intravenous infusion to adults. The intravenous solution is infused over a one-hour period to asymptomatic patients and over six to eight hours to those who have symptoms. The solution should be well diluted to avoid the thrombophlebitis that occurs at high concentrations. The drug is given to children and to patients with lead encephalopathy by intramuscular injection. The local anesthetic *procainamide hydrochloride* may be added to the intramuscular dosage to minimize the pain that occurs at the site of the drug injection. The daily intravenous dosage is divided for infusion at 12-hour intervals, and the daily intramuscular dosage is divided for administration at four- or six-hour intervals.

The dosage of the drug, which is the same for intramuscular or intravenous administration, depends on the severity of intoxication as indicated by the blood lead concentrations. Adults and children with blood levels of 50 to 100 mcg/100 ml and mild symptoms of intoxication are given 1 gm/M^2/day for three to five days, and those with higher blood lead levels are given 1.5 gm/M^2 daily for three to five days. Dimercaprol 4 mg/kg may be given concurrently at separate injection sites to increase the rate of lead excretion, lower mortality, and decrease brain damage when the blood levels are high and there is evidence of encephalopathy. Children may receive more than two courses of treatment. The treatment of adults is usually limited to two courses of therapy.

Adults with lead nephropathy and a serum creatinine concentration of 2 mg/100 ml may be given calcium EDTA at a dosage of 1 gm/day for five days; those with a serum creatinine of 2 to 3 mg/100 ml are given 500 mg/day for five days. The same dosage is given but the intervals between administration are lengthened when the patient's creatinine levels are higher than 3 mg/100 ml to avoid the symptoms of gout that occur when lead is mobilized in excess of the amount that can be excreted. The courses of treatment are repeated at one-month intervals until the lead excretion is reduced to near-normal levels.

Calcium EDTA may be administered to children and adults at a dosage of 25 mg/kg of body weight to a maximum of 1 gm for the diagnosis of lead poisoning. The drug is given by intramuscular injection or it may be infused intravenously over a one-hour period. When the 24-hour urine specimen contains more lead than 500 mcg/liter, the person is treated to remove the excess lead burden from the tissues. Calcium EDTA may be given orally to ambulatory adults as a dosage of

4 gm/day and to children at a daily dosage calculated on the basis of 65 mg/kg of body weight. Those daily dosages are divided for administration three to four times per day.

Approximately 5 to 10 percent of the drug is absorbed after oral administration. The oral route is used infrequently because it is considered to increase the absorption of lead. The excretion of chelated lead begins within one hour after intravenous administration of calcium EDTA, and the peak excretion occurs within 24 to 48 hours. An average of 3 to 5 mg of lead is excreted in the urine after the parenteral administration of 1 gm of the drug to patients with acute lead poisoning or high concentrations of lead that are readily mobilized from the soft tissues. The colic caused by lead poisoning may disappear within two hours, and the muscular weakness and tremors disappear after four to five days of treatment with calcium EDTA.

The absorbed drug is widely distributed in the extracellular fluids with the exception of the cerebrospinal fluids. The half-life of the drug is 20 to 60 minutes after intravenous infusion and one to five hours after intramuscular administration. The unchanged drug and the metal chelates are rapidly excreted from the kidneys by glomerular filtration. Approximately 50 percent of the intravenous dose appears in the urine within one hour and 95 percent of the drug is excreted in 24 hours.

Lead levels greater than 40 mcg/100 ml of blood indicate excess exposure to lead. Mild clinical symptoms are usually present when the levels reach 50 to 79 mcg/100 ml, and therapy usually is planned for the patient. Severe lead poisoning is considered to be present at blood concentrations of 80 to 100 mcg/100 ml, and encephalopathy is associated with levels in excess of 100 mcg/100 ml. Therapy does not eliminate the risk of permanent severe residual brain damage.

Adverse Effects.   Some of the adverse effects of the drug are potentially fatal. The most serious toxic manifestation is renal tubular necrosis, which is related to excessive daily dosage levels. The drug may be given on an intermittent schedule to avert the renal toxicity. The renal toxicity

produces the same symptoms as those associated with renal damage caused by lead poisoning (i.e., proteinuria, microscopic hematuria). The blood urea nitrogen levels (BUN) and a daily urinalysis are evaluated before and during each course of therapy to allow early detection of the toxicity. Therapy is interrupted when anuria is present to avoid the toxic effects of high concentrations of the chelates on the damaged renal tissues.

Anorexia, nausea, vomiting, headache, numbness, tingling, myalgia, arthralgia, hypercalcemia, and hypotension may occur when the drug is administered parenterally. There have been reports of histamine-like reactions (sneezing, nasal congestion, lacrimation) that appeared four to eight hours after the intravenous infusion of the drug. The cardiac conduction patterns should be monitored during parenteral administration because electrocardiographic changes (i.e., T wave inversion) may occur. Muscle cramps, weakness, fatigue, malaise, and sudden chills, fever, or excessive thirst occur occasionally.

Edetate Disodium (DISOTATE, ENDRATE, SODIUM VERSENATE)

The drug (EDTA) chelates divalent and trivalent metals (i.e., magnesium, zinc, and trace metals), but it has the greatest affinity for calcium. It forms a stable, soluble complex with calcium ions, and the chelate is readily excreted by the kidneys.

Therapy Considerations.   The drug is given to adults with hypercalcemia by intravenous infusion at a dosage calculated on the basis of 50 mg/kg of body weight (maximum 3 gm/24 hours). The daily intravenous dosage for children is calculated on the basis of 40 to 70 mg/kg of body weight. The intravenous infusion is given slowly over a three-to-four-hour period. The frequency and duration of treatment are based on the serum calcium levels. Patients should remain in bed for a few minutes after the infusion is finished to avoid postural hypotension.

The drug is also occasionally given to children or adults for the treatment of ventricular arrhythmias associated with acute, severe digitalis toxicity. The intravenous dosage is calculated on the basis of 15 mg/kg/hour to a maximum dosage of 60 mg/kg/day. Electrocardiographic monitoring allows termination of the infusion when the desired effect is attained.

The patient's status is monitored closely, and calcium for injection should be available in a syringe during the infusion. The drug can reduce the serum calcium levels rapidly and produce symptoms of hypocalcemia (i.e., tetany, convulsions, severe cardiac arrhythmias, respiratory arrest). When the person's blood pressure is taken, the inflation of the cuff causes pressure on the nerves and the blood vessels that produces carpopedal spasm (Trousseau's sign) in the presence of hypocalcemia.

EDTA exerts a negative inotropic effect on the heart. The hypocalcemia it induces may have a transient effect that antagonizes the inotropic and chronotropic effects of digitalis glycosides. Slow intravenous infusion of the chelating drug allows calcium to move from the bones to maintain the serum calcium levels, and symptoms are less acute than those occurring with rapid intravenous administration. The serum potassium levels are also monitored during therapy with the drug because it lowers the serum levels by an undetermined mechanism. EDTA chelates magnesium, zinc, and other essential trace metals, and the serum levels may be low.

The drug is rapidly excreted, and 95 percent of the calcium chelate appears in the urine within 24 hours. The drug is not absorbed from the tissues when it is applied topically to remove calcium or lime deposits from the corneal epithelium and external layers of the stroma.

Adverse Effects. Pain and a burning sensation which often occur at the intravenous injection site after the infusion, and thrombophlebitis have been reported. EDTA frequently produces gastrointestinal symptoms (i.e., nausea, vomiting, diarrhea, abdominal cramps, anorexia). Patients may also complain of transient circumoral paresthesias, numbness, headache, and dizziness that are associated with hypotension.

The most serious potential hazard is hypocalcemia. Nephrotoxicity occurs with excessive dosages. There have been reports of calcium embolization, lassitude, malaise, thirst, fatigue, and pain, weakness, or cramps in the muscles.

Interactions. EDTA lowers the blood sugar levels and reduces the insulin requirements of diabetic patients. The basis of that action is thought to be the chelation of the zinc of the exogenous hormone preparation. EDTA activity produces hypomagnesemia, and the lowering of the serum magnesium levels decreases the activity of alkaline phosphatase and lowers the serum levels of that enzyme.

Penicillamine (CUPRIMINE)

The drug is a chelating agent and is a synthetic drug similar to the degradation products of all of the penicillins, which also lack bacterial activity. Penicillamine chelates copper, gold, mercury, lead, zinc, and other heavy metals to form stable, soluble complexes that are readily excreted by the kidneys. It also combines chemically with cystine to form *penicillamine-cystine disulfide,* which is a more soluble complex than cystine. The drug is used for the treatment of patients with cystinuria to reduce the concentration of cystine in the urine below the level that causes stone formation. During therapy with penicillamine, there is a reduction in the number and size of existing renal stones.

Therapy Considerations. The drug is administered orally. It may be used indefinitely to prevent the accumulation of copper that occurs in patients with Wilson's disease, or *hepatolenticular degeneration,* or the accumulation of cystine crystals in patients who are predisposed to cystine nephrolithiasis. The content of the penicillamine capsules can be given in 15 to 30 ml of chilled fruit juice or puréed fruit when patients are unable to swallow the capsules.

The usual dosage for adults and children is 250 mg four times per day 30 to 60 minutes before meals and two hours after the evening meal. The dosage for children is calculated on the basis of 20 mg/kg of body weight per day. One gram of penicillamine results in the urinary excretion of 2 mg of copper. The dosage adjustments are based on the quantity of copper excreted in the urine. It is considered probable that there is a negative copper balance when the 24-hour urinary copper excretion is 0.5 to 1 mg.

The dietary intake of copper is restricted to less than 2 mg/day. That diet excludes the use of chocolate, nuts, shellfish, mushrooms, liver, molasses, broccoli, and copper-enriched cereals. The person also takes 10 to 40 mg of sulfurated potash with each meal to minimize the absorption of copper from the digestive tract. Neurologic symptoms usually worsen during the initial stages of therapy. After one to three months there is noticeable improvement in the neurologic, corneal, hepatic, and psychiatric manifestations of Wilson's disease.

The usual oral dosage for adults with cystinuria is 2 gm/day, and the daily dosage for children is based on the calculation of 30 mg/kg of body weight. The daily dosage is divided for administration four times a day. A high fluid intake lowers the dosage of the drug that is needed to excrete the cystine. The person should be encouraged to drink 500 ml of fluid at bedtime and once during the night because the urine becomes concentrated and more acidic during the hours of sleep.

Dosage adjustments are based on the measurement of cystine excretion. For example, patients with a history of renal calculi may receive a dosage that maintains cystine excretion at less than 100 mg/day, and patients without a history of calculi may receive a dosage that maintains cystine excretion at 100 to 200 mg/day. Adults concurrently have a low methionine diet. The low protein content of that diet negates its use for children or pregnant women. The goal of therapy is to prevent nephrolithiasis by reducing the cystine excretion rate to near-normal levels (i.e., 40 to 80 mg/day) and maintaining the urine specific gravity below 1.010 and the urine pH at 7.5 to 8.

The oral drug is readily absorbed from the gastrointestinal tract, and peak blood levels are attained two to three hours after the drug is ingested. It crosses the placental barrier. Penicillamine is metabolized in the liver and excreted in the urine (50 percent) and feces (20 percent), primarily as the disulfides, within 24 hours.

Adverse Effects. The drug produces allergic reactions in one third of the patients. The reactions most commonly involve the cutaneous tissues (i.e., urticarial, maculopapular, erythematous rashes). The dermatologic reactions may be accompanied by pruritus, fever, arthralgia, or lymphadenopathy. The cross-sensitivity between the chelating agent and penicillin contraindicates use of the drugs by persons who have a history of a penicillin reaction.

The drug may also produce a nephrotic syndrome (i.e., massive proteinuria), hepatic dysfunction, hematologic disorders (i.e., eosinophilia, neutropenia, monocytosis, leukocytosis, leukopenia, thrombocytosis, thrombocytopenia, hemolytic anemia, bone marrow hypoplasia, and agranulocytosis). Penicillamine increases the proportions of soluble collagen in the skin and other tissues, and that effect can decrease wound healing, increase the friability of the skin at pressure sites, accelerate wrinkling of the skin, and produce white papules at injection sites.

Gastrointestinal problems also occur during therapy (i.e., anorexia, nausea, vomiting, diarrhea). There is a reversible impairment of the salt and sweet taste senses. Patients who receive the drug for other than copper chelation may be given copper (i.e., 5 to 10 gtt of a 4 percent solution of cupric sulfate in fruit juice two times a day) and that improves the taste sense.

Iron-deficiency anemia occurs in postmenopausal women and in children who are on a low-copper diet or a low-methionine diet, which is low in iron content. The administration of supplemental iron for a short period of time corrects the deficiency. There should be at least a two-hour period between the time the iron supplement is taken and the ingestion of penicillinamine because the iron binds with the chelate and decreases its absorption from the gastrointestinal tract. The drug inhibits pyridoxal-dependent enzymes and increases the body requirements for the vitamin. Patients are usually given 25 to 50 mg of pyridoxine daily during therapy with penicillamine.

Dimercaprol (BAL IN OIL)

The drug chelates antimony, arsenic, bismuth, chromium, copper, gold, lead, mercury, nickel, tungsten, and zinc. The yellow viscous drug solution has a pungent odor. Sterilization of the drug during the manufacturing process produces a small amount of sediment or flocculent material that is innocuous.

The chelate, which is formed by binding of the heavy metal with dimercaprol, forms mercaptide molecules that are excreted in the urine. The mercaptides dissociate and release the metal when the concentration of the drug declines. The dosage is planned to provide excess free drug in the body fluids to allow the binding of the metal until its excretion is completed.

Therapy Considerations. Dimercaprol is injected deeply into the muscular tissues to prevent the pain caused by the irritating effects of the drug and the sterile abscesses that occasionally occur with its administration. The usual dosage for the treatment of severe arsenic or gold salt poisoning is based on the calculation of 3 mg/kg of body weight every four hours for the first two days. The same dosage is given four times a day on the third day and two times a day for the following ten days or until recovery is complete.

The dosages for mild toxicity are usually based on the calculation of 2.5 mg/kg of body weight. The doses are given four to six times per day for the first two days and one or two times per day for a week to ten days. The patient's status is the primary factor that determines when therapy is to be terminated. Patients may receive dimercaprol ointment topically for the treatment of metal-induced dermatitis, or it may be utilized as a 5 to 10 percent oil solution for local treatment of ocular symptoms of toxicity (i.e., arsenic).

The initial drug dose for persons who are treated one to two hours after mercury poisoning is based on 5 mg/kg of body weight in an attempt to rapidly bind that metal, which causes irreversible renal tubular necrosis. Dimercaprol is effective in chronic treatment of heavy metal poisoning, but the drug is seldom employed when the metal has produced extensive tissue damage (i.e., arsenic-induced aplastic anemia, jaundice, or hemorrhagic encephalitis).

Peak blood levels of the drug are attained within 30 to 60 minutes after the intramuscular injection is given. Dimercaprol is slowly absorbed through the tissues when it is applied topically. The absorbed drug is distributed to all body tissues, and the highest concentrations appear in the liver and kidneys. The free, or nonchelate, drug is rapidly metabolized and excreted with the bile content of the feces or in the urine. The chelates, or mercaptides, dissociate readily in an acid medium, and alkalinization of the urine is usually planned to prevent renal tubule damage and assure that the chelate is excreted.

Adverse Effects. There may be mild and transitory adverse effects when the drug is employed at therapeutic dosages for most heavy metal poisoning. Elevation of the systolic and diastolic blood pressure is the most frequent adverse effect. The elevation usually appears within 15 to 30 minutes after the drug is given, and the pressure levels gradually return to the normal range in two hours. The pressure elevation is dose related and may be more severe when the drug is given at high dose levels (i.e., 5 mg/kg). High dosages also produce vomiting, convulsions, stupor, and coma in 50 percent of the patients within 30 minutes after the injection is given. The person usually recovers within one to six hours.

The drug produces an unpleasant breath odor, pain in the teeth, and a burning sensation of the lips, mouth, throat, eyes, and penis. Dimercaprol occasionally produces nausea, vomiting, headache, sweating, weakness, and a sensation of tightness or constriction of the throat and chest.

There have also been reports of muscular aches, pain, or spasm, and tingling of the extremities. The drug also produces hemolytic anemia in persons with an inherited glucose-6-phosphate dehydrogenase (G-6-PD) deficiency. Topical application of dimercaprol may produce erythema and edema of the local tissues. Fever frequently occurs after the first two to three doses of the drug are given to children, and they may also have a transient reduction in polymorphonuclear leukocyte levels. Many of the symptoms may be relieved by the use of an antihistamine.

Interactions. The drug interferes with the normal accumulation of iodine in the thyroid gland. Dimercaprol forms a toxic complex with iron, and supplemental iron therapy is withheld until 24 hours after therapy with the chelating agent is terminated.

Alcohol Deterrent

Disulfiram (ALCOPHOBIN, ANTABUSE, RO-SULFINRAM)

The drug produces a hypersensitivity to alcohol that induces vomiting when the alcohol is ingested after the drug is taken. That disulfiram-alcohol interaction is a useful approach to the maintenance of an abstinence plan by consenting, motivated alcoholics.

Disulfiram inhibits the enzymatic oxidation of acetaldehyde to acetate in the liver. The interference with the natural pathway for the catabolism of alcohol produces a marked elevation in the blood concentration of acetaldehyde when alcohol is ingested. The sensitivity to alcohol increases during prolonged therapy with disulfiram.

Therapy Considerations. The drug is initially taken orally at least 12 hours after the last drink of alcohol. The maximum initial dosage is 500 mg, which is taken every morning for a period of one to two weeks. The dosage is then adjusted to the maintenance dosage level of 125 to 500 mg/day. The drug may be taken at bedtime by persons in whom the drug produces drowsiness.

Disulfiram is rapidly absorbed from the gastrointestinal tract. The initial toxic reaction to alcohol can occur 3 to 12 hours after the drug initially is taken. The reaction occurs when the quantity of alcohol that is ingested raises the blood alcohol concentration to 5 to 10 mg/100 ml, and the reaction is at its peak when the blood alcohol content is 50 mg/100 ml. Approximately 20 percent of an absorbed dose of disulfiram remains in the body for six days. The cumulative effects of the regular use of the drug can produce the reaction when the person drinks alcohol during a two-week period after terminating therapy with disulfiram.

The person who is taking disulfiram should be informed that the minimal amounts of alcohol that are contained in such products as cough syrups, elixirs, sauces, or vinegar, and external application of alcohol-containing liniments or lotions (i.e., aftershave lotion) can produce a reaction. Ingestion of or exposure to small amounts of alcohol can produce a reaction within 5 to 15 minutes.

The disulfiram-alcohol reaction produces copious vomiting, flushing, throbbing and pain in the head and neck, dyspnea, sweating, thirst, chest pain, palpitations, tachycardia, hypotension, syncope, vertigo, blurred vision, and confusion. The reaction is followed by a sound sleep, and the person is completely recovered on awakening. Ingestion of large amounts of alcohol that raise the blood alcohol content to 125 to 250 mg/100 ml may produce a severe reaction that progresses to respiratory depression, arrhythmias, myocardial infarction, cardiac failure, and convulsions. The reaction persists for 30 minutes to several hours, and death may occur when medical assistance is unavailable to treat the symptoms during the reaction. The person who is using disulfiram should carry an identification card that describes the reaction and the name of the physician to be contacted when a reaction occurs.

Adverse Effects. Disulfiram may produce drowsiness, fatigue, impotence, headache, dermatitis, and a garlic-like aftertaste in the mouth during the first two weeks of therapy. The problems usually subside when therapy is continued.

Interactions. Disulfiram interferes with the hepatic metabolism of alcohol, barbiturates, coumarin anticoagulants, paraldehyde, and phenytoin. The concurrent use of those drugs may increase the plasma levels and produce toxic effects. Persons receiving isoniazid during therapy with disulfiram may show behavioral changes, incoordination, or unsteady gait. Concurrent use of metronidazole produces acute psychoses and confusion in some patients who concurrently are taking disulfiram. The tricyclic antidepressant amitriptyline enhances the disulfiram-alcohol reaction.

Potassium-Removing Resin

Sodium Polystyrene Sulfonate (KAYEXALATE)

The drug is a cation-exchange resin employed for the treatment of patients with persistent hyperkalemia. Elevation of serum potassium levels (>6 mEq/L) most commonly occurs as a consequence of acute renal failure. Chronic renal failure also produces a retention of nitrogenous wastes, and dialysis is planned to remove the potassium and other metabolic wastes that accumulate in those patients.

Therapy Considerations. Sodium polystyrene sulfonate is usually administered orally, but it may be administered rectally as a retention enema when oral administration is not feasible (i.e., persistent vomiting, paralytic ileus). The oral dosage of 15 gm is gently mixed with 150 to 200 ml of water and administered one to four times per day. The concurrent administration of a 70 percent solution of *sorbital* at a dosage of 10 to 20 ml usually is planned with the use of the cation-exchange resin. The hyperosmotic effect of sorbital in the intestinal tract maintains the liquid content of the feces, and that action counteracts the constipating effects of the exchange resin. Sorbital usually is given every two hours during the initial period of therapy, and that dosage schedule may be adjusted when the patient has the desired two loose stools per day.

The solution that is administered as a high retention enema contains 30 to 50 gm of sodium polystyrene sulfonate in 100 ml of an aqueous vehicle such as 10 percent dextrose, 1 percent methylcellulose, or 10 percent sorbitol solution. The enema is retained as long as possible (i.e., six to ten hours) to provide maximum intraintestinal cation exchange. A cleansing enema is given after each retention enema treatment period. Each gram of resin optimally will remove about 1.37 mEq of potassium ions.

The exchange process begins in the stomach after the oral resin is ingested. The drug is converted from the sodium to the hydrogen form in the stomach, and it liberates the hydrogen in the colon in exchange for the potassium ions, which are present in high concentrations. Excretion of the resin in the feces removes the potassium ions from the body. The intraintestinal exchange process gradually causes the movement of additional potassium ions from the circulating fluids to the intestinal secretions, and they become bound to the resin in the intestinal lumen. The resin has a high affinity for potassium ions, but other cations may also be removed by the exchange process (i.e., calcium, ammonium, magnesium). During therapy with the exchange resin, the serum electrolyte levels are monitored, and treatment is interrupted when the potassium levels reach the normal range of 4 to 5 mEq/L. The calcium levels are also monitored when therapy is continued for periods longer than three days and replacement therapy is planned to correct hypocalcemia. Patients with cardiac arrhythmias associated with hyperkalemia and those concurrently receiving digitalis are usually placed on a cardiac monitor during the period of therapy.

The drug may produce anorexia, nausea, vomiting, hypokalemia, hypocalcemia, and constipation. The release of sodium in the stomach by the exchange resin can elevate the serum sodium levels during prolonged treatment with the exchange resin. The subsequent overhydration associated with sodium and water retention can produce congestive heart failure.

Drugs Controlling Hyperuricemia

The uricosuric agents *probenecid* and *sulfinpyrazone* reduce elevated blood urate levels by blocking the renal tubule reabsorption of uric acid. *Allopurinol* inhibits the action of the enzyme, which is required for the formation of uric acid. The drugs are employed for treatment of persons with gout and for prevention of crystal or stone formation in persons with elevated serum urate levels. Alkalinization of the urine increases the solubility of uric acid crystals, and a fluid intake of at least 2 to 3 liters/day assures excretion of the uric acid.

Probenecid (BENEMID, PROBALAN, PROBENIMEAD, ROBENECID)

The drug is a sulfonamide derivative that acts as a renal tubular blocking agent. It competes with uric acid for the active reabsorption sites in the proximal convoluted tubules. That action reduces the serum urate levels by inhibiting reabsorption of uric acid. There is a consequent increase in the quantity of uric acid that is excreted in the urine. Probenecid concurrently reduces the plasma protein binding of urate, and that action also increases the uric acid excretion rate.

Therapy Considerations. Probenecid is administered orally with meals or with an antacid to decrease gastric irritation. The initial dosage for the treatment of patients with gout is 250 mg twice daily during the first week of therapy. The dosage is then increased to 500 mg two times per day. The therapeutic dosage usually relieves the patient's symptoms and produces a marked increase in the urinary output of uric acid (>700 mg/24 hours). The dosage is increased in increments of 500 mg at four-week intervals, when the therapeutic response is inadequate, until the maximum daily dosage of 2 gm is reached. Therapy is continued indefinitely, but dosage reductions may be planned when symptoms are well controlled after a period of six months.

The competitive action of probenecid at the renal tubule sites also is used to therapeutic advantage during treatment with drugs that are secreted by the renal tubules (i.e., penicillin and other weak acids). The use of probenicid with such drugs reduces their excretion and provides the higher plasma levels that are desired for treatment of the patient. That therapeutic use and dosage of probenecid are discussed in detail in the text with the discussion of the drugs with which it is employed concurrently for therapy.

The drug is rapidly absorbed from the gastrointestinal tract. Approximately 75 percent of the circulating drug is bound to plasma proteins. The drug crosses the placental barrier. Maximal renal clearance of uric acid occurs within 30 minutes after the drug is administered.

Probenecid is slowly metabolized in the liver to metabolites that possess some uricosuric activity. The drug is primarily secreted by the proximal tubules. Reabsorption is nearly complete in an acid urine. Alkalinization of the urine decreases reabsorption of the drug without modifying its activity as a uricosuric agent. Alkalinization of the urine also increases the solubility of uric acid and reduces stone formation. Probenecid produces a false positive reaction when cupric sulfate reagents (Benedict's Qualitative Reagent, CLINITEST, or Fehling's Solution) are used for tests of glycosuria. The glucose oxidase reagents

(CLINISTIX, TES-TAPE) should be used for the urine tests.

Treatment with probenecid is usually started when the serum urate levels are higher than 9 mg/100 ml to prevent movement of the urates into the joints and to prevent formation of renal crystals or stones that are associated with higher serum urate levels. When therapy is planned for a patient with an acute gout attack, the initial use of the drug is postponed until two to three weeks after the attack subsides. The postponement avoids the flareup of symptoms that occurs when probenecid is given during the painful, inflammatory phase of gouty arthritis. There may be an increased frequency of acute gout attacks during the first 6 to 12 months of therapy with probenecid. Colchicine may be given concurrently to prevent the attacks. Probenecid is also frequently employed to promote uric acid excretion when patients have hyperuricemia during treatment with diuretics, pyrazinamide, or ethambutol.

Adverse Effects. There is a low incidence of adverse effects during therapy with probenecid. Headache, anorexia, nausea, and vomiting are the most frequent adverse effects. There have also been reports of dizziness, flushing, sore gums, frequent urination, and anemia. Hemolytic anemia may occur in patients with an inherited glucose-6-phosphate dehydrogenase (G-6-PD) deficiency. Allergic reactions, which rarely occur, include dermatitis, pruritus, fever, hypotension, and anaphylaxis. The increased concentrations of uric acid in the renal tubules may produce stone formation, and the resulting renal colic is manifested as flank pain and hematuria.

Interactions. Probenecid blocks the renal secretion of nitrofurantoin, and that action reduces its effectiveness in the control of urinary tract infections and may also increase its toxicity. Probenecid may also inhibit the renal tubule secretion of oral sulfonylurea hypoglycemic agents and prolong their duration of action. By inhibiting the secretion of aminosalicylic acid, dapsone, or indomethacin, probenecid may increase the plasma levels and promote the toxic effects of those drugs. It also inhibits the sodium-excreting effects of furosemide and ethacrynic acid and increases the excretion of calcium, magnesium, and citrate during thiazide diuretic therapy.

The uricosuric actions of probenecid and salicylates are mutually antagonistic. An alternate nonsalicylate drug should be used when an analgesic, anti-inflammatory, or antipyretic agent is required during therapy with the uricosuric drug. The effects of allopurinol and probenecid are additive, and the drugs are used concurrently to therapeutic advantage.

Sulfinpyrazone (ANTURANE)

The drug provides a uricosuric action similar to that of probenecid. It is infrequently employed for treatment of patients with gout or hyperuricemia because it can produce bone marrow depression.

Therapy Considerations. Sulfinpyrazone is taken orally with meals at a dosage of 100 to 200 mg two times per day during the first week of therapy. Dosage is then increased to the maintenance level of 200 to 400 mg twice daily or the dosage that is required to maintain serum urate levels within normal limits. The drug is rapidly absorbed from the gastrointestinal tract. Peak plasma levels are attained within one to two hours. The duration of action is four to ten hours. The circulating drug is approximately 98 percent bound to plasma proteins. Sulfinpyrazone has a plasma half-life of three hours. It is rapidly metabolized in the liver, and the N^1-*p-hydroxyphenyl* metabolite possesses uricosuric activity. The drug is secreted primarily by the renal tubules. Approximately 90 percent of the unchanged drug is excreted in the urine and the remainder is excreted as the active and inactive metabolites. Approximately 5 percent of the unchanged drug is excreted in the feces after a 48-hour period.

Adverse Effects. Gastrointestinal disturbances frequently occur during therapy with sulfinpyrazone (i.e., nausea, dyspepsia, gastrointestinal pain and bleeding, and the reactivation of peptic ulcers). Although blood dyscrasias occur very rarely, they include anemia, leukopenia, agranulocytosis, and thrombocytopenia.

There have been reports of skin rash, dizziness, vertigo, tinnitus, and edema. The high concentrations of uric acid in the urine may produce renal stones during the early weeks of therapy, and a high fluid intake is essential during that period.

Interactions. Because of their similar mode of action, sulfinpyrazone interacts with other agents in a manner similar to that of probenecid. There are indications that colchicine acts synergistically with sulfinpyrazone in the production of acute myeloblastic leukemia and multiple myeloma. Cholestyramine can bind sulfinpyrazone and delay its absorption from the gastrointestinal tract. Administration of sulfinpyrazone one hour before or four to six hours after the administration of cholestyramine prevents the intraintestinal binding.

Allopurinol (ZYLOPRIM)

The drug is employed for the treatment of patients with hyperuricemia or gout. Its mode of action differs from that of the uricosuric agents.

Allopurinol inhibits the action of the enzyme *xanthine oxidase* that catalyzes the conversion of *hypoxanthine* to *xanthine* and the conversion of *xanthine* to *uric acid*. By blocking the enzymatic activity that is required to convert the oxypurines to uric acid, allopurinol decreases the serum and urine levels of uric acid. The action of the drug increases the renal excretion of hypoxanthine and xanthine. Those products are independently soluble, but excretion of large quantities of the xanthine compounds can cause crystal formation in the nephrons. Concurrent alkalinization of the urine increases the solubility of the purines and can decrease the incidence of crystalluria. The drug also decreases the serum urate levels by increasing the incorporation of hypoxanthine and xanthine into the cellular *deoxyribonucleic acid* (DNA) and *ribonucleic acid* (RNA).

Therapy Considerations. Allopurinol initially is administered as a single oral dose of 100 to 200 mg/day. The drug is taken after eating to decrease gastric irritation. The dosage is usually increased in increments of 100 mg each week until the maximum dosage of 800 mg/day is reached or the serum urate levels are reduced to less than 6 mg/100 ml. Dosages above 300 mg are given in divided doses. When the drug is used for the treatment of patients with gout, the drug is taken indefinitely.

The drug may be employed to prevent uric acid nephropathy in patients who are receiving antineoplastic drugs or drugs that periodically increase serum urate levels (i.e., aluminum nicotate, diazoxide, diuretics, mecamylamine, pyrazinamide). A dosage of 600 to 800 mg/day may be used for two to three days with a copious fluid intake to reduce the high levels of serum urates that are produced by drug-induced destruction of malignant tissues. Children six to ten years of age may receive 300 mg of allopurinol per day and children under six years of age may receive 150 mg/day for 48 hours during antineoplastic drug therapy. The dosage is adjusted according to the patient's response. The lower dosages avert the allopurinol-induced inhibition of azathioprine or mercaptopurine oxidation by *xanthine oxidase*, which can occur when the drug is given at dosages of 300 to 600 mg/day. Decreased oxidation of the antineoplastic drugs potentiates their bone marrow depression effects. Allopurinol therapy is usually started one to two days after the antineoplastic drug therapy, and continuation of allopurinol administration beyond two to three days is dependent on the patient's blood urate levels.

Approximately 80 percent of the drug is absorbed from the gastrointestinal tract. Peak plasma levels are attained within two to six hours. The serum urate concentrations begin to decline within 24 to 48 hours. Continual mobilization of urate deposits from the joints and tophaceous deposits maintains the elevated serum urate levels, and it may be one to three weeks before the serum urate levels reach their lowest point, or nadir.

Allopurinol is distributed in all body fluids. The drug is metabolized in the liver, and the active metabolite *alloxanthine,* which has a much longer half-life than allopurinol, also inhibits the activity of the enzyme *xanthine oxidase.* The unchanged drug and its active metabolite are excreted in the urine. Creatinine clearances are evaluated periodically to allow dosage adjustments when renal function is compromised.

During the first 6 to 12 months of therapy there may be an increased frequency of attacks of acute gout. Colchicine may be administered for the first three to six months to reduce the incidence and severity of the gout attacks.

Adverse Effects. The most common adverse effect is a pruritic, maculopapular skin rash. Although the incidence of adverse effects is low, there may be a variety of dermatologic problems (i.e., exfoliative dermatitis, and urticarial, erythematous, hemorrhagic, or purpuric rashes). Drug therapy is discontinued when a rash occurs. Fever, malaise, alopecia, and fu-runculosis also occur and usually respond to a reduction in dosage. There occasionally are gastrointestinal disturbances (i.e., nausea, vomiting, dyspepsia, peptic ulceration, pancreatitis, abdominal pain, diarrhea), retinopathy, lymphadenopathy, hyperlipemia, drowsiness, vertigo, and tachycardia. There have been a few reports of idiosyncrasies that produced fever, leukopenia, eosinophilia, or arthralgias.

Interactions. Allopurinol increases the incidence of bone marrow depression when it is given concurrent with cyclophosphamide. Allopurinol potentiates the anticoagulant effect of dicumarol by inhibiting the hepatic microsomal enzymes. The concurrent use of thiazide diuretics or ethacrynic acid may increase the serum levels of the metabolite *alloxanthine* and increase the toxicity of allopurinol. The concurrent use of allopurinol and chlorpropamide may produce hypoglycemia because tubular excretion of the oral hypoglycemic drug is blocked by allopurinol.

Drugs That Reduce Blood Ammonia Levels

The intestinal hydrolysis of urea by bacterial enzymes and bacterial deamination of ingested proteins and other nitrogenous substances produces ammonia, which diffuses from the intestine into the portal blood. When the blood passes through the liver, the ammonia is removed and it is resynthesized to urea or glutamine before entering the hepatic venous blood.

In the presence of chronic liver disease, substantial quantities of ammonia-carrying portal blood can enter the systemic circulation through collateral blood vessels, intrahepatic communications, or surgical portosystemic shunts. The presence of ammonia in the blood that perfuses the cerebral tissues produces irritation and neurologic symptoms may become severe as the blood ammonia level rises. The blood ammonia concentration, which normally is 40 to 70 mcg/100 ml, may rise as high as 250 mcg/100 ml in severe portosystemic encephalopathy.

DRUG THERAPY

Neomycin sulfate and *lactulose* are the drugs that are administered orally to reduce the production of ammonia in the intestine. The drugs are an important aspect of the therapeutic plan for reduction of protein in the gastrointestinal tract (i.e., dietary protein restriction, removal of old blood from the tract).

Neomycin Sulfate

Less than 3 percent of the orally administered drug is absorbed from the intestinal tract. The antibiotic drug acts within the intestinal lumen to decrease the quantity of bacteria that are available for the synthesis of ammonia. Neomycin sulfate (MYCIFRADIN, NEOBIOTIN) usually is administered to adults at a dosage of 4 to 12.5 gm/day in four divided doses. The course of therapy usually is limited to five or six days to avoid the occurrence of ototoxicity, nephrotoxicity, and suprainfections that are associated with prolonged therapy. Administration of the drug for more than one week also is reported to induce the malabsorption of proteins and to contribute to the adverse catabolic effects of protein restriction.

Lactulose

The drug is a synthetic disaccharide that is employed for short- or long-term treatment of patients with portosystemic shunting of blood associated with chronic hepatic disease.

Action Mode. Lactulose is metabolized by colon bacteria and the intestinal content is acidified by the increased levels of lactic and acetic acids that are produced by lactulose degradation. The diffusible ammonia in the colon couples with hydrogen ions in the acidic colonic content and nondiffusible ammonium is formed. The osmotic laxative action of the lactulose metabolites increases the rate at which the ammonium ions are excreted with the feces.

Therapy Considerations. The usual daily adult dosage of lactulose (CEPHULAC) is 90 to 150 ml and that dosage is divided for administration three to four times per day. The dosage usually is adjusted to produce two or three soft stools per day. It is desirable that the stools show a pH 5 during therapy with lactulose. When the blood ammonia levels are markedly elevated, the drug may be given orally or by nasogastric tube at hourly intervals to produce a rapid effect. The dosage intervals are lengthened to a three-to-four-dose per day schedule when the laxative effect is attained.

The drug is a sweet-tasting syrup that some patients find unpalatable. The taste can be disguised by mixing the syrup with citrus fruit juice. The syrup contains lactulose (10 gm/15 ml) and small amounts of galactose and fructose. The orally administered syrup is poorly absorbed from the intestine and only 3 percent of the drug is excreted in the urine.

Lactulose reduces the blood ammonia levels by 25 to 50 percent in three fourths of the persons treated. There usually is an increased tolerance to protein and the dietary intake of protein may be increased to a level that maintains a positive nitrogen balance during therapy with lactulose.

Some improvement in the patient's status may appear within 24 hours but maximum beneficial effects may require up to seven days of therapy. Decreased arterial blood ammonia levels and normal electroencephalographic studies provide objective evidence of improvement. Qualitative assessment of the improvement in mental status can be determined by asking the patient to subtract serial sevens, write his name, identify the day and date, or name the President of the United States.

Adverse Effects. Severe diarrhea occasionally occurs and the drug therapy is discontinued to avoid the fluid and potassium losses that can contribute to encephalopathy. Patients also occasionally have abdominal distention and cramping, flatulence, anorexia, nausea, or vomiting.

Interactions. Concurrent use of neomycin or other anti-infective drugs can interfere with the bacterial degradation of lactulose in the colon and prevent the acidification of the colonic contents that is essential for the drug effect. The concurrent use of laxatives may falsely indicate that the dosage of lactulose is adequate to produce the desired number of stools per day.

Biliary Stone Dissolution Agent

Most gallstones are composed primarily of cholesterol that has precipitated from a cholesterol-saturated bile, crystallized, and developed into stones. Chenodiol, or *chenodeoxycholic acid,* which is a primary bile acid, is being investigated in national clinical trials to determine its efficacy in decreasing the precipitation, or increasing the solubility, of biliary cholesterol in patients with gallstones. In early clinical trials, the action of the drug prevented the formation of new cholesterol-containing stones and gradually dissolved existing gallstones in members of the study population.

Small gallstones are dissolved in 3 to 12 months when the drug is taken at a dosage of 10 to 15 mg/kg of body weight each day. Large stones may take as long as three years to dissolve completely. The gallstones tend to recur when drug therapy is terminated. Diarrhea is a frequent adverse effect in persons taking the drug.

Review Guides

1. Describe the nursing intervention that would be indicated when apomorphine hydrochloride is given to produce emesis in a young adult.
2. Outline the factors that would be included when counseling the patient who is receiving penicillamine for the control of persistent cystine levels.
3. Describe the assessments that would be planned and the duration of the monitoring period when a child is receiving deferoxamine mesylate for the treatment of acute iron intoxication.
4. Explain briefly the methodology employed for diagnosis of lead poisoning.
5. Describe the observations that would be planned when a child is receiving intramuscular injections of edetate calcium disodium for treatment of chronic lead poisoning.
6. Explain the rationale for placing the patient with a history of congestive heart failure on a cardiac monitor when edetate disodium is being administered.
7. Describe the difference in the mode of action between probenecid and allopurinol.
8. Explain briefly the rationale for use of allopurinol when a child is receiving antineoplastic drugs for treatment of leukemia.
9. Describe briefly the rationale for use of probenecid during therapy with penicillin.

Additional Readings

Alvares, Alvito P.; Fischbein, Alf; Sassa, Shigeru; Anderson, Karl E.; and Kappas, Attallah: Lead intoxication: effects of cytochrome P-450-mediated hepatic oxidations. *Clin. Pharmacol. Ther.*, **19**:183, February, 1976.

Aronow, Regine, and Fleishmann, Larry E.: Mercury poisoning in children. *Clin. Pediatr.*, **15**:936, October, 1976.

Baehler, Richard W., and Galla, John H.: Conservative management of chronic renal failure. *Geriatrics,* **31**:46, September, 1976.

Barzel, Uriel S.: The changing face of hyperparathyroidism. *Hosp. Pract.*, **12**:89, November, 1977.

Cohen, Donald J.; Johnson, Warren T.; and Caparulo, Barbara K.: Pica and elevated blood lead level in autistic and atypical children. *Am. J. Dis. Child.*, **130**:47, January, 1976.

Conley, Dean R., and Goldstein, Leonard I.: Pathogenesis and therapy of cholesterol gallstones. *Med. Clin. North Am.*, **59**:1025, July, 1975.

Croft, Harriet, and Frenkel, Sallie: Children and lead poisoning. *Am. J. Nurs.*, **75**:102, January, 1975.

Dailey, G. W., and Deftos, L. J.: Differential diagnosis of hypercalcemia. *Hosp. Med.*, **11**:30, February, 1975.

Fadel, Hossam E.; Northrop, Grelajo; and Misenhimer, H. Robert: Hyperuricemia in pre-eclampsia. *Am. J. Obstet. Gynecol.*, **125**:640, July 1, 1976.

Francone, Carol A.: "My battle against Wilson's disease." *Am. J. Nurs.*, **76**:247, February, 1976.

Freedman, Philip, and Smith, Earl C.: Acute renal failure. *Heart Lung*, **4**:873, November–December, 1975.

Greenblatt, David J.; Allen, Marcia D.; and Koch-Weser, Jan: Accidental iron poisoning in children. *Clin. Pediatr.*, **15**:835, September, 1976.

Hecht, Arthur; Gershberg, Herbert; and St. Paul, Henry: Primary hyperparathyroidism. *J.A.M.A.*, **233**:519, August 11, 1975.

Hunter, Gary R., and Gaisford, Walter D.: Guide to

the diagnosis and management of obstructive jaundice. *Hosp. Med., 13*:82, June, 1977.

Iser, John H.; Dowling, R. Hermon; Mok, H. Y. I.; and Bell, G. D.: Chenodeoxycholic acid treatment of gallstones. *N. Engl. J. Med., 293*:378, August 21, 1975.

Jonides, Linda K., and Heindl, Mary C.: Difficulties in treating lead poisoning. *Pediatr. Nurs., 1*:24, September–October, 1975.

Juliani, Louise: Assessing renal function. *Nursing 78, 8*:34, January, 1978.

Kao, Ing; Drachman, Daniel B.; and Price, Donald L.: Botulinum toxin: mechanism of presynaptic blockade. *Science, 193*:1256, September 24, 1976.

Kappas, Attallah, and Alvares, Alvito P.: How the liver metabolizes foreign substances. *Sci. Am., 232*:22, June, 1975.

Kelley, William N.: Current therapy of gout and hyperuricemia. *Hosp. Pract., 11*:69, May, 1976.

Kolb, Felix O.: Medical management of the patient with renal stones. *Primary Care, 2*:317, June, 1975.

Landgrebe, Albert R.; Myhan, William L.; and Coleman, Mary: Urinary tract stones resulting from the excretion of oxypurinol. *N. Engl. J. Med., 292*:626, March 20, 1975.

Levinsky, Norman G.: Pathphysiology of acute renal failure. *N. Engl. J. Med., 296*:1453, June 23, 1977.

Lilis, Ruth, and Fischbein, Alf: Chelation therapy in workers exposed to lead. *J.A.M.A., 235*:2823, June 28, 1976.

Lovejoy, Frederick H., Jr., and Berenberg, William: Poisoning in children under age 5. *Postgrad. Med., 63*:79, March, 1978.

Lowenthal, David T.: The treatment of hyperuricemia. *Am. Fam. Physician, 14*:98, July, 1976.

Max, Martin: Acute hypercalcemic crisis. *Heart Lung, 5*:624, July–August, 1976.

Mayer, Bernard W., and Schlackman, Neil: Organophosphates—a pediatric hazard. *Am. Fam. Physician, 11*:121, May, 1975.

Mennear, John H.: The poisoning emergency. *Am. J. Nurs., 77*:842, May, 1977.

Mofenson, Howard C., and Greensher, Joseph: Keeping up with changing trends in childhood poisonings. *Clin. Pediatr., 14*:621, July, 1975.

Mooty, Joyce; Ferrand, Charles F., Jr.; and Harris, Paul: Relationship of diet to lead poisoning in children. *Pediatrics, 55*:636, May, 1975.

Morgan, J. M.: Problems in the diagnosis of lead poisoning. *Clin. Med., 82*:14, June, 1975.

Nugent, C. A.: Answers to questions on the differential diagnosis of hypercalcemia. *Hosp. Med., 14*:106, February, 1978.

O'Dorisio, Thomas M.: Hypercalcemic crisis. *Heart Lung, 7*:425, May–June, 1978.

Propper, Richard D.; Shurin, Susan B.; and Nathan, David G.: Reassessment of desferrioxamine B in iron overload. *N. Engl. J. Med., 294*:1421, June 24, 1976.

Reigart, J. R., and Whitlock, N. H.: Relationship between free erythrocyte porphyrins and whole blood lead. *Pediatrics, 57*:54, January, 1976.

Rinear, Charles E., and Rinear, Eileen: Emergency! Part 3: care for aspiration, burns, and poisoning. *Nursing 75, 5*:40, April, 1975.

Silbergeld, Ellen K., and Chisolm, J. Julian, Jr.: Lead poisoning: altered urinary catecholamine metabolites as indicators of intoxication in mice and children. *Science, 192*:153, April 9, 1976.

Simon, Norman M.; Lennon, Roslyn G.; and Johnson, Marianna Kiefer: Chronic renal failure. Part I: Pathophysiology and medical management. *Cardiovasc. Nurs., 12*:7, March–April, 1976.

Talbott, John H.: Gouty arthritis and hyperuricemia. *Hosp. Med., 13*:44, June, 1977.

Tripp, Alice: Hyper and hypocalcemia. *Am. J. Nurs., 76*:1142, July, 1976.

Verhulst, Henry L.; Peterson, William; and Trissel, Lawrence: How to treat overdosages of drugs and common poisons. *Pharm. Times, 41*:46, March, 1975.

Waldman, Judy M.; Mofenson, Howard C.; and Greensher, Joseph: Evaluating the functioning of a poison control center. *Clin. Pediatr., 15*:75, January, 1976.

Walser, Mackenzie: Treatment of renal failure with keto acids. *Hosp. Pract., 10*:59, June, 1975.

Walsh, Francis M.; Crosson, Francis J.; Bayley, Marianne; McReynolds, John; and Pearson, Barry J.: Acute copper intoxication. *Am. J. Dis. Child., 131*:149, February, 1977.

Wedeen, Richard P.; Maesaka, John K.; Weiner, Barry; Lipat, Gregoro A.; Lyons, Michael M.; Vitale, Leonard F.; and Joselow, Morris M.: Occupational lead nephropathy. *Am. J. Med., 59*:630, November, 1975.

Wilson, Douglas R.: Renal calculi: diagnosis and medical management. *Primary Care, 5*:41, March, 1978.

22

Diarrhea and Constipation

The intestinal tract provides a vital link between the body fluids and the food supply from the environment. Elimination of the waste products of ingested foods is essential to the natural function of the digestive tract.

Most individuals have a relatively regular habit pattern for bowel elimination that occurs in a cyclic pattern in relation to the foods ingested. Disruptions in that pattern can cause abdominal discomfort and adversely affect the appetite and the intake of nutrients.

Physiologic Correlations

INTESTINAL FLUID AND NUTRIENT ABSORPTION

The primary function of the small intestine is absorption of nutrients from the intraluminal contents. Although the combined length of the small intestine (duodenum, jejunum, ileum) is approximately 660 cm (22 ft), the absorption surface of the lumen is far greater than is indicated by that longitudinal measurement. The villi that project into the lumen markedly increase the epithelial contact surface for the absorption of nutrients.

Intestinal Fluid Secretion

The single layer of columnar epithelium that lines the intestinal lumen is interspersed with *crypts of Lieberkühn*. Those crypts secrete a fluid that is similar to the extracellular fluids. Distention of the small intestine or the presence of irritating substances in the intestinal lumen stimulates the local *myenteric reflexes* that cause the secretion of copious amounts of fluids from the crypts. Those secretions dilute and facilitate the absorption of the chyme and other substances from the intestinal lumen. The villi rapidly reabsorb the secretions along with the intestinal intraluminal substances.

Intestinal Contraction

The digestion and absorption of foods in the small intestine are accomplished by an interrelated series of events that involve hormonal secretion (i.e., cholecystokinin) and intestinal motility. The sight and smell of food can produce propulsive movements of the small intestine. Eating, regardless of the size of the meal, produces deep propulsive activity that lasts for one to two hours. The small intestine has a pattern of segmental annular contractions that hold food in small areas and a circular motion that churns the food. That pattern maintains the contact between the absorptive surfaces and the intraluminal content. Peristaltic waves gradually move the content toward the large intestine.

Fluid and Salt Conservation

Most of the nutrient absorption rapidly occurs in the jejunum by active transport processes. Absorption of salt and water is the most important conservation function of the intestine. That absorption occurs along the entire intestinal tract, but the principal site for reabsorption and conservation of approximately 7 liters/day of digestive secretions and about 2 liters/day of ingested fluids is the upper portion of the small intestine. Reabsorption is so efficient in the jejunum that only one sixth of the fluid volume that leaves the duodenum reaches the ileum. Sodium ions are the major cations of the intestinal content. The cations are actively absorbed and water passively follows. Chloride ions are the major anions, and they are absorbed primarily from the ileum. At the sites of chloride absorption, bicarbonate and some potassium ions are secreted.

Colon Fluid Absorption

The slower activity of the large intestine delays the movement of the intraluminal content and allows an opportunity for extraction of fluid. The colon extracts the major portion of the 1 liter of fluid that is delivered to it by the small intestine, and only 100 to 200 ml is eliminated with the feces. Unlike the small intestine, the only secretion in the large intestine is the mucus that is produced in response to direct tactile stimulation of the goblet cells by the intraluminal content or by the activity of the myenteric reflexes. The parasympathetic nerves, which supply the distal portions of the colon, can also stimulate the secretion of copious quantities of mucus from the goblet cells. That stimulation also markedly increases colon motility.

Pathophysiologic Correlations

DIARRHEA

Diarrhea is defined as an abnormal frequency and fluidity of the stools in relation to the person's customary bowel habits. High-volume diarrhea, which is of small-intestine origin, may occur as a consequence of intraluminal factors that irritate the epithelial lining or interfere with the reabsorption of the fluid that is secreted by the crypts. It may also occur when the osmolality of the intraluminal content is altered by foods that escape absorption (i.e., lactose) and remain in the lumen to cause retention of fluid. In either instance, the intraluminal fluid is increased as a consequence of the secretory processes, and the concurrent distention with fluid produces an increased motility of the intestine.

Many irritants provoke diarrhea by stimulating *adenyl cyclase* and the consequent activity of *cyclic 3',5'-adenosine monophosphate* (cAMP). The activity of cAMP increases the quantity of crypt secretions. Factors that cause diarrhea by irritation (i.e., chemicals, drugs, bacterial or viral infections) produce a continuous diarrhea unrelated to the ingestion of foods and unrelieved by fasting. Infectious diarrhea in adults generally is of bacterial origin, and in children it tends to be of viral origin.

The diarrhea that is reduced by fasting is usually related to an agent that initially caused the osmotic movement of fluid. The diluting effects of the crypt secretions and the increased intestinal motility can effectively propel the substance through the bowel and terminate its diarrhea-producing effect.

Bacteria and virus infections are frequently the cause of irritation in the large intestine. The enteritis causes an increase in the secretion of water, electrolytes, and mucus from the epithelial cells. The fluids and mucus provide a protective action by diluting the irritant. The increased peristalsis that accompanies the enteritis may also shorten the period of contact with the irritant. Psychogenic factors can also cause an increase in parasympathetic nerve stimulation that increases the motility and the production of secretions in the colon.

CONSTIPATION

Constipation is defined as a decrease in the frequency of bowel movements, difficult passage of a hard stool, lengthy periods of straining to pass the stool, and a feeling of incomplete evacuation after the bowel movement. Constipation can be an acute or a chronic health problem. Hospitalized patients frequently are constipated as a consequence of decreased activity or immobility, changes in diet, drugs, dehydration, or psychologic interference with the ability to defecate in an unnatural position. Each of the foregoing factors can slow the movement of the feces through the large intestine and increase the reabsorption of fluid from the stool. The hard and dry fecal material can become a mass that is larger than the anal opening that is provided by relaxation of the internal and external sphincters.

Attempts to defecate and remove a hard, dry stool from the intestine require straining. That process can exhaust the patient and can jeopardize the health of patients with chronic heart failure. The *Valsalva maneuver,* which is used to strain at stool, involves taking a deep breath, closing the glottis, and contracting the abdominal muscles. That combination of maneuvers raises the intrathoracic pressure and thereby compresses the mediastinal structures (Fig. 22–1). The compression of the major blood vessels at initiation of the maneuver may cause dizziness or fainting. At the termination of the maneuver, the sudden influx of blood into the right atrium and ventricle from the previously compressed inferior and superior vena cava can provide a blood volume overload that distends the heart chambers and exceeds the pumping ability of the decompensated heart.

Chronic constipation can occur as a consequence of the irregular bowel habits that often are associated with inattention to the urge to defecate. Ignoring of that stimulus reduces the sensitivity of the defecation reflex. At a subsequent time, the movement of fecal material into the rectum may provide a defecation stimulus, but there often is less effective emptying of the lower intestine.

Antidiarrheal Drugs

DRUG THERAPY

Diarrhea may be a short-term problem that is associated with the irritation of foods, toxic agents, or drugs. Antibiotic-induced suppression of the normal bacterial flora of the intestine is also a common cause of diarrhea. In those instances, withdrawal of the offending agent and the use of drugs to control the excess intraluminal fluid or the intestinal motility may limit the problem to a short episode. The antidiarrheal agents also provide control of the recurrent or persistent diarrhea that is associated with pathology of the intestinal tract (i.e., regional enteritis, ulcerative

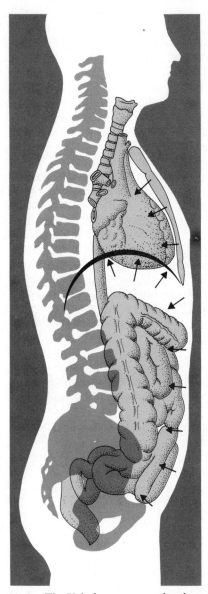

Fig. 22–1. The Valsalva maneuver involves deep inhalation, closing of the glottis, and contraction of the abdominal muscles. That manuever raises the intra-abdominal and intrathoracic pressures. The increased pressure on the intestine facilitates bowel evacuation.

colitis, diverticulitis) while other therapeutic measures are being employed to control the disease process.

The antidiarrheal drugs are nonspecific agents that control the diarrhea without specifically treating the underlying cause of the problem. The drugs include the *gastrointestinal motility inhibitors, adsorbents,* or *intestinal bacillus.* The decision to employ a particular drug is based on the status of the patient and the cause, characteristics, and duration of the diarrhea.

Gastrointestinal Motility Inhibitors

The drug group includes *diphenoxylate hydrochloride, loperamide hydrochloride,* and the *opium preparations.* The drugs are the primary agents for the control of diarrhea of short duration. Their addiction potential limits their use for long-term control of diarrhea in most situations. They are subject to control under the Federal Controlled Substances Act of 1970.

Action Mode. The gastrointestinal motility inhibitors increase the contraction of the circular movement of the intestinal tract and that action increases the contraction of the bowel segments and reduces the forward propulsion that contributes to the diarrhea. They also reduce the production of secretions in the tract. The slower transit time of the intraluminal content allows reabsorption of the fluid and reduces the fecal volume.

Diphenoxylate Hydrochloride. Therapy Considerations. The drug is a synthetic narcotic that is available in combination with atropine sulfate as an oral tablet or solution (LOMOTIL). The atropine sulfate that is contained in the formulation is provided at a subtherapeutic level (25 mcg/tablet), and it acts as a deterrent to abuse of the drug by addicts without producing the anticholinergic effects that are natural to atropine.

The initial adult dosage of the drug is 15 to 20 mg/day, and that dosage is divided for administration three to four times per day. Children

2 to 12 years of age initially may receive the liquid preparation at a dosage calculated on the basis of 0.3 to 0.4 mg/kg/day. That dosage may be divided for administration five times per day. The drug is provided in an oral solution with a calibrated dropper that allows accurate calculation of the children's dosage. After the acute diarrheal episode is relieved, the maintenance dosage usually is decreased to one fourth the level of the initial dosage.

The oral drug is well absorbed from the gastrointestinal tract, and peak serum drug levels are attained within two hours. It has a plasma half-life of approximately 215 hours. The onset of action appears within 45 minutes, and that effect lasts three to four hours. The drug is metabolized in the liver, and the active metabolite *diphenoxylic acid* has a plasma half-life of 4.4 hours. The metabolites slowly enter the feces with the bile. Some of the drug is excreted in the urine.

Adverse Effects. High dosages may produce narcotic effects, which include euphoria and suppression of the narcotic abstinence syndrome. Side effects that may occur during therapy include gastrointestinal disturbances (i.e., nausea, vomiting, abdominal discomfort, distention, paralytic ileus), central nervous system effects (i.e., restlessness, insomnia, sedation, dizziness), and allergic reactions (i.e., pruritus, angioedema, urticaria). When the drug is administered to children under two years of age, there may be effects that are attributable to the anticholinergic action of the atropine content of the preparation (i.e., dryness of the skin and mucous membranes, thirst, urinary retention, flushing).

The drug seldom is given to children younger than two years of age because of the low therapeutic margin in that age group. Persons who are taking the drug for the control of diarrhea should be cautioned to keep the drug out of the reach of children. Overdosage of the tablets produces symptoms of atropinism and symptoms of acute toxicity that are produced by the narcotic analgesics (i.e., central nervous system depression). There have been fatalities in children who have taken relatively few tablets.

Loperamide Hydrochloride (IMODIUM). *Therapy Considerations.* The initial adult dosage of the oral capsule is 4 mg, and subsequent doses of 2 mg are given after each loose, unformed stool to a maximum of 16 mg/day. The dosage for children is based on the calculation of 240 mcg/kg/day, divided for administration two to three times per day. The dosage is usually reduced to approximately one half the initial dosage level for maintenance therapy after the initial acute symptoms are controlled.

The oral drug is readily absorbed and peak plasma drug levels are attained in four hours. The drug has a plasma half-life of approximately 40 hours. The unchanged drug and its metabolites enter the feces with the bile. A minimal amount of the drug is excreted in the urine.

Adverse Effects. The most frequent adverse effects are gastrointestinal disturbances (i.e., epigastric or abdominal pain and distention, constipation, dry mouth, nausea, vomiting), drowsiness, fatigue, and skin rashes. Overdoses of the drug can cause constipation, central nervous system depression, and gastrointestinal irritation. It is often difficult to separate the symptoms from those associated with diarrhea.

Opium Preparations. *Opium tincture,* which contains 1 percent morphine anhydrous, is the most commonly prescribed preparation for the control of acute episodes of diarrhea. It is a deodorized opium tincture and is frequently referred to as DTO. *Paregoric,* which contains 0.04 percent morphine anhydrous, is a camphorated opium tincture that is also frequently used for the control of diarrhea. Both drugs are administered orally.

Therapy Considerations. The usual adult dosage of *opium tincture* is 0.6 to 1 ml. That dosage may be given four or more times per day to a maximum daily dosage of 6 ml.

The usual adult dosage of *paregoric* for the control of diarrhea is 5 ml to 10 ml one to four times per day. The dosage for children is based on the calculation of 2 to 4 ml/M² of body surface area after each loose stool. The drug is mixed with a small quantity of water for administration. The mixture has a milky appearance that is caused by the separation of the anise oil and camphor.

The oral drug is well absorbed from the gastrointestinal tract. It is rapidly metabolized in the liver, and plasma levels of morphine are low. Approximately, 75 percent of the drug is excreted in the urine within 48 hours.

Adverse Effects. Persons taking the drug occasionally become nauseated and may have other gastrointestinal disturbances. Overdose of the drug can cause depression of the central nervous system.

Adsorbents

Kaolin and *bismuth salts* are employed primarily for their adsorbent action in the control of diarrhea. Aluminum hydroxide, activated charcoal, or magnesium trisilicate may also be used occasionally for their adsorption action in the control of diarrhea. The drugs may be employed as single agents but more frequently are used in combination with opium preparations for the control of acute diarrhea.

Kaolin. The drug is a hydrated aluminum silicate. It frequently is employed in combination with the carbohydrate product *pectin.* Although the mechanism of action of pectin is unclear, the combination provides an adsorption and demulcent effect that controls diarrhea when it is given after each loose stool. The usual oral dosage of kaolin and pectin mixture (KAOPECTATE) is 15 to 30 ml. The drug mixture is scheduled for ad-

ministration two hours before or after the oral antibiotic *lincomycin* because adsorption of the antibiotic can reduce the serum drug levels.

Bismuth Salts. The bismuth salts (subcarbonate, subgallate, subsalicylate) have adsorbent and mild antacid properties. The salts are incorporated into many antidiarrheal mixtures. The drug salts are also available as a suspension with camphorated opium tincture.

Intestinal Bacteria

Lactobacillus acidophilus replaces the natural acid-producing bacteria when the normal bacterial flora has been modified by the use of antibiotics. The antibiotic-related diarrhea is controlled by the reestablishment of the normal physiologic and bacterial flora.

The drug is available as capsules that also contain the bulk-forming product *carboxymethylcellulose sodium* (BACID). Two of the capsules are taken two to four times per day for the control of diarrhea.

Lactobacillus acidophilus is also available as granules or tablets that contain *Lactobacillus bulgaricus.* That bacterium is able to ferment carbohydrates, and the lactic acid formed in the process enhances the growth of the normal intestinal bacteria. Three to four of the combination tablets (LACTINEX) or one packet of the granules is used three or four times per day. The tablets are taken with one-half glass of milk or tomato juice. The granules may be sprinkled on cereal or other food.

Laxatives

DRUG THERAPY

Drugs may be employed to maintain regular patterns for bowel elimination, to relieve constipation, or to prepare the intestinal tract for diagnostic or surgical procedures. The groups of laxatives are *bulk-forming agents, lubricants, saline cathartics, stimulants,* and *wetting agents.*

Bulk-Forming Agents

The laxatives are employed primarily for the control of bowel elimination when the person is confined to bed for prolonged periods of time or when the person's bowel activity is too weak to provide the peristalsis required for evacuation. Laxatives commonly are employed to maintain bowel function in elderly patients. The group of drugs includes *carboxymethylcellulose sodium,* *methylcellulose,* and *psyllium hydrophilic mucilloid.*

Action Mode. The drugs expand in the intestine when they absorb the intraluminal fluid. The increased bulk in the intestinal lumen stimulates the myenteric reflexes, and that provides the increased motility required to move the bowel content toward the anal route for evacuation.

Carboxymethylcellulose and Methylcellulose. The two drugs have a similar mode of action. *Methylcelluose* (CELLOTHYL, HYDROLOSE) is soluble in gastric juices, but *carboxymethylcellulose sodium* (CMC CELLULOSE GUM) is insoluble. Both drugs are available as liquids and tablets for oral use. When the drug is taken with water, it forms a colloidal solution that loses water when it mixes with the feces. The resulting gel increases the bulk of the stool.

The usual adult dosage is 2 to 6 gm/day, which may be divided for administration two to four times a day (Table 22–1). Children over six years of age may be given 1 to 1.5 gm/day. The liquid forms of the drugs are usually employed for children because chewing of the tablets can cause the formation of bulk in the esophagus. Drinking at least one full glass of fluid when taking the drug is essential to assure that there is adequate moisture to avoid impaction by the drug and the fecal contents in the intestine.

Psyllium Hydrophilic Mucilloid. Fifty percent of the drug is the mucilaginous portion of the psyllium seeds *Plantago ovata* and 50 percent is dextrose. Use of the drug leads to formation of a natural, soft, water-retaining, gelatinous fecal material. The drug powder is thoroughly mixed in a full glass of cool fluid and a second glass of liquid is taken. That procedure assures that the drug is cleared from the esophagus and that it arrives in the intestinal tract before it expands. The drug (Table 22–1) is usually given one to three times per day

Table 22–1.
Laxatives

Drug	Single Oral Dose (Adult)
Bulk-Forming Agents	
Carboxymethylcellulose sodium (CMC CELLULOSE GUM)	1–1.5 gm
Methylcellulose (CELLOTHYL, HYDROLOSE)	1–1.5 gm
Psyllium hydrophilic mucilloid (EFFERSYLLIUM, METAMUCIL)	4–7 gm
Lubricant	
Mineral oil	15–45 ml
Saline Cathartics	
Magnesium citrate	200 ml
Magnesium sulfate	10–30 gm
Milk of magnesia	15–30 ml
Sodium phosphate	3.6–7.2 gm
Stimulants	
Bisacodyl (DULCOLAX)	10–30 mg
Cascara sagrada	120–325 mg
Castor oil	15–60 ml
Danthron (DORBANE, MODANE)	37.5–150 mg
Senna fruit (SENOKOT)	326–374 mg
Sennosides A and B (GLYSENNID)	12–24 mg
Wetting Agents	
Dioctyl calcium sulfosuccinate (SURFAK)	50–240 mg
Dioctyl sodium sulfosuccinate (COLACE, COMFOLAX, DOXINATE)	50–200 mg
Poloxamer 188 (POLYKOL)	500–750 mg

Lubricants

Mineral oil, or liquid petrolatum, lubricates the gastrointestinal tract and prevents the dehydration of fecal material in the intestine. The drug is often used as an emulsion or in combination with milk of magnesia (i.e., HALEY'S M-O) at bedtime to facilitate early-morning defecation. Most persons take the mineral oil with fruit juice to rapidly move the oil from the oral tissues.

Prolonged use of the lubricant can cause a deficiency of the fat-soluble vitamins A, D, E, and K. Small amounts of the oil are absorbed and transported throughout the body as foreign substances.

The drug is contraindicated for persons with a weak swallowing reflex because passage of the oil into the lungs can produce lipoid pneumonia. Continual use also causes anal leaking of the oil and consequent soiling of the clothing or bedding.

The drug is also employed as a rectal retention enema to facilitate the passage of feces when there is a fecal impaction in the rectum. Retention of the oil in the rectum for a period of 20 to 30 minutes softens the dried and impacted fecal mass and allows its passage or its removal by digital manipulation. A cleansing enema usually is given after the fecal mass is reduced in size.

Saline Cathartics

Milk of magnesia, magnesium citrate, magnesium sulfate, and *sodium phosphate* (Table 22–1) are the saline cathartics. The drugs, with the exception of milk of magnesia, are frequently employed to purge the gastrointestinal tract of its contents prior to surgical or diagnostic procedures. The person taking the strong cathartics should be told that the urge to defecate may occur suddenly. The evacuation usually consists of a copious quantity of liquid and the explosive expulsion of flatus.

Action Mode. The laxatives increase the osmolality of the intraluminal content by providing hyperosmolar concentrations of poorly absorbed magnesium, phosphate, or sulfate ions. The increased amount of fluid in the intestinal lumen provides the myenteric reflex that increases the motility of the gut. The fecal material rapidly moves toward the anal region where it stimulates the defecation reflex.

The saline cathartics are also thought to stimulate the release of the hormone *cholecystokinin-pancreozymin* from the small intestinal mucosa. That enzyme provides a motor and secretory ef-

fect in the small intestine that increases the cathartic action of the drugs.

Milk of Magnesia. Milk of magnesia, or magnesia magma, is the most gentle and slow acting of the saline cathartics. It is the most commonly used over-the-counter laxative. The drug (Table 22–1) is taken at the time of retiring at night and usually produces a natural bowel movement when the added stimulus of food at breakfasttime activates the gastrocolic and duodenocolic reflexes. The preparation contains 7 to 8.5 percent magnesium hydroxide. The antacid action of its ingredients makes the drug useful as a gastric antacid when it is used at lower dosage (i.e., 5 to 10 ml).

Milk of magnesia is frequently used as an emulsion that contains mineral oil. The emulsion should be stored at room temperature because refrigeration causes aggregation of the colloids and the drug is less effective as a laxative.

Magnesium Citrate. The pleasant-tasting lemon-flavored preparation contains potassium bicarbonate and magnesium carbonate, which provides an effervescent effect. Liberation of magnesium oxide in the intestine produces the cathartic action. Chilling of the drug before it is taken increases its palatability.

Magnesium Sulfate. Magnesium sulfate, or epsom salt, is a bitter-tasting powder or granules. The drug is taken when the stomach is empty. Dissolving the drug with a full glass of iced liquid (240 ml) partially masks the disagreeable taste. Each 15 gm of the drug retains about 400 ml of fluid in the intestine, and within one to two hours there is an urgent need to defecate. The bowel movement consists of a fluid or semifluid evacuation. Patients usually complain of feeling exhausted after completion of the bowel evacuation.

Sodium Phosphate. The drug is more pleasant tasting and less drastic in action than magnesium sulfate. It produces a liquid or semiliquid bowel movement within one hour after it is taken. The drug is most effective when taken on an empty stomach with a full glass of warm water.

Stimulants

The stimulants are the most commonly used and misused of the laxatives. The drugs are readily available as over-the-counter preparations, and persons can use them to provide regular evacuation patterns that are in excess of those natural to their food intake patterns. Continued use of the stimulants reduces the natural reflex responses to fecal distention of the bowel. The group of drugs includes *bisacodyl, oxyphenisatin acetate, castor oil,* and the anthraquinone derivatives *danthron, cascara sagrada,* and *senna preparations.*

Bisacodyl. Action Mode. The drug stimulates the sensory nerve endings in the mucosa of the colon. That action stimulates the parasympathetic motor nerves that provide the increased peristalsis and secretions required for movement of fecal material toward the anus.

Therapy Considerations. Bisacodyl is available as an enteric-coated oral tablet (Table 22–1) and also as a rectal suppository. The usual adult dosage of the oral tablet is 10 to 15 mg. The higher dosage (30 mg) may be employed when it is desirable to evacuate the bowel for diagnostic procedures. The oral dosage for children is 5 to 10 mg. The enteric-coated tablet is swallowed whole to avoid gastric irritation. Water or fruit juice is usually taken with the drug because ingestion of milk or an antacid within one hour of the time the drug is taken can cause gastric disintegration of the tablet.

The suppositories are used for individuals who have difficulty swallowing the tablets. They may be employed at a specific time (i.e., 6 A.M.) on alternate days to provide the stimulus to evacuation when a bowel regularity plan is being established. The suppositories are also used for bowel evacuation for patients two hours before the onset of the second stage of labor.

One 10-mg suppository may be used for adults and children over two years of age. One half that dosage (5 mg) is used for children or infants under two years of age. Prolonged use of the suppositories can cause rectal irritation.

The drug is often given orally at bedtime and as a suppository in the morning when bowel evacuation is required for diagnostic examinations. Addition of tannic acid to the bisacodyl powder increases its solubility, and a 1-liter solution containing a 2.5-gm packet of bisacodyl tannex (CLYSODRAST) may be employed as an enema or as a radiopaque enema adjuvant in the barium sulfate suspension that is used for colonic fluoroscopic examinations.

The oral drug produces a soft, formed stool and a gentle bowel movement within 6 to 12 hours. The higher dosages (i.e., 20 to 30 mg) may produce several loose, unformed stools. The rectal suppository usually produces a soft, formed stool within 10 to 120 minutes. When the suppositories are given in the early morning (i.e., 6 A.M.) to establish a regular bowel evacuation regimen, an opportunity is provided for the patient to use the bedpan or commode within 15 minutes after breakfast is eaten.

The oral drug primarily acts locally on the intestinal mucosa, and approximately 95 percent of the drug is excreted with the feces. The 5 percent of the drug that is absorbed from the intestine is metabolized in the liver and excreted in the urine. Absorption of the drug from the suppositories or the enema solution is negligible. Although abdominal cramps, tenesmus, nausea, vertigo, or diarrhea occasionally occurs, the drug seldom causes sufficient discomfort to negate its use.

Castor Oil. The drug undergoes saponification in the small intestine, and that process releases the irritating *ricinoleic acid,* which induces peristalsis. The purging effect of the drug provides the emptying of the bowel that is required for endoscopic or fluoroscopic examination of the bowel or of the kidneys, ureters, and bladder. The catharsis occurs within a period of two to six hours, and there may be an explosive emptying of the fecal contents of the bowel. Patients usually complain of exhaustion and cramping during the bowel evacuation period.

The drug is available as a liquid, capsules, or a 36 or 60 percent flavored aromatic emulsion of *castor oil* (ALPHAMUL, NEOLOID). The unpleasant taste can be masked by serving the chilled drug with fruit juice or coffee. The emulsion is the more palatable of the liquid formulations.

Anthraquinone Derivatives. Danthron, cascara sagrada, and the *senna preparations* are the drugs that are anthraquinone derivatives. Rhubarb and aloe are also members of the anthracene group. The drugs provide a laxative effect by release of the active principles, which stimulate propulsive movements in the large intestine. The drugs produce a gentle evacuation within 8 to 12 hours. They usually are administered at bedtime as a single dose (Table 22–1) to provide an after-breakfast bowel movement.

Danthron is excreted in the milk of nursing mothers and may produce a laxative effect in the nursing infant. It may also impart a pink or red color to an alkaline urine.

Cascara sagrada is available as tablets, as fluid-extract, and as an aromatic fluidextract. The drug is the mildest of the anthracene derivatives. The sweetened, debittered, aromatic fluidextract is more palatable, but it is considered to be less effective as a laxative than the fluidextract. The drug produces a soft or formed stool within six to eight hours with little cramping pain.

Senna preparations are available as *senna leaf powder,* fluidextract, or syrup; as *senna fruit* (SENOKOT) granules, tablets, and suppositories or granules (X-PREP); and as *sennosides A and B* (GLYSENNID) tablets. The senna products are converted to active anthraquinoidal aglycones by the enzymatic action of bacteria in the colon. The aglycones stimulate the myenteric reflexes that increase the propulsive movements of the intestine. Some of the drug is absorbed from the intestine, and the presence of the substances in the urine may impart a yellowish-brown color to acid urine or a reddish-violet color to alkaline urine. The drugs are usually administered at bedtime.

The early-morning evacuation is sometimes accompanied by abdominal cramps.

Wetting Agents

The drugs are utilized to produce a softer, bulkier stool that is easier to evacuate for patients who have hemorrhoids or perineal surgery, and for patients with cardiac problems or other bed patients who have hard, dry, dehydrated feces that are difficult to evacuate. The wetting agents include *dioctyl sulfosuccinate salts* and *poloxamer 188.*

Action Mode. The orally administered drugs lower the surface tension at the oil-water interface of the fecal material in the intestinal lumen. That action allows the water and fat to penetrate the fecal material, and the feces are softer and more moist.

Dioctyl Sulfosuccinate Salts. The drug is available as *dioctyl calcium sulfosuccinate* capsules, *dioctyl sodium sulfosuccinate* capsules, powder, solution, syrup, and tablets. It also is available as *dioctyl potassium sulfosuccinate* rectal solution with glycerin (RECTALAD). The drug is included in many formulations that contain laxatives.

The fecal-softening action of the drug initially is evident within 24 to 48 hours after drug therapy is instituted. Use of the drugs seldom causes adverse effects other than occasional mild cramping pains.

The oral *dioctyl sodium sulfosuccinate* solutions should be given in milk or fruit juice to mask the bitter taste. The wide range of dosage (Table 22–1) represents the variation in the quantity of the drug required to produce the desired stool-softening effect. The usual daily dosage of dioctyl sodium sulfosuccinate for children 6 to 12 years of age is 40 to 120 mg; for children three to six years of age, the usual dosage is 20 to 60 mg; and for younger children the dosage is 10 to 40 mg. The usual dosage of *dioctyl calcium sulfosuccinate* for children is 50 to 150 mg/day.

Poloxamer 188. The drug is a surface-active agent with emulsifying and wetting properties similar to those of dioctyl sulfosuccinate salts. The dosage for children over 12 years of age is the same as the adult dosage (Table 22–1). Children 3 to 12 years of age may be given 200 to 600 mg/day. Infants or children under three years of age are given 100 to 400 mg/day. The dosage may be reduced after the initial stool-softening effect is established. The total daily dosage may be given as a single dose or as divided doses.

NURSING INTERVENTION

The maintenance of elimination patterns frequently is the focus of attention in the nursing care of hospitalized patients. Drugs that are employed for the control of varying health problems can contribute to the incidence of diarrhea or constipation. Because of the complexity of modern health care, it is customary to maintain a daily record of the evacuation patterns of patients to assure that problems with constipation are identified promptly.

Care of the Patient with Diarrhea

It is essential to record the frequency, amount, and characteristics of all diarrheal movements. The fluid losses are estimated and recorded with the fluid output data. Diapers are weighed when infants have persistent diarrhea to allow accurate replacement of the fluid and electrolyte losses.

The physiologic status of infants, young children, and elderly or acutely ill patients can be jeopardized by relatively short periods of persistent diarrhea. The losses of fluid readily cause dehydration, and the intraluminal secretion of bicarbonate can produce metabolic acidosis.

The drugs employed for suppression of intestinal motility usually are effective in decreasing the peristaltic rushes, abdominal cramping pain, and output of liquid stools. The enteritis

that initiated the diarrhea can continue to cause the production of fluid and mucus from the intestinal crypts and glands and that fluid may be sequestered in distended loops of bowel. Those fluid losses may continue to contribute to the extracellular fluid dehydration. Examination of the abdominal contour for evidence of bowel distention and gently placing the stethoscope on the abdomen to listen for bowel sounds aid in assessing the bowel status. External pressure may precipitate peristalsis when the bowel is irritable, and the examination must be done with a light touch to avoid that stimulation.

Parenteral fluid replacement may be required when the intestine remains irritated. During an acute episode of diarrhea, fasting and bed rest are indicated. Wetting the lips with cool water may help to alleviate the thirst associated with fluid losses. Small amounts of sugar-containing liquids may be given after the acute phase has subsided because those substances are absorbed from the stomach. The amount of fluid must be small (i.e., 30 ml) to avoid the stimulus to the gastrocolic or duodenocolic reflexes that can precipitate peristaltic movements and the return of diarrhea. The person should be informed of the rationale for fluid restriction because the thirst and feeling of gastrointestinal emptiness often make the individual eager to eat and drink after the diarrhea is relieved.

The chronic diarrhea that is associated with organic diseases of the intestine (i.e., ulcerative colitis) also produces dehydration and electrolyte imbalances. When the diarrhea is persistent, the continual presence of fecal material in the anal region produces skin redness and excoriation. Application of petrolatum or zinc oxide ointment is soothing to the tissues and provides a barrier to fecal contact.

The hypermotility of the intestinal tract decreases the absorption time for nutrients, and the patient can become malnourished. Patients in that situation often require parenteral feedings to provide the required nutrients and to promote healing of the surface tissues that are excoriated by the fecal material. Although the antidiarrheal drugs provide some control of the hypermotility of the intestine, there often is "breakthrough" diarrhea until the organic disease is controlled by therapy that is specific for the disease process.

Antibiotic therapy frequently causes suppression of the intestinal bacterial flora in children, and diarrhea can occur about the fourth day of therapy. The fecal material is greenish, mucus containing, and foul smelling. Termination of the antibiotic treatment and institution of antidiarrheal drug therapy, fasting, and rest usually resolve the problem. It is important to instruct the parent about the planned schedule for use of the motility suppressants to assure that they are aware that the dosage should not be increased above the level that is prescribed. That practice in well-meaning parents has led to drug toxicity in children taking diphenoxylate hydrochloride with *atropine sulfate* (LOMOTIL) for the control of diarrhea. The parent should also be informed that there may be a change in the regular bowel habits for 24 to 48 hours after the diarrhea episode. Alerting them that there may be a short period of time before food residue produces a formed stool may allay their concern about constipation.

Counseling

A significant proportion of the population seems to be preoccupied with their bowel movements, and many people have misconceptions about normal bowel function. The continual use of laxatives to maintain a preconceived pattern for daily evacuation can lead to a reduced sensitivity of the defecation reflex. Elderly patients quite frequently have the misconception that a daily bowel movement is essential to health. Their concern for healthful bowel function can provide a constructive basis for health teaching.

The assessment of each person's dietary patterns, daily fluid intake, activity, and bowel evacuation patterns provides the baseline data for the health teaching. The most common cause of constipation is ignoring the defecation urge that is caused by the distended rectum. When the individual subsequently uses a laxative to relieve the ignored defecation urge, the resulting bowel evacuation is followed by a period of two to three days when there is insufficient fecal material in the colon to stimulate the defecation reflex. A vicious cycle is established when the person again takes a laxative because of concern with strict evacuation schedules. Encouraging the person to establish a food-initiated pattern of regularity can break that cycle and retain the natural sensitivity of the bowel to fullness.

Including bulk-forming foods in the diet and increasing the daily intake of fluids (>2000 ml) are primary factors in restoring or maintaining regularity patterns. When elderly persons are living on a marginal income, the cost of suggested foods should be carefully considered. An increase in the intake of fresh fruit and vegetables may be the ideal, but the lower cost of whole-grained cereals may make those foods the better choice for the elderly person. The dietary intake of bran, which contains 20 percent cellulose, provides an indigestible residue that is distended by intestinal fluid and provides a natural, bulky stool.

Regularity of eating and maintenance of physical activity within the capabilities of the individual are also important aspects in establishment of a natural and healthful bowel regimen. The bowel is relatively inactive during the hours of sleep. Upon arising, the force of gravity and movement of the abdominal muscles produce some bowel activity. When the person has a warm drink or breakfast, the stimulus to the gastrocolic and duodenocolic reflexes produces peristaltic rushes that move the fecal content toward the rectum. The person who attends to that stimulus usually can evacuate the lower bowel easily. The discussion of that sequence of events with the individual may help him correct poor hygienic practices that have contributed to ineffective or laxative-dependent control of bowel function. Laxatives are most effective when used discriminately for the periodic control of constipation. They can produce a hypotonic bowel when they are used continually. Individuals should also be made aware that the use of laxatives in the presence of abdominal pain is contraindicated. The motility that is induced by the drugs can cause rupture of an inflamed appendix or other abdominal lesion that is the source of the pain.

Review Guides

Describe the following:
1. The primary factor that affects long-term use of the intestinal motility suppressants.
2. The adverse effects of diphenoxylate hydrochloride with *atropine sulfate* (LOMOTIL).
3. The primary difference between opium tincture and paregoric.
4. The rationale for the use of *Lactobacillus acidophilus*.
5. The factors that must be considered when administering carboxymethylcellulose.
6. The differences in the stools that are produced by magnesium sulfate and bisacodyl.
7. The rationale for administering milk of magnesia in the evening and castor oil in the daytime.
8. The mode of action of senna fruit.

Additional Readings

Alexander, Mary M., and Brown, Marie Scott: Physical examination: part 13. *Nursing 76,* **6:**65, January, 1976.

Bass, Linda: More fiber—less constipation. *Am. J. Nurs.,* **77:**154, February, 1977.

Benson, John A.: Simple chronic constipation: pathophysiology and management. *Postgrad. Med.,* **57:**55, January, 1975.

Buhac, Ivo, and Balint, John A.: Diarrhea and constipation. *Am. Fam. Physician,* **12:**148, March, 1977.

Copeland, Lucia: Chronic diarrhea in infancy. *Am. J. Nurs.,* **77:**461, March, 1977.

Corman, Marvin L.; Veidenheimer, Malcolm C.; and Coller, John A.: Cathartics. *Am. J. Nurs.,* **75:**273, February, 1975.

Donata, Sam T.: Changing concepts of infectious diarrheas. *Geriatrics,* **30:**123, March, 1975.

Erle, Henry R.: Constipation. *Primary Care,* **3:**301, June, 1976.

Franklin, John E., Jr.: The infectious diarrheas. *Primary Care,* **3:**83, March, 1976.

Harvey, R. F., and Read, A. E.: Mode of action of the saline purgatives. *Am. Heart J.,* **89:**810, June, 1975.

Jeejeebhoy, K. N.: Symposium on diarrhea 1. Definition and mechanisms of diarrhea. *Can. Med. Assoc. J.,* **116:**737, April 9, 1977.

McIntosh, Henry D., and DuPont, Herbert L.: "Turista"—it's not a single disease. *Heart Lung,* **5:**636, July–August, 1976.

Nahmias, A. J.; Gomez-Barreto, J.; Kohl, S.; Oleske, J.; and Flax F.: Newer microbial agents in diarrhea. *Hosp. Pract.* **11:**75, March, 1976.

Olhney, Larry: Constipation in childhood. *Am. Fam. Physician,* **13:**85, March, 1976.

Phillips, Sidney P.: Diarrhea: pathogenesis and diagnostic techniques. *Postgrad. Med.,* **57:**65, January, 1975.

Portnoy, Benjamin L.; DuPont, Herbert L.; Pruitt, David; Abdo, Julio A.; and Rodriquez, Jorge T.: Antidiarrheal agents in the treatment of acute diarrhea in children. *J.A.M.A.,* **236:**844, August 16, 1976.

Schuster, Marvin M.: Disorders of the aging G.I. system. *Hosp. Pract.,* **11:**95, September, 1976.

Walker, W. Allan: Host defense mechanisms in the gastrointestinal tract. *Pediatrics,* **57:**901, June, 1976.

Wasserman, Gary S.; Green, Vernon A.; and Wise, George W.: Lomotil ingestions in children. *Am. Fam. Physician,* **11:**93, June, 1975.

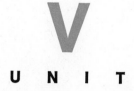

U N I T

Drugs Used to Maintain Rest, Activity, and Emotional Equilibrium

23

Depression, Psychosis, Anxiety States

CHAPTER OUTLINE

Changing concepts in the biopsychosocial sciences have provided the basis for modern patterns of treatment for persons with emotional problems. Those treatment plans gradually have transferred patient care from impersonal large institutions to ambulatory care facilities and psychiatric units in general hospitals. Those are the most widely publicized and obvious changes that have occurred in the treatment of emotional problems during the past two decades. The current understanding of the interrelatedness of the psyche and the soma is also evident in the broader and more personalized approaches to the acute or long-term health care of individuals with co-existing physical and emotional problems.

There are many unanswered questions about the functions of the human brain, and modern research is directed at clarifying the relationship of genetic inheritance, organic disease, and neuronal transmission to the onset, duration, and severity of emotional problems.

Physiologic Correlations

The subcortical and cortical projections of the limbic system control the behavior associated with emotions, subconscious motor and sensory responses, and intrinsic feelings of pain or pleasure. The intercommunications between neuronal pathways in the brain provide an extensive and intricate network for distribution of stimuli.

STRESS RESPONSES

An experience, or stress, provides the stimulus that is transmitted to the limbic system, hypothalamus, cerebrum, and cerebellum. The distribution of the stimulus to the cortical areas of the brain allows decoding through the scanning of stored experiences, language, and memory patterns. That interpretation of perceptions, associations, and recall patterns contributes to the formulation of a physical or an emotional response to the situation. The neural centers may elicit responses that involve distinct patterns of autonomic and somatic stimuli. Most of the decoding occurs at the unconscious level, and there may be a peripheral response without a correlative emotional response to the stimulus.

NEUROTRANSMITTERS IN THE BRAIN

The neural network of the brain provides a direct neuron-to-neuron pathway for the trans-

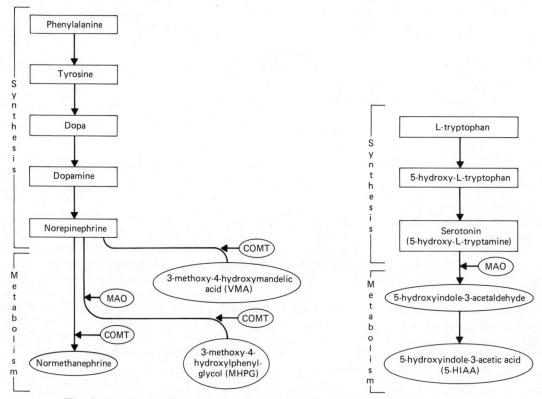

Fig. 23–1. Simplified diagram of the biosynthesis and metabolism of norepinephrine and serotonin.

mission of impulses. The primary neurotransmitters involved in the neuronal relay of impulses are *acetylcholine, dopamine, norepinephrine,* and *serotonin.* Like other neural pathways in the body, the transmission of an impulse causes the release of the neurotransmitter from the activated presynaptic neuron. The transmitter substance travels across the synaptic cleft to act on the receptors of the postsynaptic neuron.

Biosynthesis and Metabolism

Dopamine, norepinephrine, and serotonin are synthesized by a series of enzymatic conversions in the brain tissues (Fig. 23–1). The neurotransmitter is released from storage granules when the presynaptic neuron is activated. After it activates the postsynaptic receptors, some of the neurotransmitter may remain in the synaptic cleft where

it is inactivated by enzymes. The inactivated metabolites (MHPG, VMA, 5-HIAA) pass into the circulating plasma and are excreted in the urine.

The neurotransmitter that is not inactivated in the synaptic cleft is taken up by the presynaptic neuron. After its uptake, the transmitter may be inactivated by enzymes in the neuron or it may reenter the storage granules. For example, norepinephrine is released from the presynaptic neuron, and those molecules that remain in the cleft are inactivated by the enzyme *catechol-O-methyl transferase* (COMT). The norepinephrine that is taken up by the presynaptic neuron is inactivated by the enzyme *monoamine oxidase* (MAO), or it may enter the storage granules from which it can be released for subsequent neural transmission.

Acetylcholine is also synthesized in the brain tissues. After its liberation and the stimulation of

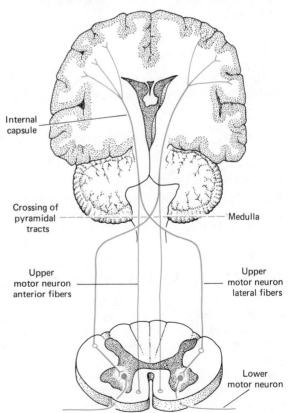

Internal capsule

Crossing of pyramidal tracts

Medulla

Upper motor neuron anterior fibers

Upper motor neuron lateral fibers

Lower motor neuron

Fig. 23–2. The pyramidal tract fibers, which travel from the motor cortex to the anterior horn cells of the spinal cord, provide the impulses for voluntary movements of the skeletal muscles.

the postsynaptic receptors, acetylcholine is inactivated by *acetylcholinesterase*. Unlike dopamine, norepinephrine, and serotonin, the acetylcholine is thought to be completely inactivated in the synaptic cleft.

Tissue Responses

At the central nervous system tissues that control body function, the stimulation activates the enzyme *adenyl cyclase*. The enzyme is the hormonal messenger for the conversion of *adenosine triphosphate* (ATP) to *cyclic adenosine 3′, 5′-monophosphate* (cAMP). That conversion provides the energy for the neural transmission required for stimulation of organic responses. For example, the stimulus at the cerebral motor strip activates the neural impulses that travel through the pyramidal tracts to the skeletal muscle tissue receptors.

Pyramidal Tract Transmission

The control of voluntary muscle movement and muscle tone is dependent on transmission of stimuli through the neural pathways of the pyramidal tracts (Fig. 23–2). The passage of stimuli through the subcortical pathway of the tract is dependent on the activity of the neurotransmitters (i.e., dopamine, norepinephrine) in the brain.

The subcortical fibers travel through the internal capsule to the medulla where most of the fibers cross (70 to 90 percent). Approximately 55 percent of the pyramidal fibers end at the anterior horn cells of the cervical cord, 20 percent in the thoracic cord, and 25 percent in the lumbosacral segments of the spinal cord. That distribution provides greater control over the volitional movements of skeletal muscles of the upper extremities than the lower limbs.

The impulses that are conveyed to the spinal cord by the fibers of the tract provide the stimulus to the lower motor neurons that innervate the skeletal muscle. Pyramidal tract neural transmission is essential to the intricate individual movements of the muscles (i.e., fingers, hands). Damage to the tract or changes in the activity of the neurotransmitters cause the loss of volitional muscle movements and superficial reflexes. They also cause increased deep tendon reflexes and muscle spasticity.

Pathophysiologic Correlations

Emotional problems are often manifested in behavioral responses and physiologic disturbances. For example, depression produces the correlative physiologic, behavioral, and psychologic responses that affect the bodily functions, actions, and feelings of the person (Fig. 23–3).

NEUROTRANSMITTER ABNORMALITIES

Depression is believed to be related to the absence or deficiency of norepinephrine or serotonin at functionally important sites in the brain. Excess norepinephrine activity has been linked with manic episodes, and excess dopamine has been associated with schizophrenia. Some evidence for the role of the neurotransmitters in the pathogenesis of emotional disorders has been obtained from the differing urinary concentrations of the neurotransmitter metabolites during the acute illness and changes in those levels during drug-induced remissions.

Abnormally high or low concentrations of neurotransmitters in the brain and the imbalance between those transmitters producing opposing effects are thought to be basic to most emotional problems. Those problems may range from temporary lapses in the individual's ability to cope with stress to temporary, intermittent, or prolonged periods when the person is out of touch with reality.

Therapy Plans

Therapy varies with the extent of the disruption of functional patterns. Individuals with problems

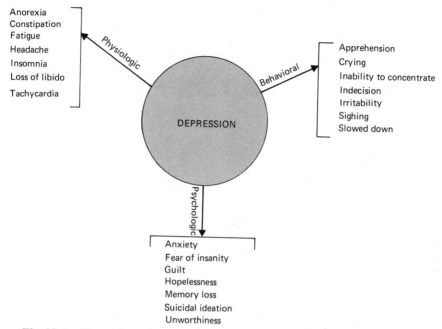

Fig. 23–3. Depression affects the functions, actions, and feelings of the person.

in their life situations that exceed their ability to cope may benefit from the objective counsel of a professional who can assist them to reorient their goals and to establish priorities for management of their problems.

In many situations the use of antidepressant, antipsychotic, or antianxiety drugs is useful for the control of acute or transient emotional problems. The drugs are also invaluable adjuncts to psychotherapy for persons with severe emotional disturbances. Drug therapy often provides the control required for the person to be amenable to psychotherapy and to move toward resocialization.

Antidepressant Drugs

DRUG THERAPY

The varying modes of therapy for depression are selected on the basis of the manifestations of the emotional problem. Psychotherapy, electroconvulsive therapy, and antipsychotic, antianxiety, or antidepressant drugs may be employed alone or in varying combinations for the differing disorders associated with depressions of endogenous or exogenous origin. The drugs contribute to rehabilitation and resocialization by accelerating the rate of improvement and by decreasing the danger of suicide and reducing the severity of symptoms.

The antidepressants are employed primarily to relieve behavioral and physiologic problems that interfere with the person's ability to function. Antidepressants provide the control of emotional responses by increasing the neurotransmitter levels (i.e., norepinephrine, serotonin) at the synapse of neurons in the brain. The drugs employed for treatment of depression include *lithium carbonate, cerebral stimulants, tricyclic drugs,* and *monoamine oxidase inhibitors.*

Lithium Carbonate

The drug is employed for treatment of acute manic episodes and is also utilized prophylactically for treatment of patients with recurrent manic and depressive episodes. Lithium decreases the intensity of the cyclic manic-depressive reactions rather than their frequency. That modification in behavioral responses often averts the need for hospitalization.

Action Mode.   Lithium is believed to provide an antimanic and antidepressive effect by blocking the release of norepinephrine and stimulating its uptake at the neural synapse. It is also thought to alter the sodium ion activity in the membranes of brain tissues.

Therapy Considerations.   The drug is administered orally (Table 23–1) and is rapidly absorbed from the intestinal tract. It appears in the serum within 15 to 30 minutes; peak serum drug levels are attained in one to three hours. The circulating drug is widely distributed in body fluids and readily moves into the tissues of the liver, spleen, and kidneys. There is a time lag of approximately six to ten days before equilibrium is attained between serum levels and the concentrations in the cellular fluids of the brain and other tissues (i.e., skin, muscle, bone, adrenals, intestine, heart, lungs, and pancreas). That time lag correlates with the four-to-ten-day period before control of manic episodes occurs in 80 percent of the patients receiving the drug.

The drug crosses the placental barrier. It also

Table 23–1.
Antidepressants

Drug	Route	Daily Dosage* (mg)	Number of Divided Doses
Lithium carbonate (ESKALITH, LITHANE, LITHONATE)	Oral	900–3600	3
Stimulants			
Deanol acetamidobenzoate (DEANER)	Oral	25–100	1
Methylphenidate (RITALIN)	Oral	20–60	2–3
Pemoline (CYLERT)	Oral	56.25–75	1
Tricyclics			
Amitriptyline (ELAVIL)	Oral	75–300	3–4
	IM	80–120	4
Desipramine (NORPRAMIN, PERTOFRANE)	Oral	50–200	2–3
Doxepin (SINEQUAN)	Oral	30–300	3
Imipramine (TOFRANIL)	Oral/IM	50–300	1–3
Nortriptyline (AVENTYL)	Oral	75–100	3–4
Protriptyline (VIVACTIL)	Oral	45–160	3–4
Monoamine Oxidase Inhibitors			
Isocarboxazid (MARPLAN)	Oral	10–30	1
Phenelzine (NARDIL)	Oral	15–45	1–3
Tranylcypromine (PARNATE)	Oral	20–30	3

* Dosages in the upper half of the range are used for hospitalized patients; dosages in the lower half of the range are used for ambulatory patients.

appears in glandular secretions (i.e., sweat, salivary glands) and in the milk of nursing mothers. The circulating drug appears in the cerebrospinal fluid within two hours after it is ingested, and within 24 hours the drug concentration reaches 30 to 60 percent of the serum levels.

Approximately 50 percent of the drug is eliminated in the urine within 24 hours, and about 75 to 95 percent is excreted by the end of a 72-hour period. The urinary excretion of lithium is lower during acute manic episodes and rises at the termination of that period. The drug elimination rate is also slower in the elderly and in persons with a low daily dietary intake of sodium chloride or high salt losses (i.e., diaphoresis).

There are many indications that lithium ions substitute for sodium ions in the body when sodium ion levels are reduced. A low sodium intake may decrease the serum sodium levels and thereby increase the reabsorption of the lithium ions at renal tubules. That action can elevate the serum drug concentrations. Persons taking the drug should be instructed to maintain a dietary sodium chloride intake at a normal level (5 gm/day) and to maintain a fluid intake of approximately 3 liters/day. Supplementary salt may be required to replace the losses that occur when sweating during prolonged periods of elevated environmental temperatures.

The dosage level may be at the maximum levels of the therapeutic range (i.e., 1500 to 2500 mg/day) when lithium is administered to a hospitalized patient during an acute manic episode. The serum drug concentrations are evaluated every two to three days to assure that the serum concentration is maintained at the effective therapeutic level of 0.9 to 1.4 mEq/liter. The maximum therapeutic serum drug concentration during intensive therapy is 2 mEq/liter. At the time of improvement in the patient's mania seven to ten days), the dosage usually is reduced to 50 percent of the initial quantity to avoid toxic serum drug concentrations (i.e., > 2 mEq/L).

During maintenance therapy, the serum drug levels are evaluated at weekly intervals until they stabilize between 0.5 to 1.2 mEq/liter. Subsequent evaluations are planned at one- or two-month intervals. The blood samples are usually drawn before the drug is taken in the morning to allow an 8-to-12-hour time lapse after the previous dose of the drug.

Adverse Effects. Gastrointestinal disturbances (i.e., transient nausea, gastric pain) commonly occur during the initial days of therapy but usually subside after several days. The fine tremor of the hands, thirst, and frequent urination that occur early in the period of therapy may persist throughout the time that the person is taking the drug. Excess weight gain is frequently a problem during prolonged therapy. Other problems that occur are dryness of the mouth and the hair (with thinning), diminished cutaneous sensation or anesthesia, impaired proprioception, blurred vision, tinnitus, headache, lethargy, pruritus, acneform eruption, metallic taste in the mouth, incontinence of urine, hypothyroidism, and T wave abnormalities.

Toxicity. Diarrhea, vomiting, drowsiness, weakness, muscle fasciculations, and lack of coordination are early signs of lithium toxicity and require a reduction of the dosage. The person who is taking the drug and a family member should be informed of the necessity of withholding the drug and informing the physician when those problems appear. At a serum drug concentration above 2 mEq/liter, the adverse effects include severe problems with cardiac arrhythmias, hypotension, hyperactive reflexes, convulsions, somnolence, coarse tremor, muscle twitching, and dysarthria. Later evidence of the high serum drug concentration (i.e., >2.5 mEq/L) are neurologic problems that include coma, increased deep tendon reflexes, and hypertonicity of the muscles of the extremities. The severity of the problems may necessitate the use of osmotic diuretics to reduce the levels of the drug in the body tissues and fluids.

CEREBRAL STIMULANTS

The drugs commonly employed for central nervous system stimulation are *methylphenidate* and *pemoline* (Table 23–1). *Deanol acetamidobenzoate* less frequently is employed as a stimulant. The drugs have similar pharmacologic actions, which also include respiratory stimulation and sympathomimetic activity. They are used for the control of hyperkinetic behavior disorders associated with minimal brain dysfunction in children.

Action Mode

The drugs are thought to increase the release of norepinephrine and its utilization by subcortical structures (i.e., limbic and reticular tissues). The drug action contributes to restoration of balance between norepinephrine and acetylcholine at central neural receptors. That action improves productivity by decreasing psychomotor activity and excessive responses to environmental stimuli. The outcome for hyperkinetic children is an improvement in the ability to concentrate, and that has a positive effect on learning and on interpersonal relationships.

Therapy Considerations

The drugs are administered orally to children over six years of age. There has been considerable controversy about the misuse of the drugs on a relatively broad scale to decrease the "hyperactivity" of schoolchildren. The drugs are intended for use in conjunction with psychologic, educational, and social measures that are employed in situations where the child is evaluated and supervised closely. Drug therapy may be interrupted periodically to allow evaluation of the child's improvement.

Adverse Effects

Nervousness and insomnia are the most frequent adverse effects, but the symptoms often subside with continuation of drug therapy. Other effects include gastrointestinal disturbances (i.e., anorexia with associated weight loss, nausea, dryness of the throat, diarrhea), mild depression, dizziness, insomnia, headache, irritability, fatigue,

or hallucinations. Allergic reactions that may occur during therapy include urticaria, fever, arthralgia, skin rash, and serious dermatologic reactions (i.e., exfoliative dermatitis, erythema multiforme).

Tolerance and psychologic dependence have been reported. The patient or a family member may increase the dosage when tolerance develops, and that can cause symptoms of overdosage (i.e., tachycardia, hallucinations, excitement, agitation, restlessness).

TRICYCLIC ANTIDEPRESSANTS

The drugs are employed primarily for the treatment of moderate or severe endogenous depression. The tricyclics have sedative and antianxiety properties that enhance their effect in the treatment of depression. Those patients who respond to therapy with the drugs show a decrease in morbid preoccupation, mood elevation, increased voluntary physical activity, and an improvement in eating and sleep patterns.

Amitriptyline, desipramine, doxepin, imipramine, nortriptyline, and *protriptyline* are the tricyclics employed for treatment of depression. Imipramine hydrochloride is also used for treatment of children with enuresis. During the period of drug therapy, the child is more readily aroused by the stimulus of a full bladder and bed wetting is reduced.

Action Mode

The drugs block the uptake of norepinephrine and serotonin at presynaptic neurons in the brain and prolong the sympathetic activity of those neurotransmitters. Concurrent anticholinergic activity also may contribute to the maintenance of equilibrium between the brain neurotransmitters.

Therapy Considerations

The drugs are usually administered orally (Table 23–1) and are readily absorbed from the intestine. There is considerable individual variation in the rate of hepatic metabolism of the drugs. Most of the circulating drug and its active metabolites are rapidly bound to plasma and tissue proteins. The drugs are distributed to the brain, heart, lung, and liver tissues and they cross the placental barrier. Some of the drug undergoes enterohepatic recycling. That process returns the drug to the gastrointestinal tract from which it is reabsorbed. Recycling of the drug adds to the duration of action and increases its metabolism in the liver. More of the metabolites are excreted in the urine and fewer metabolites are excreted with the bile content in the feces.

There is a time lag of five days to three weeks before a consistent improvement in the state of depression is evident. During that time interval there may be transient episodes of mood elevation or severe depression. The initial recovery is associated with an increase in the level of psychomotor activity, which usually is evident to the family before the emotional state allows the depressed person to perceive the improvement.

The person usually is too apathetic during the depression to organize a suicide attempt, but when the emotional status improves, the individual is capable of implementing a successful suicide plan. The family usually relaxes their surveillance when improvement is evident, and they should be informed of the necessity to continue their supervision until there are additional indicators of improved psychosocial status. Drug therapy may be continued for a period of six months after remission to reduce the potential for relapse.

There are differences in the responses of individuals to the tricyclic preparations that are available. For example, there seem to be imipramine responders and amitriptyline responders. The urinary excretion of norepinephrine metabolites differs between individuals responding to each of the drugs. Those persons who respond to imipramine therapy have low levels of *3-methoxy-4-hydroxylphenyl glycol* (MHPG) in the urine, while those responding to amitriptyline excrete normal or high levels of the metabolite. The excretion rate of the tricyclics is also affected by the pH of the urine. Alkalinization of the tubular urine increases reabsorption of the drug, while acidification of the urine hastens renal excretion of the drug.

Preparations Available

Amitriptyline Hydrochloride. The drug is rapidly absorbed after oral or parenteral administration (Table 23–1), and the peak serum drug concentrations occur within 2 to 12 hours. The plasma half-life of the drug ranges from 10 to 50 hours. Approximately 25 to 50 percent of the inactive metabolites are excreted in the urine within 24 hours.

Desipramine Hydrochloride. The oral drug is readily absorbed from the intestine, and peak serum drug levels occur within four to six hours after the drug is taken (Table 23–1). The plasma half-life of the drug ranges from 7 to 60 hours.

Doxepin Hydrochloride. The oral drug (Table 23–1) is readily absorbed from the intestine, and the peak plasma drug levels occur within two hours after it is taken. The plasma half-life of the drug is six to eight hours.

Imipramine. The drug is available as *imipramine hydrochloride* tablets for oral administration and as a solution for intramuscular injection (Table 23–1). *Imipramine pamoate* capsules are available for oral administration.

The oral formulations are completely absorbed from the intestinal tract, and peak serum drug concentrations occur within one to two hours after the drug is taken. The peak plasma drug levels occur within 30 minutes after the drug is injected intramuscularly. The plasma half-life ranges from 8 to 16 hours, and 70 percent of the metabolites are excreted in the urine within 72 hours.

Nortriptyline Hydrochloride. The drug may be the agent of choice when stimulation of the patient is desirable. The oral drug is slowly absorbed from the intestinal tract, and peak plasma levels occur within seven to eight and one-half hours after the drug is taken. The plasma half-life ranges from 16 to 90 hours, and approximately one third of the inactive metabolites are excreted in the urine within 24 hours. Persons taking the drug frequently complain of an unpleasant taste in the mouth.

Protriptyline Hydrochloride. The oral drug is completely absorbed from the intestine, and peak plasma levels occur within 24 to 30 hours. The metabolites are slowly excreted in the urine, and it requires approximately 16 days for one half of the drug to be eliminated.

The initial dosage is usually low. Increments in the dosage are made slowly because the drug causes greater restlessness and insomnia than other tricyclics.

Adverse Effects

There may be central nervous system or anticholinergic effects within a few hours after the drugs are taken. The problems usually are transient and tolerance to them develops with continuation of drug therapy. The adverse effects are less distressing to the person when the drug dosage initially is given at the lower level of the therapeutic range. That plan allows a gradual increase in the dosage to the level that is planned for maintenance therapy. Excess weight gain and an absence of taste or an unpleasant taste in the mouth are the problems that the person frequently finds distressing during therapy with the drug.

Central Nervous System Effects. The central nervous system effects include agitation, fine tremors, and exacerbation of the depression, states of anger, mania, delusions, hallucinations, or schizophrenic excitement. Paresthesias, dysarthria, or drowsiness may also occur. The patient and a family member should be informed of the necessity of avoiding hazardous situations to prevent falls or injury when drowsiness is present. Elderly persons frequently become confused and disoriented when taking the drugs. The drugs lower the convulsive threshold, and seizures may occur in persons with epilepsy or a history of seizures.

Anticholinergic Effects. The anticholinergic activity of the drugs frequently causes dryness of the mouth, visual problems (i.e., blurred vision that results from mydriasis and cycloplegia), sweating, impotence, or constipation. The problems most often occur during therapy with protriptyline. The effects on the cardiovascular system include postural hypotension, tachycardia, and arrhythmias.

Overdosage. The drug may be utilized by the patient in a suicidal attempt, and as little as ten times the daily dosage of the drug can be lethal. The toxic levels cause severe anticholinergic and central nervous system effects. When the person is conscious, emetics may be used to remove the unabsorbed drug from the stomach. Drug therapy may be required to reverse the effects of the absorbed drug (i.e., physostigmine, neostigmine). The patient is observed for a four-day period because there may be a recurrence of the symptoms of toxicity after a 72-hour period.

Interactions

The anticholinergic activity of the drugs may potentiate the action of other drugs with similar properties (i.e., atropine, phenothiazines). The drugs may also produce additive effects when central nervous system depressants are administered concurrently (i.e., alcohol, sedatives, hypnotics). The tricyclics antagonize the antihypertensive effects of guanethidine.

Concurrent use of monoamine oxidase inhibitors can cause convulsions, hyperpyretic crisis, and death. A 14-day interval is planned after termination of therapy with the monoamine inhibitors before therapy with a tricyclic is started.

MONOAMINE OXIDASE INHIBITORS

The drugs are employed primarily for treatment of patients with phobic-anxiety states. They are considered alternates to the tricyclic antidepressants for initial therapy of most depressed patients. Although their secondary placement as therapeutic agents relates partially to their lower clinical efficacy, the serious adverse effects that can occur during therapy have contributed to that status. *Isocarboxazid* and *phenelzine* may be employed for treatment of ambulatory patients, but *tranylcypromine* is used only for hospitalized patients who are closely monitored for adverse effects of the drug.

Action Mode

The enzyme monoamine oxidase acts at central and peripheral nerves to catalyze the decomposition of the bioamines norepinephrine, epinephrine, and serotonin within the presynaptic neuron ending. Inhibition of that activity at central neuron sites increases the concentrations of free norepinephrine and serotonin at the brain tissue receptors. There is a latent period, which varies from two days to three weeks, before the peak antidepressant effect of the drugs occurs. That latency also affects the duration of action after therapy is terminated.

Adverse Effects

The most frequent adverse effects are gastrointestinal disturbances (i.e., nausea, vomiting, constipation, anorexia, dryness of the mouth), restlessness, insomnia, drowsiness, dizziness, weakness, headache, postural hypotension, urine retention, transient impotence, and skin rash. Dosage adjustments may be required to ameliorate the symptoms. Ocular damage with changes in the fundus, visual fields, and color perception (i.e., red-green vision) may occur. Hepatocellular damage is a serious problem that has occurred during therapy.

Interactions

The addition of reserpine or guanethidine to the drug therapy regimen can cause severe hypertension. Concurrent administration of a tricyclic antidepressant can produce a toxic reaction manifested as agitation, delirium, convulsions, elevation of the body temperature, and an increase in the pulse and respiration rates. A two-to-three-week drug-free period is usually planned to avoid the adverse effect when the treatment is to be changed to the use of a tricyclic drug.

A life-threatening acute hypertensive crisis may be precipitated when the person who is taking the drug ingests foods with a high tyramine or tryptophan content. Foods that can precipitate the crisis include those that require bacteria or molds for their preservation or preparation (i.e., pickled herring, alcoholic beverages, broad bean pods, chicken livers, aged or natural cheese). The crisis occurs as a consequence of the increased synthesis of norepinephrine at a time when the enzyme *monoamine oxidase* is unavailable for its metabolism. The tyramine-related syndrome is characterized by occipital headache, palpitations, stiffness of the neck muscles, vomiting, sweating, photophobia, and arrhythmias. Ambulatory patients who are taking the drugs should be informed of the problem, and a written list of tyramine-containing foods should be provided for their reference at home. The patients should be informed that excessive use of caffeine (i.e., coffee) or chocolate also can precipitate a crisis.

The monoamine oxidase inhibitors decrease the metabolism of other drugs in the liver. That action may potentiate the activity of general anesthetics, barbiturates, narcotics, alcohol, or corticosteroids. The drugs also potentiate the action of anticholinergic drugs, the hypertensive effects of sympathomimetics, and the hypotensive effects of meperidine.

Antipsychotic Drugs

The primary difference between the antipsychotic drugs and other psychotropic drugs employed for the treatment of emotional problems lies in their capacity to modify the symptoms of schizophrenia. There are qualitative and distinct planned therapeutic effects and a predictable mode of action that differ from those of the antianxiety drugs. Although the term *antipsy-*

chotic best describes their therapeutic use, they are commonly referred to as *major tranquilizers.*

DRUG THERAPY

The drugs are widely used to control the emotional problems (i.e., hallucinations, delusions, distorted perceptions, withdrawal, paranoia) that cause agitation, combativeness, hyperactivity, or hostility. The use of the drugs contributes to elimination of the thought disorder and decreases the high expenditure of energy associated with the behavioral manifestations of the emotional disturbances.

The *phenothiazines* include drugs described as *aliphatic* to designate their structural relationship to the group. Those drugs have open chains of carbons in their structure rather than the rings that are characteristic of the *piperidine* and *piperazine* derivatives of phenothiazine. In addition to the phenothiazines, the antipsychotic drugs include *butyrophenones, dibenzoxazepines, oxoindoles,* and *thioxanthenes.*

The antipsychotic drugs have similar pharmacologic actions. Their classification according to structure provides a framework for comparisons of the frequency and severity of the adverse effects that occur during therapy. Most of the drugs have *extrapyramidal effects* that cause skeletal muscle dysfunction, and they also have *anticholinergic effects.* Many of the antipsychotic drugs cause *adrenergic-blocking effects, drowsiness, photosensitivity, cholestatic jaundice, blood dyscrasias,* and *metabolic* or *endocrine changes.* The frequency of their occurrence is presented with the description of the individual drugs.

Action Mode

The antipsychotic drugs affect many biochemical processes in the central nervous system, but the specific modifications of most of those processes is unclear. Recent evidence suggests that the drugs produce antipsychotic effects by decreasing the activity of the neurotransmitter in the subcortical structures of the brain. The drugs block the receptors of the postsynaptic neurons

in the limbic system, basal ganglia, and substantia nigra. Their action on the medullary chemoreceptor trigger zone, or vomiting center, provides control of persistent vomiting.

Adverse Effects

Extrapyramidal Tract Effects. The blocking of dopamine at the dopaminergic receptors, which normally inhibits the activity of the striatal neurons, causes increased peripheral muscle activity. The problems are manifested as *pseudoparkinsonism, akathisia, dystonias* and *dyskinesias,* or *tardive dyskinesia.*

Pseudoparkinsonism characteristically involves rigidity, tremor, and complete or partial loss of muscle movement (akinesia). The problems occur most frequently in elderly persons on long-term therapy. The shuffling gait, masklike facies, tremor that subsides during intentional muscle movement, and pill-rolling movements of the fingers typify pseudoparkinsonism.

Akathisia, or motor restlessness, is described by patients as a feeling of restlessness and muscle quivering. The intense anxiety caused by immobility leads to continual involvement in moving around without sitting to rest.

Impairment in muscle tone, or *dystonia,* and defects in muscle movement, or *dyskinesia,* cause an inability to coordinate voluntary muscle movement. The difficulty with control of the tongue and facial muscles may affect speech and swallowing. Clonic contraction or spasms of the muscle groups can involve the eye, face, mouth, neck and back muscles, or the peripheral musculature. The problems may occur in the early days of therapy and seem to be more prevalent in young male patients.

Tardive dyskinesia is the term commonly used to describe the syndrome because it manifests itself months or years after therapy is initiated. The syndrome is characterized by facial tics, grimacing, vermicular movements of the tongue, side-to-side movements of the chin, and choreoathetoid movements of the trunk or limbs. The slow, rhythmic, stereotyped movements may be generalized or may be limited to single muscle groups (i.e., buccofaciomandibular, buccolingual). Although the problems may occur in children or adults after a few weeks of therapy, they more frequently occur during long-term therapy as a late irreversible extrapyramidal syndrome. The condition has been called *persistent dyskinesia* because it continues unchanged for years after therapy is terminated.

Anticholinergic Effects. The central and peripheral action of the drugs can interfere with most of the natural parasympathetic activities in a manner similar to that of atropine. During therapy with the drugs there may be dryness of the mouth, mydriasis and cycloplegia (with associated blurring of vision), urine retention, decreased gastrointestinal motility, and tachycardia. At high dosages the drugs can cause delirium. The anticholinergic effects cause many problems for patients taking the drugs. For example, dryness of the mouth predisposes the buccal membranes to *Candida* infections, teeth become loosened, or dentures fit poorly. Constipation is often a problem in patients who are emotionally disturbed, and the antipsychotic drug effect intensifies that problem. Adequate hydration provides some relief of oral dryness and constipation. Sugarless lozenges also may reduce the dryness of the mouth.

Adrenergic-Blocking Effects. Hypotension with an associated dizziness may occur as a consequence of the blocking of norepinephrine activity on the peripheral arteriole and venule receptors. Peripheral pooling of blood may cause dizziness on arising from a supine position in the morning (postural hypotension). Prevention of sudden position changes and the wearing of elastic stockings modify the problem. There is a gradual development of tolerance to the hypotensive effects as therapy continues. Parenteral administration of the antipsychotic drugs may cause a sudden sharp drop in blood pressure. When possible, it is advisable for the patient to remain in a supine position for a period of one-half hour after the drug is administered to allow time for the return of hemodynamic equilibrium.

Drowsiness. Sedation commonly occurs during therapy with the drugs, and that effect initially led to the description of the drugs as *major tranquilizers*. The problem can be modified by administration of the daily dosage at bedtime in some instances. Oversedation may necessitate a reduction in dosage of the drug. During prolonged therapy the sedative effects are less intense and are better tolerated.

Photosensitivity. Sensitivity reactions that occur during therapy with the antipsychotic drugs are *photoallergic reactions* and *phototoxic reactions*. Exposure to intense ultraviolet rays (i.e., sunlight, fluorescent lighting) can cause the cutaneous eruptions of the photoallergic reaction. Minimal or brief exposure to the heat of the sun can cause an intense erythema of the superficial tissues that is a phototoxic reaction. The use of a sun-screening lotion, umbrella, sunshade, or extra clothing may decrease the problems for persons who cannot avoid the exposure.

Cholestatic Jaundice. Edema of the biliary structures, which may occur during the first four weeks of therapy, interferes with the flow of bile into the duodenum. Frequent examination of the sclera of the eyes allows early detection of the jaundice that is associated with the biliary obstruction. Although the entity is considered to be a benign hypersensitivity reaction, therapy is usually interrupted when the problem arises.

Blood Dyscrasias. Agranulocytosis rarely occurs, but it is potentially fatal. The problem usually appears during the third to the eighth week of therapy and is most common in elderly women. The patient or a family member should be instructed to withhold the drug when there is a fever, sore throat, or weakness and to inform the physician promptly. That response to the early evidence of leukocytosis can avert the progression of bone marrow toxicity.

Metabolic or Endocrine Changes. Drug suppression of hypothalamic and pituitary function commonly causes weight gain. Female patients may have menstrual irregularities, flow of breast milk after cessation of nursing (galactorrhea), or gynecomastia. Male patients may have problems with impotence and decreased libido.

The effects of the drugs on the thermal receptors of the hypothalamus may cause an elevated or subnormal body temperature level. The concurrent anticholinergic inhibition of sweating may contribute to hyperpyrexia in children, but the problem seldom occurs in adults.

PHENOTHIAZINES

The phenothiazines that are employed for their antipsychotic effects include the aliphatic derivatives, *chlorpromazine, promazine,* and *triflupromazine;* the piperidine derivatives, *mesoridazine, piperacetazine,* and *thioridazine;* and the piperazine derivatives, *acetophenazine, butaperazine, carphenazine, fluphenazine, perphenazine, prochlorperazine,* and *trifluoperazine* (Table 23–2).

Therapy Considerations

The phenothiazines are well absorbed from the intestinal tract and from the parenteral injection sites. The drugs are readily distributed in most body tissues, and high concentrations appear in the brain tissues. The drugs are metabolized primarily in the liver, and the metabolites appear in the lungs, liver, kidneys, and spleen. Some of the metabolites have effects similar to those of the parent compounds. The drugs cross the placental barrier. The unchanged drugs and their metabolites are excreted in the urine, bile, and feces, and in the milk of nursing mothers. The unchanged drugs and their metabolites may be excreted slowly in the urine over a period of six months after the termination of therapy.

In addition to their frequent use for control of emotional problems, the drugs are employed for the control of persistent vomiting. The pheno-thiazines are also used for prelabor or preoperative preparation of selected patients.

Chlorpromazine Hydrochloride

The drug is an aliphatic derivative that is available in forms for oral or parenteral administration (Table 23–2). In acute situations it may be administered as a single dose (i.e., 25 to 50 mg) by intravenous injection. *Chlorpromazine* is also available as a suppository that is employed at a dosage of 150 to 400 mg/day divided in three to four doses.

The initial daily oral dosage for children is calculated on the basis of 2 to 2.5 mg/kg of body weight, divided for administration four to six times per day. The maximum dosage for severely disturbed older children is 200 mg per day and the maximum dosage for younger children is 100 mg/day. The initial daily rectal dosage for children is calculated on the basis of 3.3 to 4.4 mg/kg of body weight. The intramuscular dosage is calculated on the basis of 1.5 to 2 mg/kg of body weight. Those daily doses are divided for administration six to eight times per day. The maximum dosage for children 5 to 12 years of age is 75 mg/day and for younger children it is 40 mg/day. Higher dosages for children are calculated on an individualized basis.

The onset of action of the oral drug is 30 to 60 minutes, and the duration of action is four to six hours. The oral drug is also available as an extended-release formulation that provides a similar onset of action but has a 10-to-12-hour duration of action. The rectal suppositories are slowly absorbed, and the onset of action is later than that of other forms of the drug. The duration of action after their absorption is three to four hours. The intramuscular drug is readily absorbed, and the onset of action occurs within 30 minutes. The duration of action is three to four hours.

The drug solution is highly irritating to the tissues. Changing the needle after filling the syringe protects the tissues of the intramuscular injection tract from excess drug contact. Nurses who prepare the drug sometimes have dermatitis

Table 23–2.
Antipsychotic Drugs

| Drug | Daily Dosage Range (Adult) | | | Incidence of Adverse Effects (Frequency) |
	Route	Dosage* (mg)	Number of Divided Doses	
Phenothiazines: Aliphatics				*High:* Drowsiness, hypotension, anticholinergic effects.
Chlorpromazine (THORAZINE)	Oral	30–1000	2–4	
	IM	100–2400	4–6	*Moderate:* Parkinsonism, dystonia, galactorrhea, photosensitivity, men-
Promazine (SPARINE)	Oral/IM	40–1200	4–6	strual changes, cholestatic jaundice,
Triflupromazine (VESPRIN)	Oral	20–150	2–6	rashes, convulsions, ECG changes.
	IM	60–150	2–6	*Low:* Blood dyscrasias, lenticular deposits and opacities
Phenothiazines: Piperidines				*High:* Drowsiness, hypotension, anticholinergic effects, weight gain,
Mesoridazine (SERENTIL)	Oral	30–400	2–3	inhibition of ejaculation.
	IM	25–200		
Piperacetazine (QUIDE)	Oral	20–160	2–4	*Moderate:* Parkinsonism, akathisia
Thioridazine (MELLARIL)	Oral	150–800	3–4	menstrual changes, photosensitivity, ECG changes, galactorrhea
				Low: Blood dyscrasias, pigmentary retinopathy, cholestatic jaundice, dystonia, convulsions, rashes
Phenothiazines: Piperazines				*High:* Parkinsonism, akathisia,
Acetophenazine (TINDAL)	Oral	40–80	3	dystonia, anticholinergic effects
Butaperazine (REPOISE)	Oral	15–100	3	*Moderate:* Postural hypotension,
Carphenazine (PROKETAZINE)	Oral	25–400	2–3	photosensitivity, galactorrhea,
Fluphenazine (PERMITIL, PROLIXIN)	Oral	1–20	3–4	menstrual changes, drowsiness,
	IM	2.5–10		anorexia, rashes
Perphenazine (TRILAFON)	Oral	12–64	3–4	*Low:* Blood dyscrasias, cholestatic
	IM	5–30		jaundice, lenticular deposits and
Prochlorperazine (COMPAZINE)	Oral	15–150	3–4	opacities, ECG changes, decreased
	IM/IV	40–120	4–6	libido, convulsions
Trifluoperazine (STELAZINE)	Oral	2–30	2	
	IM	4–10	4–6	
Butyrophenones				*High:* Parkinsonism, akathisia, dystonia
Droperidol (INAPSINE)	IM	2.25–10		*Moderate:* Blood dyscrasias,
Haloperidol (HALDOL)	Oral	1–15	2–3	postural hypotension, sedation,
	IM	6–30	3–6	menstrual changes, galactorrhea
				Low: Cholestatic jaundice, photosensitivity, rashes, weight gain, convulsions, impotence, neurotoxicity
Dibenzoxazepines				*High:* Parkinsonism, akathisia,
Loxapine succinate (LOXITANE)	Oral	20–250	2–4	oculogyric crisis, drowsiness
				Moderate: Dystonia, hypotension, hypertension, convulsions, anticholinergic effects
				Low: Rashes, edema, hyperpyrexia, paresthesias

Table 23–2 (*Continued*)

Drug	Daily Dosage Range (Adult)			Incidence of Adverse Effects (Frequency)
	Route	Dosage* (mg)	Number of Divided Doses	
Oxoindoles Molindone (MOBAN)	Oral	15–225	3–4	*High:* Parkinsonism, akathisia, anticholinergic effects, drowsiness *Moderate:* Dystonia, postural hypotension, menstrual changes, anorexia, rashes *Low:* Leukopenia, ECG changes
Thioxanthenes Chlorprothixene (TARACTAN)	Oral IM	75–600 75–200	3–4	*High:* Drowsiness, hypotension, anticholinergic effects *Moderate:* Parkinsonism, dystonia, galactorrhea, photosensitivity, menstrual changes, cholestatic jaundice, rashes, convulsions, ECG changes, weight gain *Low:* Blood dyscrasias, lenticular deposits and opacities
Thiothixene (NAVANE)	Oral IM	6–60 8–20	2–3 2–4	*High:* Parkinsonism, akathisia, dystonia, anticholinergic effects *Moderate:* Postural hypotension, galactorrhea, photosensitivity, menstrual changes, drowsiness, anorexia, rashes *Low:* Blood dyscrasias, cholestatic jaundice, lenticular deposits and opacities, ECG changes, decreased libido, convulsions

* Dosage at the upper half of the range usually is used for hospitalized patients who are under close supervision.

from contact with the solution. The dermal irritation can be avoided by wearing rubber gloves or by thorough handwashing to remove drops of the solution from the hands immediately after preparing the drug.

Chlorpromazine is metabolized in the liver and kidneys. The drug is excreted primarily in the urine.

The deposits of metabolites in the lens and cornea are clinically insignificant. They occasionally appear in the skin and cause cosmetically objectionable skin pigmentation. When they are identified early, a change to another antipsychotic drug can be planned.

Promazine Hydrochloride

The drug is available in forms of oral use and as solutions for intramuscular injection (Table 23–2). Promazine may be administered slowly as an intravenous injection to severely agitated patients at a dosage within the range of 50 to 150 mg. An additional dose of the drug may be given by intravenous injection within five to ten minutes when it is required to control behavioral responses. The maximum total dosage of the parenteral drug is 300 mg. Administration by the oral route is usually planned after the acute episode has subsided.

Triflupromazine Hydrochloride

The drug is an aliphatic derivative that is available for oral or parenteral administration (Table 23–2). In acute situations, it may be administered to adults as a single intravenous injection of 2 to 6 mg. The drug is also available as *triflupromazine* suspension that may be used for children or adults who have difficulty swallowing the tablets or for patients who sequester the tablets in the buccal pouch.

The daily oral drug dosage for children is based on the calculation of 2 mg/kg of body weight to a maximum of 150 mg. The daily intramuscular dosage for children is calculated on the basis of 200 to 250 mcg/kg of body weight to a maximum of 10 mg. The daily dosage is divided for administration three times per day.

The incidence of extrapyramidal and sedative effects is higher with triflupromazine than with chlorpromazine, but hypotension, dry mouth, and blurred vision occur less frequently. The drug is a more effective antiemetic than chlorpromazine.

Mesoridazine Besylate

The drug is a piperidine derivative that is available in forms for oral use or for intramuscular injection (Table 23–2). The adult dosage provides the guidelines for the dosage for children over 12 years of age. The drug is not recommended for younger children.

Piperacetazine

The drug is a piperidine derivative that is available in tablets for oral use (Table 23–2). The adult dosage provides the guidelines for the dosage for children over 12 years of age. The drug is not recommended for younger children.

Thioridazine Hydrochloride

The drug is a piperidine derivative that is available as tablets or liquid for oral use (Table 23–2). The dosage for children 2 to 12 years of age is 20 to 40 mg/day. That dosage may be divided for administration two to four times per day.

Acetophenazine Maleate

The drug is a piperazine derivative that is available for oral administration (Table 23–2). The drug is used primarily for treatment of ambulatory patients. It is not recommended for administration to children.

Butaperazine Maleate

The drug is a piperazine derivative that is available for oral administration (Table 23–2). It is more effective as an antiemetic than chlorpromazine or prochlorperazine. The dosage for children over 12 years of age is similar to the adult dosage. The drug is not recommended for younger children.

Carphenazine Maleate

The drug is a piperazine derivative that is available for oral use (Table 23–2). The onset of action occurs within one-half to one hour after it is taken, and the duration of action is four to six hours.

Fluphenazine

The drug is a piperazine derivative that is available as *fluphenazine hydrochloride* in the form of an elixir, tablets, extended-release tablets, and a solution for injection (Table 23–2). The daily oral dosage range for children is 0.25 to 3.5 mg, divided for administration six to eight times per day. The concentrated oral solution of fluphenazine hydrochloride may be administered as a diluted solution by mixing it with water, sodium chloride solutions, carbonated beverages, or fruit juices. After administration of the oral drug, the onset of action occurs within one hour and that action persists for six to eight hours.

Fluphenazine decanoate and *fluphenazine enanthate* are available in sesame oil vehicles for subcutaneous or intramuscular injection. The formulations are slowly released from the adipose tissues, and they have an onset of action within 24 to 72 hours. The average duration of action is two weeks. The drugs are usually administered to adults or to children over 12 years of age at a dosage within the range of 12.5 to 100 mg at two-to-six-week intervals. The extrapyramidal tract adverse effects may appear from two to three days after the drug is given, and those effects persist for five days. The drug may be given at lower dosage initially to reduce the high incidence of the problems that occur during the early days of therapy.

In addition to the adverse effects of the phenothiazine group, the drug causes nausea, polyuria, headache, glaucoma, and peripheral edema. Mental depression is also a common adverse effect of fluphenazine.

Perphenazine

The drug is a piperazine derivative that is available in forms for oral or parenteral administration (Table 23–2). The drug may be administered as a single intravenous injection of 5 mg in an acute situation.

The daily oral dosage for children from one to six years of age is 4 mg; for children 6 to 12 years of age it is 6 mg; and for older children the dosage range is 6 to 12 mg/day. The daily dosage is divided for administration three times per day.

Prochlorperazine

The drug is a piperazine derivative that is available as *prochlorperazine edisylate* syrup or liquid concentrate for oral administration. It is also available as solutions for parenteral administration (Table 23–2).

Prochlorperazine suppositories may also be used as an alternate method of administering the drug. The daily dosage is 50 mg, which may be divided for administration two times per day.

Prochlorperazine maleate is available as tablets and extended-release capsules for oral use.

The daily oral dosage for children 2 to 12 years of age is 5 to 7.5 mg. The maximum dosage for children two to five years of age is 20 mg/day and that for children 6 to 12 is 25 mg/day. The daily dosage is divided for administration two to three times per day. The intramuscular dosage for children under 12 years of age is calculated on the basis of 130 mcg/kg of body weight. The drug is usually administered as a single deep intramuscular injection, and subsequent doses are given orally.

The onset of action after oral administration occurs within 30 to 40 minutes and the action persists for three to four hours. The extended-release formulations provide an action onset within 30 to 40 minutes, and the action persists for 10 to 12 hours. The rectal suppository provides an onset of action within 60 minutes, and the action persists for three to four hours. Intramuscular injection of the drug provides an onset of action within 10 to 20 minutes, and the action persists for three to four hours.

Trifluoperazine

The drug is a piperazine derivative that is available for oral use or for intramuscular injection (Table 23–2). The daily oral dosage range for children from 6 to 12 years of age is 1 to 15 mg. The higher dosage may be divided for administration two times per day. The daily intramuscular dosage for children ranges from 1 to 2 mg, and the higher dosage may be divided for administration two times per day.

BUTYROPHENONES

The drug group includes *droperidol* and *haloperidol*. The drugs are closely related to the piperazine derivatives of phenothiazine.

Droperidol

The drug is administered intramuscularly as a preoperative agent (Table 23–2), and it is administered intravenously during the induction and maintenance of anesthesia for its antianxiety, sedative, and antiemetic effects. The preoperative intramuscular dosage for children 2 to 12 years of age is calculated on the basis of 100 to 150 mcg/kg of body weight.

The onset of action is evident within three to ten minutes after administration by either of the parenteral routes and the duration of action is six to eight hours. The selective use of the drug limits the adverse effects that are predictable for the structural group. The partial block of post-ganglionic alpha-adrenergic receptors and direct vasodilator action of droperidol may cause mild to moderate hypotension and tachycardia within three to ten minutes after the drug is administered.

Haloperidol

The drug is available in forms for oral and intramuscular administration (Table 23–2). The oral drug is absorbed well. The peak plasma levels are attained within two to six hours after oral administration and within ten minutes after the drug is administered intramuscularly. The physiologic effect is evident within 30 to 45 minutes. The drug is metabolized in the liver. Approximately 40 percent of the drug is excreted in the urine within five days. About 15 percent of the unchanged drug and its metabolites enter the feces with the bile. The drug appears in the milk of nursing mothers. Haloperidol is excreted slowly over a 28-day period.

DIBENZOXAZEPINES

Loxapine Succinate

The drug is administered orally (Table 23–2) and is absorbed rapidly from the intestinal tract. The drug is metabolized rapidly in the liver, and the major metabolites, *8-hydroxyloxapine* and *7-hydroxyloxapine,* have activity similar to that of the parent drug. The serum levels of the unchanged drug and the active metabolites decline in a biphasic manner. The initial half-life of the drug is five hours and that during the second

phase is 19 hours. The sedative effect of the drug appears within 20 to 30 minutes of the time that it is administered, and the duration of that effect is 12 hours. The drug is widely distributed in body tissues and crosses the placental barrier. Approximately 50 percent of the active and inactive metabolites are excreted in the urine and feces within 24 hours. The drug may also appear in the milk of nursing mothers.

OXOINDOLES

Molindone Hydrochloride

The drug is available for oral administration (Table 23–2). The dosage for children over 12 years of age is based on the dosage for adults. Children from three to five years of age may be given single daily doses of 1 to 2.5 mg.

The drug is rapidly absorbed from the gastrointestinal tract, and peak plasma levels occur within one hour. The plasma half-life of molindone is 1.5 hours. The drug has a duration of action of 24 to 36 hours. Almost all of the drug is metabolized in the liver. Approximately 90 percent of the inactive metabolites are excreted in the urine and feces within 24 hours. The drug appears in the milk of nursing mothers.

THIOXANTHENES

Chlorprothixene and *thiothixene* are the drugs in the chemical grouping. The drugs are structurally and pharmacologically related to the aliphatic and piperazine derivatives of phenothiazine.

Chlorprothixene

The drug is available in forms for oral use and for intramuscular injection (Table 23–2). The daily oral dosage for children over six years of age is 30 to 100 mg. The dosage is usually divided for administration three to four times per day. The drug is not recommended for children under six years of age. When the oral liquid is used, it may be made more palatable by mixing it with milk, fruit juices, or carbonated beverages.

The oral drug is absorbed partially from the gastrointestinal tract. The injected drug is rapidly absorbed and its effects are evident within 10 to 30 minutes. The drug is metabolized in the liver and the metabolites are excreted in the urine. The unabsorbed drug is excreted in the feces.

Thiothixene

The drug is available as *thiothixene* capsules. *Thiothixene hydrochloride* is available as an oral liquid concentrate and as a solution for intramuscular injection (Table 23–2). The daily adult dosage range is used as a guide for adjustment of the dosage for children over 12 years of age. The drug is not recommended for younger children.

The drug is absorbed readily when it is administered by the oral or parenteral route. The therapeutic response may be evident within one to six hours after the drug is given by intramuscular injection and within a few days to several weeks after oral use of the drug. The drug is widely distributed in body tissues. It is metabolized in the liver, and the unchanged drug and the metabolites enter the feces with the bile.

Antianxiety Drugs

The drugs are widely used for the control of emotional responses when individuals experience high levels of stress in their life situations. They are also employed for modification of anxiety associated with neuroses and depression. Although studies of their effectiveness as compared to placebo are conflicting, persons taking the drugs attest to an improved ability to control psychomotor activity and to tolerate emotional problems in their daily living.

The antianxiety drugs include the *antihistamines, benzodiazepines,* and *carbamates.* Although the term *antianxiety drugs* best describes their therapeutic use, the drugs commonly are referred to as *minor tranquilizers.* Other drugs that have sedative effects (i.e., barbiturates) occasionally are employed for treatment of patients who have high anxiety levels, but the persistent daytime sedation associated with their use often interferes with the functional ability of the individual.

ANTIHISTAMINES

The antihistamines employed for the control of anxiety include *buclizine* and *hydroxyzine.* The drugs are used as short-term or long-term therapy for ambulatory or hospitalized patients. Hydroxy-zine is used more frequently than the other drugs in the antihistamine group.

Action Mode

The antihistamines provide mild sedation and control of anxiety by depressing neurotransmission in the hypothalamus and the brainstem reticular formation. The drugs also have skeletal muscle relaxant, anticholinergic, antiemetic, and some analgesic activity.

Hydroxyzine

The drug is employed for the symptomatic treatment of anxiety states and for the control of persistent vomiting. It is also used for preoperative and postoperative medication to reduce the anxiety that often increases the requirements for analgesics.

Therapy Considerations. *Hydroxyzine hydrochloride* is the drug form that is available for oral use (tablets, syrup) and for intramuscular injection. *Hydroxyzine pamoate* is available in capsules and as a suspension for oral administration (Table 23–3).

Hydroxyzine pamoate is converted to the

Table 23–3.
Antianxiety Drugs

Drug	Route	Dosage (mg)	Number of Divided Doses	Incidence of Adverse Effects (Frequency)
				Daily Dosage Range (Adult)
Antihistamines				*High:* Ataxia, drowsiness, hangover, anticholinergic effects
Buclizine (SOFTRAN)	Oral	50–150	1–3	*Moderate:* Dizziness, nausea, depersonalization, increased anxiety
Hydroxyzine (ATARAX, VISTARIL)	Oral	75–400	3–4	
	IM	100–600	4–6	*Low:* Convulsions, gastrointestinal disturbances, allergic reactions
Benzodiazepines				*High:* Ataxia, drowsiness
Chlordiazepoxide (LIBRIUM)	Oral	15–300	3–4	*Moderate:* Dizziness, confusion, excitement
	IM/IV	75–300	4–6	
Chlorazepate (TRANXENE)	Oral	15–60	2–4	*Low:* Hypotension, blood dyscrasias, jaundice, allergic reactions
Diazepam (VALIUM)	Oral	4–40	2–4	
Lorazepam (ATIVAN)	IM	4–90	3–6	
	Oral	1–10	2–3	
Oxazepam (SERAX)	Oral	30–120	3–4	
Prazepam (VERSTRAM)	Oral	20–60	1–3	
Carbamates				*High:* Ataxia, drowsiness, dizziness
Chlormezanone (TRANCOPAL)	Oral	700–800	3–4	*Moderate:* Hypotension, cardiac arrhythmias, vomiting, paresthesias, seizures, allergic reactions
Meprobamate (EQUANIL, MILTOWN)	Oral	1200–2400	3–4	
Tybamate (SOLACEN)	Oral	750–2000	3–4	*Low:* Blood dyscrasias, blurred vision, Stevens-Johnson syndrome, bullous dermatitis, syncope, exacerbation of porphyria

hydrochloride in the gastric acid. The oral formulations are absorbed well from the gastrointestinal tract, and the onset of action occurs within 15 to 30 minutes after the drug is ingested.

The daily oral dosage for children under six years of age is 50 mg/day and for children over that age it is 50 to 100 mg/day. The daily dosage is divided for administration three or four times a day.

The dosage for single intramuscular injection (i.e., preoperatively) for children is calculated on the basis of 1.1 mg/kg of body weight. The injection should be given into the midlateral muscles of the thigh when the drug is administered to children or adults. The intramuscular dosage for adults may also be injected into the upper outer quadrant of the gluteal muscle. The drug is irritating to the tissues, and marked discomfort often occurs at the site of the injections. Alternating the sites modifies the problem when repeated injections are required.

Adverse Effects. There is a high frequency of drowsiness during the initial period of therapy. The sedative effects are less pronounced after the drug has been taken for a few days. Dosage reduction may be required when the drowsiness interferes with the person's ability to function.

The anticholinergic effects of the drug include dryness of the mouth, mydriasis and cycloplegia (with an associated blurring of vision), urine retention, decreased gastrointestinal motility, and tachycardia. The problems are more severe when the drug is administered parenterally than when it is given orally.

Buclizine Hydrochloride

The drug has antihistaminic, central nervous system depressant, antiemetic, and antispasmodic activity. It has been used alone or in combination with other drugs for the control of motion sickness and other problems that precipitate vomiting.

The drug is available in tablet form for oral administration (Table 23–3). The duration of action ranges from 12 to 24 hours after ingestion. The dosage for children over three years of age is 25 to 50 mg, and that dose may be divided for administration two times per day. The drug causes adverse effects similar to those of other drugs in the antihistamine group.

BENZODIAZEPINES

The drugs in the benzodiazepine group frequently are employed as antianxiety agents. Patients demonstrate an increase in vigor and express a feeling of well-being while taking the drugs. The low suicidal potential of the drugs is an advantage because they are used primarily by ambulatory persons who can intentionally take an overdose of the drug.

The structurally and pharmacologically similar drugs in the group includes *chlordiazepoxide, chlorazepate, diazepam, lorazepam, oxazepam,* and *prazepam*. During the past few years, the national listing of all of the prescription drugs according to their frequency of use has shown diazepam to be the first drug on the list.

Action Mode

The drugs provide a therapeutic effect by depressing neurotransmission in the limbic system and other subcortical structures of the brain and in the polysynaptic reflex arcs of the spinal cord.

The drug action produces sedative, anticonvulsant, and skeletal muscle relaxant effects.

Diazepam

Therapy Considerations. The drug is available for oral use and for intramuscular injection (Table 23–3). In acute situations, the drug may be administered slowly (i.e., 5 mg/min) as a single intravenous injection. The intravenous dosage ranges from 5 to 15 mg. That route of administration usually is employed for limited time periods because tolerance has been reported during intravenous use of the drug. The daily oral dosage range for children over six months of age ranges from 3 to 10 mg, which is divided for administration three or four times per day.

The oral drug is absorbed well from the gastrointestinal tract. The onset of action occurs within one-half to one hour, and the peak plasma levels of the drug appear within two hours after the oral drug is ingested. The onset of action after intramuscular injection of the drug is 15 to 30 minutes. The drug is irritating to the tissues, and there may be desquamation at the muscular sites of the injections. Alternation of the injection sites decreases the pain and reduces the tissue injury. The intravenous injection provides a rapid onset of action, and the effects persist for approximately three hours.

Diazepam is metabolized in the liver. The principal metabolite is chemically similar to *oxazepam*. The plasma half-life of the drug is 20 to 40 hours. That time period represents an initial seven-to-ten-hour half-life of the drug and prolongation of that half-life by addition of the active metabolite *oxazepam*. The long half-life maintains a therapeutic effect when the drug is taken two times per day.

The drug crosses the placental barrier and appears in the milk of nursing mothers. Metabolites of the drug are excreted in the urine and feces.

Adverse Effects. Diazepam produces adverse effects that are common to the benzodiazepine group of drugs (Table 23–3). Overdosage of the drug causes somnolence, confusion, coma, diminished reflexes, and minimal respiratory and cardiac depression. The long plasma half-life of the drug prolongs the effect of the drug that is absorbed at the time of the overdosage.

Chlordiazepoxide

Therapy Considerations. The drug is available as *chlordiazepoxide* tablets for oral use. It is also available as *chlordiazepoxide hydrochloride* capsules for oral use and as solutions for parenteral injection (Table 23–3). The daily oral dosage for children over six years of age is 10 to 30 mg, which may be divided for administration two to four times per day. The intramuscular dosage for children over 12 years of age is 25 to 50 mg. The drug is usually given as a single intramuscular injection, and the oral route is usually utilized for subsequent drug administration.

The oral drug is well absorbed from the gastrointestinal tract. The drug appears in the plasma within one-half to one hour, and peak plasma levels occur in four hours. The onset of action following intramuscular injection of the drug is 15 to 30 minutes and that following intravenous injection is 3 to 30 minutes.

The drug is widely distributed in body tissues and crosses the placental barrier. The plasma half-life of chlordiazepoxide is 6 to 30 hours. It is metabolized in the liver and the metabolites are excreted in the urine and feces.

Adverse Effects. The drug can cause the same adverse effects as other drugs in the benzodiazepine group (Table 23–3). It may also cause a paradoxic increase in irritability, hostility, hyperexcitability, and hallucinations. The problem may occur within the first few weeks of therapy with the drug. Overdosage of the drug may cause confusion, somnolence, diminished reflexes, and coma.

Chlorazepate Dipotassium

The drug is available in capsules for oral administration (Table 23–3). It is decarboxylated in the stomach, and the active metabolite *nordiazepam* is absorbed from the intestinal tract. Peak plasma levels of the metabolite are attained within one hour. The long plasma half-life of the metabolite (about 24 hours) provides therapeutic levels when the drug is taken two times per day. Nordiazepam is metabolized in the liver, and 80 percent of the metabolites are excreted in the urine and feces within ten days. The metabolites may also appear in the milk of nursing mothers. The adverse effects and manifestations of overdosage are similar to those of other benzodiazepines.

Lorazepam

The drug is available as scored tablets for oral administration (Table 23–3). Approximately 90 percent of the oral drug is absorbed within one hour, and the peak plasma concentration occurs in about two hours. Lorazepam has a plasma half-life of 12 hours. Steady-state serum concentrations of the drug are attained within two to three days after therapy is initiated. The drug is metabolized in the liver, and the inactive metabolites are excreted in the urine (88 percent) and in the feces. The adverse effects and manifestations of overdosage are similar to those of other benzodiazepines. When dosage increments are required, the evening dosage is increased before the daytime dosage to reduce the incidence of adverse effects of the drug.

Oxazepam

The drug is useful when the individual's status indicates the need for a short-acting, nonaccumulating antianxiety agent (i.e., a single acute anxiety-provoking episode). The oral drug (Table 23–3) is well absorbed from the gastrointestinal tract, and peak plasma levels appear within four to six hours. The plasma half-life ranges from 3 to 21 hours. The drug is metabolized in the liver, and the glucuronide conjugates are excreted in the urine. Oxazepam can cause the same adverse effects as other drugs in the benzodiazepine group.

Prazepam

The drug has the same action mode, therapeutic uses, and adverse effects as other benzodiazepine compounds. The usual daily dosage of 30 mg may be given as a single dose at bedtime. A divided dosage schedule is used when higher doses are required for the control of anxiety, and increments in dosage are made by increasing the bedtime dose.

CARBAMATES

The drugs are employed to control anxiety and tension in psychoneurotic states and in other situations where the person's ability to function interferes with living patterns. The drug group includes *chlormezanone, meprobamate,* and *tybamate.*

Action Mode

Like other antianxiety drugs, the carbamates are thought to act on the limbic system, thalamus, and hypothalamus to provide control of emotional responses to environmental stimuli. The person's behavioral responses are less aggressive and hostile during therapy with the drug. Concurrent depression of neural transmission in the polysynaptic arcs of the spinal cord provides a very mild skeletal muscle relaxant effect.

Chlormezanone

Therapy Considerations. The drug is administered orally (Table 23–3) and is rapidly absorbed from the gastrointestinal tract. It produces an effect in 15 to 30 minutes that lasts for approximately four to six hours. The drug appears in highest concentrations in the kidney, liver, muscle, heart, and body fat. The unchanged drug and the metabolites are excreted in the urine.

The daily oral dosage for children 5 to 12 years of age is 150 to 400 mg. That dosage is divided for administration three to four times per day. Drowsiness is the most common adverse effect.

There is a moderate incidence of dizziness, flushing, nausea, depression, edema, and weakness. There have also been a few reports of reversible jaundice.

Meprobamate

Therapy Considerations. The drug is usually administered orally (Table 23–3) and is well absorbed from the intestinal tract. The usual oral sedative dosage for children 6 to 12 years of age is based on the calculation of 25 mg/kg of body weight per day, divided for administration two to three times per day.

Peak plasma levels of the drug are attained within one to three hours. The sedative effects of the drug occur within less than one hour after it is taken orally. The plasma half-life of meprobamate averages from 10 to 11 hours. The drug is distributed in all body tissues and crosses the placental barrier. Meprobamate is metabolized rapidly in the liver, and the unchanged drug and its inactive metabolites are excreted in the urine. The concentration of the drug that is excreted in the milk of nursing mothers may be two to four times that of the maternal plasma drug levels.

Adverse Effects. The most frequent adverse effects of the drug are ataxia, drowsiness, and dizziness (Table 23–3). Seizures may be precipitated in patients with epilepsy who receive the drug. The occurrence of allergic or hypersensitivity reactions (i.e., rash, urticaria, pruritus, Stevens-Johnson syndrome, bullous dermatitis) necessitates the termination of therapy.

Tybamate

Therapy Considerations. The drug is administered orally (Table 23–3) and is absorbed well from the intestinal tract. The daily oral dosage for children over 6 to 12 years of age is calculated on the basis of 20 to 35 mg/kg of body weight, divided for administration three to four times per day.

Peak plasma levels are attained within one-half to two hours, and those levels persist for four to six hours. The plasma half-life of the drug is four to four and one-half hours. The drug is metabolized in the liver, and the metabolites are excreted in the urine.

NURSING INTERVENTION

Acutely psychotic patients who are apathetic, withdrawn, and disinterested in their personal welfare require the assistance of the nurse to meet their physical health needs (i.e., nutrition, elimination, sleep). Although the effect that the consistent ministrations of the nurse has on the emotional status of the patient initially may be difficult to measure, the meaning to the family is more tangible. Their perceptions of the interaction patterns of the nurses can bolster their efforts to establish meaningful personal communications with the emotionally disturbed patient.

Nothing touches the family more than the mental illness of one of its members, and they need assistance to cope with the emotional impact of that illness. The psychiatrist and the nurse can provide the counsel and guidance that are required to help the family members to function in their vital role in the patient's treatment plan and to maintain their own emotional equilibrium.

The control of behavioral responses that is provided by drug therapy often allows the patients to remain in familiar community surroundings during the treatment period. The plans for rehabilitation are initiated when there is an improvement in the patient's level of communication, purposeful activity, interest in the environment, and ability to concentrate and plan. Drug therapy, psychotherapy, and group experiences usually are continued throughout the period of rehabilitation. Progress often is slow, and there are periods of regression during the protracted period of rehabilitation.

Noncompliance with the drug therapy plan may contribute to the patient's lack of progress. The emotionally disturbed patient often neglects to take the prescribed drugs. The attitudes of family members also affect the therapy plan. Their impatience with the prolonged period of therapy may cause them to accelerate the patient's use of the drugs. It is not unusual for a family member to terminate the drug therapy plan at the earliest sign of improvement in the person's behavioral status. It is important that they understand that the drugs are controlling the patient's behavior and that such interruptions can retard the recovery and rehabilitation process.

Emotional problems exist on a continuum from schizophrenic psychosis to isolated episodes of acute anxiety. The following outline provides basic guidelines that can be employed when planning nursing intervention for patients with differing emotional problems. The outline can be used to *establish baselines for assessing the patient's emotional status, plan measures to maximize the effect of the drug therapy and minimize the level of emotional stress,* and *prepare the patient for assessing the progress for the drug therapy plan.*

Guidelines for Nursing Intervention

I. Establish baselines for assessing the patient's emotional status.
   A. Obtain the patient's statement of the problem and the functional limits caused by the problem.
   B. Obtain information about psychosocial factors affecting the resolution of the problem (i.e., health history, health care practices, compliance with prescribed therapies, previous problems with drugs, interpersonal relationships).
   C. Identify the factors that evoke behavioral manifestations of emotional stress.
      1. Observe the patient's behavior (i.e., coping mechanisms, adaptive behavior).
      2. Elicit factors that the patient defines as stressors (i.e., loss of

something valued, injury or threat of injury, frustration of drives, financial burdens).

3. Ascertain whether misinformation or lack of information is a source of anxiety.

4. Observe the patient's behavioral responses during social interactions (i.e., family, visitors, professional personnel).

D. Examine the patient for physiologic manifestations of emotional stress.

1. Observe changes in cardiovascular status.

a. Elevation of systolic blood pressure.

b. Changes in heart rate and rhythm (i.e., increased rate, force, irregularities).

c. Increased rate and depth of respirations.

2. Observe the muscles for tension.

a. Tension of large voluntary muscles.

b. Tremor of fine voluntary muscles.

3. Palpitate the abdomen to determine whether there is distention of the urinary bladder or bowel.

4. Listen with the stethoscope for sluggish or absent bowel sounds.

5. Observe the skin for decreased perfusion of superficial tissues (i.e., pallor, decreased temperature).

6. Observe the pupils for dilation.

II. Plan measures to maximize the effect of the drug therapy and minimize the level of emotional stress.

A. Modify the environment to decrease disruptive sensory stimuli.

B. Utilize measures to improve physical comfort (i.e., showers, back rub).

C. Utilize periods of receptivity to maximize voluntary involvement in planned therapeutic activities (i.e., counseling, interpersonal relationships, physical activities).

D. Implement prescribed therapies to alleviate emotional stress (i.e., antidepressant, antianxiety, or antipsychotic drugs).

E. Act as patient advocate to obtain specialty services required for the relief of those problems identified as stressors (i.e., social services, counseling).

F. Plan for the consistency of professional contact persons and of the care provided by those persons.

III. Prepare the patient for assessing the progress of the drug therapy plan.

A. Translate the therapy plan into the patient's language, environment, and life-style and specify the patient's responsibilities in implementing the plan.

B. Interpret the plan to significant others who will be assisting the patient with implementation of the therapy plan.

C. Describe to the patient and a family member the problems requiring physician contact (i.e., status changes, adverse effects of the drugs).

D. Provide written instructions for use at home (i.e., schedules for taking medications, date and time of group sessions or appointments for evaluation of progress).

E. Reassess the patient's readiness to maintain the drug therapy plan at home.

Review Guides

1. Outline a plan for observing the patient during a clinic visit, for evidence of adverse effects of the chlorpromazine that he has been taking for three months.

2. Prepare a list of questions that could be used during a clinic visit to elicit information about functional problems resulting from adverse effects of the fluphenazine the elderly patient has been taking since leaving the hospital two months previously.
3. Formulate a teaching plan for the patient who is being discharged from the hospital with a prescription for lithium carbonate after partial remission of a manic episode.
4. Outline the factors that would be included in a teaching plan for the ambulatory patient who is to take isocarboxazid at home.
5. Formulate a care plan that could be utilized for the hospitalized patient who is receiving amitriptyline hydrochloride.
6. Describe the assessments that should be made immediately after the patient is given haloperidol intramuscularly.
7. Outline a plan for assessment of the patient when the intramuscular administration of haloperidol is changed to oral administration of the drug.

Additional Readings

Allen, Robert E., and Stimmel, Glen L.: Neuroleptic dosage, duration, and tardive dyskinesia. *Dis. Nerv. Syst.,* **38**:385, May, 1977.

Appleton, William S.: Third psychoactive drug usage guide. *Dis. Nerv. Syst.,* **37**:39, January, 1976.

Åsberg, Marie; Ringberger, Vivi-Ann; Sjöquist, Folke; Thorén, Peter; Thäshman, Lil; and Tuck, J. Richard: Monoamine metabolites in cerebrospinal fluid and serotonin uptake inhibition during treatment with chlorimipramine. *Clin. Pharmacol. Ther.,* **21**:201, February, 1977.

Athinarayanan, Pakski; Pierog, Sophie H.; Nigam, Sarvesh K.; and Glass, Leonard: Chlordiazepoxide withdrawal in the neonate. *Am. J. Obstet. Gynecol.,* **124**:212, January 15, 1976.

Ballard, Joyce E.; Boileau, Richard A.; Sleator, Esther K.; Massey, Ben H.; and Sprague, Robert L.: Cardiovascular responses of hyperactive children to methylphenidate. *J.A.M.A.,* **236**:2870, December 20, 1976.

Biggs, John T.: Clinical pharmacology and toxicology of antidepressants. *Hosp. Pract.,* **13**:79, February, 1978.

Carroll, Bernard J.; Curtis, George C.; and Mendels, Joseph: Neuroendocrine regulation in depression. 1. Limbic system—adrenocortical dysfunction. *Arch. Gen. Psychiatry,* **33**:1039, September, 1976.

Carter, Roy G.: Psychotolysis with haloperidol: rapid control of the acutely disturbed psychotic patient. *Dis. Nerv. Syst.,* **38**:237, April, 1977.

Creese, Ian; Burt, David R.: and Snyder, Solomon H.: Dopamine receptor binding predicts clinical and pharmacological potencies of antischizophrenic drugs. *Science,* **192**:481, April 30, 1976.

Dunner, David L.; Stallone, Frank; and Fieve, Ronald R.: Lithium carbonate and affective disorders. *Arch. Gen. Psychiatry,* **33**:117, January, 1976.

Gittelman-Klein, Rachel, and Klein, Donald F.: Methylphenidate effects on learning disabilities. *Arch. Gen. Psychiatry,* **33**:655, June, 1976.

Haddad, Lester M.: Management of hallucinogen abuse. *Am. Fam. Physician,* **14**:82, July, 1976.

Hall, Richard C. W., and Kirkpatrick, Brian: The benzodiazepines. *Am. Fam. Physician,* **17**:131, May, 1978.

Hollister, Leo E.: Clinical use of tricyclic antidepressants. *Dis. Nerv. Syst.,* **37**:17, March, 1976.

Janson, Paul A.; Watt, J. Brooks; and Hermos, John A.: Doxepin overdose. *J.A.M.A.,* **237**:2632, June 13, 1977.

Jellinek, Theodore: Mood elevating effect of trihexyphenidyl and biperiden in individuals taking antipsychotic medication. *Dis. Nerv. Syst.,* **38**:353, May, 1977.

Johnson, Judith J.: An ambulatory mental health clinic. *Nurs. Clin. North Am.,* **12**:571, December, 1977.

Kielholz, P.: Treatment for masked depression. *Psychopharmacol. Bull.,* **11**:31, January, 1975.

Kobayaski, Ronald M.: Drug therapy of tardive dyskinisia. *N. Engl. J. Med.,* **296**:257, February 3, 1977.

Lerer, Robert J., and Lerer, M. Pamela: The effects of methylphenidate on the soft neurological signs of hyperactive children. *Pediatrics,* **57**:521, April, 1976.

Marjerrison, G.: Psychotherapy and tricyclic antidepressants. *Dis. Nerv. Syst.,* **37**:15, March, 1976.

McAfee, Heidi Ann: Tardive dyskinesia. *Am. J. Nurs.,* **78**:395, March, 1978.

Mendels, J.; Stern, S.; and Frazer S.: Biochemistry

of depression. *Dis. Nerv. Syst.*, **37**:3, March, 1976.

Osborn, Gerald G., and York, Jonathan L.: Psychoactive drugs in the treatment of the aged. *Practical Psychol. Physicians*, **4**:20, April, 1977.

Post, Robert M., and Goodwin, Frederick K.: Time dependent effects on phenothiazines on dopamine turnover in psychiatric patients. *Science*, **190**:488, October 31, 1975.

Preskorn, Sheldon H.: Benzodiazines and withdrawal psychosis. *J.A.M.A.*, **237**:36, January 3, 1977.

Prien, Robert F., and Caffey, Eugene M., Jr.: Guidelines for antipsychotic drug use. *Resident Staff Physician*, **21**:165, September, 1975.

Rifkin, Arthur; Quitkin, Frederic; and Klein, Donald F.: Akinesia. *Arch. Gen. Psychiatry*, **32**:672, May, 1975.

Shader, R. I.: Problems of polypharmacy in depression. *Dis. Nerv. Syst.*, **37**:30, March, 1976.

Sider, Roger C.: Economizing with psychotropic drugs. *Primary Care*, **3**:137, March, 1976.

Snyder, Solomon H.: Biochemical factors in schizophrenia. *Hosp. Pract.*, **12**:133, October, 1977.

Stephenson, Carol A.: Stress in critically ill patients. *Am. J. Nurs.*, **77**:1806, November, 1977.

Stimmel, Glen L.: Neuroleptics and the corpus striatum: clinical implications. *Dis. Nerv. Syst.*, **37**:219, April, 1976.

Stokes, Peter E.; Kocsis, James H.; and Arcuni, Orestes J.: Relationship of lithium carbonate dose to treatment response in acute mania. *Arch. Gen. Psychiatry*, **33**:1080, September, 1976.

Strayhorn, Joseph M., and Nash, James L.: Severe neurotoxicity despite "therapeutic" serum lithium levels. *Dis. Nerv. Syst.*, **38**:107, February, 1977.

Swanson, James M., and Kinsbourne, Marcel: Stimulant-related state-dependent learning in hyperactive children. *Science*, **192**:1354, June 25, 1976.

Taylar, Charles E.: Psychoactive drugs: uses, misuses, and abuses. *Primary Care*, **2**:135, March, 1975.

Tsuang, Ming T.: Lithium therapy: practical aspects. *Dis. Nerv. Syst.*, **37**:282, May, 1976.

Viederman, Milton, and Rusk, Gary H.: Appropriate use of psychotropic drugs in physical illness. *Primary Care*, **4**:601, December, 1977.

Williams, James G.: Common errors in the treatment of depression. *Am. Fam. Physician*, **14**:60, August, 1976.

Winsberg, Bertrand G.; Yepes, Luis E.; and Bialer, Irv: Pharmacologic management of children with hyperactive/aggressive/inattentive behavior disorders. *Clin. Pediatr.*, **15**:471, May, 1976.

24

Sleeplessness

The natural activity patterns of most individuals follow a relatively consistent schedule from day to day. At the termination of the day's activities, a period of sleep restores the physical energy required for continuation of activities during the following day.

The demands of work and the personal role of the individual are the primary determinants of the hours of activity, and the circadian, or 24-hour, rhythms are adjusted by the individual's mode of living. Once they are established, those rhythms become a major determinant of the person's peak mental and physical efficiency periods.

The circadian rhythms of neural, hormonal, and metabolic functions are synchronized with the sleep-wakefulness cycles of the individual. For example, there is a reduced production of adrenocortical hormones during the initial hours of sleep when environmental stresses, which naturally precipitate the release of those hormones, are least likely to occur. The production of those hormones is high during the latter hours of the sleep period (i.e., 4 A.M. to 8 A.M.), and their activity readies the physiologic environment for the work of the hours of wakefulness.

Physiologic Correlations

Sleep studies have demonstrated that identifiable patterns of neurophysiologic and biochemical changes occur during the sleep periods. Objective measurements of those changes have facilitated analysis of the stages of sleep. Although there is a considerable difference between the sleep patterns of individuals, the time period of each stage is consistent for the same person on different nights.

STAGES OF SLEEP

The sleep patterns are divided into *nonrapid eye movement* (nonREM) *sleep* and *rapid eye movement* (REM) *sleep* periods. The nonREM sleep includes four stages that collectively are described as the vegetative states of sleep.

A latent period after retiring is the "settling-in" period. The length of time involved in the latent period varies among individuals, but it is generally about 30 minutes. At the termination of the latent period there is a brief period of somnolence (i.e., three to five minutes), which is described as nonREM stage 1, when the person has fleeting thoughts and can be awakened easily. When aroused the person usually states, "I wasn't asleep."

The latent period and nonREM stage 1 occur immediately after retiring. The sleep patterns that follow that time period are the nonREM stages 2, 3, and 4, and REM sleep. Although the duration of those stages varies in length during the period of sleep, the progression follows the same sequence. Activity, age, health status, and the stages of growth and development influence the duration of the sleep patterns and the total sleep period (Fig. 24–1).

NonREM Stage 2 Sleep

Sleep spindles appear on the electroencephalographic (EEG) recordings that are taken during nonREM stage 2 sleep. The ocular movements are slow, rolling, or asynchronous gliding movements. The person can be awakened easily and, when aroused, usually will describe having been in deep thought or reverie.

NonREM Stage 3 Sleep

The dreams that occur during stage 3 and continue into stage 4 sleep are short, thoughtlike, and life experience centered. The muscles are more relaxed, the vital signs are lower, and it is more difficult to waken the person from stage 3 than from stage 2 sleep.

NonREM Stage 4 Sleep

Stage 4 is the period of deep sleep. The muscles are very relaxed and the person rarely moves. This stage of sleep is affected by the daily activities of the individual and is longest in the first cycle of the sleep period. When aroused, the person responds slowly.

The 80-to-90-minute period of deep sleep in the first sleep cycle of children is related to their high physical activity during the waking hours. Their deep sleep makes them less responsive to the stimulus of a full bladder, and nocturnal enuresis can occur during stage 4 sleep. There is also a high incidence of somnambulism and loud outcry (night terror syndrome), which are unrelated to dreams, and sleep talking, teeth grinding (bruxism), and snoring during stage 4 sleep.

The metabolic rate, oxygen consumption, and carbon dioxide production are at a low normal level. The blood pressure, pulse, respirations, urine volume, and plasma volume are also at a low normal level.

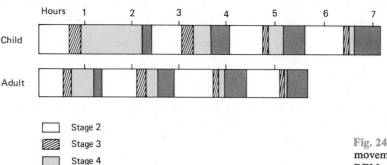

Stage 2
Stage 3
Stage 4
REM

Fig. 24–1. The duration of rapid eye movement (REM) sleep and the nonREM stages of the sleep cycle of children differs from that of adults.

REM Sleep

The name of the sleep stage describes the bursts of fast, binocular, synchronous movements of the eyes in all directions. Those movements may be seen by observing the eyeball movement under the person's closed eyelids.

The dreams that occur during the initial REM sleep are short and dull and have aspects of the day's activities in them. During subsequent REM sleep, the dreams become longer, vivid, and colorful, and they are less concerned with the events of daily life.

REM sleep is a time of sympathetic nerve excitement, hormone release, and metabolic acceleration. It is a period of activated light sleep during which it is difficult to waken the person. The respiratory rate may be increased 7 to 20 percent and the heart rate may be increased 5 percent over the person's baseline level. Both the respirations and pulse rate may be irregular. The systolic blood pressure is elevated (i.e., 30 mm Hg above the baseline). The mean pressure may fluctuate widely. There is decreased muscle tone but there may be some "breakthrough" body movements. The metabolic activity is accompanied by an increase in the secretion of adrenocortical and medullary hormones and posterior pituitary hormones.

The REM sleep of infants constitutes 50 to 80 percent of the sleep time. REM sleep occurs shortly after the onset of sleep, and the cycle between REM periods is short. During the infant's REM sleep there is almost continual stretching, grimacing, sucking, and vocalization. The total REM sleep during the night declines rapidly, and it comprises two to three hours of the total sleep period by the time the child is five years of age.

Pathophysiologic Correlations

SLEEP DEPRIVATION

The quality of sleep is as important as the duration of the sleep period. Psychogenic or environmental factors that disrupt the natural progression through the stages of sleep can effect physical and mental performance and behavior during the waking hours. For example, the parent who is aroused frequently by the cries of an infant or sick child and the patient whose sleep is disturbed by required treatments, pain, or respiratory distress usually show evidence of the sleep loss on the following day. Those persons usually have adequate stage 2 and stage 3 sleep but show signs of stage 4 and REM sleep deprivation.

Stage 4 Sleep Deprivation

Persons who are deprived of stage 4 sleep waken feeling physically uncomfortable. Their concern over vague physical problems and changes in bodily feelings is evident in depressed or resigned statements throughout the waking hours. Such persons are withdrawn and less aggressive throughout the day. During the succeeding undisturbed sleep period a significant increase in stage 4 sleep occurs at the expense of the other sleep stages.

REM Sleep Deprivation

Persons who are deprived of REM sleep during one sleep period may show no signs of decreased mental or physical efficiency. When the deprivation is secondary to a strong psychogenic stimulus (i.e., student preparing for an examination, the bride-to-be, the novice traveler, the expectant father), the hormonal level during the waking hours may compensate for the sleep deprivation. When the deprivation continues to disrupt the sleep periods (i.e., five to seven nights of deprivation), the person becomes irritable and anxious. There are obvious problems with motor coordination and the ability to concentrate. The person is less integrated and less interpersonally effective. There may be signs of confusion, suspicion, withdrawal, insecurity, introspection, and an inability to derive support from others. When undisturbed sleep is allowed, the REM time is increased up to 50 percent over the baseline level, and the psychomotor problems are minimal or absent during the subsequent hours of wakefulness. The person may recall details of the vivid, colorful, and bizarre dreams that seem to have filled the night of undisturbed sleep.

INSOMNIA

There is considerable variation in the sleep requirements of individuals. The person's alertness and readiness for the day's activities within one hour after arising may be used as a guideline for determining the adequacy of the period of sleep. The sleep time is inadequate when the person feels tired after that one-hour period.

Insomnia, which is the abnormally prolonged inability to sleep, can be produced by emotional disequilibrium or it can cause emotional disequilibrium. Restlessness and the inability to relax prolong the latent period of the sleep pattern. The tossing and turning in search of a comfortable sleep position are frustrating and tiring to the person who retired to obtain needed rest at the end of a day's activities. A prolonged latent period raises the anxiety level of the individual. That sequence of events, when repeated for several nights, is the reason that 25 to 50 percent of individuals over 40 years of age use drugs (i.e., alcohol, sedatives, hypnotics) to induce and maintain sleep patterns.

Change, challenge, or threat may disturb the circadian rhythms and disrupt sleep-wakefulness cycles of the individual. Each of those factors can deprive the hospitalized patient of stage 4 and REM sleep. Many patients, when asked if they slept well, will state that they were awake most of the night, while the night nurse reports that they were asleep during each of the regularly scheduled periods of observation. That contradiction in perceptions occurs when the person's sleep pattern involves only nonREM stage 2 and stage 3 sleep cycles.

Drug-controlled sleep is often planned for the hospitalized patient because the unfamiliar environment and the illness present the problems of change, challenge, and threat that disrupt sleep patterns. The natural activity on the hospital unit during the night prolongs the patient's period of latency and disrupts the sleep stages. Drugs are not a panacea for the patient because many of the sedative-hypnotic drugs reduce the nonREM stage 4 and REM sleep periods.

Sedative-Hypnotic Drugs

DRUG THERAPY

The dosage of the drug determines whether it will produce a sedative or hypnotic effect. The *sedative dosage* ideally alleviates anxiety and tension without causing drowsiness or lethargy. The drug usually is taken two to four times during the daytime. The *hypnotic dosage* induces sleep and usually is taken 15 to 30 minutes before bedtime. The hypnotic dosage may also be administered 60 to 90 minutes before intrusive diagnostic studies or surgery to provide the relaxation and drowsiness desirable prior to those anxiety-provoking procedures.

The sedative-hypnotic drugs include the *barbiturates* and other drugs that are collectively described as the *nonbarbiturate sedative-hypnotics* and *nonbarbiturate sedatives*. The drugs represent the most widely prescribed group of drugs in the world. Despite their wide use, the sedative-hypnotic drugs are not innocuous agents. During 1977 they were implicated in approximately 5000 drug-related deaths in the United States. That figure represents 35 percent of the total number of drug-related deaths. Overdoses of barbiturates caused 900 of those fatalities.

BARBITURATES

The drugs are frequently used for their sedative and hypnotic effects. Some of the barbiturates are used as anticonvulsants (i.e., mephobarbital, metharbital, phenobarbital). The barbiturates sometimes are administered parenterally (i.e., amobarbital, pentobarbital, secobarbital) for the control of acute convulsive episodes.

Action Mode

The barbiturates act in part at the level of the thalamus where they inhibit the ascending conduction pathways in the multisynaptic midbrain reticular formation. That action raises the arousal threshold and interferes with transmission of impulses from the thalamus to the cerebral cortex.

The drugs produce central nervous depression, which can progress as the dosage level is increased (i.e., sedation, hypnosis, sleep, deep stage 4 sleep, anesthesia, coma, death). The degree of depression depends on the dosage, route of administration, and pharmacokinetics of the particular barbiturate and the patient's age and physical status. The concurrent use of other drugs (i.e., alcohol) also effects the level of central nervous system depression.

Therapy Considerations

At therapeutic dosage levels the barbiturates depress cerebrocortical sensory and motor activity and produce sedation and drowsiness. The drugs frequently produce paradoxic excitement and hyperactivity when they are given to children. Elderly patients often become excited, noisy, confused or depressed. The effects that occur in elderly patients are thought to be related to drug-induced depression of the inhibitory centers of the cerebral cortex.

The barbiturates suppress REM sleep, but tolerance to the REM-suppressant effects of the drugs develops with continued use. Withdrawal of the drug after it has been used for a prolonged period of time may produce a marked increase in dreaming, nightmares, or insomnia during several subsequent drug-free sleep periods. The sleep pattern disturbance that follows the termination of therapy is known as REM rebound effect.

The depression of impulse transmission in the autonomic ganglia that is produced by sedative doses of the barbiturates reduces the tone and motility of the gastrointestinal tract, and constipation may be a problem. Although the hypnotic dosage of the drugs has a depressant effect on the medullary respiratory centers, the level of respiratory depression is similar to that naturally occurring during sleep.

The circulating drug is rapidly distributed to all body tissues and fluids. The highest concentrations are attained in the brain and liver tissues. The lipid affinity of the drugs is a primary factor in their duration of action at brain sites. The drugs cross the placenta, and the fetal blood concentrations rapidly equilibrate with those of the maternal blood. The drugs are slowly metabolized by the hepatic microsomal enzymes, and the unchanged drug or the metabolites are excreted in the urine. The drugs are secreted in the milk of nursing mothers, and traces of the drug also appear in the feces and saliva.

Adverse Effects

The barbiturates may produce gastrointestinal disturbances (i.e., nausea, vomiting, diarrhea), severe central nervous system depression, drowsiness, lethargy, vertigo, headache, mental depression, and myalgic, neuralgic, or arthralgic pain. Hypnotic doses of the drug frequently produce residual sedation or "hangover" during the following morning, and the inefficient psychomotor performance may persist for hours.

Allergic reactions include urticaria, angioedema, rashes, fever, and serum sickness. The drugs may sensitize the skin to ultraviolet rays, and exposure to the sun may produce a severe sunburn. Although the incidence of exfoliative dermatitis is rare, drug therapy is terminated when there is evidence of high fever, severe headache, stomatitis, conjunctivitis, rhinitis, urethritis, or balanitis that precedes the cutaneous lesions. Early identification of the problems is essential to allow termination of drug therapy. The continued tissue release of drug may cause progression of the irreversible and fatal stage of the dermatologic reaction.

The hematologic status of the person is evaluated periodically during prolonged therapy with the barbiturates because there have been a few reports of agranulocytosis, thrombocytopenic purpura, and megaloblastic anemia. The person who is taking the drug is instructed to inform the physician promptly when there is a sore throat, fever, easy bruising, petechiae, epistaxis, or other signs of infection or bleeding.

The drugs seldom are administered intravenously for sedation or hypnosis, but the nurse should be aware that intravenous administration of the drugs may produce severe respiratory depression, apnea, laryngospasm, bronchospasm, coughing, vasodilation, and hypotension. Those problems can occur as a delayed response up to six hours after the drug has been administered intravenously (i.e., during a minor surgical procedure), and the patient may be returned to the unit within that six-hour period.

Drug Interactions

There are many known interactions between phenobarbital and other drugs, and other barbiturates may interact in a similar manner. The barbiturates may induce activity of the hepatic microsomal enzymes and thereby increase the rate of metabolism of coumarin, digitoxin, corticosteroids, tricyclic antidepressants, or doxycycline. That action decreases the serum drug concentrations of the drugs, and a higher dosage may be required to provide the desired therapeutic effect when a barbiturate is added to the drug therapy plan. The dosage is decreased to avoid toxicity when the barbiturate is withdrawn from the therapy plan.

The barbiturates interfere with the absorption of griseofulvin and dicumarol from the gastrointestinal tract. They also interfere with the production of adrenocorticotropic hormone from the anterior pituitary gland.

The central nervous system depressant effects of the barbiturates are potentiated by drugs that have similar effects (i.e., sedatives, hypnotics, antihistamines, antipsychotics, antianxiety drugs, alcohol). The administration of ketamine for anesthesia after the patient has received a barbiturate can produce profound respiratory depression.

Monoamine oxidase inhibitors or disulfiram can decrease the metabolism of barbiturates. The interaction can prolong the effect of the barbiturate and produce toxic levels of the drug.

Acute Toxicity

The toxic doses of the barbiturates vary, but, in general, severe toxic reactions occur with the ingestion of five to ten times the usual hypnotic dose. Ingestion of 15 to 20 times the toxic dose or concurrent ingestion of other central nervous system depressants is potentially fatal. The American Academy of Clinical Toxicology has developed a standardized reporting form that allows rapid estimation of the severity of intoxication with barbiturates (Table 24–1).

Therapeutic measures are instituted promptly after the initial rapid evaluation of the person's

Table 24–1.

Classification System for Estimating the Severity of Intoxication

	Level of Functional Decompensation
0	None: no effect on function
1	Slight: functions without assistance
2	Grossly incompetent but ambulatory
3	Stupor or delirium but responds to verbal stimuli
4	Unconscious: responds to light pain
5	Unconscious: responds to deep pain only
6	No pain response; respiration adequate
7	Respiration inadequate or apneic
8	Constant instrument-maintained heart rate; isoelectric EEG
9	Death

status. A health team member usually is assigned to obtain information from friends or relatives, when they are with the unconscious patient, about the particular drug or drugs that were ingested. When the person is comatose, vital signs are taken, an endotracheal tube is inserted, and gastric lavage is performed. Activated charcoal is used in the lavage solution because it is an effective adsorbent for the barbiturates that are retained in the stomach. Assisted ventilation, intravenous fluids, cardiac monitoring, monitoring of the urine output, and dialysis are usually included in the plan for treatment of the comatose patient. Those measures are employed selectively when the level of functional decompensation is less than that of level four on the classification scale.

Chronic Toxicity

The barbiturates are subject to control under the Federal Controlled Substances Act of 1970. The problems of psychologic and physical dependence frequently occur when the drugs are used for prolonged periods of time (i.e., > eight weeks). The withdrawal symptoms usually appear when the barbiturate-dependent person has an 8- to 12-hour period of abstinence. The withdrawal syndrome includes problems that progressively increase in severity: anxiety, sleep disturbances, nausea and vomiting, irritability, restlessness, tremulousness, postural hypotension, seizures, withdrawal psychosis, hyperpyrexia, and death. The seizures that occur in the barbiturate-dependent person characteristically are major motor, or tonic-clonic, seizures, and status epilepticus is a potential problem.

Termination of drug therapy of the barbiturate-dependent person involves a plan for gradual withdrawal of the drug. A stabilizing dosage of the barbiturate is given, and that dosage is reduced in small decrements each day.

Preparations Available

Amobarbital. *Amobarbital* provides an intermediate duration of action when it is administered orally for sedation or hypnosis (Table 24–2). The same dosages are used when *amobarbital sodium* is administered orally or by deep intramuscular injection. It also may be given as a slow intravenous injection (i.e., 100 mg/min of a 10 percent solution) in emergency situations (i.e., convulsions). The adult intravenous dosage ranges from 0.065 to 1 gm.

The oral sedative dosage for children is based

Table 24–2.
Barbiturate Dosages Employed for Sedative or Hypnotic Effect in Adults

Drug	Controlled Substance Schedule	Daily Sedative Dosage (Oral)	Single Hypnotic Dosage (Oral) (mg)	Therapeutic Effect	
				Onset of Sedation (min)	Duration (hr)
Amobarbital (AMYTAL)	II	60–150 mg ÷ 3	65–200	20	4–6
Aprobarbital (ALURATE)	III	120 ÷ 3	40–160	20	4–6
Butabarbital sodium (BUTISOL)	III	45–120 mg ÷ 3–4	50–100	30	6–8
Hexobarbital (SOMBULEX)	III	250–750 mg ÷ 2	250–500	5–10	3–4
Pentobarbital (NEMBUTAL)	II	80–120 mg ÷ 3–4	100–200	10–15	2–4
Phenobarbital (LUMINAL)	IV	32–128 mg	50–320	60–120	6–10
Secobarbital (SECONAL)	II	60–150 mg ÷ 2–3	100–200	10–15	2–4
Talbutal (LOTUSATE)	III	—	120	20	4–6

on the calculation of 6 mg/kg of body weight, divided for administration orally in two to three divided doses. The single intramuscular or intravenous hypnotic dosage for children 6 to 12 years of age is based on the calculation of 5 mg/kg of body weight. The intramuscular drug primarily is employed for the control of seizures.

Aprobarbital. The drug is an intermediate-acting agent that is available as an elixir primarily used for sedation or treatment of mild or pronounced insomnia (Table 24–2). The dosage for children has not been established.

Butabarbital Sodium. The drug is used orally to provide sedation or sleep (Table 24–2). The sedative dosage for children is based on the calculation of 6 mg/kg of body weight, divided for administration three times per day. The hypnotic dosage for children has not been estabilshed.

Hexobarbital. The drug is used primarily as an ultra-short-acting hypnotic, but it also is employed as a sedative prior to diagnostic or minor surgical procedures and to provide postoperative sedation (Table 24–2). It is useful for restoration of sleep when the person's sleep is interrupted during the night. The dosage for children has not been established.

Pentobarbital. *Pentobarbital* is a short-acting drug that is administered orally (Table 24–2). *Pentobarbital sodium* is administered orally, rectally, or by deep intramuscular injection. The drug is also administered as a slow intravenous injection for the induction of anesthesia or in emergency situations.

The rectal suppositories may be employed to provide the hypnotic dosage. The dosage for adults is 120 to 200 mg. Children from 12 to 14 years of age receive 60 to 120 mg; those 5 to 12 years of age receive 60 mg; those one to four years of age receive 30 to 60 mg; and infants over two months of age receive 30 mg of the drug.

The intramuscular hypnotic dose for adults is 150 to 200 mg. The dosage for children is based

on the calculation of 3 to 5 mg/kg of body weight to a maximum dosage of 100 mg.

The oral or rectal sedative dosage for children is based on the calculation of 6 mg/kg of body weight, which is divided for administration three times per day. The drug usually is administered orally or rectally to children to provide preanesthetic sedation.

Phenobarbital. The oral drug is absorbed slowly from the gastrointestinal tract. The delayed onset of action negates its routine use as an oral hypnotic agent. *Phenobarbital* is administered orally for its long-acting sedative effects. *Phenobarbital sodium* is administered orally, rectally, or by subcutaneous or intramuscular injection. The drug may also be administered as a slow intravenous injection (i.e., 60 mg/min) to a maximum total daily dosage of 600 mg.

The oral drug may be given as a single daily dose to provide a sedative effect because it has a long serum half-life (two to five days). It is frequently given in two to three divided doses (Table 24–2). The daily oral sedative dosage for children is based on the calculation of 2 mg/kg of body weight, which may be divided for administration three to four times per day. The parenteral anticonvulsant dosage for children is based on the calculation of 1 to 6 mg/kg of body weight. The hypnotic or anticonvulsive dosage that is used for administration of the drug rectally to children is based on the calculation of 6 mg/kg/day, and that dosage is divided for administration in three doses.

Secobarbital. *Secobarbital* is a short-acting drug that is administered orally (Table 24–2). *Secobarbital sodium* is administered orally, rectally, or by deep intramuscular injection. It may also be administered intravenously for control of convulsions in emergency situations.

The intramuscular hypnotic dosage for adults is the same as the oral dosage (100 to 200 mg). The intramuscular hypnotic dose for children is based on the calculation of 3 to 5 mg/kg of body weight to a maximum dose of 100 mg.

The oral preoperative sedative dosage for children is 50 to 100 mg, and that same dosage may be given as a rectal suppository or as a solution to children over three years of age. The dosage for rectal administration may also be calculated on the basis of 4 to 5 mg/kg of body weight.

Talbutal. The drug is an intermediate-acting agent that is administered orally (Table 24–2). It is used primarily for its hypnotic effect in the treatment of simple insomnia. The dosage for children has not been established.

NONBARBITURATE SEDATIVE-HYPNOTICS

The drugs are widely used for their hypnotic effects in the control of simple insomnia. Administration of the drugs 15 to 30 minutes before retiring decreases sleep latency and provides a restful sleep pattern. The drugs are also utilized as daytime sedatives to decrease anxiety and tension. They may be given as a single dose 60 to 90 minutes before intrusive diagnostic procedures or surgery to provide a sedative-hypnotic effect.

The nonbarbiturate sedative-hypnotic drugs are *chloral hydrate, chloral betaine, triclofos, paraldehyde, glutethimide, methaqualone, methyprylon, ethchlorvynol, ethinamate, flurazepam hydrochloride,* and *promethazine hydrochloride.* The drugs, with the exception of *paraldehyde, promethazine,* and *triclofos,* are subject to control under the Federal Controlled Substances Act of 1970.

Action Mode

The drugs are clinically effective in producing the central nervous system depression required for a sedative or hypnotic effect, but the specific mode of action of most of the drugs has not been determined. The drugs, like the barbiturates, act at the level of the thalamus where they inhibit the ascending multisynaptic midbrain reticular formation. That action raises the arousal threshold and interferes with transmission of impulses from the thalamus to the cerebral cortex.

Chloral Hydrate and Chloral Betaine

The pharmacologic properties of chloral hydrate are shared by chloral betaine, which dissociates immediately after ingestion to chloral hydrate and betaine. The central nervous system depressant effects of chloral hydrate are provided principally by the active metabolite *trichloroethanol.* That metabolite is also the primary active principle of *triclofos sodium.* Chloral hydrate provides a prototype of the actions and effects of those closely related drugs.

Therapy Considerations. Hypnotic doses of the drug produce quiet, deep sleep that closely resembles normal physiologic sleep. The higher levels of the dosage range suppress stage 4 sleep, but the drug has no effect on other phases of the sleep cycles.

Chloral hydrate is administered in the same dosages orally or rectally, and chloral betaine is administered orally at a slightly higher dosage level (Table 24–3). The drug is very irritating to the gastric mucosa, and the liquid-containing capsules should be taken with a full glass of fluid (i.e., water, milk, ginger ale, fruit juice, formula). The syrup should be diluted with liquid before it is ingested. The sedative dosage of chloral hydrate is given three times per day after meals to avoid gastric irritation.

The hypnotic dose for children is based on the calculation of 50 mg/kg of body weight to a maximum single dose of 1 gm. The daily sedative dose for children is based on the calculation of 24 mg/kg of body weight, which is divided for administration three times per day. The maximum daily sedative dosage is 1.5 gm/day. A single dose based on the calculation of 20 to 25 mg/kg may be given to children prior to electroencephalographic evaluations.

The drug is absorbed rapidly from the gastrointestinal tract after oral or rectal administration. Drowsiness occurs within 15 minutes after the hypnotic dose is taken. The drug and the active metabolite *trichloroethanol* cross the blood-brain barrier and the placental barrier. The metabolite has a plasma half-life of about 8 to 11 hours. The

Table 24–3.
Nonbarbiturate Sedative-Hypnotics: Dosage and Therapeutic Effect in Adults

Drug	Controlled Substance Schedule	Daily Sedative Dosage (Oral)	Single Hypnotic Dosage (Oral)	Onset (min)	Duration (hr)
Chloral betaine (BETA-CHLOR)	IV	0.87–1.74 gm	0.87–1.74 gm	30–60	6–8
Chloral hydrate (AQUACHLORAL, NOCTEC, SOMNOS)	IV	750 mg ÷ 3	0.5–1 gm	30–60	4–8
Ethchlorvynol (PLACIDYL)	IV	—	0.5–1 gm	15–60	5
Ethinamate (VALNID)	IV	—	0.5–1 gm	20–30	4–5
Flurazepam (DALMANE)	IV	—	15–30 mg	15–30	4–8
Glutethimide (DORIDEN)	IV	0.5–1 gm	250–500 mg	15–30	4–8
Methaqualone (QUAALUDE, SOPOR)	II	225–300 mg ÷ 3–4	150–300 mg	10–30	3–4
Methyprylon (NOLUDAR)	III	—	200–400 mg	30–60	5–8
Paraldehyde	IV	5–15 ml	15–30 ml	10–20	6–8
Promethazine (PHENERGAN, QUADNITE)		25–50 mg	—	20	2–6
Triclofos (TRICLOS)		—	1.5 gm	20–40	6–8

drug is metabolized, in the liver and the erythrocytes, to an active and an inactive metabolite. The metabolites are excreted in the urine. They produce a false positive reaction when Benedict's Qualitative Reagent is used to test for glycosuria. Some of the metabolites are secreted with the bile and eliminated with the feces. Minimal quantities of the active metabolites are excreted in the milk of nursing mothers.

Adverse Effects. The most frequent adverse effects are nausea, vomiting, and diarrhea. In contrast to other sedatives (i.e., barbiturates), residual early-morning lethargy and discomfort, or "hangover," occur infrequently. Ataxia, dizziness, and skin rashes (i.e., urticaria, angioedema, eczema, erythema multiforme) occur occasionally. A reduction in the total white blood count and relative eosinophilia may occur.

Drug Interactions. The drug can potentiate the central nervous system depressant effects of other drugs. When chloral hydrate is combined with alcohol, the combination, which is known as a "Mickey Finn" or "knockout drops," causes a sudden loss of consciousness. When the drug is taken after ingestion of alcohol, the person may experience tachycardia, palpitations, facial flushing, and dysphoria that occur as a consequence of vasodilation.

Administration of furosemide intravenously to a person who has taken chloral hydrate within a period of 24 hours produces diaphoresis, flushing, a feeling of uneasiness, and variable blood pressure changes (i.e., hypertension). The inactive *trichloroacetic acid* metabolite of chloral hydrate can displace the coumarins from their plasma albumin-binding sites. That action can produce a transient increase in the hypoprothrombinemic effect of the anticoagulant.

Toxicity. Overdosage of chloral hydrate produces symptoms similar to those that occur with barbiturate overdoses (i.e., hypotension, coma, respiratory depression, cardiac arrhythmias, and hypothermia). There may also be evidence of miosis, vomiting, areflexia, or muscle flaccidity. The treatment, like that for barbiturate overdosage, is based on the level of functional decompensation. Death, as a consequence of respiratory depression, has occurred after ingestion of 4 gm of chloral hydrate.

Prolonged use of the drug can produce tolerance, and that may cause the person to increase the dosage to a toxic level in an attempt to obtain the hypnotic effects of the drug. At the termination of therapy the dosage is reduced gradually to avert the symptoms of delirium tremens and hallucinations that are characteristic of the chloral hydrate withdrawal syndrome in drug-dependent persons.

Triclofos Sodium

Therapy Considerations. The central nervous system depressant effects of the drug are similar to those of chloral hydrate and the barbiturates. The drug is administered orally (Table 24–3) for its hypnotic effects in the treatment of simple insomnia. The hypnotic dosage of the drug for children over 12 years of age is based on the adult dosage. The drug is not used as a routine hypnotic drug for younger children. The single dosage for children who are being prepared for electroencephalographic evaluation is based on the calculation of 22 mg/kg of body weight. Drowsiness occurs approximately 20 minutes after the drug is taken.

Triclofos is absorbed rapidly from the gastrointestinal tract. It is rapidly dephosphorylated in the intestinal lumen, intestinal wall, and in the blood to the active metabolite *trichloroethanol*, which is also the active metabolite of chloral hydrate. The metabolite may produce a false positive reaction when Benedict's solution is used for tests for glycosuria. The drug is minimally effective as a hypnotic after a two-week period of regular use.

Adverse Effects. Triclofos frequently produces residual sedation in the early-morning hours ("hangover"), motor incoordination, and dizziness. Gastric irritation (i.e., nausea, vomiting, flatulence), "bad taste" in the mouth, eosinophilia, and leukopenia occur occasionally. There have been a few reports that excitement and urticaria have occurred. The drug interactions and toxic effects that occur during therapy with triclofos are similar to those that were described as occurring with the use of chloral hydrate.

Paraldehyde

Most drugs are prepared in forms that disguise their odor, but the commonly used liquid form of paraldehyde has a characteristic penetrating odor that unavoidably permeates the medication preparation area. Because it readily decomposes on exposure to light and air to form a highly toxic *acetaldehyde,* it is stored in a tightly stoppered amber glass bottle or vial.

Therapy Considerations. The drug produces sedative and hypnotic effects similar to those of chloral hydrate, alcohol, and the barbiturates. It is thought to depress the ascending reticular activating system. That action causes an imbalance between the inhibitory and facilitory mechanisms.

Paraldehyde is administered orally. It is occasionally administered intramuscularly or intravenously to adults in emergency situations (i.e., delirium tremens). The oral drug is available in capsules or as a liquid. Paraldehype is occasionally administered in oil as a retention enema. That route of administration has an irregular rate of absorption, which has made it nearly obsolete.

The oral liquid (Table 24–3) is diluted in milk or iced fruit juice to disguise the taste and odor and to decrease the gastric irritation. The drug is commonly used for treatment of the alcohol withdrawal syndrome. Adults are given an oral dose of 5 to 10 ml, and alcoholics seem unaffected by the disagreeable, burning taste of the liquid.

The drug is absorbed rapidly from the gastrointestinal tract. The cerebrospinal fluid drug concentrations reach their maximum level within 30 to 60 minutes after the drug is administered, and they are 25 to 30 percent of the blood concentrations. The hypnotic effect is attained within 5 to 15 minutes when the drug is administered by the oral route. The drug crosses the placenta. The serum half-life of the drug ranges from 3.5 to 9.5 hours.

The drug is metabolized primarily in the liver (80 to 90 percent). A significant amount of the unchanged drug crosses the alveolar membranes and is excreted on expiration. The exhaled drug has a penetrating odor similar to that of the liquid drug.

Adverse Effects. The most frequent adverse effects are an unpleasant taste in the mouth that lasts until excretion of the unchanged drug has been completed, gastric irritation, residual sedation on awakening ("hangover"), dizziness, and ataxia. Occasionally the drug produces confusion or paradoxic excitement.

Toxicity. The drug infrequently is abused. The overdosage is usually at a level that prolongs the sleep of the person without causing respiratory depression. At higher dosage the symptoms and their treatment are similar to those of chloral hydrate overdosage. Fatalities have occurred with oral dosages of 25 ml.

Chronic use of the drug can produce toxic hepatitis, nephrosis, and metabolic acidosis. Paraldehyde-dependent persons may consume large quantities daily (i.e., 120 ml), and abstinence or sudden withdrawal can produce delirium tremens and hallucinations.

Glutethimide

The drug is related structurally to methyprylon, methaqualone, and the barbiturates. Glutethimide has central nervous system effects similar to those of the barbiturates.

Therapy Considerations. The hypnotic dosage levels (Table 24–3) produce quiet, deep sleep. There is a significant decrease in nonREM stage 4 and REM sleep. Tolerance develops to the REM sleep suppression, but at the termination of therapy the REM rebound may cause a marked increase in dreaming, nightmares, or insomnia during several subsequent sleep periods. The drug becomes ineffective as a hypnotic after 14 days of continued use.

The anticholinergic effects of the drug may produce mydriasis, inhibition of glandular secretions (i.e., decreased salivation), and reduced intestinal motility. The oral drug is irregularly absorbed from the gastrointestinal tract. The circulating drug is widely distributed in adipose tissue, liver, kidneys, brain, and bile. It crosses the placental barrier and appears in the milk of nursing mothers. The drug is metabolized in the liver. A small amount of the unchanged drug (<2 percent) and the metabolites is excreted in the urine.

Adverse Effects. There is a high incidence of skin rashes. Residual sedation in the morning, ataxia, and dizziness are frequent adverse effects of the drug. Gastrointestinal disturbances (i.e., nausea, vomiting, anorexia) and hypotension occasionally occur. There have been a few reports of blurred vision, exfoliative dermatitis, paradoxic excitement, acute hypersensitivity reactions, blood dyscrasias (i.e., thrombocytopenia, aplastic anemia, leukopenia, megaloblastic anemia), and porphyria.

Drug Interactions. The concurrent use of other central nervous system depressants produces additive sedative effects. The concurrent use of drugs with anticholinergic effects (i.e., phenothiazines, tricyclic antidepressants, belladonna alkaloids) produces effects that are additive with those of glutethimide (i.e., dryness of the mouth, blurred vision, constipation, urine retention).

The induction of hepatic microsomal enzymes by the drug increases the metabolism of coumarin anticoagulants. That action decreases the therapeutic effectiveness of the anticoagulants unless the dosage is increased.

Toxicity. Overdosage with glutethimide produces symptoms similar to those caused by barbiturate overdosage. The toxic doses produce high levels of the active metabolite *4-hydroxy-2-ethyl-2-phenylglutarimide* (4-HG) in the plasma and tisues. The action of the metabolite and the slow release of the drug from the adipose tissues prolong the comatose state. The person may be comatose for several days. The irregular pattern of release of the drug from the adipose tissues provides an uneven and somewhat unpredictable improvement and regression in the person's status. For example, after treatment of the comatose state, the person may be responding, alert, walking about, and then in a comatose state. Overdosage with 10 gm of the drug is usually fatal.

Toxic symptoms that may appear with overdosage or prolonged use include problems with anticholinergic effects of the drug (i.e., dryness of the mouth, widely dilated and fixed pupils, adynamic ileus, urinary bladder atony). The drug is usually withdrawn gradually when the person is glutethimide dependent to avoid the severe symptoms of the withdrawal syndrome (i.e., nausea, vomiting, nervousness, tremulousness, tachycardia, abdominal cramps, fever, chills, numbness of the extremities, dysphagia, delirium, hallucinations, and major motor seizures).

Methaqualone and Methaqualone Hydrochloride

The drug has central nervous system depressant effects similar to those of glutethimide, methyprylon, and the barbiturates. The hypnotic dosage of the drug produces cerebral depression that provides quiet, deep sleep. It significantly depresses REM sleep, but tolerance develops to the REM suppression. There is a REM rebound effect at the termination of therapy. The effectiveness of the drug as a hypnotic is low after 14 days of regular use.

Therapy Considerations. *Methaqualone* and *methaqualone hydrochloride* are administered orally. The adult hypnotic dosage of methaqualone hydrochloride is 200 to 400 mg, which is higher than that of methaqualone (Table 24–3). The dosage for pediatric patients has not been established.

The drug is rapidly absorbed from the gastrointestinal tract. It is distributed in the adipose tissues, liver, kidneys, heart, brain, spleen, cerebrospinal fluid, and skeletal muscles. It is metabolized in the liver, and the inactive metabolites are excreted in the urine, bile, and feces.

Adverse Effects. The most frequent adverse effects are headache, residual sedation, dizziness, and paresthesias. Occasionally the drug produces gastrointestinal disturbances (i.e., dry mouth, anorexia, vomiting), tachycardia, diaphoresis, bromhidrosis, paradoxic excitement, and allergic reactions (i.e., urticaria, rashes). There have been a few reports of agranulocytosis and aplastic anemia.

Drug Interactions. The concurrent use of other central nervous system depressants produces sedative effects that are additive with those of methaqualone. The drug induces hepatic microsomal enzymes, but the effect on coumarin anticoagulant metabolism is clinically insignificant.

Toxicity. The drug has been widely abused. Its popularity is related to the rapid onset of action and the long duration of the state of relaxation and euphoria. Mild toxicity produces symptoms similar to those of barbiturate overdosage. Ingestion of 2.4 gm of methaqualone produces coma that is accompanied by pyramidal signs (i.e., hypertonia, hyperreflexia, myoclonia, convulsions). There may also be pupillary dilation, tachycardia, delirium, and spontaneous vomiting. Ingestion of 8 gm has caused death.

The drug dosage is reduced gradually when the individual is methaqualone dependent to avoid the symptoms of the withdrawal syndrome (i.e., nausea, vomiting, anorexia, abdominal cramps, diaphoresis, nervousness, tremulousness, headache, anxiety, confusion, weakness, insomnia, nightmares, hallucinations, major motor seizures).

Methyprylon

The drug has central nervous system depressant effects similar to those of glutethimide, methaqualone, and the barbiturates. The hypnotic dosage of the drug produces a quiet, deep sleep that is similar to natural physiologic sleep patterns. The drug suppresses REM sleep. Tolerance develops to that suppression, but at the termination of therapy there is an REM rebound effect.

Therapy Considerations. Methyprylon is administered orally (Table 24–3). The hypnotic dosage for children over three months of age is 50 to 200 mg. The daily sedative dosage for children is 150 to 200 mg, which is divided for administration three to four times per day.

The drug is fairly well absorbed from the gastrointestinal tract. Sleep occurs within one hour after the hypnotic dose of drug is taken, and the duration of that sleep is five to eight hours. The drug is metabolized in the liver; the metabolites are secreted in the bile and subsequently reabsorbed from the intestine. The primary route of excretion is the urine.

Adverse Effects. The most frequent adverse effects are residual sedation and dizziness. Gastrointestinal disturbances (i.e., nausea, vomiting, esophagitis, diarrhea) occasionally occur. There have been a few reports of paradoxic excitement, rashes, and blood dyscrasias. As with other central nervous system depressants, the concurrent use of alcohol or other depressants increases the sedative effects of methyprylon.

Toxicity. The symptoms of overdosage are similar to those that occur with overdosage of barbiturates. Doses higher than 6 gm produce deep coma that is accompanied by marked hypotension and respiratory depression. Persons sometimes have episodes of excitation, convulsions, delirium, and hallucinations when recovering from methyprylon intoxication.

The drug dosage is reduced gradually in methyprylon-dependent persons to avoid the symptoms of withdrawal syndrome, which is similar to the barbiturate withdrawal syndrome. There may also be confusion, marked nervousness, insomnia, diaphoresis, polyuria, hyperreflexia, delirium, hallucinations, and convulsions.

Ethchlorvynol

The drug has central nervous system effects similar to those of chloral hydrate and the barbiturates. Like those drugs, it produces a quiet, deep sleep and it suppresses REM sleep. At the termination of therapy there may be a REM rebound effect.

Therapy Considerations. Ethchlorvynol is administered orally to adults (Table 24–3). The pediatric dosage has not been established. The drug is absorbed rapidly from the gastrointestinal tract. The hypnotic effect occurs within 15 to 60 minutes, and the duration of sleep is five hours.

The circulating drug is distributed in the liver, kidneys, spleen, brain, bile, cerebrospinal fluid, and it is highly localized in body lipids. It crosses the placental barrier. The drug is metabolized in the liver and kidneys, and small amounts (<0.1 percent) of the unchanged drug and the metabolites are excreted in the urine in 24 hours.

Adverse Effects. The most frequent adverse effects are residual sedation, ataxia, dizziness, and hypotension. The drug occasionally produces vomiting, blurred vision, paradoxic excitement, confusion, and urticaria. There have been a few reports of amblyopia, cholestatic jaundice, and thrombocytopenia.

Drug Interactions. Additive central nervous system depression may occur when the drug is administered concurrent with other drugs having sedative effects. That depression may also occur when it is administered concurrent with monoamine oxidase inhibitors. Use of the drug with amitriptyline can produce transient delirium. Ethchlorvynol induces the hepatic microsomal enzymes, and that action can accelerate the metabolism of the oral anticoagulants.

Toxicity. The symptoms of overdosage are similar to those of barbiturate overdosage. Mydriasis, areflexia, and bradycardia may also occur. Ingestion of 7 gm of ethchlorvynol has caused death.

The dosage of the drug is reduced gradually at the termination of therapy in ethchlorvynol-dependent persons to prevent the onset of the withdrawal syndrome, which includes symptoms of anxiety, confusion, perceptual distortions, memory loss, irritability, agitation, severe hallucinations, delirium, and major motor seizures. During the abstinence period there may also be anorexia, nausea, vomiting, weakness, dizziness, diaphoresis, muscle twitching, and weight loss.

Ethinamate

The drug has central nervous system depressant effects similar to those produced by the barbiturates. The hypnotic dose of the drug rapidly produces sedation and induces sleep.

Therapy Considerations. The drug is administered orally (Table 24–3). The pediatric dosage has not been established. Ethinamate is rapidly absorbed from the gastrointestinal tract. The hypnotic dosage induces sleep within 15 to 20 minutes, and the sleep period lasts for three to five hours. The drug has a serum half-life of 2.5 hours. It is metabolized rapidly in the liver and the metabolites are excreted in the urine.

Adverse Effects. The most frequent adverse effects are residual sedation, ataxia, and dizziness. Confusion and rashes occasionally occur. There have been a few reports of thrombocytopenic purpura and drug fever. As with other central nervous system depressants, the concurrent use of drugs with similar effects may produce excessive sedation.

Toxicity. The symptoms of overdosage are similar to those that occur with barbiturate overdoses. The central nervous system depression that is produced by ethinamate is of shorter duration than that of other hypnotics. Hepatic function may be impaired, and there may be transient evidence of jaundice. Ingestion of 15 gm of ethinamate can be fatal.

The dosage is reduced gradually at the termination of therapy of ethinamate-dependent persons to avoid the symptoms of the withdrawal syndrome. The syndrome includes tremulousness, hyperactive reflexes, severe insomnia, agitation, syncopal episodes, confusion, disorientation, severe hallucinations, and major motor seizures.

Flurazepam Hydrochloride

The drug is a benzodiazepine similar to the group of drugs commonly employed as antianxiety drugs. The National Institute on Drug Abuse (NIDA) in its 1977 report "Sedative-Hypnotic Drugs: Risks and Benefits" concludes that the benzodiazepines are generally the preferred sedative-hypnotic drugs. The characteristics of the drugs that lead to that conclusion are
1. Their relative safety,
2. Less additive effect with alcohol,
3. Relatively little interaction with other drugs,
4. Relatively little effect on liver enzyme production,
5. Less rapid development of tolerance and physical dependence,
6. Relatively little influence on REM sleep,
7. Less possibility of causing death from accidental or intentional overdose.

Action Mode. Flurazepam acts at the limbic and subcortical levels of the central nervous system. That action produces sedation, skeletal muscle relaxation, and anticonvulsant effects. The reduction of emotional activity that results from depression of the limbic system facilitates the induction of sleep. REM sleep is unaffected by the usual hypnotic doses of flurazepam. There is a marked decrease in stage 3 and stage 4 sleep periods.

Therapy Considerations. The drug is administered orally (Table 24–3). The adult dosage is used for children over 15 years of age; the dosage for younger children has not been established. The drug is absorbed rapidly from the gastrointestinal tract. The rapid action of the drug provides sleep induction within 15 to 30 minutes; the duration of the sleep period is seven to eight hours. The drug is more effective on the second and third nights than on the first night.

The circulating drug is 75 percent bound to plasma proteins, and the drug is widely distributed throughout the body tissues. It is rapidly metabolized in the liver. Approximately 80 percent of the metabolites is excreted in the urine and 10 percent is eliminated in the feces within 72 hours.

The active metabolite *N-1-hydroxyethylfluraze-pam* has a serum half-life of two hours, and *N-1-desalkylflurazepam* has a serum half-life of 19 hours. The metabolites contribute significantly to the therapeutic and toxic effects of the drug.

Adverse Effects. The most frequent adverse effects are residual sedation or drowsiness, and ataxia. The drug occasionally produces a bitter taste in the mouth, confusion, paradoxic excitement, and dizziness. There have been a few reports of hypotension, blood dyscrasias, jaundice, and immediate allergic reactions. The concurrent use of other central nervous system depressants can increase the sedative effects of flurazepam.

Toxicity. The benzodiazepines are the sedatives most often involved in suicide attempts. Overdosage with flurazepam can produce somnolence, confusion, and coma.

Promethazine Hydrochloride

The drug is an ethylamino derivative of phenothiazine. Therapeutic doses of the drug produce central nervous system depression. The drug also has antihistaminic, antiemetic, anticholinergic, and local anesthetic effects.

Therapy Considerations. Promethazine is administered orally, rectally, or by intramuscular or slow intravenous injection (i.e., 25 mg/min). The dosage (Table 24–3) is the same for each of the routes of administration. The single dose for sedation of children (i.e., preoperatively or postoperatively) is based on the calculation of 0.5 to 1.1 mg/kg of body weight.

The oral drug is well absorbed from the gastrointestinal tract and from the parenteral administration sites. The onset of the sedative effects occurs within 20 minutes after oral, rectal, or intramuscular administration of the drug and within three to five minutes after it is given intravenously. The duration of the sedative effects is two to six hours. The drug is widely distributed in body tissues. It is metabolized in the liver, and

the metabolites are slowly excreted in the urine and feces.

Adverse Effects. The anticholinergic effects of the drug may produce dryness of the mouth and blurring of vision. Confusion, disorientation, and dizziness may also occur. There have been a few reports of restlessness, akathisia, irregular respirations, and photosensitivity that caused severe sunburn.

Drug Interactions. Like other central nervous system depressants, the concurrent administration of drugs with similar effects can produce an additive sedative effect. Promethazine reverses the vasopressor effect of epinephrine.

Toxicity. Overdosage with promethazine produces a deep sleep and coma. Children may have a paradoxic reaction that includes hyperexcitability, abnormal movements, nightmares, and respiratory depression.

NONBARBITURATE SEDATIVES

The drugs are administered parenterally to relieve the anxiety, apprehension, and emotional tension associated with pain. They may be used to relieve anxiety and tension and to produce sleep during labor or prior to surgery. The drugs are *methotrimeprazine hydrochloride* and *propiomazine hydrochloride*.

Methotrimeprazine Hydrochloride (LEVOPROME)

Action Mode. The drug, a propylamino derivative of phenothiazine, shares the pharmacologic actions of that group of drugs, which commonly are employed as antipsychotic agents. Its primary action is depression of the subcortical area of the brain. Its action at the level of the thalamus, hypothalamus, and the reticular and limbic systems results in suppression of sensory impulses, reduction of motor activity, sedation, and tranquilization. It can also alter temperature regulation and produce amnesia. It has antihistaminic, local anesthetic, antiemetic, and weak anticholinergic effects. It is used primarily for its sedative and analgesic effects in the treatment of bedfast patients.

Therapy Considerations. The drug is administered as a deep intramuscular injection into a large muscle mass to reduce the irritating effects. The patient is instructed to remain in bed for at least six hours after the intramuscular injection to avoid the orthostatic hypotension, fainting, weakness, and dizziness that may occur. Hypotension, which occurs within 10 to 20 minutes after the drug is administered, may continue for 4 to 12 hours during the initial period of therapy. Tolerance to the effect gradually occurs, and the drop in blood pressure is less severe after several doses of the drug have been given.

The analgesic dose of 40 to 120 mg is divided for administration four to six times per day. That dosage provides a sedative and analgesic effect in 20 to 40 minutes that may persist for four to five hours. The preoperative dose for sedation is 2 to 20 mg, and it is administered 45 minutes to three hours before surgery. The dosage for children younger than 12 years of age has not been established.

The absorbed drug crosses the placenta and enters the cerebrospinal fluid. Insignificant amounts of the drug appear in the milk of nursing mothers. The drug is metabolized in the liver, and the metabolites are excreted slowly in the urine and feces.

Adverse Effects. The most common adverse effect is orthostatic hypotension, which occurs during the initial period of therapy. Drowsiness, excessive sedation, and amnesia also occur frequently. The drug occasionally produces disorientation, euphoria, headache, weakness, slurring of speech, nausea, vomiting, chills, and palpitations. The anticholinergic effects of the drug produce abdominal discomfort, dryness of the mouth, nasal congestion, tachycardia or bradycardia, and urine retention. There have been a few reports of blood dyscrasias with long-term use of the drugs.

Drug Interactions. Additive sedative effects can occur when other central nervous system depressants are administered concurrent with methotrimeprazine. The drug may potentiate the action of other anticholinergic agents, skeletal muscle relaxants, or antihypertensive drugs. It also reverses the vasopressor effect of epinephrine.

Propiomazine Hydrochloride (LARGON)

The drug is an ethylamino derivative of phenothiazine. Although the exact mechanism of its sedative action is unknown, the drug produces central nervous system depression at therapeutic dosage levels. It also has antihistaminic, antiemetic, and anticholinergic effects.

Therapy Considerations. The drug is administered to adults at a dosage of 10 to 40 mg by intramuscular or intravenous injection. The dosage may be repeated at three-hour intervals. The single preoperative or postoperative dosage for children weighing less than 27 kg (60 lb) is based on the calculation of 0.55 to 1.1 mg/kg of body weight.

The drug is well absorbed from parenteral injection sites, and peak sedative effects appear within 40 to 60 minutes after the drug is administered intramuscularly and within 15 to 30 minutes after intravenous administration. The duration of the sedative effects is three hours; the effects decline rapidly after that time. The drug is widely distributed in body tissues and fluids. It is metabolized in the liver and excreted in the urine and in the bile.

Adverse Effects. Dryness of the mouth is the most frequent adverse effect. The drug occasionally produces tachycardia, gastrointestinal disturbances, and skin rashes. Elderly patients may have dizziness, confusion, or amnesia.

Drug Interactions. The sedative effects are additive when other central nervous system depressants are administered concurrently. Propiomazine can reverse the vasopressor effect of epinephrine.

NURSING INTERVENTION

Sleeplessness generally is described as *simple insomnia* to differentiate it from the disruption in sleep patterns that is associated with severe emotional disturbances. Simple insomnia can usually be ameliorated by modification of sleep-disturbing factors and use of sedative-hypnotic drugs.

There are three common patterns of sleep disruption, and those types of insomnia provide a framework for assessing the person's specific sleep problem:

Initial insomnia: Prolonged periods of sleep latency.

Intermittent insomnia: Recurrent periods of wakefulness

Terminal insomnia: Early waking and an inability to return to sleep.

Nursing Assessment

Sleep requirements vary between individuals, and the quality may be more important than the quantity of sleep. Nursing assessment is essential to definition of the person's sleep requirements and the specific sleeplessness problem. The data that are obtained provide the baselines, or framework, for planning nursing intervention *to decrease the person's requirements for sedative-hypnotic drugs or to maximize the effects of those drugs that are administered.*

When an opportunity is provided for the patient to identify the adequacy of sleep periods or factors that are causing insomnia, the patient usually provides very explicit information. Initial insomnia is the most common problem, and environmental factors are the most frequently identified cause of that insomnia. Patients often describe the talking at the nurses' station, the moaning of the patient nearby, the lights in the room, and the room temperature as factors that make it difficult to get to sleep.

Those factors may be contributing to the problem, but personal psychologic factors are the most common cause of initial insomnia. In addition to discussing plans for modifying the noise, lights, and room temperature, it is important to obtain further information about psychologic factors that may also be contributing to sleep latency (i.e., anxiety about the family, illness, surgery, finances).

Problems are often out of proportion with reality during the presleep hours. The nurse can help the patient return the problem to its natural importance. The time that is spent with the patient also provides an opportunity to identify the nursing measures that can be employed to resolve realistic problems. The nurse, in the role of listener and consultant, is often instrumental in providing the relaxation that is essential to the onset of sleep.

Physical factors are common causes of initial or intermittent insomnia. Pain, cough, and pruritus are the most common sleep-disrupting problems. Administration of a hypnotic drug has no effect on pain, and in many instances the patient's discomfort becomes more evident when the drug is administered in the presence of pain. Drug-induced suppression of the inhibitions that influence behavior allows the patient to more freely express the physical discomfort through vocalization and body movements. The relief of pain is a priority consideration, and the hypnotic drug can be administered concurrently or at a later time to induce sleep.

The nursing measures that promote relaxation and relieve discomfort (i.e., back rub, providing fresh bedclothing or bedding) have a positive effect on the induction of sleep. The use of prescribed therapies for the relief of cough or pruritus also contributes to the patient's relaxation and decreases the initial or intermittent insomnia.

There are several light sleep periods in the natural sleep pattern, and discomfort during those periods is the primary cause of intermittent insomnia. For example, the stimulus of wet bedding can prevent progression of the sleep cycles and maintain the sleep at the stage 2 level. Changing the bedding may waken the patient, but the subsequent periods of sleep will follow the natural cycles.

Intermittent insomnia can be produced by several physical factors (i.e., hunger, thirst, snoring, sleep apnea, fullness of the bladder). Identification of the specific factors that most frequently waken the individual allows planning for the resolution of those problems. The disturbing factors are highly individual. For example, the person's initial insomnia or intermittent insomnia may be related to sleeping in a dark, quiet environment that contrasts with the familiar environment of a home on a busy city street. The resolution of the problem depends on its cause. In the foregoing situation the monotonous sound of the radio may induce and maintain the person's sleep. Most patients, when asked, state that they can't wait to get home to sleep in their own bed. Although part of that statement is related to the perception of that period of time as related to the absence of illness, it is at least partially related to the return of familiar, long-established rituals (i.e., changing of attire) and environmental preparation for sleep (i.e., modification of the lighting, sound, temperature).

Terminal insomnia is a common problem in elderly patients and in persons whose circadian rhythms are markedly different from the sleep-wakefulness cycles of the hospital environment. The insomnia of elderly patients is often related to early retiring, daytime inactivity, and napping. Nurses often employ a planned program of daytime stimulation that includes frequent contact with the patient and encouraging the person to sit in the chair or to ambulate frequently. That plan often meets with resistance from the patient but does improve the sleep patterns of the elderly person.

Persons who maintain regular patterns of activity and sleep that are different from the hospital sleep-wakefulness schedule may initially have some minor difficulty with daytime psychomotor function. The acutely ill person usually has sufficient sleep deprivation to allow the transition to the hospital routine. The person with a short-term illness more often retains, at least partially, the cycles that are natural to the established biologic rhythms.

Planned monitoring of the patient's status is affected by the sleep cycles. Monitoring of the vital signs during REM sleep will not waken the patient, but the recordings will be affected by the accelerated autonomic nervous system activity. Relaxation of the neck muscles, which usually causes the head to fall into an uncomfortable-looking position, can be used as one of the guides to the presence of REM sleep. Vital signs can be taken at the termination of that sleep period when the patient corrects the unnatural position.

The effectiveness of the hypnotic drugs is enhanced by the use of nursing measures, and the patient enjoys the psychosomatic benefits of sleep. Most of the hypnotic drugs are less effective after they have been used regularly for a 14-day period. The sleep-inducing effects of the drugs can be maintained when there are interruptions in that pattern of regular use. On nights when the environment is quiet and the patient is pain free and tired, the use of comfort measures may induce sleep without the use of the drugs.

The drugs that alter stage IV or REM sleep periods are potentially insomnia-producing agents, and abrupt cessation of their use can cause disturbances in the sleep patterns. For example, the person may have an increased REM sleep time when the use of hypnotics is terminated after a prolonged period of regular use. The vivid dreams that are remembered for a short period of time on waking may be distressing to the patient. After the regular use of hypnotics in the hospital, the person who experiences the REM rebound effect during sleep at home may continue to take a hypnotic drug to obtain "dreamless sleep." That misuse of the drugs may be averted by their judicious use during the period of hospitalization and by informing the patient that the dreaming episodes, or REM rebound effect, decrease during each subsequent sleep period.

Review Guides

Describe the following:

1. The restrictions on the use of drugs subject to the controls of the Federal Controlled Substances Act of 1970.
2. The timing of nursing measures to prepare the patient for sleep when secobarbital is to be given.
3. The events of the sleep stages that affect the monitoring of vital signs during the night.
4. The nursing care of the patient after administration of the preoperative dose of secobarbital.
5. The factors that should be considered when preparing liquid chloral hydrate for administration to the patient.
6. The primary factors that differentiate flurazepam from other hypnotic drugs.
7. The precautions that should be taken when administering paraldehyde intramuscularly.
8. The relationship between the distribution in adipose tissue that occurs with glutethimide and methaqualone and the severity and duration of toxicity.
9. The nursing measures that should be planned for the patient with level 2 functional decompensation after an overdose of phenobarbital.
10. The factors that should be considered when the patient who is receiving coumarin, digitoxin, or phenobarbital refuses to take the sedative each time it is offered during the day.

Additional Readings

Aschoff, J. Juergen: Circadian systems in man and their implications. *Hosp. Pract.,* **11:**51, May, 1976.

Bassler, Sandra Furman: The origins and development of biological rhythms. *Nurs. Clin. North Am.,* **11:**575, December, 1976.

Bowers, Joan E.: Caring for the elderly. *Nursing 78,* **8:**42, January, 1978.

Cohen, Sidney: Sleep and insomnia. *J.A.M.A.,* **236:** 875, August 16, 1976.

Emde, Robert N.; Swedberg, Jay; and Suzuki, Bruce: Human wakefulness and biological rhythms after birth. *Arch. Gen. Psychiatry,* **32:**780, June, 1975.

Greenblatt, David J., and Miller, Russel R.: Rational use of psychotropic drugs, 1. Hypnotics. *Am. J. Hosp. Pharm.,* **31:**990, October, 1974.

Greenblatt, David J.; Shader, Richard I.; and Koch-Weser, Jan: Flurazepam hydrochloride. *Clin. Pharmacol. Ther.,* **17:**1, January, 1975.

Hansen, Alfred R.; Kennedy, Katherine A.; Ambre, John J.; and Fischer, Lawrence J.: Glutethimide poisoning. *N. Engl. J. Med.,* **292:**250, January 30, 1975.

Jenkins, Betty Lou: A case against "sleepers." *J. Geriatr. Nurs.,* **2:**10, March/April, 1976.

Kales, Anthony; Bixler, Edward O.; Scharf, Martin; and Kales, Joyce D.: Sleep laboratory studies of flurazepam: a model for evaluating hypnotic drugs. *Clin. Pharmacol. Ther.,* **19:**577, May, 1976.

Kochansky, Gerald E.; Hemenway, Thomas S., III.; Salzman, Carl; and Shader, Richard I.: Methaqualone abusers: a preliminary survey of college students. *Dis. Nerv. Syst.,* **36:**348, July, 1975.

Lanuza, Dorothy M.: Circadian rhythms of mental efficiency and performance. *Nurs. Clin. North Am.,* **11:**583, December, 1976.

Myers, Robert R., and Stockard, James J.: Neurologic and electroencephalographic correlates in glutethimide intoxication. *Clin. Pharmacol. Ther.,* **17:**212, February, 1975.

Natalini, John J.: The human body as a biological clock. *Am. J. Nurs.,* **77:**1130, July, 1977.

Norris, Catherine M.: Restlessness: a nursing phenomenon in search of meaning. *Nurs. Outlook,* **23:**103, February, 1975.

Pagel, James F., Jr.: Sleep disorders and insomnia. *Am. Fam. Physician,* **17:**165, February, 1978.

Pappenheimer, John R.: The sleep factor. *Sci. Am.,* **235:**24, August, 1976.

Saario, I.; Linnoila, M.; and Mäki, M.: Interaction of drugs with alcohol on human psychomotor skills related to driving: effects of sleep deprivation or two weeks' treatment with hypnotics. *J. Clin. Pharm.,* **15:**52, January, 1975.

Sinal, Sara H., and Crowe, James E.: Cyanosis, cough and hypotension following intravenous administration of paraldehyde. *Pediatrics,* **57:**158, January, 1976.

Smith, David E., and Wesson, Donald R.: *Diagnosis and Treatment of Adverse Reactions to Sedative-Hypnotics.* National Institute on Drug Abuse, Rockville, Md., 1974.

Smith, Jackson A., and Renshaw, Doreena C.: A clinical study of insomnia. *Am. Fam. Physician,* **71:**140, March, 1975.

Teutsch, Giete; Mahler, Donald L.; Brown, Colin R.;

Forrest, William H., Jr.; James, Kenneth E.; and Brown, Byron W.: Hypnotic efficacy of diphenhydramine, methapyrilene, and pentobarbital. *Clin. Pharmacol. Ther.,* **17:**195, February, 1975.

Tom, Cheryl K.: Nursing assessment of biological rhythms. *Nurs. Clin. North Am.,* **11:**621, December, 1976.

Vogel, Gerald W.: A review of REM sleep deprivation. *Arch. Gen. Psychiatry,* **32:**749, June, 1975.

Wang, Richard I. H.; Stockdale, Susan L.; and Hieb, Elizabeth: Hypnotic efficacy of lorazepam and flurazepam. *Clin. Pharmacol. Ther.,* **19:**191, February, 1976.

Zelechowski, Gina Pugliese: Helping your patient sleep: planning instead of pills. *Nursing 77,* **7:**62, May, 1977.

25

Pain and Hyperpyrexia

Pain is a common human experience, and its presence may temporarily or consistently interfere with the person's ability to function. Relief of the persistent pain that is associated with chronic disease states (i.e., terminal cancer, amputation, extensive joint inflammation or degeneration) has been the focus of many clinical investigations. Recent reports of trials with operant conditioning, hypnosis, acupuncture, autogenic training, bio-feedback, meditation, electrical stimulation, and controlled relaxation-breathing techniques indicate that, to some degree, all of the methods aid in the control of pain or improvement in the person's ability to manage the pain experience. Each of the methodologies offers a viable alternative, for carefully selected patient populations, to the use of strong analgesics for the control of pain.

Physiologic Correlations

Sensory-Motor Reflexes

The unmyelinated sensory nerve ending receptors that detect pain send impulses along the afferent sensory myelinated or unmyelinated (visceral afferent) nerve fibers from the tissues to the spinal cord. The fibers pass through the posterior nerve root ganglion, and some of the impulses from the sensory cell bodies of the ganglion are relayed to the spinal cord reflex arc. They return as efferent motor impulses to the site of stimulation to produce a physical muscular action directed at avoidance of the pain source (Fig. 25–1).

Pain Perception

Other pain impulses, which enter the posterolateral horn from the ganglion sensory cell bodies, cross the spinal cord to the contralateral anterior horn cells and ascend through the spinothalamic tract to the brainstem. Those ascending reticular projections arrive at the posteroventral lateral nucleus of the thalamus where the stimulus

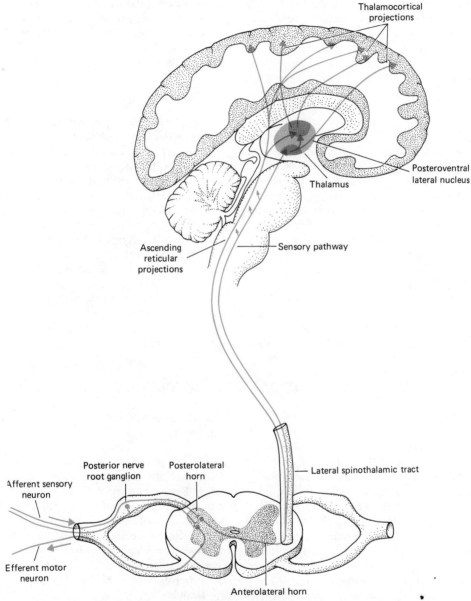

Fig. 25–1. Some of the sensory stimuli are relayed to the reflex arc, and efferent neurons stimulate motor responses in the periphery. Other sensory impulses cross to the opposite lateral spinothalamic tract and travel to the thalamus. Relay of the impulses to the cerebral cortex allows interpretation of the pain.

is grossly interpreted as a generalized painful sensation. The passage of the stimulus to the cortical neurons allows definitive recognition, localization, and quantitation of the pain stimulus. Efferent fibers from the cerebral cortex produce skeletal, psychic, and autonomic nervous system responses to the pain stimulus.

Pain Stimulus Suppression

Neurobiologist investigators have discovered natural endogenous peptides in the brain that are described as depressing the responses to pain impulses. The peptides, which are produced primarily in the pituitary gland and other subcortical structures, are called *endorphins* because they mediate a state of indifference or an emotional detachment from pain stimuli that is similar to that produced by morphine.

When the brain centers are directly stimulated (i.e., by electrode or probe), the *endorphins* combine with specific receptors on nerve cells and alter their function. Impulses that travel down the spinal cord intercept or block incoming pain impulses before they reach the thalamic or cortical centers, and pain perception is blunted or aborted. It is possible that the differing levels of neurotransmission by the *endorphins* contribute to the variation in responses to pain between individuals.

Temperature Regulation

The internal body temperature is regulated primarily by the central thermoreceptive areas of the anterior hypothalamus. An elevation in the temperature of the blood that perfuses the hypothalamus or afferent impulses from the peripheral and visceral thermoreceptors can precipitate the hypothalamic-directed sympathetic nerve stimulation of the sweat glands and the peripheral blood vessels that is required for dissipation of heat from the body surfaces. The vasodilation and increased secretion of sweat accelerate the processes of radiation, convection, and evaporation of heat that lower the body temperature. Concurrent sympathetic nerve stimulation of the cardiac and respiration rate is an adjunct to the heat dissipation processes.

Pathophysiologic Correlations

Hyperpyrexia

Pyrogenic substances which are released by leukocytes at the site of tissue injury or pathogen invasion, act on the hypothalamic heat-regulating centers to reset the thermostatic controls to a higher level of internal temperature. Peripheral vasoconstriction reduces the circulation of blood to the superficial tissues, which allows the internal temperature to rise to a level that satisfies the thermostat setting. Shivering occurs as the skin temperature drops below that of the environment and the increased muscle activity produces internal heat. When the internal temperature reaches the thermostatic control level, sympathetic stimuli produce vasodilation and sweating to dissipate the excess heat. Temperature elevations above 42° C (107.6° F) are considered to be destructive to body tissues.

Pain Recognition, Localization, and Quantitation

Pain is a physiologic protective mechanism that provides a warning signal when tissues are injured. Spinal reflexes provide the motor nerve stimuli that lead to immediate withdrawal of peripheral tissues from noxious or destructive stimuli. Concurrent neural impulses transmitted to the cerebral tissues provide the recognition and discrimination patterns that produce the behavior patterns for avoidance of a similar pain-provoking stimulus.

Pain is a subjective experience that is highly personal and difficult to describe to another. When asked to quantitate the pain experience, the person may describe it as mild, severe, intolerable pain that occurs gradually, suddenly, intermittently, or persistently without relief. Those variables provide relatively clear-cut determinants of the amount of discomfort experienced by the individual.

Patients may characterize the pain as a dull ache, sharp or stabbing, burning, pressing, gnawing, or shooting. They can often pinpoint the location of the pain when it is in an extremity or superficial site. The organization of the nerve tracts from visceral sites sometimes makes localization difficult. The convergence of sensory fibers from one organ with those of other organs or with pain fibers from the skin may cause the pain to be referred to sites apart from the affected organ. For example, patients with angina pectoris have referred pain in the left arm, shoulder, and jaw.

The descriptions offered by the person are reflections of the way the pain is perceived by that individual. They also reflect the tolerance to pain, which in turn is affected by life experiences and factors in the immediate environment. Acute pain, or the fear of pain in persons conditioned by prior experiences, can distort the person's perceptions, judgments, and actions. For example, the person may cry uncontrollably or show cringing withdrawal behavior when a simple procedure is to be performed (i.e., intramuscular injection).

Pain Responses

Superficial Pain. Severe superficial pain precipitates sympathetic nerve stimulation that produces sweating, tachycardia, and an elevated blood pressure as a consequence of peripheral vasoconstriction. When those physiologic effects appear, they provide measurable parameters for evaluation of the pain status of the person. Con-

current generalized muscle tension, restlessness, facial expressions, or the refusal to change position can be evaluated to differentiate between pain-related sympathetic nerve activity and other factors that precipitate similar physiologic responses. In most situations, the patient's statement of discomfort and pain can be the primary clue, but the objective assessment is invaluable when planning care for the stoic person who seldom provides adequate information for evaluation of the pain status.

Deep Visceral Pain. Deep pain in the bones or in the abdominal or thoracic viscera is often described by the patient as dull, aching, or diffuse in character. The emission of impulses from the pain source, or trigger zone, can provide spinal reflex motor activity that causes muscle spasm, vasospasm, and profuse sweating, or *hyperhidrosis.* The analysis of pain in movable body parts at the conscious level may cause the individual to splint the part to reduce the painful stimulus that is caused by motion. Protracted periods of high-level sensory input can lead to long-lasting reflex disorders (i.e., contractures) that become added sources of pain, discomfort, or disability for the individual.

Disruption of physiologic processes is highest with deep visceral pain, and patients are often anorexic, weak, pale, nauseated, and sweating. Hypotension and bradycardia also are common problems. Chronic pain states can interfere with patterns of living, limit interpersonal relationships, distort reality, and cause psychologic abnormalities. It is not uncommon for those persons to reach the point where they question the value of their existence.

Analgesics

Analgesics in varying forms have been employed for centuries for the relief of pain. In most households there is a small supply of aspirin or acetaminophen (TYLENOL) that is used for control of pain or fever. In general, individ-

uals seek medical assistance for control of pain when the familiar remedies (i.e., an analgesic, rest, eating, cold or warm compresses) fail to relieve their pain.

DRUG THERAPY

There is considerable diversity in the pharmacologic agents that are employed for pain control. The selection of the drug is influenced by the cause, location, severity, and duration of the sensory stimulus and its effect on the individual's ability to function. Although drugs may be utilized as the only therapeutic measure, they are often prescribed as part of a multidimensional therapy plan for removing, modifying, or blocking the precipitating stimulus. Those measures can range from surgical intervention or the injection of a local anesthetic to the use of heat, massage, or splints. Physical, chemical, and pharmacologic agents are important aspects of pain control, but, from the sufferer's point of view, one of the most meaningful aspects is that something is being done to alleviate the discomfort. That aspect often contributes a great deal to the effectiveness of the adjunctive measures that are employed.

Analgesics are commonly employed for the control of existing pain or they may be used prior to pain-inducing procedures (i.e., dressing changes, surgical procedures). Some of the analgesics have properties (i.e., antipyretic, anti-inflammatory) that make them useful for alleviation of the basic pathophysiologic process in addition to modifying the discomfort caused by that problem. The analgesics include the *addictive analgesics,* which are utilized for the control of moderate to severe pain; *salicylates* and *nonsalicylate mild analgesics,* which are utilized for the control of mild to moderate pain; *anti-inflammatory analgesics,* which are employed for the control of gout or arthritic pain; and miscellaneous analgesics.

ADDICTIVE ANALGESICS

The drugs employed for the control of moderate to severe pain, with the exception of pentazocine, are narcotics, and their use is restricted by their inclusion as Schedule II Controlled Substances under the federal Comprehensive Drug Abuse Prevention and Control Act of 1970. That statute restricts their use because the drugs have a high potential for abuse, which may lead to severe psychologic or physical dependence. Although pentazocine has not been included under the restrictions of the statute, it also causes physical and psychologic dependence in some persons. The common characteristic of the drugs is the occurrence of a withdrawal, or abstinence, syndrome when use of the agent is interrupted.

The drugs are highly effective in the control of acute pain, and they frequently are prescribed pre- and postoperatively or during labor. They are also utilized for the control of pain for patients with myocardial infarction, pulmonary edema, and severe injuries. Their administration is usually prescribed as "p.r.n.," and their judicious use is based on assessment of the patient by the nurse prior to preparing the drug for administration.

The addictive analgesics are seldom employed as initial therapy for the control of pain in situations where their use predictably will be required for protracted periods of time (i.e., terminal cancer, multiple fractures). It is usual for those patients to receive a nonaddicting agent or a weaker narcotic when such agents provide pain relief. That plan of therapy allows use of the strong analgesics for episodes of acute pain unrelieved by the more regularly administered drugs. It also allows for the progression to the use of addictive analgesics when severe pain becomes more frequent. Whenever it is possible, regular around-the-clock administration of addicting analgesics is avoided. To provide the required pain relief, nonaddicting drugs may be alternated with the analgesics at irregularly spaced intervals when the patient has pain. That plan for interruption of regularly spaced administration of the narcotics lessens the addicting potential of the drugs and also reduces the incidence of tolerance to their analgesic effects.

Action Mode

The addictive analgesics include naturally occurring opioids, semisynthetic or synthetic agents with effects comparable to those of the prototype *morphine sulfate.* The drugs are thought to act at multiple cortical and subcortical receptors. The sensory cortex of the frontal lobes is a central nervous system drug action site that produces the analgesia without a concurrent loss of consciousness. The euphoria, mood changes, and mental-clouding effects of the drugs produce a state of indifference or an emotional detachment from the pain stimulus.

Concurrent with their analgesic effects, the drugs act on the pons and medulla and on the musculature of the eye and the gastrointestinal tract to produce effects other than the planned therapeutic effects. There is variation in the frequency, intensity, and duration of the problems caused by the drugs, but each strong analgesic has a potential for some disruption of physiologic function when it is employed for the alleviation of pain.

Adverse Effects

Respiratory Depression. The drug action on the respiratory control centers in the medulla decreases their sensitivity to the natural carbon dioxide stimulus. That action disrupts the normal respiratory rhythm and decreases the rate and depth of respirations. The retention of carbon dioxide produces cerebral vasodilation with a consequent increase in the blood flow to cerebral tissues and an increase in the production of cerebrospinal fluid. Those effects constitute a contraindication to the use of the addictive analgesics for patients with brain surgery or trauma. Elderly patients frequently have a marked decrease in the rate and depth of respirations when they receive the drugs. Because the drugs frequently cause respiratory depression, it is standard practice to withhold them when the pre-administration count of respirations is below 15/minute. Respiratory assistors or narcotic antagonists may be required when the respirations are severely depressed (i.e., <10/minute).

Cough Suppression. Depression of the cough centers of the medulla occurs during therapy with the drugs. Weaker narcotics (i.e., codeine sulfate) may be utilized for that antitussive property, and narcotics are included in some cough preparations. The retention of secretions consequent to a depressed cough reflex can adversely effect the respiratory status of an acutely ill individual who is receiving the addictive analgesics for pain relief.

Nausea. The initial irritating effects on the chemoreceptor trigger zone of the medullary vomiting center may precipitate vomiting, but the depressant effects on the center usually decrease that problem during subsequent drug administration. Nausea may be a persistent problem during therapy. Although the nausea may be partially related to a continued effect on the medullary centers, ambulatory patients may be nauseated as a consequence of the orthostatic hypotension and vestibular sensitivity caused by the drugs.

Hypotension. The hypotension that occurs in ambulatory patients may be partially related to the bradycardia and peripheral vasodilation that occur consequent to the action of the drug on the cardiac and vasomotor control centers of the medulla. The drug-induced histamine release may also contribute to the hypotension. Histamine release also produces flushing, pruritus, redness of the eyes, and sweating in some patients. Hypotension is evident when the patient rises to a sitting position after the analgesic is administered. It is a relatively common problem when patients are given an analgesic (i.e., meperidine hydrochloride) prior to being transferred from the surgical recovery room to the unit. The position changes involved in the movement from the stretcher to the bed often result in a drop in blood pressure as well as profuse perspiration and nausea. The patient's temperature may also be subnormal because the drugs decrease the hypothalamic response to impulses from the peripheral thermoreceptors.

Miosis. The opium alkaloids and their semi-synthetic derivatives (Table 25–1) produce contraction of the pupils, or miosis. They also in-

Table 25–1.
Analgesics Employed for Control of Moderate to Severe Pain

Drug	Route	Adult Dosage	Pain Relief Period Duration (hr)
Alphaprodine*† (NISENTIL)	SC	0.4–1.2 mg/kg	1.5–2
	IV	0.4–0.6 mg/kg	0.5–1
Anileridine*† (LERITINE)	Oral	25–50 mg	2–3
	SC/IM	25–100 mg	2–3
Fentanyl*† (SUBLIMAZE)	IM	0.05–1 mg	1–2
Hydromorphine*‡ (DILAUDID)	Oral	2 mg	4–5
	SC/IM } IV	1–4 mg	4–5
Levorphanol*† (LEVO-DROMORAN)	Oral	2–3 mg	4–5
	SC	2–3 mg	6–8
Meperidine*† (DEMEROL)	Oral } SC/IM	50–150 mg	2–4
Methadone*† (DOLOPHINE)	Oral	5–15 mg	3–5
	SC/IM	2.5–10 mg	4–6
Morphine*§	SC/IM	5–20 mg	4–5
	IV	2.5–15 mg	
Oxymorphone*‡ (NUMORPHAN)	SC/IM	1–1.5 mg	3–6
Opium alkaloids, concentrated*§ (PANTOPON)	SC/IM	5–20 mg	3–7
Pentazocine† (TALWIN)	Oral	50–100 mg	2–4
	SC/IM/IV	30–60 mg	2–3

* Narcotic.
† Synthetic addictive analgesics.
‡ Semisynthetic opium derivative.
§ Opium alkaloid.

crease accommodation and sensitivity to light and decrease intraocular pressure. Observations of pupil size ("pinpoint" pupils) are useful when monitoring the residual effects of the opioids before administering the drug. Meperidine and related agents have little effect on the pupils and sometimes cause dilation.

Auditory and Olfactory Acuity Losses. The addictive analgesics also affect auditory and olfactory nerve acuity. Although the slight depression of hearing may present few problems, the close interrelationship between smell and taste can have an adverse effect on the patient's desire to eat.

Smooth Muscle Tonus. Digestion of foods may be delayed or incomplete because the drugs slow gastric emptying and decrease the secretion of gastric and pancreatic enzymes and bile. The drugs also increase the tone of the smooth muscles of the gastrointestinal tract. The tonus inhibits the natural waves of peristalsis, and segments of the tract may periodically be in spasm. Constipation and gaseous distention are common problems when the drugs are utilized for pain relief.

A comparable effect on the musculature of the urinary tract may cause urine retention. The drugs increase the tone of the lower portions of the ureters, the detrusor muscle, and the vesicular sphincter. The tonus of the detrusor muscle may cause urgency in the patient who has received an analgesic, but the tonus of the vesicular sphincter may make voiding difficult. The tone of the ureters and the drug-induced release of antidiuretic hormone (ADH) from the pituitary gland decrease the bladder urine volume, and the urine output may be low.

The cholinergic effects on the gastrointestinal and urinary tract are usually evident when the opium alkaloids and their semisynthetic derivatives are administered. The synthetic analgesics (i.e., meperidine hydrochloride) may produce anticholinergic effects that cause dryness of the mouth, tachycardia, palpitations, muscle tremors, delirium, or hallucinations.

Interactions

The addictive analgesics may potentiate the central nervous system depressant effects of other drugs (i.e., general anesthetics, tranquilizers, sedatives, hypnotics, or alcohol). The drugs also enhance the effects of neuromuscular blocking agents and drugs with skeletal muscle relaxant properties (i.e., kanamycin).

Abstinence Syndrome

The physiologic problems of the addicted person often reflect the common adverse effects of the drug. The gastrointestinal effects cause loss of appetite, weight loss, marked constipation, coated tongue, and halitosis. Constricted pupils, tremors, and poor speech coordination reflect the central nervous system effects of the addictive analgesics.

The narcotics are commonly abused, and the chronic user gradually develops tolerance to the analgesia and euphoria and to some of the adverse effects of the drugs. The emergence of tolerance necessitates higher dosage to obtain the same analgesia and euphoria that formerly occurred with lower dosage. There is cross-tolerance to the narcotics, and the addict may use varying drug combinations to produce the desired effects. Withdrawal of the addictive analgesics causes an abstinence syndrome that varies in severity according to the quantity of the drug used and the duration of the drug abuse.

The abstinence syndrome, which may appear within 12 to 14 hours after the last dose of the drug, includes yawning, lacrimation, rhinorrhea, sneezing, and perspiration. Those problems become more severe, and there is a gradual onset of tremors, dilated pupils, and "gooseflesh." Within a period of 36 hours the person may have uncontrollable twitching of the muscles and cramps in the legs, abdomen, and back. Vomiting and diarrhea frequently appear, and there is elevation of the temperature, pulse, respirations, and blood pressure.

The painful physiologic disruptions reach a peak level in approximately 48 hours and may remain at that level for a 72-hour period. There is a gradual remission of the problems over the following five to ten days. The behavior of the person during the abstinence syndrome is an indication of the suffering imposed by abstinence (i.e., surly, pessimistic, fault finding, irritable, restless, impulsively destructive, or abusive).

Neonate Withdrawal Symptoms. Most newborn infants exhibit withdrawal symptoms when the mother is a narcotics addict. When the mother has abstained from taking the drug for a week prior to the labor period, the violent in utero kicking of the fetus is an indication of its withdrawal status. After delivery that infant may be asymptomatic.

Many addicted mothers take a large dose of the drug at the onset of labor, and their infants usually have respiratory distress at the time of birth. Additional problems in the neonatal addict may appear within the first 24 hours after birth. Overt signs of withdrawal include yawning, sneezing, stretching, sweating, nasal stuffiness, and lacrimation.

The infants usually are described as "jittery" or "jumpy." Central nervous system irritability in the infants causes restlessness, inability to sleep, excessively shrill crying when slightly disturbed or when hungry, rigid muscles, markedly hyperactive reflexes, muscle tremors when undisturbed, and respirations at the rate of 76 to 95/minute.

The infants often have a low birth weight. They may suck on their fists as though starving, but they nurse or take their formula poorly. Their nutritional status is jeopardized further by vomiting, regurgitation, and explosive diarrhea that may occur more than eight times a day. Dehydration, emaciation, and excoriation of the skin caused by thrashing movements (i.e., nose, ears, bony prominences) are common problems. Hyperpyrexia may accompany severe withdrawal symptoms.

Treatment of the infants requires control of the symptoms and administration and gradual withdrawal of weak narcotics. The addiction is a physiologic problem without a psychologic component, and that facilitates control of the addiction of the surviving infants.

Opium Alkaloids

Morphine sulfate and *opium alkaloids, concentrated,* are the opium alkaloids employed for control of moderate to severe pain. Other opium alkaloids are utilized for control of lesser pain, diarrhea, or cough. The semisynthetic opium alkaloids are *hydromorphone* and *oxymorphone.*

Morphine Sulfate. The drug is the most frequently prescribed agent for control of severe pain. The usual routes for administration are subcutaneous or intramuscular injection, but it may be administered intravenously for an immediate effect in selected acute situations.

The peak analgesic effect varies with the route of administration, but the onset of action occurs within 20 minutes. Subcutaneous injection of morphine provides a peak analgesic effect within 50 to 90 minutes; intramuscular injection, within 30 to 90 minutes; and intravenous injection, within 20 minutes. The duration of analgesia ranges from four to seven hours.

The effect on respirations also reflects the varying absorption rates from the injection sites. Subcutaneous administration of morphine produces a maximum depressant effect on respirations in 90 minutes; intramuscular injection, within 30 minutes; and intravenous administration, within seven minutes. The duration of respiratory effects is two to three hours. The predictable effects on respirations serve as a guide for monitoring patients who have borderline respiration rates (<15/minute)

at the time of drug administration. Administration of oxygen and use of respiratory assistors may be required when the patient has a marked decrease in respiratory rate after administration of the drug.

The drug is often prescribed for administration "as required" (p.r.n.) at four-hour intervals. The dosage for adults varies with the intensity of the pain (Table 25–1). The subcutaneous dosage for children is calculated on the basis of 100 to 200 mcg/kg of body weight to a maximum dosage of 15 mg.

Opium Alkaloids, Concentrated. The drug (PANTOPON) represents a concentration of the opium alkaloids as they occur naturally. The hydrochloride preparation employed for control of moderate to severe pain contains 50 percent anhydrous morphine, and the drug is administered parenterally (Table 25–1). The peak analgesic effects and the duration of action are similar to those of morphine.

Hydromorphone Hydrochloride. The primary advantage of the semisynthetic opium derivative is that the dose can be administered orally, parenterally, or as a rectal suppository (3 mg) for the control of pain (Table 25–1). Although there is some variation according to the route of administration, the usual onset of analgesic action is within 15 to 30 minutes after administration. That effect peaks in 30 to 90 minutes and is maintained for four to five hours.

Nausea, vomiting, constipation, and euphoria occur somewhat less frequently with the use of hydromorphone than with morphine. *Hydromorphone hydrochloride* is available in forms for administration orally, subcutaneously, intramuscularly, intravenously, or rectally. *Hydromorphone sulfate* is available for administration parenterally (SC, IM, IV). During the slow intravenous infusion of the drug, the patient's respirations and blood pressure are monitored frequently.

Oxymorphone Hydrochloride. The semisynthetic opium alkaloid is administered parenterally, or the dosage (2 to 5 mg) may be administered by rectal suppository (Table 25–1). Although it less frequently causes constipation, it more frequently causes nausea, vomiting, and euphoria than does morphine.

The rectal suppository provides an onset of analgesic action within 15 to 30 minutes; subcutaneous or intramuscular injection, within 5 to 10 minutes; and intravenous injection, within two to five minutes. The intravenous dosage is 500 mcg, which may be increased gradually to attain analgesia. The duration of action when the drug is administered parenterally ranges from three to six hours (Table 25–1).

Synthetic Addictive Analgesics

The synthetic analgesics include *levorphanol, meperidine, alphaprodine, anileridine, fentanyl, methadone,* and *pentazocine* (Table 25–1). The actions and adverse effects of the drugs are comparable to those of morphine. Levorphanol is closely related in chemical structure to the opium alkaloids. Alphaprodine, anileridine, fentanyl, and meperidine have a similar *phenylpiperidine* chemical structure.

Levorphanol Tartrate. The drug is administered orally or subcutaneously for control of moderate to severe pain. It produces less nausea, vomiting, and constipation but more sedation and smooth muscle stimulation than does morphine. Subcutaneous administration of levorphanol produces an initial effect within 60 minutes and a peak effect within 60 to 90 minutes. The analgesia lasts approximately six to eight hours.

Meperidine Hydrochloride. The drug is commonly employed for the control of moderate to severe pain. It produces approximately the same degree of respiratory depression as that of morphine, but the depression may be somewhat shorter in duration. At the dosage level employed for analgesia, meperidine produces antitussive effects. It has no appreciable effects on gastrointestinal motility and seldom causes constipation. The drug causes corneal anesthesia that decreases the corneal reflex. Particles can collect on the cornea (i.e., dust) in the absence of the natural protective blinking reflex.

The analgesia produced by the oral drug may be less than one half that attained by parenteral administration, but the ease of administration makes the oral drug useful for ambulatory patients. The orally administered drug produces a peak analgesic effect within one hour that lasts for two to four hours. When the oral syrup is utilized for oral administration, it is diluted in 120 ml (4 oz) of water to avoid the slight topical anesthesia of the mucous membranes that is caused by the syrup.

Meperidine can be injected subcutaneously or intramuscularly, but the irritation and inflammation of subcutaneous tissues caused by the drug make the intramuscular injection the favored method of administration. The peak analgesic effect is attained within 40 to 60 minutes after subcutaneous injection and within 30 to 50 minutes after intramuscular injection of the drug. The duration of analgesia is similar to that attained with the use of the oral drug (two to four hours).

The drug may be administered every three to four hours for control of pain (Table 25–1). The dosage for children is calculated on the basis of 1 to 1.8 mg/kg of body weight to a maximum of 100 mg when the drug is to be given orally, subcutaneously or intramuscularly. The drug is a weak base, and the excretion rate is higher when the urine is acid than when it is slightly alkaline.

Concurrent administration of a monoamine oxidase inhibitor may cause central nervous system stimulation with sweating, rigidity, and hypotension or hypertension that can be fatal. When meperidine is administered with atropine sulfate, the interaction at receptor sites enhances the effect of the atropine.

Meperidine (50 to 150 mg) may be administered slowly as a well-diluted intravenous injection in emergency situations when immediate analgesia is required. Respiratory support equipment should be available when the drug is administered intravenously.

Alphaprodine Hydrochloride. The drug produces an analgesic effect within five to ten minutes after subcutaneous injection and within one to two minutes after the dosage is administered intravenously (Table 25–1). The onset of action is more rapid but the duration of the analgesic effect is shorter than that of meperidine.

Anileridine. The drug has antitussive activity in addition to its analgesic action. Like meperidine, the drug produces little constipation. It produces nausea and vomiting more frequently than does meperidine. It causes less sedation, and the depression of respirations is shorter than that caused by meperidine. The analgesic effects occur within 15 minutes after the drug is absorbed from the oral, subcutaneous, or intramuscular administration routes.

Anileridine hydrochloride is administered orally. *Anileridine phosphate* is available in solution for parenteral administration. The drug may occasionally be administered as a slow intravenous injection in emergency situations when an immediate analgesic action is required.

Fentanyl Citrate. The drug is frequently administered intravenously during the induction and maintenance of anesthesia. Intravenous injection of the drug frequently produces muscle rigidity that interferes with expansion of the thoracic cage and causes bronchospasm, laryngospasm, or apnea.

The short duration of action of fentanyl limits its usefulness for recurring pain. When it is administered intramuscularly (Table 25–1) for control of acute pain, patients frequently complain of pain at the injection site. Like the opium alkaloids, the drug may cause miosis. The incidence of nausea is lower with use of fentanyl than with use of the opium alkaloids.

Methadone Hydrochloride. The drug is employed for control of pain, and it is widely used in FDA-approved maintenance programs for narcotic addicts. In those programs the drug is employed to convert the drug habit from drug injection to the less health-threatening oral route of drug use. Concurrent therapies (i.e., psychosocial) are planned to assist the addict with efforts toward rehabilitation.

The absorbed drug becomes firmly bound to tissue proteins, and the cumulative effects can produce sedation when the drug is administered regularly. Repeated oral use (i.e., methadone maintenance therapy) provides a prolonged period of action (i.e., 22 to 48 hours). The central nervous system effects (i.e., respiratory depression) may continue for 48 hours after an overdose of the drug.

Methadone has antitussive activity in addition to its analgesic action. The drug produces less euphoria and constipation but a somewhat greater degree of respiratory depression than the opiates. The onset of action of the parenterally administered drug is similar to that of morphine. The duration of action of a single oral dose ranges from three to five hours and that of a parenteral dose from four to six hours (Table 25–1).

Pentazocine. The drug is a nonnarcotic analgesic. It has a weak narcotic antagonist action in addition to its analgesic activity. That property limits the periodic use of the drug with narcotic analgesics for the control of chronic pain because the introduction of pentazocine into the plan can cause withdrawal symptoms. Although long-term use of the drug causes physiologic and psychologic dependence, its addicting potential is considerably less than that of the other addictive analgesics. The drug produces less respiratory depression, but the hypnotic effects and suppression of gastrointestinal motility are similar to those produced by morphine.

The oral drug is slowly absorbed from the intestinal tract, and analgesia is attained much later and persists longer than that attained with parenteral administration (Table 25–1). Subcutaneous or intramuscular injection of the drug can cause tissue irritation, and prolonged use of the drug can cause ulceration, necrosis, or fibrosis of the tissues. Parenteral injections provide an analgesic effect within 10 to 30 minutes, and that effect lasts for two to three hours. The short duration of analgesia necessitates administration of the parenteral drug at three-hour intervals for control of persistent pain.

Cross-tolerance between pentazocine and the other addictive analgesics occurs infrequently. That probably is related to the chemical structure, which is different from that of other analgesics. The drug causes adverse effects similar to those of the opium alkaloids. It may also produce severe neuropsychiatric effects (i.e., confusion, hallucinations, bizarre dreams, depression, nervousness, agitation, extreme euphoria, psychosis). Appearance of the behavioral problems necessitates cessation of therapy with the drug.

Pentazocine hydrochloride is the drug form for oral administration. *Pentazocine lactate* is employed for the subcutaneous or intramuscular injections.

Narcotic Antagonists

The drugs are employed to counteract the severe respiratory depression that is produced by excess doses of narcotic analgesics. The narcotic antagonists are *naloxone hydrochloride, levallorphan tartrate,* and *nalorphine hydrochloride.*

Action Mode. The drugs compete with the narcotic analgesics at central nervous system receptors to decrease the respiratory depression, coma, and convulsions that are caused by the narcotics. They also antagonize the cardiovascular, gastrointestinal, analgesia, and pupillary responses that are produced by the analgesics.

The action of the drugs on the respiratory center receptors in the medulla lowers the threshold for the carbon dioxide stimulus to respiration. There is an increase in the respiratory rate and minute volume, and the blood carbon dioxide levels are decreased.

Therapy Considerations. The drugs are utilized primarily for treatment of individuals who have narcotic-induced respiratory depression. Small doses are used to avoid the withdrawal symptoms that can be precipitated when the drugs are given to a narcotic-dependent individual. When the duration of action of the narcotic is longer than that of the narcotic antagonist, respiratory depression can recur unless an additional dose of the narcotic antagonist is administered.

The antagonists may be given intravenously to the mother before the delivery of her infant when it is evident that she has recently taken a narcotic. The drug is more frequently injected into the umbilical vein when there is respiratory depression in the narcotic addict's newborn infant.

Naloxone, the newest of the narcotic antagonists, is the drug of choice for treatment of suspected narcotic-induced respiratory depression. Unlike the other antagonists, it is also effective in counteracting the effects of pentazocine. It has no agonist properties and does not cause respiratory depression.

Nalorphine and *levallorphan* have similar antagonist actions and also have agonist activities. In the absence of a narcotic their agonist properties produce morphine-like effects.

Naloxone Hydrochloride (NARCAN). The drug is administered parenterally. The intravenous route is used in emergency situations. The initial intravenous dose for adults is 400 mcg, and that dose may be repeated at two-to-three-minute intervals when necessary. Children may receive an initial dose of 10 mcg, which may be repeated at two-to-three-minute intervals. When respiratory depression persists after three doses, it is considered that a factor other than a narcotic or pentazocine is causing the problem.

The dosage for narcotic-induced respiratory depression in the newborn is 10 mcg/kg of body weight, and that dose is injected into the umbilical vein of the infant. The dosage may be repeated at two-to-three-minute intervals.

Naloxone and methadone (METHENEX) are available in a tablet form that is used in narcotic withdrawal programs. The naloxone is rapidly metabolized when the oral tablet is taken, and it has no effect on respirations. When the person dissolves the tablet and injects the drug, the action of naloxone counteracts the effects of the methadone and may produce withdrawal symptoms in the addict. The tablet is a useful deterrent to the injection of methadone.

The onset of action of the drug occurs within one to two minutes after intravenous administration and within two to five minutes after subcutaneous or intramuscular injection of the drug. The duration of action following intravenous injection is approximately 45 minutes. The drug crosses the placental barrier.

Naloxone is rapidly metabolized in the liver. Approximately 60 to 70 percent of the drug is excreted within 72 hours after it is injected.

Tremor and hyperventilation may be associated with the abrupt return to consciousness after the drug has been administered for narcotic overdosage. There are few reports of adverse effects when the drug is given at the therapeutic dosage level.

Levallorphan Tartrate (LORFAN). The drug usually is administered intravenously but can also be administered by subcutaneous or intramuscular injection. The initial dosage for adults with narcotic-induced respiratory depression is 1 mg. One to three additional doses of 500 mcg to 1 mg may be given at 10-to-15-minute intervals to a maximum total dose of 3 mg. The initial dose for children is based on the calculation of 20 mcg/kg of body weight. The subsequent dose, which may be administered in 10 to 15 minutes, is based on the calculation of 10 to 20 mcg/kg of body weight.

The dosage for the treatment of narcotic-induced respiratory depression in the newborn is based on the calculation of 20 mcg/kg of body weight, and that dosage is diluted to 2 ml with isotonic sodium chloride for injection into the umbilical vein of the infant. The dosage is repeated in five to ten minutes if necessary.

The effects of the drug on narcotic-induced respiratory depression are evident within one to two minutes after it is injected intravenously. The duration of action is two to five hours. Acute withdrawal symptoms may be precipitated in narcotic-dependent persons within 5 to 15 minutes after the drug is injected subcutaneously. The drug crosses the placenta.

The drug can produce effects similar to those of morphine when the respiratory depression is unrelated to narcotics. There may be analgesia,

respiratory depression, sedation, moderate bradycardia, slight decrease in systolic blood pressure, and miosis. The drug can also produce anxiety, transient dysphoria or hallucinations. The adverse effects that occasionally occur are sweating, dizziness, lethargy, pallor, nausea, gastric upset, and a sense of heaviness in the limbs. Irritability and increased crying may appear in neonates.

Nalorphine Hydrochloride (NALLINE). The drug is administered parenterally. The initial adult intravenous dose is 5 to 10 mg; additional doses may be given at 10-to-15-minute intervals to a maximum of three doses. Children may receive an initial dose of 100 mcg/kg of body weight intravenously or intramuscularly, and that dose may be repeated in 15 minutes if necessary.

The dosage for narcotic-induced respiratory depression in the newborn is 200 to 500 mcg, and that amount is diluted with isotonic sodium chloride for injection into the umbilical vein of the infant. The same dosage can be used for subcutaneous or intramuscular injection.

When the person has narcotic-induced respiratory depression, the drug effects are apparent within one to two minutes after parenteral administration. The duration of action is 1.5 to 4 hours. The drug precipitates acute withdrawal symptoms within 5 to 20 minutes after it is administered subcutaneously to narcotic-dependent persons. The drug readily crosses the placenta.

The agonist activity of the drug may produce effects similar to those of morphine or levallorphan when the respiratory depression is not related to narcotics. Adverse effects of nalorphine are similar to those produced by levallorphan.

SALICYLATES

The salicylates are synthetic derivatives of *salicylic acid*. The drugs are hydrolyzed to salicylic acid before absorption from the gastrointestinal tract. The parent compound is a component in ointments or lotions, and the pleasant wintergreen-smelling counterirritant is briskly massaged into the skin to provide the heat required for relief of muscle or joint pains.

The oral salicylates may be prescribed for control of pain or hyperpyrexia, but they are readily available as nonprescription over-the-counter (OTC) drugs. There are more than 100 clearly identified salicylates and 300 OTC preparations that contain salicylates. Selection of a particular salicylate for pain or temperature control is often based on the personal preference of the purchaser. That preference may be affected by the gastric irritation caused by some formulations, or it may be influenced by advertising claims of differences in solubility and effectiveness.

Action Mode

The salicylates have antipyretic, analgesic, anti-inflammatory, and antirheumatic activity. The antipyretic action of the salicylates results from lowering of the central hypothalamic thermostat level. That lower setting provides the stimulus for peripheral vasodilation and the increased peripheral blood flow required for heat dissipation from the skin surface. The concurrent increase in sweating accelerates heat dissipation. The antipyretic action of the salicylates is rapid and effective in most febrile persons.

The salicylates provide pain relief by a selective depressant action at subcortical brain sites. Their effectiveness in relief of headache, myalgia, and arthralgia is related, at least partially, to the blocking of prostaglandin synthesis at sites of inflammation or irritation.

Therapy Considerations

The salicylates are administered orally (Table 25–2). The drug is dissolved and partially absorbed in the stomach, and the remainder is rapidly absorbed from the small intestine. Approximately 50 to 80 percent of the circulating drug is bound to plasma proteins. The drug is rapidly distributed to all body tissues. Peak plasma drug concentrations are attained within one to two hours, and the levels are maintained for four to six hours. The salicylates are hydrolyzed in the liver and the metabolites are excreted in the urine. There may be minor changes in the color of the urine and a false positive reaction when Benedict's Qualitative Reagent is utilized for tests of glycosuria.

The antipyretic effect of the drug is beneficial when there is a temperature elevation. Maintenance of a relatively normal temperature during round-the-clock administration for control of pain or inflammation can concurrently control fever that provides the warning sign when there is an infection.

The serum drug concentration required for an

Table 25–2.
Dosage of Salicylates Employed to Control Pain or Hypyrexia

Drug	Adult (gm)	Child	Number of Divided Doses
Aspirin (acetylsalicylic acid)	2.4–5.2	14–100 mg/kg	4–6
Aluminum aspirin	—	600–900 mg	4–6
Calcium carbaspirin (CALURIN)	1.8–3.6	1.2–2.4 gm*	6
Carbethyl salicylate (SAL-ETHYL CARBONATE)	2.4–3.6	14–100 mg/kg	4–6
Choline salicylate (ARTHROPAN)	3.4–7.7	0.63–2.52 gm	6
Magnesium salicylate (MAGAN)	1.8–4.8	14–100 mg/kg	4–6
Salicylamide (AMID-SAL, SALRIN)	1.4–3.6	14–100 mg/kg	4–6
Salsalate (DISALCID)	2.4–3.6	14–100 mg/kg	4–6
Sodium salicylate	1.4–3.9	14–100 mg/kg	4–6

* Dosage for 6-to-12-year-olds.

optimum anti-inflammatory effect may overlap with that at which ototoxicity occurs. It is common practice for the dosage level of the salicylate to be increased gradually to that producing tinnitus, or a buzzing, tingling sensation in the head that persists for five minutes. The dosage is then adjusted downward (i.e., <600 mg) for maintenance dosage at the subtinnitus level. Elderly persons have a decreased ability to hear high-frequency tones (i.e., tinnitus), and the serum drug levels are utilized as guides to their dosage adjustments and for other individuals with high-frequency hearing loss. The serum drug levels required for treatment of rheumatoid arthritis range from 15 to 30 mg/ml. At that therapeutic range, the ototoxicity causes a 20-to-30-decibel hearing loss in most patients receiving an adequate anti-inflammatory dose of the salicylates. The hearing loss does not affect the ability to hear normal conversational tones and is reversible when therapy is terminated.

Each of the drugs included in Table 25–2 has an analgesic effect equivalent to that of aspirin. Although salicylamide is chemically similar to aspirin, it is much less effective as an antipyretic agent than aspirin and the other salicylates. Salicylamide provides an alternate drug for control of pain or inflammation when patients are allergic to aspirin.

Sodium salicylate (Table 25–2) also is available as a solution for intravenous administration. It seldom is necessary to administer the salicylates parenterally because the drugs are available in the form of rectal suppositories that provide effective control of hypyrexia or pain in patients who are unable to take oral drugs. The suppositories are irritating to the rectal mucosa when they are employed at frequent intervals.

Adverse Effects

Gastric Irritation. The drugs often cause epigastric distress or painless occult bleeding by their irritating effects on the gastric mucosa. Retention of drug particles in the convolutions, or *rugae,* of the stomach contributes to the irritating effects of the salicylates. Compounds with small particles cause less irritation. The gastric irritation can be modified by administration of the drug shortly after meals, with a snack or a full glass of milk or water. Gastric irritation is common when the drugs are taken in large doses on a regularly scheduled basis or when other drugs having ulcerogenic effects (i.e., glucocorticoids) are administered concurrently. It is usual to test the stools for occult blood content (i.e., guaiac testing) when individuals are receiving the aspirin under those circumstances.

It is estimated that 70 percent of the patients have occult bleeding during therapy with aspirin, and the average blood loss is approximately 4 ml/day. Persons are instructed to inform their physician when the stools are black or when gastric distress is persistent (i.e., epigastric pain, decreased tolerance to familiar foods, eructation). The enteric-coated formulations may be employed to allow continuance of therapy.

Buffered formulations may shorten the dissolution time of the salicylates by increasing the pH at the surface of the drug particles. The reduced quantity of undissolved particles in the stomach may lessen gastric irritation. The sodium content of some buffered tablets must be considered when the individual's sodium intake is to be restricted. For example, ALKA-SELTZER contains 521 mg of sodium per tablet.

Nausea and Vomiting. Gastric disturbances may be caused by vagus nerve stimulation that is precipitated by irritation of receptors in the gastric mucosa. The salicylates also cause nausea and vomiting by their irritating effects on the chemoreceptor trigger zone of the vomiting center in the medulla.

Allergic Reactions. Anaphylactic reactions have occurred during therapy with the salicylates. Reactions commonly are asthmatic in character, and the decreased ventilation can be life threatening. The drugs are not given to children or adults with a history of asthma, hay fever, or nasal polyps. Skin rashes may also appear during therapy with the salicylates.

Bleeding Time Prolongation. Aspirin is the only salicylate identified as decreasing the adhesiveness of platelets thereby prolonging the bleeding time. The concurrent use of anticoagulants requires frequent monitoring of the coagulation status of the patient.

At therapeutic dosage levels the salicylates inhibit the renal tubule secretion of urates. That action may increase the plasma levels of those metabolic wastes.

Salicylism. Large dosage or prolonged therapy with salicylates can cause toxicity, or *salicylism.* Mild salicylate poisoning is characterized by headache, dizziness, tinnitus, dimness of vision, confusion, lassitude, drowsiness, sweating, thirst, nausea, vomiting, diarrhea, hyperventilation, and tachycardia.

Acute salicylate poisoning causes rapid progression of the same symptoms and evidence of cerebral hyperactivity (i.e., excitement, talkativeness, incoherent speech, restlessness, hallucinations, convulsions). The symptoms progress to increased central nervous system depression, stupor, and coma. The outcome is fatal when the problems progress to cardiovascular collapse, respiratory insufficiency, and convulsions. Treatment of toxicity is symptomatic. Hemodialysis may be performed to remove the excess drug when serum levels are high.

The incidence of accidental ingestion and associated toxicity in children has decreased appreciably since the introduction of the "childproof" cap on drug bottles. Persons who are taking the drugs for arthritis have the prerogative of requesting that the drug be in bottles with standard caps when they have difficulty manipulating the newer closures. Those persons should be reminded to keep the drugs out of the reach of children who may enter the household.

Interactions

The salicylates can displace drugs from their plasma protein-binding sites and enhance their therapeutic effect. Salicylates compete for binding sites with the oral anticoagulants, sulfonyl-ureas, methotrexate, penicillin, and phenytoin. The salicylates also antagonize the uricosuric activity of probenecid and sulfinpyrazone by competing for their renal tubule sites of activity.

NONSALICYLATE MILD ANALGESICS

The group of drugs identified as nonsalicylates include drugs that are employed primarily for the control of mild to moderate pain. The drugs are used alone or in combination with salicylates for pain relief. They also provide effective therapy for persons who are hypersensitive to salicylates or for whom those drugs are contraindicated.

Acetaminophen, phenacetin, codeine, etho-heptazine citrate, mefenamic acid, and propoxy-phene are drugs employed primarily for their analgesic activity. The drugs may be utilized for short-term control of pain or they may be used intermittently with stronger analgesics for treatment of chronic pain.

Acetaminophen

The drug is one of the most frequently used agents for the control of pain or hyperpyrexia. It is a valuable alternate drug for persons for whom salicylates are contraindicated. For example, individuals with a history of peptic ulcers or allergies and persons who are taking oral anticoagulants benefit from the availability of acetaminophen.

Action Mode. Like the salicylates, acetaminophen acts at subcortical sites to interrupt the neural stimuli that travel to cortical areas of the brain. The antipyretic activity is produced by depression of the hypothalamic temperature control centers. That action lowers the thermostatic setting, and the subsequent release of autonomic nervous system stimuli causes vasodilation and increased peripheral blood flow.

Therapy Considerations. The drug is rapidly absorbed from the gastrointestinal tract. Peak serum drug levels are attained within 10 to 60 minutes, and the drug has a plasma half-life of 75 minutes. Approximately 25 percent of the circulating drug is bound to plasma proteins. The drug is rapidly distributed to body tissues and fluids.

Acetaminophen is metabolized in the liver. One of the metabolites, *para-aminophenol,* can cause methemoglobinemia, but there have been no reports of that problem. Most of the drug (85 percent) is excreted by the kidneys as the glucuronide within 24 hours after ingestion.

Adverse Effects. Acetaminophen is relatively nontoxic at therapeutic dosage levels (Table 25–3). Hepatic necrosis and death have occurred with overdosage (i.e., >10 gm). Treatment of toxicity is symptomatic, and supportive measures are employed for the maintenance of the respiratory, fluid, and electrolyte status of the person.

Phenacetin

The drug, like acetaminophen, is a *para-aminophenol* derivative, and it has the same actions and therapeutic indications as that drug. Phenacetin infrequently is used alone but it is a component of several compounds that are employed for the control of pain (i.e., aspirin, phenacetin, and caffeine, EMPIRIN COMPOUND).

Therapy Considerations. The drug is rapidly absorbed from the gastrointestinal tract, and peak plasma levels are attained in one to two hours. The drug has a plasma half-life of 45 to 90 minutes. Approximately 25 percent of the circulating drug is bound to plasma proteins. Although phenacetin is widely distributed in body tissues it passes less freely into the cerebrospinal fluid than acetaminophen.

Hepatic metabolism by the microsomal enzymes produces the active metabolite *acetaminophen.* That metabolite provides most of the activity of the drug, but the unchanged drug may also contribute to the antipyretic and analgesic effects. A small amount of the drug is converted to *N-hydroxyphenetidin,* which can cause methemoglobinemia. Persons with a genetic deficiency of the hepatic enzymes required for conversion of the drug to acetaminophen may have an excess production of the methemoglobin-inducing metabolite. Approximately 66 percent of the unchanged drug and its metabolites are excreted in the urine within 24 hours.

Adverse Effects. The drug can induce changes in hemoglobin and in the sulfhydryl groups that destroy the erythrocytes. That effect on the red

Table 25–3.

Nonsalicylates Employed for Control of Mild to Moderate Pain

Drug	Route	Dosage			Other Properties	
		Adult (Single Dose) (mg)	Child	Number of Doses Daily	Anti-pyretic	Anti-inflammatory
Acetaminophen (DATRIL	Oral	325–650	162.5–325 mg†	6	+	0
LIQUIPRIN, NEBS, TEMPRA)	Rectal	125–600		3–4		
Codeine*	Oral ⎫					
	SC ⎬	30–60	3 mg/kg	4–6	0	0
	IM ⎭					
Ethoheptazine citrate						
(ZACTANE)	Oral	75–150	—	3–4	0	0
Mefenamic acid						
(PONSTEL)	Oral	250–500	—	4	+	+
Propoxyphene (DARVON,						
DOLENE)	Oral	65–100		4–6	0	0

* Narcotic.
† Dosage for 7-to-12-year-olds.

blood cells and the associated hemolytic anemia occur most frequently in individuals with a deficiency of the enzyme *glucose-6-phosphate dehydrogenase* (G-6-PD). Renal damage has been associated with prolonged chronic use.

Codeine

The drug, a narcotic that is derived from opium, is a Schedule II Controlled Substance. It is employed for the control of mild to moderate pain and is also useful alone or as a component of cough mixtures to suppress persistent nonproductive cough. Although the drug has actions and adverse effects similar to those of the addictive analgesics that are employed for severe pain, the usual analgesic dosage causes few problems.

Therapy Considerations. The drug is often administered orally (Table 25–3), and the oral tablet is well absorbed from the intestine. Although parenteral administration provides approximately one third more analgesia, the onset of action (15 to 30 minutes) and action duration (four to six hours) are similar when the drug is administered by the oral or subcutaneous routes. The drug is metabolized in the liver, and the conjugates are excreted in the urine.

Codeine phosphate is available in forms for oral or parenteral administration and *codeine sulfate* is administered orally. The oral drug commonly is administered with aspirin; the difference in the mechanisms of action of the two drugs provides an additive analgesic effect. Codeine is also available in combination with a variety of other drugs that are prescribed for pain control. Oxycodone, a synthetic derivative similar to codeine, is also available as a component of compounds that are utilized for the control of mild to moderate pain (i.e., oxycodone, aspirin, phenacetin, and caffeine PERCODAN).

Adverse Effects. The most common problems during therapy with codeine are nausea and persistent itching in the perinasal tissues, which sometimes necessitate termination of therapy. The drug has an addiction potential, but it is not one of the commonly abused drugs. The same precautions against regularly scheduled long-term administration should be observed with the use of codeine as with other addictive analgesics.

Ethoheptazine Citrate

The drug is chemically related to meperidine, but it lacks the addictive potential of that drug. The drug (Table 25–3) infrequently is employed alone for control of pain but is a component in compounds containing aspirin (ZACTIRIN) or other analgesics.

Gastrointestinal disturbances (i.e., nausea, vomiting, epigastric distress), dizziness, or pruritus may occur during therapy. When combination tablets are employed, the adverse effects of each of the components of the formulation must be considered.

Mefenamic Acid

The drug has analgesic, antipyretic, and anti-inflammatory activity (Table 25–3). It is infrequently utilized for the control of pain but provides effective control of mild to moderate pain in selected acute situations. It is also employed for its anti-inflammatory effects.

Therapy Considerations. The drug is absorbed slowly from the intestinal tract. Peak plasma drug levels are attained within two to four hours, and the analgesia persists for six hours. The drug is metabolized in the liver. Approximately 50 percent of the unchanged drug or its metabolites are excreted in the urine within 24 hours. Some of the drug is also excreted in the feces.

Adverse Effects. The most common adverse effects are gastrointestinal disturbances (i.e., nausea, vomiting, dyspepsia, constipation). Those problems can be modified by administration of the drug with meals. Diarrhea occurs with prolonged use or high dosage, and the problem may persist until therapy with the drug is terminated. Therapy is also discontinued when there is evidence of an allergic reaction (i.e., facial edema, dyspnea, urticaria).

Neurologic effects include drowsiness, dizziness, vertigo, nervousness, or headache. Reduction of the dosage may alleviate the problems, but persistent neurologic problems necessitate cessation of therapy.

Interactions.   The gastric irritation of the drug can potentiate the ulcerogenic effects of other drugs (i.e., glucocorticoids, phenylbutazone, indomethacin, salicylates). The drug may also increase the hypoprothrombinemia of patients who are receiving oral anticoagulants concurrent with mefenamic acid. The insulin requirements of diabetic patients are reported to be increased during therapy with mefenamic acid.

Propoxyphene

The drug is a synthetic analgesic structurally similar to methadone. The high incidence of propoxyphene abuse led to its inclusion as a Schedule IV Controlled Substance in 1977. That designation identifies a low potential for abuse that can cause physical or psychologic dependence.

Action Mode.   The drug is employed for its effective control of mild to moderate pain. The site of action is thought to be similar to that of the addictive analgesics, which interfere with transmission of the pain stimulus to the cortical areas of the brain.

Therapy Considerations.   The drug is available as *propoxyphene hydrochloride* and as *propoxyphene napsylate* for oral administration. Both forms are also available in combination tablets containing salicylates or other analgesics. The usual dosage of propoxyphene hydrochloride is 65 mg and that of propoxyphene napsylate is 100 mg (Table 25–3).

The oral drug is absorbed from the upper segments of the small intestine, and analgesia is attained within 15 to 60 minutes. Peak plasma drug levels are attained within two to three hours; the analgesic effect persists for four to six hours. The serum half-life of propoxyphene is 12 hours. The drug is widely distributed in body fluids and it enters the cerebrospinal fluid.

The drug is metabolized in the liver. Approximately 25 percent of the unchanged drug and the metabolites are excreted in the urine within 48 hours after the drug is administered.

Adverse Effects.   The central nervous system effects that may occur during therapy include dizziness, headache, sedation, somnolence, insomnia, and paradoxic excitement. Propoxyphene may also cause skin rashes and gastrointestinal disturbances (i.e., nausea, vomiting, abdominal pain, constipation). The symptoms of overdosage are similar to those that occur with addictive analgesic drug toxicity, but convulsions appear more frequently with overdoses of propoxyphene than with the narcotics.

ANTI-INFLAMMATORY ANALGESICS

The drugs employed for the control of arthritic pain also have anti-inflammatory activity. With the exception of colchicine, the drugs have antipyretic activity, but they are seldom employed for the control of fever (Table 25–4). The drugs include *colchicine, hydroxychloroquine sulfate, gold compounds,* and drugs that are structurally similar, as well as pyrazolone and arylacetic acid derivatives. The pyrazolone derivatives include *phenylbutazone, oxyphenbutazone,* and *dipyrone,* which are structurally and pharmacologically related drugs. The arylacetic acid derivatives include two groups of pharmacologically related drugs: *fenoprofen calcium, ibuprofen,* and *naproxen,* which are closely related, and *indomethacin* and *tometin sodium,* which are pharmacologically similar.

Action Mode

The clinical effectiveness of the drugs has been established, but the physiologic basis for their effects remains unclear. Blocking of the synthesis

Table 25–4.

Drugs Employed for Control of Gout and Arthritic Pain

Drug	Route	Dosage Adult Daily Dose (mg)	Number of Doses Daily	Other Properties Anti-pyretic	Anti-inflammatory
Colchicine	Oral	0.5–1.2	6–8	—	Weak
	IV	1–2			
Fenoprofen calcium (NALFON)	Oral	300–600	4	+	+
Hydroxychloroquine sulfate (PLAQUENIL)	Oral	200–600	1–2	+	+
Ibuprofen (MOTRIN)	Oral	300–400	3–4	+	+
Indomethacin (INDOCIN)	Oral	25–200	3	+	+
Naproxen (NAPROSYN)	Oral	250–500	1–2	+	+
Oxyphenbutazone (OXALID, TANDEARIL)	Oral	100–400 mg	3–4	+	+
Phenylbutazone (AZOLID, BUTAZOLIDIN)	Oral	100–400 mg	3–4	+	+
Tolmetin sodium (TOLECTIN)	Oral	400 mg	3–4	+	+

of prostaglandins is considered to contribute to their effectiveness in the control of the peripheral inflammation that produces arthritic pain, but the exact mode of that action has not been delineated.

Colchicine

Action Mode.   The drug is employed primarily for its antigout activity. The drug-induced reduction of inflammation is thought to occur as a consequence of interference with the natural leukocyte response to the irritation caused by urate crystals in the tissues of the joints. The inhibition of leukocyte activity lessens the painful inflammatory response in the tissues.

Therapy Considerations.   Colchicine can be administered intravenously for acute attacks, but it is usually given by the oral route (Table 25–4). The absorbed drug travels to the liver where it is partially metabolized, and the unchanged drug and the metabolites are secreted with the bile into the duodenum. The drug and metabolites are reabsorbed from the small intestine and returned to the circulation. That recycling process provides a delayed rise in the plasma drug levels after the initial levels have declined. The double peak in plasma drug levels is an important factor when toxic effects occur.

The drug is distributed to most body tissues (i.e., kidneys, liver, spleen, intestinal tract), and there is a high concentration of the drug in the leukocytes. Most of the unchanged drug and its metabolites are excreted in the feces, but a small amount is excreted in the urine.

In the treatment of acute gout, the drug dose may be administered once every hour until diarrhea appears. Within 48 hours after initiation of therapy there is usually a marked reduction in the inflammation and pain. Diarrhea often occurs approximately 12 to 24 hours after that improvement is evident. The improvement confirms the diagnosis of gout.

In the treatment of chronic recurrent gouty arthritis, the drug may be given prophylactically at low dosage. The person is instructed to increase the dosage at the onset of joint inflammation and pain.

Adverse Effects.   Gastrointestinal disturbances are the most common adverse effects (i.e., nausea, abdominal cramps, vomiting, diarrhea). The onset of symptoms necessitates interruption of therapy until the gastrointestinal disturbances subside.

Therapy can usually be reinstituted in one to two days.

Overdosage, intravenous administration, or prolonged use can produce symptoms of bone marrow depression (i.e., agranulocytosis, aplastic anemia, reversible leukopenia, thrombocytopenia), alopecia, hepatic dysfunction, peripheral neuritis, myopathy, or gastrointestinal hemorrhage. Some of the pathologic problems may be associated with the decreased mitotic activity of rapidly proliferating tissues caused by colchicine (i.e., bone marrow depression, epidermal changes, gastrointestinal disturbances). Acute toxicity may cause death due to respiratory depression.

Hydroxychloroquine Sulfate

The drug has analgesic, anti-inflammatory, and antipyretic activity (Table 25–4). It is an antimalarial agent, and, in addition to its clinical use for the treatment of patients with rheumatoid arthritis, it is employed for discoid and systemic lupus erythematosus therapy.

Therapy Considerations. Hydroxychloroquine is administered to adults at a dosage of 200 to 400 mg one or two times per day. The dose is taken with meals or with a glass of milk to reduce the incidence of gastric irritation. The therapeutic response is usually evident in 4 to 12 weeks. The dosage is usually reduced when the person's arthritis improves to lessen the hazard of retinopathy that occurs with the prolonged use of high doses. Salicylates and corticosteroids are often used in conjunction with the drug. The dosage of those drugs is also gradually reduced, or they are eliminated at the time of improvement in the person's status. Concurrent acidification of the urine increases the renal excretion of hydroxychloroquine by 20 to 90 percent.

Adverse Effects. The gastrointestinal disturbances that occur during therapy include anorexia, nausea, vomiting, abdominal cramps, and diarrhea. An acute attack or exacerbation can occur when patients with psoriasis or porphyria are given the drug. Retinopathy appears to be dose-related and may not present visual symptoms when it occurs. There have been reports of hemolytic anemia in patients with an inherited *glucose-6-phosphate dehydrogenase* (G-6-PD) deficiency. Other adverse effects that are produced by the drug include irritability, headache, dizziness, vertigo, tinnitus, nerve deafness, emotional changes, and muscular weakness.

Phenylbutazone

The drug is usually employed for short-term treatment of pain associated with acute gout, active stages of arthritis, and musculoskeletal disorders (i.e., bursitis, tendonitis). Although the drug has analgesic properties, the primary indication for its use is the anti-inflammatory activity of the drug.

Therapy Considerations. Phenylbutazone is absorbed rapidly from the gastrointestinal tract. The onset of action occurs within 30 to 60 minutes after the drug is taken, and the peak plasma drug levels are obtained in two hours. The drug has a plasma half-life of 72 hours, and the long duration of action (three to five days) produces a steady-state plateau of the circulating drug in three to four days when the drug is taken regularly each day. Approximately 98 percent of the drug is bound to plasma proteins.

The circulating drug is widely distributed in body tissues, and it crosses the placental barrier. Phenylbutazone is metabolized slowly by the hepatic microsomal enzymes to *oxyphenbutazone* and an inactive metabolite. The metabolites and minimal amounts of the unchanged drug are excreted in the urine.

Adverse Effects. The drug frequently causes serious adverse effects. It is very irritating to the gastric mucosa, and patients frequently have problems with nausea, vomiting, and epigastric discomfort. Administration of the drug with meals usually is planned to modify the gastric irritation. The drug may cause ulcerations in the epithelial lining at varied sites in the gastrointestinal tract (i.e., mouth, esophagus, stomach, duodenum, large intestine). The person who is to take the drug should be informed of the adverse effects and instructed to withhold the dosage and inform the physician when there is evidence of dyspepsia, epigastric pain, gastrointestinal bleeding (i.e., black or tarry stools), or the excess fatigue that may be associated with anemia.

Phenylbutazone may also cause serious hematologic toxicity. Potentially fatal aplastic anemia or agranulocytosis may occur during therapy or several weeks after therapy is terminated. Leukopenia, thrombocytopenia, and pancytopenia also may occur as manifestations of the toxic effects of the drug.

Prolonged therapy usually includes a plan for regularly scheduled evaluation (i.e., every one to two weeks) of the person's hematologic status. Patients are instructed to withhold the drug dosage and inform their physician when they have chills, fever, sore throat, inflammation or ulceration in the oral tissues, or excessive fatigue unrelated to other obvious causes. Drug therapy is terminated when those signs of hematologic toxicity appear.

Allergic reactions, which usually are dermatologic problems, may occur during therapy. Because the skin reactions can progress to serious tissue destruction (i.e., exfoliative dermatitis, erythema multiforme), the drug is discontinued when reactions occur. Fluid retention may also occur during therapy with phenylbutazone.

Interactions. The drug may potentiate the action of oral anticoagulants, insulin, oral sulfonylurea hypoglycemic agents, or sulfonamides. The dosage of those drugs may require reduction during therapy with phenylbutazone.

Oxyphenbutazone

The drug is an analog of phenylbutazone and has the same therapeutic effects, adverse effects, and drug interactions as that drug. There seems to be a slightly lower incidence of gastric irritation with the use of oxyphenbutazone than with the parent drug. The dosage of the drug is the same as that of phenylbutazone (Table 25–4).

Dipyrone

Dipyrone (NARONE, PYRILIGIN), like phenylbutazone and oxyphenbutazone, is a *pyrazolone* derivative. It has not been approved for general use in the United States. It is used only in selected situations for control of life-threatening hyperpyrexia when other drugs are ineffective. In those situations it may be administered orally, intramuscularly, or intravenously. The oral or parenteral antipyretic dose for adults is 0.5 to 1 gm to a maximum daily dosage of 3 gm. The dosage range for children is 250 to 500 mg to a maximum daily dosage of 1 gm for children younger than six years of age and 2 gm for children 6 to 12 years of age. The drug may be administered to adults or children at intervals of three to four hours. The limited quantity of the drug that is administered for the control of hyperpyrexia reduces the incidence of adverse effects common to the pyrazolone group of drugs.

Fenoprofen Calcium

The drug has analgesic, antipyretic, and antiinflammatory activity (Table 25–4). The drug is employed for symptomatic treatment of persons with acute and chronic rheumatoid arthritis.

Therapy Considerations. The orally administered drug is rapidly and completely absorbed from the stomach and the small intestine. The drug is usually administered 30 minutes before or two hours after meals. Food delays its absorption without affecting the total amount that is absorbed.

Peak therapeutic plasma drug levels are attained within one-half to two hours after the drug is administered, and those levels are maintained by regularly scheduled drug administration. The plasma half-life of the drug is 2.7 hours. Enterohepatic recycling may contribute to the steady plasma drug levels. Approximately 99 percent of the circulating drug is bound to plasma proteins. Fenoprofen is metabolized in the liver, and 90 percent of the unchanged drug and the inactive metabolites are excreted in the urine within 24 hours. The drug is also excreted in the milk of nursing mothers.

Adverse Effects. Gastrointestinal disturbances commonly occur within the first month of drug therapy (i.e., anorexia, dyspepsia, nausea, vomiting, abdominal pain, constipation, diarrhea, peptic ulcers, hemorrhage). Central nervous system effects include headache, drowsiness, dizziness, fatigue, tremor, insomnia, mental depression, and nervousness. Ophthalmic problems (i.e., blurred vision) and auditory problems (i.e., tinnitus, hearing loss, deafness) may occur during therapy with fenoprofen calcium. Pruritus, rash, sweating, or palpitations also may occur.

Interactions. Concurrent administration of aspirin or phenobarbital decreases the serum levels of fenoprofen. The drug may potentiate the action of warfarin, dicumarol, sulfonamides, sulfonylureas, hydantoins, or salicylates by displacing the drugs from protein-binding sites. Fenoprofen decreases the aggregation of platelets, and that action may enhance the effects of anticoagulants.

Ibuprofen

The drug has analgesic, anti-inflammatory, and antipyretic activity (Table 25–4). It has the same therapeutic uses, adverse effects, and drug interactions as fenoprofen calcium.

Therapy Considerations. Most of the oral drug (80 percent) is absorbed from the gastrointestinal tract. The drug (Table 25–4) is usually administered one-half hour before or two hours after meals because the presence of food in the stomach slows its absorption. Peak plasma drug levels are attained within one to two hours. There is a time lag of a few days to two weeks before the therapeutic response is evident. The drug is metabolized in the liver, and approximately 70 percent of the unchanged drug and the inactive metabolites are excreted in the urine within 24 hours.

Naproxen

Naproxen has the same therapeutic uses, adverse effects, and drug interactions as fenoprofen calcium and ibuprofen. The drug is employed for symptomatic treatment of acute and chronic rheumatoid arthritis.

Therapy Considerations. The drug (Table 25–4) is completely absorbed from the gastrointestinal tract. The presence of food delays absorption of the drug but has no effect on the quantity of the drug absorbed.

Peak plasma drug levels are attained within two to four hours after the drug is taken, and the plasma half-life is 11 to 20 hours. About 99 percent of the circulating drug is bound to plasma proteins. The drug crosses the placental barrier. Naproxen is metabolized in the liver, and 97 percent of the unchanged drug and the inactive metabolite are excreted in the urine within five days after the drug is taken. A small amount of the drug is excreted in the milk of nursing mothers.

Indomethacin

The drug has analgesic, antipyretic, and anti-inflammatory activity (Table 25–4). It is employed for the symptomatic treatment of acute and chronic rheumatoid arthritis and has been used to suppress inflammation and increased vascular permeability at other tissue sites (i.e., pericardial inflammation).

Therapy Considerations. Indomethacin is administered orally after meals or with a snack, milk, or an antacid because the drug is irritating to the gastric mucosa. The drug is absorbed readily from the gastrointestinal tract, and peak plasma drug levels are attained within one-half to two hours after the drug is administered. The activity of the drug is maintained for four to six hours. Approximately 90 percent of the circulating drug is bound to plasma proteins.

The drug is metabolized in the liver; 65 percent of the metabolites is secreted into the urine by renal tubules and the remainder of the drug (35 percent) is excreted in the feces. Within 24 hours, 90 percent of the drug is eliminated. A small quantity of the drug is excreted in the milk of nursing mothers.

The dosage is reduced gradually over a two-day period when the drug therapy is terminated after less than a week. The patient is observed for the recurrence of pain and a rise in the body temperature during the two-day period.

Adverse Effects. Serious central nervous system and gastrointestinal effects occur frequently during therapy with indomethacin. Headache, the most common adverse effect, generally occurs in the early morning or within an hour after the drug is taken. The throbbing nature of the headache and concurrent disturbances in equilibrium may necessitate dosage reduction or cessation of therapy. Other neurologic problems that occur during the early weeks of therapy include confusion, convulsions, peripheral neuropathy, lightheadedness, and syncope. Behavioral disturbances, coma, and mental depression also may occur.

Approximately 15 percent of the persons taking the drug have gastrointestinal disturbances (i.e., nausea, vomiting, heartburn, anorexia, abdominal pain, diarrhea). The irritating effects of the drug on gastric and intestinal tissues may cause bleeding or ulcerations at varied segments of the tract. The problems often necessitate discontinuing use of the drug. The gastric disturbances sometimes persist after therapy is terminated.

Allergic reactions may occur during therapy. The problems usually are dermatologic reactions (i.e., skin rash, pruritus, alopecia, erythema nodosum). Urticaria, dyspnea, and angioedema also may occur.

There have been occasional incidents of ocular disturbances (i.e., corneal drug deposits, blurred vision, retinal pathology), bone marrow depression (i.e., leukopenia, hemolytic or aplastic anemia), and hepatotoxicity (i.e., jaundice). The multiplicity of adverse effects that can occur makes it necessary to regularly evaluate the person's physiologic status during prolonged therapy with indomethacin.

Interactions. The high plasma protein binding of the drug may cause competition for binding sites that are utilized by other drugs. The plasma levels of the displaced drug may be elevated (i.e., oral anticoagulants, sulfonamides, sulfonylureas, hydantoins, salicylates).

Tolmetin Sodium

The drug has analgesic, antipyretic, and antiinflammatory activity (Table 25–4). The drug has the same therapeutic uses and adverse effects as indomethacin.

Therapy Considerations. The drug is administered orally and is absorbed readily (75 to 100 percent) from the gastrointestinal tract. Peak plasma drug levels are attained within 30 to 60 minutes. The plasma half-life of the drug is 60 minutes. Approximately 99 percent of the circulating drug is bound to plasma proteins. The drug is metabolized in the liver, and 99 percent of the unchanged drug and the inactive metabolites are excreted in the urine within 24 hours.

Gold Compounds

The drugs, which are preparations that contain 50 percent gold, are used as an adjunct to other forms of treatment. They are most effective in slowing the progress of arthritis when they are given early in the active stage of the disease process. Their primary therapeutic effect is suppression of synovitis in active rheumatoid arthritis.

Therapy Considerations. Aurothioglucose (SOLGANAL), *gold sodium thiomalate* (MYOCHRYSINE), and *gold sodium thiosulfate with sodium thiosulfate* are administered by intramuscular injection into the gluteal muscle at weekly intervals. The initial dosage of the gold compound is 10 mg; a dosage of 25 mg may be given in the second and third weeks. Subsequent weekly dosages, which may be given for a period of 20 weeks, are 50 mg. In those persons responding to therapy, improvement usually is seen in six to eight weeks. When therapy is continued beyond a 20-week period, the dosage is usually given at two-to-three-week intervals.

The dosage of a gold compound for children is calculated proportionally on a weight basis. Children 6 to 12 years of age usually receive about one fourth of the adult dose at intervals of one or more weeks.

Adverse Effects. Most reactions to the gold compounds occur during the second or third month of treatment. The most frequent problems are cutaneous reactions (i.e., erythema, urticaria, papular or vesicular lesions, exfoliative dermatitis). The most serious effects are hematologic toxicity (i.e., aplastic anemia, agranulocytosis, leukopenia, granulocytosis). Concurrent use of antimalarials, phenylbutazone, oxyphenbutazone, or immunosuppressive agents can potentiate the incidence of blood dyscrasias.

MISCELLANEOUS ANALGESICS

The analgesics included are *ergotamine tartrate* and *dihydroergotamine mesylate,* which are used for the control of acute migraine headaches; *methysergide maleate,* which is used prophylactically for the control of vascular headaches; and *phenazopyridine,* which is used for pain in the lower urinary tract structures.

Ergotamine Tartrate (ERGOMAR, ERGOSTAT, GYNERGEN)

The drug, a derivative of ergot, has a direct effect of the intracranial blood vessels. That action decreases the vascular contraction believed to be the basic cause of migraine headaches. Use of the drug decreases the severity of the recurrent unilateral headaches, which are accompanied by nausea, vomiting, and anorexia.

Therapy Considerations. The dosage of the drug for sublingual administration is 2 mg, and that dosage may be repeated at half-hour intervals until the headache is relieved or three doses have been taken in a 24-hour period. The maximum dosage for a one-week period is 10 mg. The initial subcutaneous or intramuscular dosage is 0.25 to 0.5 mg. When the headache is unrelieved by the initial dosage, a second dosage of 0.5 mg may be given. The maximum parenteral dosage is 1 mg in a one-week period. Pain relief is usually obtained when the drug is used at the onset of the migraine headache. The maximum dosage limitations prevent the gangrenous lesions that are associated with ergot toxicity. The drug is commonly used as suppositories or tablets containing 100 mg of caffeine (CAFERGOT). The oral dose is 2 to 6 mg per attack to a maximum dosage of 10 mg/week.

Adverse Effects. Numerous adverse effects occur with large doses or prolonged use of the drug. The problems include gastrointestinal disturbances (i.e., nausea, vomiting diarrhea), neuromuscular disturbances (i.e., paresthesias of the extremities, cramping and weakness of the legs, myalgia), cardiovascular disturbances (i.e., angina-like precordial pain, sinus tachycardia or bradycardia, postural hypotension), pruritus, and localized edema. Tolerance develops with persistent use of the drug, and the person who increases the dosage to obtain pain relief may have adverse effects. Marked vasoconstriction and gangrene can occur with prolonged use of the drug.

Dihydroergotamine (D.H.E. 45)

The therapeutic indications and adverse effects of the drug are similar to those of ergotamine tartrate. Dihydroergotamine tartrate has more pronounced alpha-adrenergic-blocking effects than ergotamine. The drug is available in a solution that can be administered (1 to 2 mg) by subcutaneous, intramuscular, or intravenous injection. When the headache is unrelieved by the initial injection, a second dose may be given in one or two hours. The drug has less direct effect on the intracranial vascular smooth muscle than ergotamine tartrate but it produces fewer adverse effects. The onset of action occurs in 15 to 30 minutes and persists for three to four hours when the drug is given as an intramuscular injection.

Methysergide Maleate (SANSERT)

The drug is an ergot derivative that acts as an antiserotonin agent. The mechanism of action is unclear, but it is thought that one of its actions is an outcome of decreased serotonin-induced liberation of the prostaglandins that cause cranial arterial inflammation and constriction.

The drug is employed prophylactically at a dosage level of 4 to 8 mg/day for persons who have frequent disruptive migraine headaches. The maximum duration of therapy is six months, but therapy may be reinstituted after a drug-free period of three or four weeks. At the time of interruption of therapy, the daily drug dosage may be decreased gradually over a period of two to three weeks to avoid the appearance of "rebound headache."

Adverse effects are similar to those that occur with the use of ergotamine tartrate. Approximately 40 percent of the persons taking the drug have adverse effects, and about 20 percent have problems that necessitate termination of the drug therapy. The individual should be told to contact the physician when there is girdle, flank, or chest pain; cold, numb, or painful extremities; or leg cramps.

Phenazopyridine Hydrochloride (PYRIDIUM)

The drug is employed for its topical analgesic or local anesthetic effect on irritated urinary tract tissues. It relieves the burning, pain, or urgency that is caused by injury or irritation of the tissues. The drug is compatible with most antibacterial drugs employed for urinary tract infections.

Therapy Considerations. The usual daily adult dosage is 600 mg. The daily dosage for children is based on the calculation of 12 mg/kg of body weight. The total daily dosage is divided for administration three times a day.

The drug is excreted rapidly by the kidneys and approximately 65 percent of the unchanged drug is eliminated in the urine. The drug is an azo dye and its presence in the urine gives it an orange-red color. The drug stains on fabrics can be removed by soaking the material in a solution of sodium hydrosulfite. Persons taking the drug should be informed about the discoloration and methods for removing the stains from clothing.

When the urine is tested for glycosuria, there may be a delayed reaction with use of the glucose oxidase reagent (CLINISTIX, TES-TAPE), and it is necessary to allow for the time lag to avoid a false negative interpretation. False positive tests occasionally occur with use of TES-TAPE, and it is advisable to employ the cupric sulfate reagent (CLINITEST) for the urine test.

The only adverse effects related to use of the drug are headache, vertigo, and mild gastrointestinal disturbances. Accumulation of the drug, which occurs with renal insufficiency, can cause a yellowish tinge of the skin, and therapy should be discontinued.

NURSING INTERVENTION

Pain is personal, subjective, and difficult to interpret to another person. Whether the pain experience is acute or chronic, the individual's perceptions provide the primary data base for decisions about the use of analgesics for the control of pain. Persons in pain have a right to the relief of that distress.

Persons with chronic pain (i.e., headache, musculoskeletal problems, terminal cancer) present a challenging problem to the health professionals assisting them to maintain an ability to function. The multifaceted and interrelated physiologic, psychologic, and sociologic factors involved in chronic pain necessitate continued health team planning to meet the patient's therapy requirements. Pain clinics have been established in many areas to assist patients with management of their pain. Health team members in those clinics attempt to modify drug-taking patterns by involving the patient in therapeutic maneuvers for the prevention or alleviation of pain.

Assessing Pain Status

Pain is real. The person's perception of the intensity of the pain, observations of the physiologic effects of that distress, and the maintenance of adequate time intervals to avoid the adverse effects of the analgesic are the factors that guide the judicious use of analgesics. Fear, anxiety, and apprehension act conjointly with pain to increase sympathetic nerve stimulation. Restlessness, tachycardia, increased respiratory rate, and muscle tension may provide evidence of the psychosomatic effects of the discomfort the patient is experiencing.

Assessing Progress

Evaluation of the effectiveness of the prescribed analgesic is an essential part of the therapy plan. Responses to drugs vary, and an alternate drug may be required to provide relief for the individual who indicates that the analgesic effect is inadequate. The individual who requests pain medication at the exact time intervals allowed by the prescription is often criticized for that behavior by the nursing personnel. The problem quite frequently is inadequacy of the drug dosage. Discussion of the problem with the physician allows reevaluation of the planned therapy and the prescribing of an effective analgesic for the patient's level of pain.

It is standard practice in hospitals for the patient's narcotic prescription to be automatically canceled at the end of a 72-hour period. A new prescription is required for continued administration of the addictive analgesic. The intent of that policy is reevaluation of the need for the drug. The input of the patient and other health team members provides the basis for the physician's selection of the appropriate analgesic for the patient. When the nurse observes that the intensity of pain periodically varies, sharing that information with the physi-

cian allows prescription of a strong and a weak analgesic that can be employed according to the intensity of the pain experience.

Analgesics are often administered prior to painful procedures (i.e., extensive dressing changes, cystoscopy, surgery). That administration is timed to provide maximum analgesia before the stressful situation occurs.

The time lag between the administration of an analgesic and pain relief provides an opportunity to employ nursing measures that are additives to the analgesic. Comfort measures (i.e., changing the bed linen, back rub, positioning) should be preplanned to correlate with the administration of the drug. For example, the patient who has acute pain (i.e., first postoperative day) may be given the analgesic, and the measures can be employed immediately afterward. Delaying the administration of the analgesic allows the pain to intensify. The drugs are more effective when given at the onset of pain.

In some instances, the comfort measures and relaxation techniques can provide alternatives to the analgesic. For example, the patient who expresses the need for an analgesic on the fourth postoperative day may have adequate relief of the muscle tension that is increasing the incisional pain when the dressing is changed or a back rub or tepid bath is given. Most patients find the cutaneous stimulation of a back rub very relaxing, and the decreased muscle tension may allow the person to rest. It is also a useful practice to assist the patient with relaxation techniques when muscles are tense. Suggesting that the patient breathe slowly and deeply, while focusing on the relaxation of the big toe, often leads to relaxation of the large muscle groups.

Judicious use of addictive analgesics is the responsibility of the nurse, but those judgments are only valid when consideration is given to the patient's perception of pain. Short-term use of the drugs at regular intervals (i.e., postoperatively, posttrauma) does not cause addiction. The World Health Organization definition of addiction identifies a pattern of behavior in which there is an overwhelming involvement in obtaining and using a drug. That description seldom can be applied to a person during an acute pain-inducing illness.

The addictive analgesics can cause depression of respirations. A preliminary evaluation of the patient's respiratory status allows identification of those individuals who require close observation after administration of the drug. When respirations become slow or shallow, arousing the patient usually provides sufficient stimulation to increase the rate and depth of breathing. Pain provides a physiologic antidote to respiratory depression, and termination of the peak analgesic effect of the drug usually reverses the respiratory problem.

Assessing Hyperpyrexia Status

An elevation of the body temperature to 39° C (102.2° F) is associated with a 42 percent increase in metabolic work. That increase raises the oxygen requirements approximately 25 percent above normal, and there is a concurrent cardiac rate increase of 18 beats/minute.

Dissipation of excess heat from the body surface is facilitated when the individual is lightly covered with as much skin surface exposed to the circulating air as possible. Approximately 80 percent of the body heat is dissipated through the skin under normal basal conditions, and that amount increases appreciably when the temperature is elevated. The skin exposure is decreased when shivering occurs because the muscle activity produces heat that elevates the internal body temperature.

Administration of antipyretic drugs at regularly scheduled intervals when the temperature is elevated prevents the alternating chills and sweating associated with marked temperature changes. Use of the drugs also lessens the energy costs of the increased metabolic work. Rest is an important factor in restoration of

the reserves that are depleted by the energy expenditure of hypyrexia.

The water losses can be as high as 1500 ml when the temperature rises to 39° C. Diaphoresis also causes the loss of approximately 25 mEq of sodium and chloride. During normal metabolic activity, a fluid intake of approximately 1800 ml adequately replaces the insensible fluid losses and the urinary output, but the replacement needs are much higher (i.e., 3300 ml) when the temperature is elevated. The urine specific gravity and the quantity of the urine output provide useful guides for fluid replacement.

Patients are usually anorexic when the temperature is elevated, and it is essential that those foods or fluids that are tolerated have calories and salt for replacement of the losses. Offering carbonated beverages, or adding sugar to the warm cup of tea that the patient requests, provides calories. Bouillon, saltines, and salted popcorn often are acceptable to patients and they provide for the sodium chloride replacement.

Persistent temperature elevations above 39° C may necessitate the use of tepid sponge baths to cool the skin surface. An automatic cooling blanket or a fan may also be used to decrease the body temperature.

Children often have high temperature elevations at the onset of an infection. Some children have a low convulsive threshold, and the fever can precipitate convulsions. Tepid enemas, sponge baths, and antipyretics are employed to lower the body temperature rapidly in those children. The child's hydration status is an important factor in the safe use of antipyretics. Continued administration of the drugs when the urine output is insufficient for their elimination can lead to elevation of the serum drug concentration to a toxic level.

Counseling

Some individuals are reluctant to ask for medications for the relief of pain. Their reticence may reflect a stoic nature that makes the person hesitate to ask for help. In other individuals it may reflect a concern about drug addiction. Some patients may hesitate to ask for medication because they believe that the nurse will know when they should have the analgesic. After identifying the basic problems in each situation, a careful explanation of the rationale for the use of the drugs can increase the patient's involvement in a more constructive plan for pain control. The avoidance of pain is instinctive, and the avoidance behavior dissipates psychic and physical energy. Those individuals can be guided toward viewing the relief of pain as conserving energy for their active involvement in the therapeutic plan (i.e., deep-breathing exercises, ambulation, position changes).

The availability of aspirin and familiarity with its effectiveness in the relief of pain (i.e., headache) often interfere with the individual's use of the drug as prescribed for the control of pain and inflammation. Many persons take the drug while the pain persists, but they reserve subsequent use of the drug for pain episodes that interfere with their ability to function. The problem most frequently occurs in persons with musculoskeletal problems. A specific explanation of the rationale for therapy that includes a description of the relationship between the anti-inflammatory activity of the drug and the planned therapeutic result usually corrects the situation. The period of discussion with the individual also affords an opportunity to describe those gastrointestinal disturbances that necessitate withholding the drug and contacting the physician (i.e., intolerance to familiar foods, gastric pain, black or tarry stools).

Review Guides

1. Outline the assessments that would be made when an individual is breathing at a rate of eight times per minute when brought to the emergency room in an ambulance.
2. Formulate a plan for nursing care of the patient who had a cholecystectomy the previous day. Include the factors that would be considered in the administration of an addictive analgesic to the patient.
3. Outline the information about drug action and adverse effects that would be discussed with the person who is to take phenylbutazone after discharge from the hospital.
4. Explain the factors that determine the end point of therapy when the patient is receiving indomethacin for the control of gout. Include in the explanation the reason the patient's status must be evaluated for several hours after drug administration is terminated.
5. Outline the information about the drug that would be discussed with the parent when a young child with rheumatic fever is to receive aspirin every four hours at home.
6. Describe the factors that influence the decision to administer an addictive analgesic to the patient 72 hours after surgery.
7. Outline the predictable differences in physiologic function between a patient who is receiving morphine and one who is receiving meperidine for the control of pain.
8. Describe the explanation that would be appropriate when the patient who has methadone prescribed for the relief of persistent pain asks whether the physician has prescribed the drug because drug addiction has occurred.

Additional Readings

Babor, Thomas F.; Meyer, Roger E.; Mirin, Steven M.; and McNamee, H. Brian: Behavioral and social effects of heroin self-administration and withdrawal. *Arch. Gen. Psychiatry,* **33**:363, March, 1976.

Bartholomew, Lee E.; Rynes, Richard I.; Hedberg,

Susan A.; and Cammack, Carolyn J.: Management of rheumatoid arthritis. *Am. Fam. Physician,* **13:**116, February, 1976.

Berkowitz, B. A.; Ngai, S. H.; Yang, T. C.; Hempstead, J.; and Spector, S.: The disposition of morphine in surgical patients. *Clin. Pharmacol. Ther.,* **17:**629, June, 1975.

Blinick, George; Wallach, Robert C.; Jerez, Eulogio; and Ackerman, Bruce D.: Drug addiction in pregnancy and the neonate. *Am. J. Obstet. Gynecol.,* **125:**135, May 15, 1976.

Bremner, William J., and Paulsen, C. Alvin: Colchicine and testicular function in man. *N. Engl. J. Med.,* **294:**1384, June 17, 1976.

Calesnick, Benjamin: Use of narcotic (opiate) antagonists, *Am. Fam. Physician,* **13:**158, March, 1976.

Casterline, Charlotte L.: Intolerance to aspirin. *Am. Fam. Physician,* **12:**119, November, 1975.

Costroneo, Margaret, and Krasner, Barbara R.: Addiction, alienation and parenting. *Nurs. Clin. North Am.,* **11:**517, September, 1976.

Dinarello, Charles A., and Wolff, Sheldon N.: Pathogenesis of fever in man. *N. Engl. J. Med.,* **298:**607, March 16, 1978.

DiPalma, Joseph R.: Acetaminophen: safe aspirin substitute? *Am. Fam. Physician,* **13:**142, January 1976.

Dole, Vincent P., and Nyswander, Marie E.: Methadone maintenance treatment. *J.A.M.A.,* **236:**2117, May 10, 1976.

Easson, William M.: Understanding teenage drug abuse. *Postgrad. Med.,* **59:**173, February, 1976.

Ertel, Norman H.; Mittler, James C.; Akgun, Suat; and Wallace, Stanley L.: Radioimmunoassay for colchicine in plasma and urine. *Science,* **193:**233, July 16, 1976.

Fordyce, Wilbert E.: Evaluating and managing chronic pain. *Geriatrics,* **33:**59, January, 1978.

Frazier, Claude A.: Axioms on allergic factors in the etiology of headache. *Hosp. Med.,* **11:**106, March, 1975.

Glader, Bertil E.: Salicylate-induced injury of pyruvate-kinase-deficient erythrocytes. *N. Engl. J. Med.,* **294:**916, April 22, 1976.

Goldstein, Avram: Heroin addiction. *Arch. Gen. Psychiatry,* **33:**353, March, 1976.

Gritz, Ellen R.; Shiffman, Saul M.; Jarvik, Murray E.; Haber, Jochen; Dymond, Anthony M.; Coger; Roger; Charuvastra, V.; and Schlesinger, Joseph: Physiological and psychological effects of metha-

done in man. *Arch. Gen. Psychiatry,* **32:**237, February, 1975.

Holden, Constance: Venoms: extracting healing from the serpent's tooth. *Science,* **193:**385, July 30, 1976.

Johnson, Marion: Pain: How do you know it's there and what do you do? *Nursing 76,* **6:**48, September, 1976.

Koch-Weser, Jan: Drug therapy: acetaminophen. *N. Engl. J. Med.,* **295:**1297, December 2, 1976.

Lee, Garrett; DeMaria, Anthony N.; Amsterdam, Ezra A.; Realyvasquez, Fidel; Angel, Juan; Morrison, Stephan; and Mason, Dean T.: Comparative effects of morphine, meperidine and pentazocaine on cardiocirculatory dynamics in patients with acute myocardial infarction. *Am. J. Med.,* **60:**949, June, 1976.

Levy, Gerhard, and Yaffe, Sumner J.: Clinical implications of salicylate-induced liver damage. *Am. J. Dis. Child.,* **129:**1385, December, 1975.

Lewis, John R.: New antirheumatic agents. *J.A.M.A.,* **237:**1260, March 21, 1977.

Litt, Iris F., and Schonberg, S. Kenneth: Medical complications of drug abuse in adolescents. *Med. Clin. North Am.,* **59:**1445, November, 1975.

McCaffery, Margo, and Hart, Linda L.: Undertreatment of acute pain and narcotics. *Am. J. Nurs.,* **76:**1586, October, 1976.

MacKenzie, R. G.: Caring for the adolescent drug abuser. *Med. Clin. North Am.,* **59:**1439, November, 1975.

Mielke, C. Harold, Jr.; Heiden, David; Britten, Anthony F.; Ramos, Josefina; and Flavell, Paul: Hemostasis, antipyretics, and mild analgesics. *J.A.M.A.,* **235:**613, February 9, 1976.

Miller, R. P.; Roberts, R. J.; and Fischer, L. J.: Acetaminophen elimination kinetics in neonates, children and adults. *Clin. Pharmacol. Ther.,* **19:**284, March, 1976.

Pace, J. Blair: Helping patients overcome the disabling effects of chronic pain. *Nursing 77,* **7:**38, July, 1977.

Riordan, Charles E.; Mezritz, Marjorie; Slobetz, Frank; and Kleber, Herbert D.: Successful detoxification from methadone maintenance. *J.A.M.A.,* **235:**2604, June 14, 1976.

Roe, Robert L.: The anti-inflammatory agents used in rheumatoid disorders. *Primary Care,* **2:**259, June, 1975.

Rumack, Barry H., and Matthew, Henry: Acetaminophen poisoning and toxicity. *Pediatrics,* **55:**871, June, 1975.

Schenker, Steven; Hoyumpa, Anastacio M., Jr.; and Wilkinson, Grant R.: The effect of parenchymal liver disease on the disposition and elimination of sedatives and analgesics. *Med. Clin. North Am.,* **59:**887, July, 1975.

Scherbel, Arthur L.: Nonsteroidal anti-inflammatory drugs. *Postgrad. Med.,* **63:**69, March, 1978.

Schmitt, Mary: The nature of pain with some personal notes. *Nurs. Clin. North Am.,* **12:**621, December, 1977.

Smythe, Hugh: Nonsteroidal therapy in inflammatory joint disease. *Hosp. Pract.,* **10:**51, September, 1975.

Snyder, Solomon H.: Opiate receptors in the brain. *N. Engl. J. Med.,* **296:**266, February 3, 1977.

Stern, Robert C.: Pathophysiologic basis for symptomatic treatment of fever. *Pediatrics,* **59:**92, January, 1977.

Stewart, Elizabeth: To lessen pain: relaxation and rhythmic breathing. *Am. J. Nurs.,* **76:**958, June, 1976.

Storlie, Frances: Pointers for assessing pain. *Nursing 78,* **8:**37, May, 1978.

Turner, Robert: Aspirin and newer anti-inflammatory agents in rheumatoid arthritis. *Am. Fam. Physician,* **16:**110, July, 1977.

Weil, John V.; McCullough, Robert E.; Kline, J. S.; and Sodal, Ingvar E.: Diminished ventilatory response to hypoxia and hypercapnia after morphine in normal man. *N. Engl. J. Med.,* **292:**1103, May 22, 1975.

Welling, P. G.; Lyons, L. L.; Tse, F. L. S.; and Craig, W. A.: Propoxyphene and nonpropoxyphene: influence of diet and fluid on plasma levels. *Clin. Pharmacol. Ther.,* **19:**559, May, 1976.

Yowell, Sharon, and Brose, Carol: Working with drug abuse patients in the ER. *Am. J. Nurs.,* **77:**82, January, 1977.

Zarro, Vincent J.: New nonsteroidal anti-inflammatory drugs. *Am. Fam. Physician,* **14:**142, September, 1976.

26

Seizures

Isolated seizures may be precipitated by physical trauma to the brain tissues (i.e. head injury, brain surgery) or by physiologic factors that cause biochemical changes in the brain (i.e., hypoxia, hypoglycemia, hyponatremia, markedly elevated body temperature, drug intoxication or withdrawal). The isolated seizures usually are absent after the healing of injured brain tissue or the treatment of the causative factor.

The hallmark of epilepsy is chronic, recurring seizures. It is estimated that approximately two to four million persons in the country have epilepsy.

Physiologic Correlations

There are integrating networks throughout the brain tissues that are essential to its normal control of mental and physical function. For example, stimuli from the subcortical sites produce cerebral responses, and an integrated neural pathway between the frontal and temporal lobes coordinates the speech and hearing required for intelligible communication.

The voluntary motor responses are controlled primarily by the areas anterior to the central sulcus (Fig. 26–1). The motor areas in the left hemisphere control the responses on the right side of the body, and the right hemisphere controls those on the left side of the body. The opposite-sided control exists because the pyramidal tracts, which carry the impulses from the cerebral motor area to the peripheral structures, cross at the level of the medulla.

The cerebral voluntary motor control sites vary in the width of the neuronal areas that control motor function. The complex motor activities required for hand movements and the integrated movements of the face, tongue, and lips involved in the formation of words have larger control areas than those that control the more limited movements of the legs and trunk.

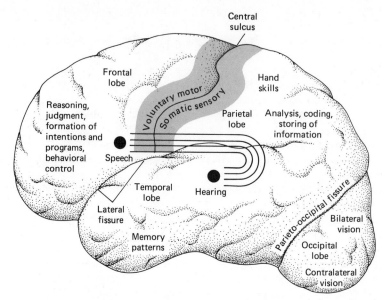

Fig. 26–1. The voluntary motor control centers are anterior to the central sulcus, and the somatic sensory control centers are located posteriorly in the parietal lobe.

Pathophysiologic Correlations

Seizures represent a wide variety of disruptions in the neural activity of the brain tissues. Isolated disruptions can represent any of the activity that commonly occurs during epileptic seizures. *Generalized seizures* involve bilateral, symmetric neuronal activity in the brain tissues. Partial seizures involve focal disruptions of the neuronal activity in the brain tissues. The following descriptions are based on the major seizure types that are included in the International Classification of Epileptic Seizures.

GENERALIZED SEIZURES

The generalized seizures include *tonic-clonic seizures, bilateral massive myoclonic seizures, absence seizures,* and *akinetic seizures.* Other descriptions of generalized seizure activity represent manifestations of similar responses in selected age groups. For example, *infantile spasms* represents the motor spasms and gradual mental deterioration that occur in infants; *clonic seizures* or *tonic seizures* represent the loss of consciousness and the rhythmic clonic muscle contractions or the rigidity of the musculature that occur in young children.

Tonic-colinc seizures were formerly called grand mal seizures. They are major convulsive episodes, or major motor seizures, that usually last one to ten minutes. An outcry may precede the loss of consciousness, which is followed by tonic spasms of all of the body musculature. The subsequent clonic phase involves synchronous, rhythmic, jerking muscle movements. At the termination of the tonic-clonic phases there is a period of cerebral depression.

The widespread firing of the cerebral neurons is followed by a period when the neurons are refractory to stimulation. The person may sleep soundly, and there may be incontinence of urine and feces.

Status epilepticus describes continuous and

uninterrupted tonic-clonic seizure activity. It represents an exhausting sequence of seizures that jeopardizes the life of the patient.

Bilateral massive myoclonic seizures are minor motor seizures that include involuntary, isolated clonic jerking contractions of the muscle groups of the trunk, head, or extremities. The person remains conscious during the 5-to-30-second episode of clonic muscle activity.

Absence seizures formerly were called petit mal seizures. During the seizure the person may have an abrupt, brief loss or clouding of consciousness and a vacuous stare with blinking of the eyelids. Although some persons have no motor activity, other persons have violent symmetric jerking of the entire body.

Akinetic seizures involve loss of consciousness and loss of muscle tone. When persons are in an erect position at the onset of an akinetic seizure, the sudden relaxation of the musculature causes them to fall.

PARTIAL SEIZURES

The person with partial seizures remains conscious and may recall distinct tastes, odors, or feelings after the seizure. *Partial seizures with elementary symptomatology* generally represent focal stimulation of the voluntary motor or somatic sensory areas of the cerebral cortex. The seizures formerly were described as jacksonian motor seizures or jacksonian sensory seizures. The motor activity may be limited to a small muscle group that represents the focal site of stimulation on the motor cortex. For example, the person may simultaneously clench the teeth and close one eye for a few seconds at frequent intervals, or there may be involuntary movements of the muscles of one limb. The sensory disturbances may also represent a focal site of stimulation of the sensory cortex, and there may be various manifestations of the neural activity.

Partial seizures with complex symptomatology are also called temporal lobe or psychomotor seizures. The stimuli usually originate in the temporal or frontal lobes of the cerebral cortex. During the three-to-five-minute seizure, the behavior of the person is confused, and there is usually some impairment of consciousness. The person's behavior may be purposeful but inappropriate to the environment in which the seizure occurs. There may be automatic, purposeless, disjointed activity and inappropriate vocalization during the seizure episode.

Antiepileptic Drugs

DRUG THERAPY

The antiepileptic drugs are employed primarily for prophylactic treatment to reduce the number or the severity of seizures. It is estimated that the currently available drugs, when used in varying combinations, can provide seizure control for 70 to 80 percent of the persons with epilepsy. The drugs also are used selectively for the prophylactic treatment of patients with severe head injuries or brain surgery to prevent the seizures associated with acute brain trauma.

The drug selected for treatment of the individual is chosen on the basis of the particular type of seizure and the known effectiveness of the drug in control of that type of seizure. Drugs that are effective in control of generalized convulsive episodes (i.e., tonic-clonic seizures) are also used for control of partial seizures (i.e., motor seizures). Those drugs that are employed for the control of generalized nonconvulsive episodes (i.e., myclonic, absence, akinetic seizures) are generally ineffective in controlling generalized convulsive episodes. The drugs may be used in varying combinations when the person has mixed seizures.

The antiepileptic drugs differ in their chemical structure but have similar pharmacologic and therapeutic properties. The drugs are chemical derivatives of *barbiturates, hydantoins, succinimides, oxazolidinediones, benzodiazepines,* and *iminostilbenes.* Valproic acid is a relatively new antiepilepsy drug. Magnesium sulfate, sodium bromide, and acetazolamide are also selectively used as anticonvulsant agents.

Action Mode

The anticonvulsants modify the bioelectrical activity at subcortical and cortical sites. That action raises the seizure threshold of the motor cortex to stimuli and limits the propagation and spread of the impulses from the foci of origin to the cortical effector sites. The drugs are thought to reduce the detonation of normal neurons by stablizing the cell membrane. That action may be related to their interference with the ionic activity (i.e., sodium, potassium, calcium, magnesium ions) at the cell membrane that is required for the conduction of nerve impulses.

Adverse Effects

Central Nervous System Effects. The most frequent adverse effects during therapy with the antiepileptic drugs are central nervous system—related problems that include ataxia, dizziness, drowsiness, dysarthria, headache, irritability, nystagmus, restlessness, and vertigo. The incidence and severity of the adverse effects are lessened when the drug dosage is lower during initial therapy. The problems generally decrease when therapy is continued.

Gastrointestinal Disturbances. Most of the drugs cause gastrointestinal disturbances (i.e., nausea, vomiting, anorexia, gastric distress, dysphagia, loss of taste sensation, constipation, diarrhea). The gastric disturbances may be decreased by taking the drugs with large quantities of fluid or with food.

Dermatologic Effects. Cutaneous reactions, which are produced by almost all of the drugs, include mild skin rashes (i.e., urticaria, scarlatiniform rash). The rash may be accompanied by fever.

There have been a few reports of exfoliative dermatitis and the Stevens-Johnson syndrome.

The person who is taking the drug should be told to withhold the drug and notify the physician when there is a high fever, severe headache, stomatitis, conjunctivitis, rhinitis, or urethritis. Those problems usually precede dermatologic evidence of the syndromes.

The person should also be told to inform the physician before taking the drug when a skin rash appears. The skin rash may be a forerunner of a potentially fatal reaction (i.e., malignant lymphoma-like syndrome, systemic lupus erythematosus). Drug therapy is terminated when the symptoms appear.

Hematologic Effects. The low folate levels that occur with most of the antiepileptic drugs can cause megaloblastic anemia. Many patients receive folic acid as prophylactic treatment while taking an antiepileptic drug. Some physicians also prescribe cyanocobalamin (vitamin B_{12}) for use concurrently with the drugs that are used for seizure control.

There have been a few reports of bone marrow depression, which is manifested as macrocytic anemia, leukopenia, thrombocytopenia, and agranulocytosis. The person should be told to withhold the drug and inform the physician when there is evidence of sore throat, fever, infection, easy bruising, epistaxis, or unusual bleeding. Drug therapy is terminated when evaluation of the blood values indicates that there is a decreased production of blood cells in the bone marrow.

Hepatotoxicity. The toxic effects of many of the drugs on the liver may initially be evident as jaundice and hepatitis-like symptoms. The person who is taking the drug should be told to inform the physician when there is evidence of dark urine, clay-colored stools, jaundice, anorexia, nausea, or other gastric or abdominal discomfort.

Nephrotoxicity. The oxazolidinediones and phenacemide have caused nephrotoxicity, and it is possible for the other drugs to produce the same problem. The toxic effects on the kidneys can cause edema, urinary frequency and burning, albuminuria, blood cells in the urine, and uremia.

Drug therapy is discontinued when there is evidence of renal toxicity.

Other Effects.   Hypocalcemia may occur when the drugs are taken at high dosage over long periods of time. Supplemental vitamin D may be prescribed for patients who are malnourished and unable to receive exposure to sunlight (i.e., institutionalized patients).

Parenteral administration of the drugs can produce severe depression of the medulla vasomotor and respiratory control centers. The problems include hypotension and respiratory depression. The patient who is receiving a parenteral drug must be monitored closely, and resuscitative equipment should be readily available.

Therapy with the antiepileptic drugs is terminated gradually to avert the seizures or status epilepticus that can occur with sudden withdrawal of the drugs. For example, drug therapy may be discontinued after a two-year seizure-free period. The withdrawal process may include a gradual reduction in drug dosage over a one-to-two-year period while the patient is observed for recurrence of seizure activity. Therapy is terminated after the dosage is at a minimal level and the person is seizure free. The plan for gradual reduction of the dosage is part of the withdrawal program for all persons regardless of the seizure-free interval that initially is used to determine that drug therapy may be terminated.

Recent evidence suggests that malformations (i.e., heart defects, facial abnormalities, mild microcephaly, hypoplasia of the distal phalanges) occur two to three times more frequently in the offspring of women taking the antiepileptic drugs than in the infants of nonepileptic mothers. The antiepileptic drug dosage may be reduced or the drug therapy may be discontinued by gradual dosage reduction in selected pregnant women, or women who plan to become pregnant. The risk of hypoxia in the mother and fetus during an episode of status epilepticus, which can occur during drug withdrawal, makes it essential that the dosage be reduced gradually and that the woman's seizure status be monitored closely during the withdrawal process. The drugs are not discontinued when pregnant epileptic women require them for the control of major seizures.

Interactions

The sedative effects of the antiepileptic drugs may be additive to the effects of other central nervous system depressants (i.e., alcohol, sedatives, antianxiety drugs). The tricyclic antidepressants can precipitate seizures, and persons who are taking an antiepileptic agent may have decreased seizure control when the drugs are used concurrently.

BARBITURATES

The long-acting barbiturates employed for their antiepileptic activity include *phenobarbital, mephobarbital,* and *metharbital.* Those barbiturates are subject to the controls of the Federal Controlled Substances Act of 1970. Also included in the group of drugs is *primidone,* which is a barbiturate analog. Other barbiturates (i.e., amobarbital, pentobarbital, secobarbital) may be administered intravenously to provide sedation for the control of status epilepticus.

Phenobarbital

Phenobarbital is the barbiturate most widely employed for the control of all types of epileptic seizures. The primary action of the drug is thought to be a reduction of the monosynaptic and polysynaptic transmission in the brain, which decreases the excitability of the nerve cells.

There are several adverse effects and drug interactions that have been reported as occurring with phenobarbital, but they have not been observed with the other barbiturates. The chemical similarity of the barbiturates makes it essential to be alert for the effects that are known phenobarbital-induced problems when the person is receiving any barbiturate.

Therapy Considerations.   The drug provides seizure prophylaxis at dosages lower than those producing hypnosis. *Phenobarbital* is administered orally, and *phenobarbital sodium* may be administered orally, rectally, or by subcutaneous, intramuscular, or intravenous injection.

The daily oral dosage of phenobarbital is frequently taken before bedtime (Table 26–1). The daily oral dosage for children is based on the calculation of 1 to 6 mg/kg of body weight.

Approximately 70 to 90 percent of the drug is absorbed from the stomach and the small intestine. Because the drug is slowly absorbed, 8 to 12 hours may be required before the peak plasma drug concentration is reached. The peak drug levels in the brain are attained within 10 to 15 hours. Approximately 20 to 45 percent of the

Table 26–1.

Adult Dosage of Oral Antiepileptic Drugs

Drug	Daily Dosage
Barbiturates (and Analogs)	
Mephobarbital (MEBARAL)	0.4–0.6 gm
Metharbital (GEMONIL)	0.1–0.8 gm
Phenobarbital	0.06–0.4 gm
Primidone (MYSOLINE)	0.25–2.0 gm
Hydantoins	
Ethotoin (PEGANONE)	1.0–3.0 gm
Mephenytoin (MESANTOIN)	0.05–0.8 gm
Phenacemide (PHENURONE)	0.75–5.0 gm
Phenytoin (DILANTIN)	0.3–0.6 gm
Succinimides	
Ethosuximide (ZARONTIN)	0.5–1.5 gm
Methsuximide (CELONTIN)	0.3–1.2 gm
Phensuximide (MILONTIN)	1.0–3.0 gm
Oxazolidinediones	
Paramethadione (PARADIONE)	0.9–2.4 gm
Trimethadione (TRIDIONE)	0.9–2.4 gm
Iminostilbenes	
Carbamazepine (TEGRETOL)	0.4–1.2 gm
Benzodiazepines	
Clonazepam (CLONOPIN)	1.5–20 mg
Diazepam (VALIUM)	4.0–40 mg
Miscellaneous Drugs	
Valproic acid	0.6–1.6 gm

circulating drug is bound to serum proteins. The drug has a plasma half-life of two to six days. The therapeutic plasma drug concentrations of 10 to 20 mcg/ml usually are reached within two to three weeks after therapy is initiated. Antiepileptic therapeutic serum drug levels range from 15 to 45 mcg/ml. Steady-state plasma drug concentrations may be achieved after three to four weeks of therapy. High concentrations of the drug are found in the brain and the liver. The drug crosses the placental barrier.

Phenobarbital is metabolized in the liver. The unchanged drug (25 percent) and its metabolite are excreted in the urine. The excretion rate of the unchanged drug is significantly increased when the urine is alkalinized. The drug is secreted in the milk of nursing mothers.

Phenobarbital sodium may be employed intravenously for the control of status epilepticus. It is administered at a dosage level of 200 to 600 mg to adults and 100 to 400 mg to children. The drug solution is highly alkaline and it should be administered with a small needle into the largest available vein to avoid the problem of thrombophlebitis, which occurs frequently. The injection rate is maintained at a maximum of 60 mg/minute to avoid the occurrence of central nervous system depression (i.e., hypotension, respiratory depression).

The onset of action occurs within five minutes when the drug is administered intravenously. Additional drug may be given when convulsions persist after the 30-minute interval required for the maximum effect of the intravenously administered drug to develop. The duration of action after parenteral administration is four to six hours.

Adverse Effects. The principal adverse effect is sedation. Nystagmus and ataxia may also occur. In addition to the adverse effects common to all of the antiepileptic drugs, phenobarbital may produce paradoxic excitement, hyperactivity, or motor restlessness when it is administered to children. The administration of the barbiturates to elderly persons can produce excitement, confusion, or depression. There have also been reports of mental dullness during continued chronic therapy with phenobarbital.

The barbiturates have produced postpartum hemorrhage and hemorrhagic disease of the newborn infant when the mother has received a barbiturate for the control of seizures. The problem, which is similar to that occurring with vitamin K deficiency, has been averted by administration of that vitamin to the infant after birth or to the mother for one month predelivery.

Phenobarbital produces mild skin rashes in 1 to 3 percent of the patients (i.e., maculopapular, morbilliform, scarlatiniform rashes). The cutaneous reactions usually fade rapidly when drug therapy is discontinued. During long-term therapy, osteomalacia has been reported.

Interactions. The barbiturates may induce the activity of the hepatic microsomal enzymes and thereby increase the rate of metabolism of coumarin, digitoxin, corticosteroids, tricyclic antidepressants, or doxycycline. That action decreases the serum concentration of the drugs, and a higher dosage may be required to provide the desired therapeutic effect when a barbiturate is added to the drug therapy plan. The dosage is decreased to avoid toxicity when the barbiturate is withdrawn from the therapy plan.

The barbiturates interfere with absorption of griseofulvin and dicumarol from the gastrointestinal tract. They also interfere with production of adrenocorticotropic hormone from the anterior pituitary gland.

Monoamine oxidase inhibitors or disulfiram can decrease the metabolism of the barbiturates. The interaction may prolong the effect of the barbiturate. It can also produce toxic levels when the person continues to take the barbiturate regularly for control of seizures.

Toxicity. Phenobarbital plasma concentrations greater than 50 mcg/ml may produce coma, and concentrations higher than 80 mcg/ml are potentially lethal. The initial signs of overdosage are central nervous system depression and apnea. Immediately after assessment of the patient's status, attempts are made to remove residual drug from the stomach. An emetic may be used to induce vomiting by the conscious person, or gastric lavage may be employed when the person is unconscious. Respiratory assistors are employed to maintain ventilation while other measures are used to correct the physiologic problems in each individual situation.

Mephobarbital

The drug is employed for prophylactic management of all types of epilepsy. It may be used as an alternate to phenobarbital when children become hyperexcitable, irritable, or hyperactive during therapy with that drug.

Therapy Considerations. The adult maintenance dosage usually is taken as a single dose at bedtime by those persons who have seizures during the night and in the morning by those who have daytime seizures (Table 26–1). Children over five years of age may receive 30 to 60 mg three to four times per day or a dosage calculated on the basis of 6 to 8 mg/kg of body weight per day. That calculated dosage may be given at bedtime as a single dose. Children younger than five years of age may be given 15 to 30 mg three or four times per day.

Approximately 50 percent of the drug is absorbed from the gastrointestinal tract. The drug is rapidly demethylated in the liver to form phenobarbital. Approximately 75 percent of the oral dose is converted to phenobarbital within 24 hours. Phenobarbital and the metabolites are excreted in the urine.

Metharbital

The drug is employed for prophylactic management of all forms of epilepsy. It, like mephobarbital, may be used as an alternate to phenobarbital when children become hyperexcitable, irritable, or hyperactive during therapy with that drug.

Therapy Considerations. The initial dosage of 100 to 300 mg is taken orally by adults one to three times per day. The dosage may be increased gradually to a level that maintains control of seizures (Table 26–1). The oral dosage for children is 50 to 100 mg one to three times per day.

The absorbed drug is metabolized by the liver to form barbital. Approximately 2 percent of the unchanged drug and 20 percent of the barbital are excreted in the urine within 24 hours.

Primidone

Primidone is employed primarily for control of psychomotor seizures. It may also be used for control of partial, autonomic, and akinetic seizures and for control of major motor seizures that are refractory to other antiepileptic drugs.

Therapy Considerations. The initial oral dosage for adults and children older than eight years of age is 50 to 125 mg/day, which is usually given at bedtime. The daily dosage may be increased in increments of 0.25 gm at two-to-three-day intervals to the maximum dosage of 2 gm/day (Table 26–1). The total daily dosage is usually divided for administration two to four times per day when the dosage level is increased above the initial level.

Children less than eight years of age initially may be given 125 mg of the drug orally at bedtime. The dosage may be increased at weekly intervals as required for seizure control to a maximum dosage of 750 mg. The maintenance dosage is divided for administration two to four times per day.

Approximately 60 to 80 percent of the drug is rapidly absorbed from the stomach and small intestine. Peak plasma drug concentrations are attained in two to four hours after a single dose is taken. The drug is slowly metabolized in the liver. A limited quantity of the drug is converted to *phenobarbital*. The metabolite *phenylethyl-malonamide,* or PEMA, which has weak anticonvulsant activity, is also formed. That metabolite is more toxic than the parent drug. During continuous oral therapy, the ratio of drug products in the urine is 15 to 25 percent of the unchanged drug, 15 to 25 percent phenobarbital, and 50 to 70 percent PEMA.

Adverse Effects. In addition to the adverse effects common to the antiepileptic drugs and to the barbiturates, there have been a few reports of psychotic reactions during therapy with primidone. The symptoms of toxicity are similar to those of the barbiturates. The crystalluria that appears with primidone toxicity facilitates the diagnosis.

HYDANTOINS

The hydantoins are the most widely used drugs for initial treatment of adults with generalized tonic-clonic, temporal lobe, and partial seizures. The drugs are thought to act at the cellular membrane to prevent accumulation of excess intracellular sodium ions during tetanic stimulation. That action decreases the posttetanic propagation of impulses. The hydantoins include *phenytoin, ethotoin, mephenytoin,* and *phenacemide.* Phenacemide is the most toxic of the group of drugs. Phenytoin is the drug most frequently used for the control of seizures.

Phenytoin

The drug is employed primarily for prophylactic therapy of grand mal and psychomotor epilepsy and is also effective in control of autonomic seizures. It is frequently used with phenobarbital or other antiepileptic drugs.

There are many adverse effects and drug interactions that have been identified as occurring with phenytoin that have not been reported with other hydantoins. It is essential to be alert for effects known to be phenytoin-induced problems when the person is receiving any of the hydantoins.

Therapy Considerations. The initial oral dosage of *phenytoin* or *phenytoin sodium* for adults is 100 mg three times per day. When additional drug is required for control of seizures, the dosage is increased in 100-mg increments at two-to-four-week intervals until seizure control is attained (Table 26–1). The maintenance dosage may be given as a single daily dosage, or two thirds of the daily dosage may be given in the morning and one third in the late afternoon.

The initial daily oral dosage for children is based on calculation of 5 mg/kg of body weight to a maximum of 300 mg. The daily dosage is divided for administration two or three times per day. The daily maintenance dosage is calculated on the basis of 4 to 8 mg/kg of body weight, and the drug is given as a single daily dose. The drug suspension must be shaken vigorously. to assure that it is resuspended before the dose is poured.

An initial loading dose of 1 gm may be given to adults to obtain an antiepileptic effect within 2 to 24 hours. That dosage is usually divided into doses of 400 mg, 300 mg, and 300 mg administered at two-hour intervals with a large glass of water or other fluid to minimize the irritating effects of the drug on the gastric mucosa. In acute situations, the drug may be given intravenously (i.e., 1 to 1.5 gm) to provide an antiepileptic effect within one to two hours. The oral loading dose for children is 500 to 600 mg, and that dosage may also be divided for administration of the total amount over a four-hour period. The maintenance dosage is started on the day following the loading dosage.

Phenytoin sodium may be given by intravenous injection for control of status epilepticus. The initial dosage of 150 to 250 mg for adults is given at a maximum rate of 50 mg/minute. Rapid intravenous injection causes marked hypotension. The solution is well diluted and is injected into the largest available vein. The drug has a pH of 12, and its irritating effect on the tissues can cause pain, inflammation, and necrosis at the injection site. A dosage of 100 to 150 mg may be given, after a 30-minute interval, when seizure activity persists. Children may be given a dosage calculated on the basis of 250 mg/M^2 of body surface area.

Differences in the dissolution and absorption between manufacturer's products affect serum phenytoin levels. Those levels are monitored regularly when the dosage form or brand is changed to avoid toxicity or loss of seizure control. The drug is well absorbed from the gastrointestinal tract. Although it may occasionally be administered intramuscularly, that is the least-favored route because the highly alkaline sodium salt is irritating to the tissues and its absorption is erratic.

The plasma half-life of the drug averages 18 to 24 hours. The therapeutic plasma level of the phenytoin generally is considered to be 7.5 to 20 mcg/ml. Therapeutic levels are usually attained after one week of therapy. The highest concentrations of the drug are found in the brain, liver, and salivary glands. Approximately 95 percent of the circulating drug is bound to plasma proteins. The drug crosses the placental barrier.

Phenytoin is metabolized in the liver, and the unchanged drug (1 percent) and the metabolites are excreted in the urine. The drug is secreted in the milk of nursing mothers.

Adverse Effects. Phenytoin frequently produces adverse effects. In addition to the adverse effects common to the antiepileptic drugs, phenytoin may produce mental dullness, blurred vision, and toxic amblyopia. When the plasma drug concentrations are at 8 to 20 mcg/ml, nystagmus may appear, and at concentrations above 30 mcg/ml, ataxia and dysarthria commonly occur. At a plasma concentration of 30 mcg/ml, there may be evidence of drowsiness and lethargy, and at a plasma concentration of 50 mcg/ml, a comatose state may occur.

Chronic use of phenytoin causes hyperplasia of the gums in approximately 20 percent of the children taking the drug. Phenytoin disrupts fibroblastic activity, and there is a gradual overgrowth of the gingival tissues around the teeth. Secondary inflammation and the associated edematous enlargement of the tissues may be prevented by meticulous oral hygiene and regular, vigorous gum massage.

Excess growth of hair (hypertrichosis) on the extremities also occurs. The hair growth occasionally becomes excessive on the trunk and face. The hypertrichosis is frequently irreversible. Overdosage causes symptoms of an acute cerebellar syndrome (i.e., ataxia) and delirium. Coma occurs rarely.

Interactions. Oral anticoagulants and disulfiram raise the plasma levels of free active phenytoin by competing with it for hepatic microsomal metabolism. Chloramphenicol, chlordiazepoxide, diazepam, estrogens, ethosuximide, methylphenidate, phenylbutazone, and some of the sulfonamides can inhibit the hepatic metabolism of phenytoin. In genetically slow acetylators, isoniazid inhibits the parahydroxylation of phenytoin in the liver. Para-aminosalicylate can further add to that effect by prolonging isoniazid blood levels. There may be as much as a 50 percent increase in the serum half-life of phenytoin when its metabolism is retarded and the person continues to take the antiepileptic drug.

Phenytoin metabolism may be accelerated by carbamazepine, folic acid, or alcohol. Phenytoin may decrease the serum levels and the half-life of dicumarol and may accelerate the metabolism of vitamin D, doxycycline, meprobamate, and dexamethasone. Phenytoin also inhibits insulin secretion from the pancreas, and the resulting hyperglycemia may increase the insulin or oral hypoglycemic drug requirements of patients who use those agents for the control of glucose levels. Large doses of aspirin can increase the activity but shorten the duration of phenytoin action by displacing it from the plasma protein-binding sites.

Ethotoin

The drug is used for prophylactic treatment of persons with major motor, focal, or psychomotor seizures. It is less toxic and less effective than phenytoin. In general, it is considered to be an alternate drug for the control of seizures and is used when seizures are refractory to control by other agents.

Therapy Considerations. The adult daily dosage is taken in four to six divided doses with food (Table 26–1). The initial dosage is usually 1 gm, which gradually may be increased to the maintenance dosage.

The initial dosage for children is usually 0.75 gm, which may be gradually increased to the maintenance level of 0.5 to 1 gm/day.

Ethotoin is metabolized in the liver. The drug and its metabolites are excreted in the urine and in the bile. Small amounts of the drug appear in the saliva.

Mephenytoin

The drug is used for prophylactic treatment of persons with major motor, focal, or psychomotor seizures. Mephenytoin has sedative properties that limit its usefulness with barbiturates, but it may be employed with other antiepileptic drugs. It is usually considered to be an alternate drug for use when seizures are refractory to control with other drugs.

Therapy Considerations. The usual initial dosage for adults and children is 100 mg, which is given as a single daily dosage for a period of one week. Increments of 50 to 100 mg may be made at weekly intervals as required for control of seizures. The maintenance dose (Table 26–1) is given in three equally divided doses per day.

The maintenance dosage for children is usually 100 to 400 mg/day in three equally divided doses. The daily dosage for children may also be calculated on the basis of 3 to 15 mg/kg of body weight.

The drug has an onset of action within 30 minutes, and that effect lasts for 24 to 48 hours. The drug is metabolized in the liver. That transformation produces an active and highly toxic metabolite (5,5-ethylphenylhydantoin), which is excreted in the urine.

Adverse Effects. The drug produces the adverse effects common to the antiepileptic drugs, but it less frequently causes the effects produced by hydantoin (i.e., ataxia, gingival hyperplasia, gastric distress, hypertrichosis). It causes blood dyscrasias more frequently than other antiepileptic drugs. The fatal dyscrasias can occur from two weeks to 30 months after therapy is started. Evaluation of the blood counts are done at two-week intervals initially. After a period of six to eight weeks blood counts are evaluated at one-to-three-month intervals. Therapy is discontinued when the neutrophil count is below the normal range. Alopecia, weight gain, edema, photophobia, and conjunctivitis may also occur during therapy with mephenytoin.

Phenacemide

The drug is considered to be a "last-resort" drug for control of seizures. It is highly toxic, and the risk-to-benefit ratio is carefully evaluated before it is used.

Therapy Considerations. The initial daily oral adult dosage is 1.5 gm, which is divided for administration in three doses. When additional drug is required for control of seizures, increments of 500 mg/dose may be made at weekly intervals until the maintenance dosage is reached (Table 26–1).

The initial oral dosage for children five to ten years of age is 250 mg three times per day. Increments of 250 mg may be made in the dosage at weekly intervals until the maintenance level is defined.

The duration of action is five hours. The drug is metabolized in the liver, and the inactive metabolites are excreted in the urine.

Adverse Effects. The drug can produce hepatotoxicity (i.e., jaundice, fatal hepatic necrosis), bone marrow depression (i.e., aplastic anemia, agranulocytosis), and severe psychologic disturbances with suicidal tendencies. It has occasionally produced nephritis. Therapy is terminated when there is evidence of the foregoing problems. Overdosage of the drug has produced drowsiness, ataxia, and coma of 24 hours' duration.

SUCCINIMIDES

The succinimides are thought to elevate the seizure threshold in the basal ganglia and in the cortex. The drugs also reduce the synaptic responses to low-frequency repetitive stimulation. They are useful agents for the control of absence, or petit mal, seizures. The succinimides include *ethosuximide, methsuximide,* and *phensuximide.*

Ethosuximide

The drug is considered to be the most useful of the antiepileptic drugs for the control of absence (petit mal) seizures in children. The drug may be used in combination with other drugs when the individual has mixed seizures.

Therapy Considerations. The initial oral drug dosage for patients over six years of age is 0.5 gm/day in two divided doses (Table 26–1). The dosage for children three to six years of age is 0.25 gm/day. The daily dosage may be adjusted in increments of 0.25 gm every four to seven days until the dosage that maintains control of seizure activity is reached. The maximum daily dosage is 1.5 gm.

Peak plasma concentrations are attained within four hours after the oral drug is ingested. It may take five days of regular use of the drug to achieve steady-state plasma drug concentrations (i.e., approximately 40 to 80 mcg/ml). The plasma half-life of the drug is approximately 60 hours in adults and 30 hours in children. The unchanged drug and its metabolites are excreted slowly in the urine. Small amounts of the drug are excreted in the feces.

Adverse Effects. Gastrointestinal disturbances, fatigue, lethargy, headache, and dizziness are relatively common. In addition to the adverse effects that are common to most of the antiepileptic drugs, the succinimides may produce hiccups, blurred vision, and diplopia. Adverse effects that have been reported with ethosuximide therapy are myopia, vaginal bleeding, and swelling of the tongue. Dyskinesias and psychiatric problems, which occasionally occur, disappear when therapy is terminated. Although toxicity rarely occurs, it produces profound central nervous system depression.

Methsuximide

The drug is employed as an alternate agent for the control of absence seizures or for psychomotor seizures. It may be used in combination with other drugs in the control of mixed seizures.

Therapy Considerations. The initial oral dosage for adults or children is 0.3 gm (Table 26–1). The dosage may be increased in 0.3-gm increments at weekly intervals to a maximum daily dosage of 1.2 gm. The daily dosage is usually divided for administration in two to three doses as the total dosage is increased.

The drug is readily absorbed from the gastrointestinal tract, and peak plasma levels are attained in one to three hours. The plasma half-life is approximately three hours. The drug is metabolized in the liver, and the active metabolite *N-demethylmethsuximide* (NDM) is thought to contribute to the antiepilepsy effect and to the central nervous system depression that is produced during therapy. The drug produces the adverse effects common to the antiepilepsy drugs and also may produce periorbital edema and hyperemia.

Phensuximide

The drug is the least effective and least toxic of the succinimides. It may be employed for short-term therapy when seizures are refractory to other drugs, but its effectiveness in the control of absence seizures tends to be reduced with prolonged use.

Therapy Considerations. The usual oral dosage for adults and children is 1 to 3 gm/day (Table 26–1). That dosage is divided for administration two to three times per day. Peak plasma drug levels are attained in one to four hours after the oral drug is ingested. The unchanged drug and its metabolite are excreted in the urine.

Adverse Effects. The drug produces the adverse effects common to the antiepileptic drugs but does not produce severe bone marrow depres-

sion. It has been reported to produce alopecia and muscular weakness.

OXAZOLIDINEDIONES

The drugs are thought to act in a manner similar to that of the succinimides to elevate the seizure threshold in the cerebral cortex and the basal ganglia. They also reduce the synaptic response to low-frequency repetitive stimulation. The drugs are utilized when absence seizures are refractory to control by ethosuximide. The oxazolidinediones include *trimethadione* and *paramethadione*. Although paramethadione is less toxic than trimethadione, it is also less effective in the control of seizures.

Trimethadione

Therapy Considerations. The initial 900-mg daily dosage of the drug for adults and children over six years of age may be increased in increments of 300 mg/day at weekly intervals until seizure control is established (Table 26–1). That dosage is given in three to four divided doses per day. The usual initial daily dosage for children two to six years of age is 600 mg and for children younger than two years of age it is 300 mg. The maintenance dosage for children is based on the calculation of 40 mg/kg of body weight, divided for administration three to four times per day.

After its absorption from the gastrointestinal tract, the drug is metabolized in the liver. The active metabolite, *5,5-dimethyl-2,4-oxazolidinedione* (DMO), has antiepileptic activity that contributes to the effectiveness of the parent drug. The plasma half-life of DMO is five to ten days, and plateau serum levels of the metabolite are attained in approximately four weeks. DMO is further metabolized and the inactive metabolites are excreted in the urine. The slow excretion of the unchanged drug (1 percent) and the metabolites is significantly increased when the urine volume is elevated or when the urine is alkaline.

Adverse Effects. The toxicity of the drug and the absence of generally available methods for determining plasma drug concentrations have limited the use of the drug. Trimethadione shares the adverse effects of the antiepileptic drugs and also has produced a myasthenia gravis-like syndrome. There have been reports of pancytopenia and fatal aplastic anemia. Drug therapy is terminated when the neutrophil count drops below 2500/cu mm. The most frequent adverse effects are drowsiness and a glare effect, or photophobia (hemeralopia). The drowsiness usually subsides during continued therapy. Hemeralopia may be reduced by wearing dark glasses or by dosage reduction. Therapy is terminated when there is evidence of blind gaps in the visual fields (scotomata). There have also been reports of alopecia, paresthesias, vaginal bleeding, and blood pressure changes during therapy with trimethadione. Toxic effects that occur with an overdose of an oxazolidinedione include nausea, drowsiness, dizziness, ataxia, and visual disturbances.

Paramethadione

Therapy Considerations. The initial 900-mg oral dosage for adults (Table 26–1) may also be given to children over six years of age. That daily dosage is divided for administration three times per day. The dosage may be increased in increments of 300 mg/day at weekly intervals until seizures are controlled.

The initial oral dosage for children two to six years of age is 600 mg, and for children younger than two years of age it is 300 mg. Those dosages may be increased gradually at weekly intervals. The daily maintenance dosage is divided for administration three to four times per day.

After its absorption from the gastrointestinal tract, the drug is metabolized in the liver. The active metabolite, *5-ethyl-5–2,4-oxazolidinedione* (DMP), has a long serum half-life, and the plateau serum DMP levels are attained within two weeks. DMP and its inactive metabolites are excreted slowly in the urine. The drug can produce the same adverse effects as those that occur during therapy with trimethadione, but they occur less frequently.

IMINOSTILBENES

Carbamazepine

Carbamazepine (TEGRETOL) is the only iminostilbene derivative that is currently used for seizure control. It is structurally related to the tricyclic antidepressants and has pharmacologic actions that are similar to those of the hydantoins. The drug is employed selectively for control of major motor and psychomotor seizures that are refractory to control by other antiepilepsy agents. The selectivity in its use is related to its high toxic potential in a small number of patients who take the drug. It is also employed for control of the pain associated with trigeminal neuralgia (tic douloureux).

Therapy Considerations. The initial adult oral dosage is 200 mg two times on the first day of therapy. The dosage may gradually be increased in 200-mg increments per day until seizures are effectively controlled (Table 26–1). At the higher dosage levels (i.e., 2.4 gm) the daily dosage is divided for use three to four times per day to minimize the adverse effects of the drug. Children may be given a maintenance dose calculated on the basis of 10 to 20 mg/kg of body weight per day, divided for administration in two to three doses.

Carbamazepine is slowly absorbed at variable rates from the gastrointestinal tract, and peak plasma drug levels are reached in two to eight hours. Approximately 75 to 90 percent of the circulating drug is bound to plasma proteins. The plasma half-life of the drug is 8 to 12 hours, and two to four days of regular use of the drug are required to attain a steady-state plasma concentration (i.e., 3 to 14 mcg/ml).

Carbamazepine is widely distributed in the body fluids and crosses the placental barrier. The drug is secreted in the milk of nursing mothers and also appears in the saliva. The metabolites and small amounts of the unchanged drug (1 percent) are excreted in the urine.

Adverse Effects. Nystagmus occurs when serum levels are below the therapeutic range. Approximately 50 percent of the persons taking the drug have adverse effects when the serum drug concentration is 8.5 to 10 mcg/ml. The most frequent adverse effects are ataxia, diplopia, drowsiness, and dizziness, which occur when the serum concentrations are above 6 mcg/ml. Like other antiepileptic drugs, carbamazepine can produce adverse effects on the neurologic, hematopoietic, cardiovascular, and hepatic systems. Many of those effects are serious during therapy with carbamazepine, and there have been reports of deaths associated with the drug-induced aplastic anemia. The anemia may be reversible if it is detected early.

The genitourinary problems that may occur with carbamazepine therapy are impotence, urinary frequency, acute urine retention, and oliguria. In addition to the gastrointestinal and dermatologic effects caused by other antiepilepsy drugs, carbamazepine can produce dryness of the mouth and oropharyngeal tissues, glossitis, stomatitis, changes in skin pigmentation, and alopecia. It may also produce diaphoresis, fever, lymphadenopathy, aching joints and muscles, leg cramps, and conjunctivitis. Overdose of the drug produces nausea, vomiting, ataxia, dizziness, drowsiness, stupor, restlessness, agitation, disorientation, tremor, involuntary movements, opisthotonos, abnormal reflexes, mydriasis, nystagmus, flushing, cyanosis, hypertension, hypotension, urine retention, and coma.

Interactions. Carbamazepine can induce hepatic microsomal enzymes, and that action may accelerate the metabolism of other drugs. It decreases the half-life of phenytoin, doxycycline, and warfarin in some patients.

BENZODIAZEPINES

Clonazepam and *diazepam* are the benzodiazepine derivatives employed for the control of epileptic seizures. Clonazepam is used primarily as an adjunct to other drugs for the control of absence, akinetic, or myoclonic seizures. The drug is subject to the controls of the Federal Controlled Substances Act of 1970.

Diazepam is considered to be the drug of choice for the control of status epilepticus and is employed parenterally for that purpose. It can also be used orally for the control of absence, akinetic, or myoclonic seizures that are refractory to treatment with other drugs. Tolerance may develop to the anticonvulsant effects of the benzodiazepines.

Clonazepam

Therapy Considerations. The usual initial oral dosage for adults and children weighing more than 30 kg is 1.5 mg in three divided doses. The dosage may be increased in increments of 0.5 to 1 mg every third day to a maximum dosage of 20 mg until seizure control is achieved (Table 26–1).

The daily oral dosage for children weighing less than 30 kg is 10 to 30 mcg/kg of body weight, divided for administration two to three times per day. The daily dosage may be increased in increments of 500 mcg every third day to a maximum daily dosage of 200 mcg/kg of body weight until the seizures are controlled.

Clonazepam is well absorbed from the gastrointestinal tract, and peak serum drug levels are attained within one to two hours after a single 2-mg oral dose. The elimination half-life of the drug is approximately 18.7 to 39 hours. The onset of action occurs within 20 to 60 minutes. The duration of action is about six to eight hours in young children and up to 12 hours in adults. The drug is metabolized in the liver. The metabolites and very small amounts of the unchanged drug are excreted in the urine.

Adverse Effects. The most frequent adverse effects during initial therapy with clonazepam are drowsiness and ataxia. Behavioral disturbances frequently occur in children during initial therapy (i.e., aggressiveness, irritability, agitation, hyperkinesis). The problems usually decrease when therapy is continued. When dosage adjustment does not reduce the severity of persistent adverse effects, drug therapy is terminated.

In addition to the adverse effects common to the antiepileptic drugs, clonazepam may produce rhinorrhea, increased salivation, excess mucus in the upper respiratory tract, and dyspnea that is associated with pulmonary congestion. The neurologic disturbances that may occur during therapy with the drug include nystagmus, diplopia, aphonia, dysarthria, slurred speech, headache, hemiparesis, choreiform movements, tremor, dizziness, vertigo, respiratory depression, and coma. Dysuria, enuresis, nocturia, urine retention, and edema of the ankles and face may also occur.

Toxicity. Overdosage of the drug may produce somnolence, confusion, ataxia, diminished reflexes, or coma. Abrupt withdrawal of the drug after long-term therapy can produce withdrawal symptoms in the drug-dependent person (i.e., severe dysphoria, irritability, restlessness, sleeplessness, hand tremors, convulsions). The long half-life of the drug may cause the symptoms to appear several days after drug therapy has been terminated.

Diazepam

Therapy Considerations. Diazepam is used orally as an adjunct to other anticonvulsants. It is more effective in chronic conditions than in acute situations. The oral dosage for adults is 2 to 10 mg two to four times per day (Table 26–1). Children may initially receive 2 to 4 mg/day in divided doses. The initial dosage is gradually increased to the level required to control seizures.

The intravenous dose of the undiluted drug that is given by infusion as an adjunct for control of status epilepticus in adults is 5 to 10 mg/minute. That dosage is infused until the seizures are controlled or a total dosage of 0.5 mg/kg of body weight has been given. Children may be given an initial intravenous dosage of 2 to 5 mg. The drug may be administered intramuscularly to children (2 to 5 mg) or to adults (5 to 10 mg) when the seizure activity interferes with intravenous injection of the drug. Maintenance therapy with an antiepileptic drug may be started concurrently with the use of diazepam. The drug produces adverse effects similar to those of clonazepam but they are less frequent and less severe. A

detailed discussion of diazepam is presented in Chapter 23.

MISCELLANEOUS ANTIEPILEPTIC DRUGS

Valproic Acid

The drug differs chemically from other anticonvulsants. It is employed for the control of simple or complex absence seizures and it is used in conjunction with other anticonvulsants for the control of refractory generalized seizures (i.e., tonic-clonic, absence, or myoclonic seizures). Valproic acid may be introduced into the therapeutic regimen to gradually replace other anticonvulsants or to allow the reduction of dosage of the drugs being used for therapy. Its precise mode of action is unknown. The brain levels of the neurotransmitter *8-gamma aminobutyric acid* (GABA) are increased during therapy with valproic acid.

Therapy Considerations. Valproic acid (DE-PAKENE) is available in capsules and as *valproate sodium* syrup. The usual daily dosage range is 600 to 1600 mg and the drug may be given in divided doses. The usual daily dosage for children is calculated on the basis of 15 to 20 mg/kg of body weight. The therapeutic serum drug level is 50 to 100 mcg/ml. The drug dosage may be higher when seizures are difficult to control (i.e., 30 mg/kg B.W.), but the dosage is adjusted to maintain the serum drug concentration below the maximum level of 200 mcg/ml.

The orally administered drug is rapidly absorbed from·the gastrointestinal tract. Approximately 90 percent of the circulating drug is bound to plasma proteins. The drug crosses the placental barrier, and it is secreted in the milk of nursing mothers. The serum half-life of the drug is 8 to 12 hours. Valproic acid is metabolized in the liver and the metabolites are primarily excreted in the urine. The ketone-containing metabolites may produce a false-positive result when the urine is tested for the presence of ketones.

Adverse Effects. Therapy may be started at a low dosage level to minimize the problems of nausea, vomiting, indigestion, and diarrhea, which commonly occur at initiation of therapy. Taking the drug with food also minimizes the gastric disturbances. The gastric symptoms usually are transient, and they subside when therapy is continued. Sedation also is a common problem during the early period of therapy, and it may be more pronounced when the drug is used in conjunction with other anticonvulsants.

Abdominal cramping, constipation, diarrhea, thrombocytopenia, and inhibition of platelet aggregation have been reported. Hepatic dysfunction has occurred in a few patients, and liver functions tests are recommended before therapy is started and at bimonthly intervals during therapy. There also have been a few reports of central nervous system disturbances (i.e., "spots before the eyes," ataxia, headache, nystagmus, incoordination, diplopia, tremor, dizziness), dermatologic problems (i.e., alopecia, rash), emotional and behavioral problems (i.e., depression, aggression, hyperactivity, psychosis), and muscle weakness.

Interactions. Valproic acid can potentiate the effects of other central nervous system depressants. An absence status was produced when the drug was used with clonazepam. The concurrent use of valproic acid with phenobarbital has produced elevated serum levels of the barbiturate.

Magnesium Sulfate

Magnesium sulfate (50 percent) is commonly employed for control of seizures that occur during preeclampsia or eclampsia. The drug is administered parenterally for control of the generalized convulsive (tonic-clonic) seizures.

Action Mode. The hypermagnesemia provided by administration of the drug controls generalized convulsions by depressing the central nervous sytem and blocking peripheral neuromuscular transmission. Although the exact mechanism of its interference with neural transmission at the motor end plate has not been identified, the drug is considered to decrease the amount of acetylcholine liberated by the motor nerve impulse. It is also an antagonist to the activity of calcium ions.

Therapy Considerations. The drug is usually administered as an intravenous infusion (i.e., 4 gm/250 ml of intravenous solution) at the rate of 150 mg/minute. A dosage of 4 to 5 gm may be injected intramuscularly into each buttock at the time the intravenous infusion is started. Additional single doses of 4 to 5 gm may be injected into the gluteal area at four-hour intervals when needed for the control of seizures. The injection sites are alternated to decrease the irritation and pain caused by the drug.

The intravenously administered drug provides an immediate onset of action that persists for 30 minutes. The onset of action occurs within one hour after intramuscular injection of magnesium sulfate, and that action persists for three to four hours. At therapeutic dosage levels the drug provides a 2.5 to 7.5 mEq/L serum magnesium concentration that is effective in the control of generalized (tonic-clonic) seizures.

Adverse Effects. The peripheral vasodilation that occurs with therapeutic doses of the drug produces flushing and sweating. At higher dosages the more extensive vasodilation produces hypotension. At serum magnesium concentrations of 4 mEq/L, the deep tendon reflexes are depressed. At concentrations of 10 mEq/L the reflexes are absent and respiratory paralysis or heart block may occur. Serum magnesium concentrations are monitored when repeated parenteral doses of the drug are required. The patellar reflexes are usually tested before each dose is administered, and the drug is withheld temporarily when the reflexes are absent.

Additional magnesium sulfate may be administered when the reflexes return and the respiration rate is at least 16/minute. A urine output less than 100 ml in four hours is also considered to be an indication for the interruption of therapy. Calcium gluconate antagonizes the action of magnesium and is administered to counteract the hypermagnesemia when toxic symptoms occur. Resuscitative equipment should always be immediately available when the drug is given by intravenous infusion. Intravenous calcium and resuscitation may be required by the newborn infant when the drug is given to the mother intravenously within two hours of delivery.

Sodium Bromide

Sodium bromide may be used for the control of major motor or myoclonic seizures in infants and preadolescent children when other drugs are unsuitable for therapy. The drug is seldom used for seizure control in adults.

Therapy Considerations. Sodium bromide is administered orally to children at a daily dosage calculated on the basis of 50 to 100 mg/kg of body weight. That daily dosage is divided for administration three times per day.

The drug is rapidly absorbed from the lower ileum, and the circulating drug is widely distributed throughout the body fluids. The bromide ions readily penetrate the red blood cells. The drug crosses the placental barrier. Sodium bromide is excreted in the sweat, feces, and urine and is secreted in the milk of nursing mothers.

Plasma drug concentrations of 20 to 25 mEq/L provide the central nervous system depression required for the control of seizures in children. Those concentrations are attained after the drug gradually accumulates over a period of several days. Maximum accumulation may require two months of continuous therapy. The plasma drug levels may remain elevated for 10 to 14 days after therapy is terminated.

The total amount of bromide plus chloride ions in the body fluids remains constant. When the plasma bromide levels become elevated by continued ingestion of the drug, the chloride ion levels are reduced by a higher rate of renal elimination. Preferential reabsorption of the bromide ions at the tubules provides the accumulation required for seizure control and increases the excretion rate of chloride ions. The plasma half-life of bromide is approximately 12 days, when the child has a normal chloride intake, as a result of its slow excretion rate. A low chloride intake is usually encouraged to allow accumulation of bromide by maintaining a high rate of renal tubule reabsorption.

Adverse Effects. The most frequent adverse effects are drowsiness and skin eruptions. Bromism, which is associated with the effects of the bromide ion, is the chronic toxicity syndrome that occurs in adults, but it seldom appears in children. The syndrome includes skin eruptions, gastrointestinal disturbances, and mental, psychic, or neurologic disturbances. Hyperkalemia also may occur.

Acetazolamide (DIAMOX)

The drug recently has been found useful as an adjunctive agent in the treatment of persons with absence and unlocalized seizures. The drug is a carbonic anhydrase inhibitor that appears to suppress abnormal or excessive discharges from the central nervous system neurons.

The usual daily dosage for adults and children is 8 to 30 mg/kg of body weight. The dosage is divided for administration two times per day. When acetazolamide is used with other anticonvulsants, the initial dosage is 250 mg/day. The adverse effects, which usually persist only for a short time, include loss of appetite, drowsiness, confusion, paresthesias, and polyuria.

NURSING INTERVENTION

A seizure history and an electroencephalogram (EEG) provide information vital to establishment of a plan for antiepilepsy drug therapy. Ambulatory and hospitalized patients should have the procedure explained to them before they go to the laboratory for the examination.

Most persons view the electronic machinery as doing something to their brain or as testing their mental capacity. It is important that those misconceptions be corrected. When patients understand that the electrical activity is in the brain and that the machine simply records that electrical activity, they more readily are able to relax and more accurate EEG recordings are obtained. The explanations of the procedure are reinforced by the technician who prepares the patient for the examination and places the EEG electrodes on the scalp at the time of the recording.

Anticonvulsants, tranquilizers, stimulants (i.e., cola, tea, coffee, cocoa) are restricted for 24 to 48 hours before the examination to assure that medications or stimulants do not influence the baseline brain activity or suppress seizure discharges. The person is told to eat regular meals the day before the examination because the hypoglycemia that results from fasting interferes with the brain wave activity. A shampoo is also required the day before the examination to assure that excess oils and hair sprays are removed. The person is instructed to go to bed late and to rise early because the short sleep period produces residual fatigue that allows the person to sleep during the examination. Sleep recordings provide essential information about brain wave activity.

Monitoring Seizure Activity

A primary concern when caring for a patient with a seizure is protection of the person from injury. Protective measures are employed judiciously according to the type of known or predictable seizure activity. For example, protective measures are not required for patients with limited focal seizures but are essential during tonic-clonic seizures.

It is standard practice to place side rails on the bed and to have a padded throat stick at the bedside of the person with a history of recent tonic-clonic seizures. On neurologic units where the potential for major motor seizures is high, an airway, padded throat stick, foam rubber–padded side rails, and suction equipment are available in each patient's unit for immediate use when needed during a seizure. During the period of highest seizure incidence (i.e., postoperatively, post-head injury), the patient's eyeglasses and dentures are removed and cigarette smoking is permitted only under direct supervision of a nurse or family member.

Children with a recent history of tonic-clonic seizures are often allowed to be ambulatory on the hospital unit during the period of diagnosis. They sometimes wear football helmets during that period to decrease the hazard of injury when they fall at the onset of a seizure. Adults who are allowed to be ambulatory require supervision to protect them against injury during a seizure.

Tonic-clonic seizures may occur without a warning sign. The patient who is standing at the onset of a seizure should be eased to a sitting position and then to a lying position on the floor. An airway can be inserted if the patient is observed before the tonic contraction of the facial muscles closes the jaw tightly. A rolled tissue or cloth can be placed between the teeth to prevent laceration of the tongue when an airway is not at hand. Ideally, gum, food, or dentures should be removed, but that is not possible when the tonic contraction of the muscles produces a tightly clenched jaw.

During the tonic phase of the seizure, which may last 10 to 15 seconds, the most important functions of the nurse are to observe the patient closely for evidence of airway obstruction and to observe the sequence of events that occur during the seizure. The only other appropriate measure is to protect the person's extremities or head from injury by placing a protective padding (i.e., towel, coat, pillow) between the patient and any structure (i.e., walls, floor) that may cause injury during the thrashing clonic movements. Restraining the person is unnecessary during the self-limiting tonic-clonic phases of the seizure.

The frothy foam that appears between the lips represents the blowing of air through the collections of mucus, and it will drain from the mouth when the person is placed in a side-lying position. The secretions become more copious during the clonic phase of the seizure, and the side-lying position prevents aspiration of the secretions that collect in the mouth. The clonic phase usually lasts for two minutes. At the termination of the muscular activity, the person may sleep briefly and then awaken somewhat dazed. A straightforward explanation that there has been a seizure usually clarifies the reason for the strange setting (i.e., the floor-lying position) for the patient. A period of natural sleep follows the major motor seizure.

A description of the seizure is entered in the patient's clinical record. The nursing note should include a detailed description of the duration, lateralization, and specific seizure activity and the patient's postseizure state of responsiveness or awareness. The tonic-clonic seizures follow a general pattern, but there are differences in the duration of the tonic and clonic muscle activity, the postseizure behavior, and the duration of the sleep period.

Other seizure types may involve activity limited to a particular body part, and a description of that involvement aids in diagnosis of the type of seizure and in the plan for treatment and health care. During the seizure, it is important that the nurse observe the movement of any part of the body, the pattern of progression of the seizure activity, positioning of the eyes, head, and extremities, responsiveness of the patient during the seizure, and the person's orientation after the event.

Counseling

There is considerable variation in the length of time that antiepilepsy drug therapy is required by patients. In general, children who have an initial epileptic seizure before adolescence will be maintained on the drugs through the adolescent period of growth and development. Therapy may be terminated after their postadolescent seizure status is evaluated.

Persons who have an epileptic seizure onset in adulthood may require lifetime therapy. The individual differences in the duration of antiepileptic drug therapy usually are managed by a conservative statement that the person will require the drugs for a relatively long period of time and that his status will be evaluated periodically to determine whether the drugs are needed.

Like other chronic health problems, it is difficult for the person to accept the need for medication when there is no seizure activity, and patients often discontinue taking the drugs. The initial information that they receive about the disease, the effectiveness of the drugs, and the measures that can be used to control or modify adverse effects may increase their compliance with the drug therapy plan. The child who is instructed about the schedule for taking the drug may be a source of support in maintenance of the therapy plan. Parents often have difficulty accepting the diagnosis and the need for prolonged antiepileptic drug therapy. Adults and adolescents often benefit from membership in the local chapter of the Epilepsy Foundation of America, which holds meetings of epileptics in the local community and periodically publishes informative newsletters about problems that are of interest to persons with epilepsy.

Specific discussion of the measures that can be used to decrease some of the problems related to care of the person with seizures may be helpful to the family. For example, a rubber sheet on the mattress prevents its being stained when incontinence occurs, and the use of a youth bed with side rails may prevent the child from falling during a nighttime seizure. Each person with epilepsy should wear an identifying bracelet or medallion to assure that appropriate care is provided when a seizure occurs. There are factors (i.e., excess fluid intake, alcohol, premenstrual edema) that lower the seizure threshold, and the person should be made aware of the potential problem. Each patient should understand that periodic laboratory tests and evaluation by the physician are essential aspects of an effective antiepilepsy drug therapy plan.

An important aspect of the care of the epileptic is to encourage continuance of a normal life pattern. Some activities must be supervised, but few activities need to be restricted. Children may participate in contact sports and may go swimming if a responsible person goes with them. Adolescents who have an informed companion can use the "buddy system" to allow their participation in some of their highly prized activities (i.e., swimming, hiking). The school nurse, who is made aware of the child's epilepsy, will instruct the teachers about the care of the child during a seizure and that practice allows the child unlimited supervised activity in the school environment.

Review Guides

1. Outline the instructions that would be given to the child and the parent when the youngster is to take ethosuximide for the control of absence seizures.
2. Outline the instructions that would be given to an adult male who is to take phenytoin for the control of tonic-clonic seizures.
3. List the hygienic measures that would be discussed with the adolescent female who is receiving phenytoin.
4. Define the instructions that would be given to the middle-aged man whose antiepilepsy drug has been changed from phenytoin to carbamazepine for the control of tonic-clonic seizures.
5. Outline the instructions that would be given to the child and the parent when the youngster is to take clonazepam for control of akinetic seizures.
6. Outline a plan for the nursing care of a pregnant woman who has received an intramuscular dose of magnesium sulfate and is receiving the drug by intravenous infusion for the control of eclampsia-related tonic-clonic seizures.

7. Outline a plan for the nursing care of the patient who is receiving diazepam for control of status epilepticus.
8. Explain the rationale for the following:
   a. The administration of phenobarbital at bedtime.
   b. The withholding of antiepilepsy drugs for 24 hours before an electroencephalogram (EEG) is to be taken.
   c. The administration of a loading dose of phenytoin.
   d. The gradual reduction in dosage when therapy with an antiepilepsy drug is to be terminated.
9. Outline a plan for monitoring the patient's status that would allow early identification of the following adverse effects that are common to the antiepilepsy drugs:
   a. Central nervous system effects
   b. Gastrointestinal disturbances
   c. Dermatologic effects
   d. Hematologic effects
   e. Hepatotoxicity
   f. Nephrotoxicity

Additional Readings

Bruya, Margaret Auld, and Bolin, Rose Homan: Epilepsy: a controllable disease. *Am. J. Nurs.,* **76:**388, March, 1976.

Buchanan, Robert A.; Kinkel, Arlyn W.; Turner, Janeth L.; and Heffelfinger, J. C.: Ethosuximide dosage regimens. *Clin. Pharmacol. Ther.,* **19:**143, February, 1976.

Butts, Priscilla: Magnesium sulfate in the treatment of toxemia. *Am. J. Nurs.,* **77:**1295, August, 1977.

Celesia, Gastrone G.: Modern concepts of status epilepticus. *J.A.M.A.,* **235:**1571, April 12, 1976.

Cooper, Clyde R.: Anticonvulsant drugs and the epileptic's dilemma. *Nursing 76,* **6:**44, January, 1976.

Crosley, Carl J.; Chee, Claire; and Berman, Peter H.: Rickets associated with long-term anticonvulsant therapy in a pediatric outpatient population. *Pediatrics,* **56:**52, July, 1975.

Fazio, Cornelio; Manfredi, Mario; and Piccinelli, Ascanio: Treatment of epileptic seizures with clonazepam. *Arch. Neurol.,* **32:**304, May, 1975.

Feldman, Robert G.: Patients with epilepsy. *Am. Fam. Physician,* **12:**135, October, 1975.

Garcia, Wanda A.: When your patient suffers a seizure. *R.N.,* **38:**45, February, 1975.

Gugler, Roland; Manion, Carl V.; and Azarnoff, Daniel L.: Phenytoin: pharmacokinetics and bioavailability. *Clin. Pharmacol. Ther.,* **19:**135, February, 1976.

Hahn, Theodore J.; Hendin, Barry À.; Scharp, Cheryl R.; Boisseau, Vincena C.; and Haddad, John G., Jr.: Serum 25-OHC and bone mass in children given anticonvulsants. *N. Engl. J. Med.,* **292:**550, March 13, 1975.

Henderson, Barry M., and Levi, J. Stuart: Febrile seizures in children. *Am. Fam. Physician,* **11:**114, January, 1975.

Hill, Michels Reba: Fetal malformations and antiepileptic drugs. *Am. J. Dis. Child.,* **130:**923, September, 1976.

Lawless, Leo M.: Understanding epilepsy. *Apothecary,* **89:**22, July/August, 1977.

Lewis, James, A.: Violence and epilepsy. *J.A.M.A.,* **232:**1165, June 16, 1975.

Li, Frederick P.; Willard, Douglas R.; Goodman, Robert; and Vawter, Gordon: Malignant lymphoma after diphenylhydantoin (Dilantin) therapy. *Cancer,* **36:**1359, October, 1975.

Livingston, Samuel; Pauli, Lydia L.; and Pruce, Irving M.: Epilepsy: diagnosis and treatment. *Pediatr. Nurs.,* **2:**23, May/June, 1976.

Livingston, Samuel, and Pruce, Irving: Petit mal epilepsy. *Am. Fam. Physician,* **17:**107, January, 1978.

Loetterle, Bridget S.; Rogers, Maisie; Valdner, Tina; Mason, Carmen; Christian, Ina; and Andreesen, Wayne: Cerebellar stimulation: pacing the brain. *Am. J. Nurs.,* **75:**958, June, 1975.

Nichol, Charles F.: Status epilepticus. *J.A.M.A.,* **234:**419, October 27, 1975.

Porter, Roger J., and Layzer, Robert B.: Plasma albumin concentration and diphenylhydantoin binding in man. *Arch. Neurol.,* **32:**298, May, 1975.

Pritchard, Jack A., and Pritchard, Signe A.: Standardized treatment of 154 consecutive cases of eclampsia. *Am. J. Obstet. Gynecol.,* **123:**543, November 1, 1975.

Pylypchuk, G.; Oreopoulos, D. G.; Wilson, D. R.; Harrison, J. E.; McNeill, K. G.; Meema, H. E.; Ogilvie, R.; Sturtridge, W. C.; and Murray, T. M.: Calcium metabolism in adult outpatients with epilepsy receiving long-term anticonvulsant therapy. *Can. Med. Assoc. J.,* **118:**635, March 18, 1978.

Rane, Anders; Höjer, Bengt; and Wilson, John T.: Kinetics of carbamazepine and its 10,11-epoxide metabolite in children. *Clin. Pharmacol. Ther.,* **19:**296, March, 1976.

Rose, James Q.; Choi, Hee K.; Schentag, Jerome J.; Kinkel, William R.; and Jusko, William J.: Intoxication caused by interaction of chloramphenicol and phenytoin. *J.A.M.A.,* **237:**2630, June 13, 1977.

Shepherd, Gordon M.: Microcircuits in the nervous system. *Sci. Am.* **238:**92, February, 1978.

Singer, Harvey S., and Freeman, John M.: Seizures in adolescents. *Med. Clin. North Am.,* **59:**1461, November, 1975.

Singsen, Bernhard H.; Fishman, Lawrence; and Hanson, Virgil: Antinuclear antibodies and lupus-like syndromes in children receiving anticonvulsants. *Pediatrics,* **57:**529, April, 1976.

Snead, C.; Siegel, N.; and Hayslett, J.: Generalized lymphadenopathy and nephrotic syndrome as a manifestation of mephenytoin (Mesantoin) toxicity. *Pediatrics,* **57:**98, January, 1976.

Swift, Nancy: Helping patients live with seizures. *Nursing 78,* **8:**24, June, 1978.

Tolman, Keith G.; Jubiz, William; Sannella, Joseph J.; Madsen, Jack A.; Belsey, Richard E.; Goldsmith, Ralph S.; and Freston, James W.: Osteomalacia associated with anticonvulsant drug therapy in mentally retarded children. *Pediatrics,* **56:**45, July, 1975.

Walson, Philip; Trinca, Carl; and Bressler, Rubin: New uses for phenytoin. *J.A.M.A.,* **233:**1385, September 29, 1975.

Waziri, Mary; Ionasescu, Victor; and Zellweger, Hands: Teratogenic effect of anticonvulsant drugs. *Am. J. Dis. Child.,* **130:**1022, September, 1976.

Wilder, B. Joe, and Ramsay, R. Eugene: Oral and intramuscular phenytoin. *Clin. Pharmacol. Ther.,* **19:**360, March, 1976.

Williams, Anne: Classification and diagnosis of epilepsy. *Nurs. Clin. North Am.,* **9:**747, December, 1974.

Wilson, J. T.; Höjer, B.; and Rane, A.: Loading and conventional dose therapy with phenytoin in children: kinetic profile of parent drug and main metabolite in plasma. *Clin. Pharmacol. Ther.,* **20:**48, July, 1976.

Zoneraich, Samuel; Zoneraich, Olga; and Siegel, Joel: Sudden death following intravenous sodium diphenylhydantoin. *Am. Heart J.,* **91:**375, March, 1976.

27

Abnormal Skeletal Muscle Function

Voluntary skeletal muscle contraction is dependent on transmission of afferent sensory and efferent motor nerve impulses through the nerve tracts between the peripheral and cerebral tissues. The functional and protective mechanisms of the musculoskeletal structures are dependent on the activity of the neurotransmitters and the integrity of the muscles and bones. The maintenance of posture, muscle tone, and coordinated movements represent complex neural interactions that provide the voluntary and involuntary controls of muscle responses. Interruption of those neural pathways can produce spasticity or flaccidity of the muscles. The excess neural stimulation produced by pain impulses from injured joints or muscles can cause contraction of the affected muscle and disrupt its functional status. The stimuli can also produce a compensatory contraction of adjacent muscle groups that interferes with bone alignment and musculoskeletal function.

Physiologic Correlations

UPPER MOTOR NEURON TRANSMISSION

Transmission of impulses from the cerebral motor cortex involves the activity of neurotransmitters along the nerve pathways, or upper motor neurons, through the brain tissues. There are complex neural circuits in the network for the central control of motor function. The circuits comprise the excitatory, or facilitory, and inhibitory feedback loops between the cortical and subcortical structures of the brain. The pyramidal and extrapyramidal tracts, which travel from the cerebral motor cortex to the spinal cord, are dependent on the neurotransmitters at cortical and subcortical sites for impulse transmission.

Neurotransmitter Activity

Dopamine, which is a precursor of norepinephrine, is primarily synthesized in the cell bodies of the melanin-containing nerve cells of the *substantia nigra.* The dopamine released from the cell bodies travels through the neural pathways to the axonal terminals in the adjacent structures of the basal ganglia, which include the *caudate nucleus, globus pallidus,* and *putamen,* and in the *red nucleus* (Fig. 27–1). Those structures and the thalamus comprise the subcortical intercommunication system and provide the neurotransmitters for impulse transmission through the brain tissues. The activity of dopamine limits the passage of impulses and prevents the spasticity of the skeletal muscles that can occur with unbridled transmission of excitatory impulses. The activity of dopamine generally decreases the tone of the extensor muscles and increases the tone of the flexor muscles.

The activity of the neurotransmitter *acetylcholine* at the subcortical receptor sites is considered to provide the excitatory control of motor nerve transmission. Balanced interaction of the

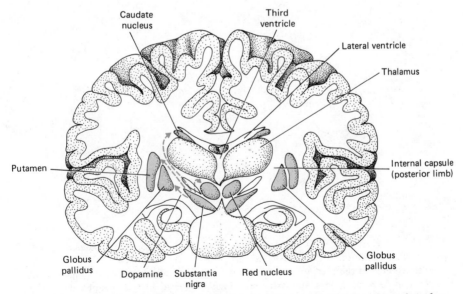

Fig. 27–1. The production and release of dopamine provide the neurotransmitter for the intercommunication system that controls motor nerve transmission at subcortical sites in the caudate nucleus, globus pallidum, putamen, and red nucleus.

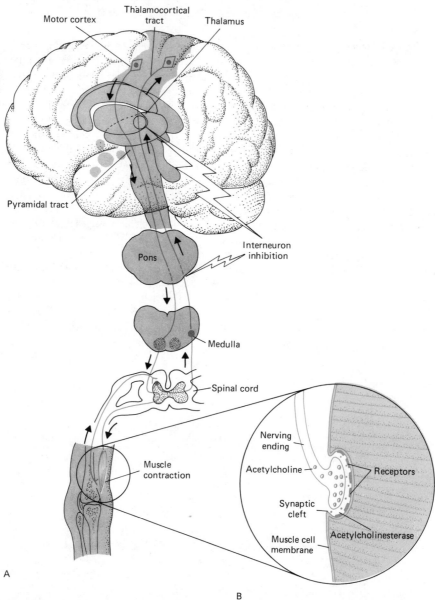

Fig. 27–2. *A.* Impulses that originate in the cerebral motor cortex are carried by the pyramidal tracts through the subcortical structures to the spinal cord. *B.* The action of acetylcholine at the receptors of the motor end plate stimulates the depolarization of the muscle fiber. Acetylcholinesterase, which is present in the synaptic cleft, inactivates acetylcholine.

hormones is the primary neurotransmitter mechanism for upper motor neuron control of smooth, coordinated contraction or relaxation of the extensor or flexor muscles.

LOWER MOTOR NEURON TRANSMISSION

The motor impulses that reach the spinal cord nerve pathways, or lower motor neurons, travel through the anterior horn cells of the spinal cord. Their passage involves complex interneuron conduction pathways, which relay the impulses to their point of exit from the cord. At the myoneural junction, or motor end plate, of the skeletal muscle fibers, the neural impulses provide the stimulus for release of the neurotransmitter acetylcholine, which is the chief chemical mediator of nerve transmission at the myoneural junction of the skeletal musculature (Fig. 27–2).

Acetylcholine Activity

The motor end plate of the skeletal muscle fibers is a complex structure with specificity for the chemical mediator. Activation of the receptor provides the stimulus for polarization of the muscle fiber. The enzyme *acetylcholinesterase,* which is present in the synaptic cleft of the motor end plate, inactivates the acetylcholine that is released into the cleft. The prompt action of the enzyme splits acetylcholine, and the inactive acetate and choline are released into the circulation.

The complex structure of the motor end plate of the skeletal muscle receptors differs from the simplistic, naked nerve structure of the visceral myoneural junction. Acetylcholine is the myoneural transmitter at the receptors of the skeletal muscular system and at the myoneural junctions of the parasympathetic nerves. Acetylcholine is also the preganglionic neurotransmitter of the sympathetic nerves, but the postganglionic neurotransmitter of the sympathetic nerves is *norepinephrine.*

Pathophysiologic Correlations

PARKINSONISM

The disruption of upper motor neuron function that occurs as a consequence of absence or depletion of dopamine and destruction of cell bodies of the neurons is described as parkinsonism. Parkinson's disease, which is also described as paralysis agitans or primary parkinsonism, represents a symptom complex similar to the disturbances associated with the postencephalitic parkinsonism that follows virus or toxin destruction (i.e., carbon monoxide, manganese) of the brain tissues. Idiopathic and postencephalitic parkinsonism represent a gradual depigmentation of the substantia nigra and the destruction of cell bodies in the cerebral cortex. The degeneration of the nuclei and intercommunicating nerve axons in the basal ganglia decreases the amount of dopamine available for the inhibitory control of upper motor nerve transmission.

Drugs can produce pseudoparkinsonism by depleting the quantity of dopamine available at subcortical receptors (i.e., reserpine) or by interfering with the responsiveness of the subcortical receptors to the activity of dopamine (i.e., phenothiazines, butyrophenones). The drug-induced inhibition of dopamine activity produces extrapyramidal symptoms similar to those that are associated with idiopathic or postencephalitic parkinsonism. Withdrawal of the drug usually leads to a gradual reversal of the symptoms.

In the absence of the inhibitory activity of dopamine, the cholinergic dominance produces an increased transmission of excitatory impulses to the skeletal musculature. The classic symptoms of tremor and rigidity are associated with absence of dopamine inhibition of impulses. The rhythmic tremor is described as a nonintention tremor because it occurs when resting. It is more rapid during stress situations but subsides during voluntary muscle movement or sleep. The tremor and rigidity become more evident as the disease progresses. There is a slowing of muscle movement (bradykinesia), akinesia, and areflexia when the cell body destruction in the brain tissues becomes extensive.

The gradual progression of muscle rigidity hampers the performance of all muscle actions and requires that considerable planning, concentration, and effort be employed by the person when doing automatic or simple tasks. There is an absence of the supportive gestures commonly associated with communication. For example, the absence of movement of the facial muscles produces a "masklike facies" that limits the viewer's ability to discern joy or sorrow when observing the person. Walking is hampered by the muscle rigidity, and the gait is hesitant, slow, and shuffling. "Propulsion gait" is used to describe the short steps and uncontrolled rapid forward movement that occur because the person cannot mobilize the muscle for braking the forward motion.

Parasympathetic nerve dominance, which occurs as a consequence of excess acetylcholine activity, produces the miosis, recession of the eyeball into the ocular orbit (enophthalmus), and partial closure of the eyelid (ptosis) characteristic of the disease. Some of the problems that add to the discomfort of the person are excess lacrimation, which is related to the absence of the blink reflex, excess flow of saliva (sialorrhea), which is related to decreased activity of the muscles involved in swallowing, persistent diaphoresis, which is unrelated to environmental or body temperature elevation, and seborrhea, which often causes skin eruptions. The concurrent slowing of gastrointestinal muscle activity produces constipation and atony of the bladder muscles, which causes frequent urination or hesitancy when the person attempts to urinate.

MYASTHENIA GRAVIS

The primary pathophysiology of myasthenia gravis is the decrease in myoneural transmission at the motor end plate of the skeletal muscle fibers or at the myoneural synapse in ocular sites. A widening of the synaptic gap and thickening of the receptor-containing membranes at the synapse reduce the response to acetylcholine stimulation. The neurotransmitter activity at the receptors may produce an initial response, but the muscle fiber contraction rapidly weakens until it ceases. After a period of rest, the muscle fiber again contracts when stimulated, but the response is generally a relatively short, rapidly fading contraction.

Although myasthenia gravis is considered to be an autoimmune disease, the relationship between the disease and the immune processes, or other pathologic processes, is unclear. The clinical entity may be limited to ocular manifestations of the disease (i.e., ptosis of the eyelids, diplopia), or it may be a generalized process affecting myoneural transmission in ocular, facial, pharyngeal, laryngeal, respiratory, and skeletal muscles. The disease is progressive, and over a period of several years the person gradually becomes more debilitated. The most disturbing functional problems are dysphagia, which causes accumulation of secretions in the oral cavity; weakness of the muscles involved in speech, which causes dysarthria that is exaggerated by the low volume of air that can be expelled to vibrate the vocal cords; and a markedly decreased vital capacity. The skeletal muscle activity may be reduced to a minimal level. The inability to expand the chest interferes with gas exchange, and death ensues when the muscles of respiration fail to respond to acetylcholine stimulation.

Antiparkinsonism Drugs

DRUG THERAPY

The drugs employed for treatment of patients with parkinsonism include *amantadine*, *levodopa*, and drugs with *central anticholinergic activity* that ideally can antagonize acetylcholine at central sites but have a limited effect on the activity of the neurotransmitter at peripheral sites.

The drugs may be used alone or in varying combinations for control of the symptoms of parkinsonism. In general, amantadine and levodopa provide objective and subjective improvement in tremor, spasticity or rigidity, bradykinesia or akinesia, sialorrhea, lacrimation, gait disturbances, and total functional ability. The anticholinergic agents are most effective in diminishing salivation, reducing the spastic contractions and involuntary movements that are characteristic of dyskinesia, and in diminishing the frequency and duration of oculogyric crises. During therapy with each of the drugs, the person usually shows an elevation in mood and greater interest in environmental activities.

AMANTADINE HYDROCHLORIDE

The drug was introduced as an antiviral agent, but it is employed for treatment of patients with idiopathic or postencephalitic parkinsonism and pseudoparkinsonism. There is subjective and objective improvement in approximately 50 percent of the patients treated with amantadine hydrochloride. The improvement in extrapyramidal symptoms generally occurs within 48 hours after therapy is started, and optimum results are evident after 2 to 12 weeks of therapy.

Action Mode

The drug is believed to provide an antiparkinsonism action by blocking the presynaptic neuron uptake of dopamine. The accumulation of dopamine in the synapses of the upper motor neuron intercommunicating pathways increases the inhibitory activity and reduces the peripheral muscular dysfunction. The near-normal balance between dopamine and acetylcholine activity also contributes to gradual improvement in the relationship of facilitory to inhibitory control of motor nerve transmission.

Therapy Considerations

Amantadine is administered orally; the usual initial dosage is 100 mg/day (Table 27-1). After a period of one week, the dosage is increased to 100 mg two times per day. The second dosage of the day is scheduled to be taken at least six hours before retiring because the drug may produce insomnia. The divided-dosage plan also decreases the incidence of adverse effects. Persons who are under close supervision may receive higher dosages (i.e., 400 mg/day), but adverse effects are dose related and their incidence and severity are

Table 27-1.

Dosage of Drugs Used for Treatment of Arteriosclerotic, Idiopathic, or Postencephalitic Parkinsonism

Drug	Usual Adult Oral Daily Dosage	
	Initial Dosage (mg)	Maintenance Dosage
Amantadine (SYMMETREL)	100	200–400 mg
Benztropine mesylate (COGENTIN)	1–4	4–6 mg
Biperiden (AKINETON)	6	5–20 mg
Chlorphenoxamine (PHENOXENE)	150	200–400 mg
Cycrimine (PAGITANE)	3.75–15	5–20 mg
Ethopropazine (PARSIDOL)	50–100	100–800 mg
Levodopa (DOPAR, LARODOPA)	500–1000	4–8 gm
Orphenadrine (DISIPAL, NORFLEX)	150 mg	200–400 mg
Procyclidine (KEMADRIN)	6–7.5	20–60 mg
Trihexyphenidyl (ARTANE, PIPANOL, TREMIN)	1–10	6–30 mg

greater when the dosage is increased. Children who are one to nine years of age are given a daily dosage calculated on the basis of 4.4 to 8.8 mg/kg of body weight to a maximum of 150 mg/day. The dosage is divided for administration two to three times per day. Children 9 to 12 years of age are given 100 mg/day, divided for administration in two doses.

Sustained improvement may last for two and one-half years before tolerance develops. The beneficial effects begin to decline in six or more weeks in 50 percent of the patients taking the drug. When decreased symptom control indicates that tolerance has occurred, the drug dosage is reduced gradually before therapy is interrupted. The gradual withdrawal is necessary to prevent exacerbation of acute symptoms of parkinsonism associated with abrupt termination of therapy when the drug has been taken for longer than 24 hours. The symptoms of the parkinsonism crises, which can occur within three days after drug therapy is terminated, include confusion, a marked increase in rigidity, urine retention, and bulbar palsy. After a period of several weeks, therapy can be reinstituted, and the drug usually provides the control that was present during the former period of treatment. Persons taking the drug should be informed of the need to maintain an uninterrupted drug-taking plan to avoid the withdrawal problems that can occur with omission of doses or unplanned cessation of drug therapy.

Amantadine is well absorbed from the gastrointestinal tract. Peak plasma concentrations are attained within one to four hours. Steady-state blood concentrations are attained after four to five days of therapy. The average half-life of the drug is 9 to 15 hours. The unchanged drug is excreted in the urine. Acidification of the urine increases the rate of excretion. Amantadine also appears in the saliva, nasal secretions, and in the milk of nursing mothers.

Use of the drug with anticholinergic agents provides additional improvement. There is greater improvement when amantadine is used with levodopa than when it is used alone. The combination also lowers the levodopa dosage requirements.

Adverse Effects

The drug produces reversible central nervous system effects (i.e., nervousness, irritability, fatigue, anxiety, insomnia, inability to concentrate, confusion, forgetfulness) and emotional problems (i.e., detachment, depression, psychosis). The adverse effects, which vary in severity, may appear within a few hours or days after therapy is started or at the time of an increase in dosage.

Persons who receive amantadine for the treatment of parkinsonism frequently have bluish mottling of the skin of the legs (livedo reticularis) after 1 to 12 months of therapy. The discoloration is reduced when the person elevates the legs. The increased capillary permeability associated with the mottling may produce edema in the cutaneous tissues of the involved areas. The mottled areas fade or change to brown spots during prolonged therapy. The lesions subside within a few weeks to months after therapy is terminated.

LEVODOPA

Action Mode

The drug is the metabolic precursor of dopamine. It crosses the blood-brain barrier and is enzymatically converted to dopamine in the basal ganglia. The drug is frequently used with the decarboxylase inhibitor *carbidopa*. When the drugs are used in combination, the activity of carbidopa prevents peripheral decarboxylation of levodopa to dopamine, and more levodopa travels into the brain tissues.

Therapy Considerations

The drug is administered orally; the usual initial dosage is 0.5 to 1 gm daily. The dosage is divided for administration two or more times per day with food. The daily dosage is usually increased by increments of 0.75 gm every three to seven days until the maximum daily dosage of 8 gm is reached. The increments often produce nausea, vomiting, anorexia, and hypotension that make it necessary to reduce the dosage or to delay increments until the person's status improves. Many stoic persons attempt to mask their discomfort to prevent the delay in dosage increases that is known to provide relief of symptoms. The optimal dosage of 3 to 6 gm/day usually is reached within six to eight weeks. The therapeutic response may be delayed for three to six months in some persons.

Significant amounts of levodopa are metabolized in the liver, lumen of the stomach, and intestines. Concurrent administration of carbidopa decreases the metabolism in the gastrointestinal tract and increases the amount of the drug that is absorbed. The unmetabolized drug is rapidly and well absorbed (40 to 70 percent) from the gastrointestinal tract.

The presence of food in the digestive tract delays absorption of the drug and produces lower peak plasma concentrations, but the drug is usually administered with food to reduce the incidence of nausea and vomiting. The tablets may be crushed or the content of the capsules may be mixed in fruit juice when patients have difficulty swallowing the solid forms of the drug. The mixture has limited stability and must be administered immediately after it is prepared.

The absorbed drug is distributed to most body tissues; the highest concentrations appear in the pancreas, liver, gastrointestinal tract, salivary glands, kidneys, and skin. More than 95 percent of the absorbed drug is decarboxylated by enzymes that are widely distributed in peripheral tissues. Less than 1 percent of the absorbed drug crosses the blood-brain barrier.

The plasma half-life of levodopa is 1 to 2.5 hours. The dopamine that is produced at brain tissues is metabolized, and the metabolites are excreted in the urine. The drug inhibits lactation and appears in the milk of nursing mothers.

Levodopa produces a false positive reaction when urinary glucose testing is done with cupric sulfate reagent (Benedict's Qualitative Reagent, CLINITEST tablets) and produces false negative reactions when glucose oxidase reagents are used (CLINISTIX, TES-TAPE). An accurate test result can be obtained by partially immersing the strip in the urine and reading the top portion, which will represent a given true color change for glucose. False positive reactions for urine ketones can occur when the tests are performed with sodium nitroprusside reagent (ACETEST, KETOSTIX, LABSTIX).

Levodopa is employed with or without carbidopa in combination with amantadine, antihistamines, and anticholinergics in the treatment of parkinsonism. The levodopa-carbidopa combination product (SINEMET-10/100, OR 25/250) expresses the carbidopa-to-levodopa ratio. The combination tablet may be employed initially but more frequently is used after the patient has received levodopa alone. The combination usually is given in the morning. The levodopa content of the combination tablet is given at 25 percent of the previous dosage because higher brain concentrations can be reached with lower doses when carbidopa reduces the peripheral metabolism of levodopa. The usual initial dosage is a 1:10 ratio or 10 mg carbidopa to 100 mg levodopa three times per day. The dosage may be increased by addition of a tablet that provides the same dosage to the daily schedule every one to two days until the maximum response is attained or a maximum dosage of 2 gm carbidopa to 200 mg levodopa has been reached. The patient is observed regularly during dosage adjustments because involuntary movements occur more rapidly with the combination than with levodopa alone.

The plasma levels of levodopa are significantly higher when the drugs are used in combination. The absorbed carbidopa is widely distributed in body tissues but does not cross the blood-brain barrier. It has a plasma half-life of one to two hours. Carbidopa doses of 70 to 100 mg/day completely inhibit peripheral dopa decarboxylase activity and markedly increase the plasma concentrations of levodopa. The plasma half-life of levodopa may be increased to three to six hours. The use of carbidopa decreases the levodopa dosage requirements by 80 to 84 percent. Although there is no change in the efficacy of levodopa, there is a reduced incidence of nausea and vomiting, and it is possible to more rapidly raise the dosage to the level that provides a therapeutic response.

Levodopa alone or in combination with carbidopa completely or partially relieves akinesia, rigidity, and tremor in 80 percent of the persons taking the drug. It also provides improvement in dysphagia, dysarthria, sialorrhea, and seborrhea, and in the gait and postural stability.

Adverse Effects

Levodopa produces numerous reversible, dose-related adverse effects. Gastrointestinal disturbances that occur less frequently than nausea and vomiting include duodenal ulcer, gastrointestinal bleeding, constipation, diarrhea, epigastric and abdominal pain, flatulence, hiccups, sialorrhea, bitter taste, dry mouth, dysphagia, changes in taste sensation, and burning of the tongue. Odoriferous sweating also occurs occasionally.

The most common serious adverse effects include choreiform, dystonic, and dyskinetic movements. Involuntary movements occur in about 50 percent of the patients on prolonged therapy (i.e., grimacing, bruxism, gnawing, chewing, vermicular movements of the tongue, rhythmic opening and closing of the mouth, bobbing movements of the head, or slow, rhythmic movements of the neck, hands, or feet). Early signs of toxicity include intermittent myoclonic body jerks during sleep, ataxia, increased hand tremor, muscle twitching, and blepharospasm.

The cardiovascular effects of the drug include flushing, hypertension, and cardiac irregularities. Orthostatic hypotension frequently occurs, but tolerance develops within a few months after therapy is instituted. Dizziness or syncope may be alleviated by the use of elastic stockings. The drug dosage may be reduced when the problems persist.

Levodopa produces many manifestations of central nervous system effects (i.e., agitation, vivid dreams, daytime somnolence, euphoria, malaise, memory loss). The appearance of serious emotional problems necessitates termination of therapy (i.e., withdrawal, depression, dementia, delirium, paranoid delusions, hallucinations, hypomania). The problems occur more frequently when the person has a history of emotional problems.

Interactions

Concurrent administration of monoamine oxidase inhibitors may cause a hypertensive crisis. Tricyclic antidepressants can augment the postural hypotension produced by levodopa. The tricyclics and anticholinergic drugs interfere with levodopa absorption from the gastrointestinal tract by delaying gastric emptying. Papaverine, phenytoin, and some antipsychotic drugs (i.e., phenothiazines, butyrophenones, and thioxanthines) antagonize the therapeutic effects of levodopa, and benzodiazepines also may decrease the control of parkinsonian symptoms. The concurrent administration of pyridoxine hydrochloride enhances the conversion of levodopa to dopamine in the brain tissues. At maintenance levels, carbidopa prevents the peripheral antagonism of pyridoxine hydrochloride.

DRUGS WITH CENTRAL ANTICHOLINERGIC ACTIVITY

The drugs employed for symptomatic treatment of idiopathic or encephalitic parkinsonism and pseudoparkinsonism are agents that provide anticholinergic activity at subcortical sites in the brain. The anticholinergic agents are *benztropine mesylate, biperiden, cycrimine, procycline,* and *trihexyphenidyl* (Table 27–1). The antihistamines *chlorphenoxamine* and *orphenadrine* and the phenothiazine *ethopropazine* also provide anticholinergic activity that is useful when the drugs are employed for treatment of persons with parkinsonism. When the drugs are used alone, they provide a maximum of 20 to 30 percent symptomatic improvement in approximately 60 to 80 percent of the patients treated. They frequently are used in combination with amantadine or levodopa to increase the therapeutic response.

Action Mode

The drugs cross the blood-brain barrier, and their blocking action decreases the activity of acetylcholine at subcortical sites. The decrease in facilitory stimuli in the intercommunicating pathways reduces the tremor and rigidity or spasticity of peripheral muscles. When the muscle spasticity is decreased, there is often a marked increase in tremors.

Therapy Considerations

Drug therapy is instituted with a low initial dosage, and that dosage is increased gradually to the level that provides relief of tremor and rigidity. The drugs are most effective when symptoms of parkinsonism are mild and the patient is young. Persons with postencephalitic parkinsonism often tolerate and require larger doses of the drugs for relief of symptoms. The drugs become less effective after prolonged periods of therapy. When therapy with the drugs is to be terminated, a gradual reduction in dosage is necessary to prevent the marked exacerbation of parkinsonism symptoms that occurs when the drugs are abruptly withdrawn.

Preparations Available

Benztropine methanesulfonate is usually administered orally four times per day (Table 27–1). It may be administered by intramuscular or intravenous injection for emergency control of acute dystonic reactions or in selected situations when the person cannot take the oral drug. The parenteral dosage is the same as the oral dosage. The maximum daily dosage of the drug is 6 mg/day. The antihistaminic properties of the drug frequently produce sedation.

Biperiden hydrochloride is usually administered orally three to four times per day (Table 27–1). *Biperiden lactate* is administered by intramuscular or intravenous injection in the emergency treatment of acute extrapyramidal disorders induced by drugs. The initial intramuscular dosage of 2

mg may be repeated every 30 minutes when symptoms persist until the maximum of 8 mg/day has been administered. The intravenous dosage of 5 mg is administered slowly and may be repeated only once in a 24-hour period.

Chlorphenoxamine hydrochloride is administered orally three times per day (Table 27–1). It is taken with meals, milk, or a snack to reduce the gastric disturbances that occur frequently.

Cycrimine hydrochloride is administered orally three times per day (Table 27–1). The drug is given with meals to decrease gastric irritation.

Ethopropazine hydrochloride is usually administered four times per day (Table 27–1). The drug is a phenothiazine and has local anesthetic, ganglionic-blocking, and weak adrenolytic activity. It produces a high incidence of adverse effects. It generally produces central nervous system depression, and in some instances cerebral stimulants have been required to alleviate the problems.

Orphenadrine is usually administered orally three times per day (Table 27–1). It may also be administered by intramuscular or intravenous injection in selected emergency situations.

Procyclidine hydrochloride is usually administered orally three times per day after meals (Table 27–1). It generally relieves muscle rigidity more effectively than tremor.

Trihexyphenidyl hydrochloride is usually given three times per day with meals and a fourth dose is taken at bedtime (Table 27–1). The drug is occasionally given before meals when there is a problem with sialorrhea.

Adverse Effects

The incidence of adverse effects of the group is dose related. The total incidence of minor adverse effects is high, and they generally represent the anticholinergic action of the drugs.

Early identification of adverse effects allows a reduction in dosage, which usually alleviates the problems. During the periods of dosage adjustment the person should be assessed for evidence of dryness of the mouth, dizziness, blurred vision, nausea, and nervousness. Other problems that may appear as manifestations of anticholinergic activity include constipation, tachycardia, urinary hesitancy or retention, drowsiness, weakness, vomiting, or headache. Central nervous system stimulation, which occasionally occurs during therapy, is usually manifested by restlessness, agitation, confusion, delirium, or hallucinations. The central effects occur most frequently in elderly persons or patients with advanced arteriosclerosis. Skin rashes rarely appear.

Anticholinesterase Drugs

DRUG THERAPY

The drugs are employed primarily for treatment of patients with myasthenia gravis. The short-acting drug *edrophonium chloride* is used for the diagnosis of myasthenia gravis, and the longer-acting anticholinesterase agents *ambenonium chloride, neostigmine,* and *pyridostigmine* are pharmacologically similar drugs used for prolonged therapy. The anticholinesterase agent physostigmine is employed primarily to increase myoneural transmission at visceral sites to improve bowel or bladder evacuation.

Individual dosage requirements vary widely, and the patient with myasthenia gravis usually regulates the dosage during prolonged therapy. To assure their readiness for that responsibility, patients are carefully counseled about the effects of the drug, the factors that affect dosage requirements (i.e., physical or emotional stress), signs of excess cholinergic activity, and the responses that indicate the need to increase the drug dosage. Those guidelines prepare the person for the assessments that are essential when individual responses require changes in the drug dosage. When the person is incapable of assuming that responsibility, a reliable family member or close associate is instructed about the use of the drug. Atropine sulfate is provided for use when overdosage produces cholinergic responses. Ephedrine sulfate or potassium chloride also may be used during therapy with anticholinesterase agents. Instructions and precautions that are appropriate to their use are included in the drug-counseling discussion to assure that they are employed as indicated to enhance muscle strength.

Action Mode

The drugs act at the myoneural junction to decrease the hydrolysis of acetylcholine by competing with the neurotransmitter for attachment sites on the enzyme *acetylcholinesterase*. The preferential hydrolysis of the drug allows acetylcholine to accumulate in the synaptic cleft, and there are higher concentrations of the transmitter available for stimulation of the receptors. The more prolonged period of acetylcholine action decreases the skeletal muscle weakness and fatigability. The drugs improve the tone and contractile response of skeletal muscles and visceral smooth muscles. The increased acetylcholinergic activity restores physiologic responses: constriction of the bronchi, increased glandular secretions (i.e., salivary and sweat glands), bradycardia, and constriction of the ureters. Those responses have a positive effect on the status of patients with myasthenia gravis.

Adverse Effects

Use of the drug in excess of the dosage required to maintain muscle strength can produce a cholinergic crisis with evidence of excess parasympathetic nerve activity. The cholinergic crisis is manifested by nausea, vomiting, diarrhea, miosis, excessive salivation and sweating, abdominal cramps, bradycardia, and bronchospasm. Hypotension, muscular weakness, cramps, and fasciculations occur. Death ensues in the unattended, untreated person. At high dosages the drugs cross the blood-brain barrier, and they can produce central nervous system stimulation that is followed by depression of the respiratory centers of the medulla.

Edrophonium Chloride (TENSILON)

The drug is employed for diagnostic purposes. When the person has myasthenia gravis, the administration of edrophonium produces a rapid improvement in the myoneural activity of acetylcholine.

The drug is also used selectively to differentiate between cholinergic crisis, which results from the depolarizing neuromuscular blockade that is caused by an overdosage of an anticholinergic drug, and myasthenic crisis, which represents inadequate acetylcholine activity at the myoneural junction. The rapid, short action of edrophonium allows discrimination between the two life-threatening entities, which have many similar characteristics, before therapy is instituted. The use of a respiratory assistor and other life support measures are required by patients before and during the test period.

Therapy Considerations. Edrophonium chloride is usually administered intravenously, but it can also be administered by subcutaneous or intramuscular injection. When the drug is employed for the diagnosis of myasthenia gravis, anticholinesterase therapy is discontinued at least eight hours before the drug is given. An assessment of muscle strength is done before the test to allow posttest comparisons of changes that occur. The edrophonium test is performed by a physician. When the initial intravenous administration of the small dose (i.e., 2 mg) of the drug produces an immediate cholinergic reaction, the test is discontinued and the patient is given a single dose of atropine sulfate (i.e., 0.4 to 0.5 mg).

Persons with myasthenia gravis require a larger dosage (i.e., 10 mg) of the drug before there is evidence of cholinergic activity. A second dose may be required after a period of 30 minutes when there is no response to the initial dosage of the drug.

The dosage for children is calculated on the basis of body weight. For example, children weighing more than 34 kg may receive the same dosages as adults, and children who weigh less than 34 kg receive one half of the adult dosage.

The intravenous dosage usually provides a response (i.e., decreased ptosis of the eyelids, increased vital capacity) within 30 seconds, and the responses occur within two to ten minutes when the drug is given by subcutaneous or intramuscular injection. When edrophonium is administered intravenously for the diagnosis of myasthenia crisis in a patient who is being treated with anticholinesterase agents, atropine sulfate is given when the injection does not produce improvement in the symptoms within 30 to 60 seconds. Those persons who do respond are given an anticholinesterase agent as soon as the improvement is evident because the edrophonium activity persists only for a period of five to ten minutes. The skeletal muscle effects may persist for 5 to 30 minutes after the drug is administered by intramuscular injection. Edrophonium chloride (i.e., 10 to 40 mg) also is used to antagonize the effects of curare overdosage.

Ambenonium Chloride (MYTELASE)

Therapy Considerations. The drug is administered orally with milk or food. The usual initial dosage is 5 mg three to four times per day, and that dosage is increased at two-day intervals until the daily dosage produces the maximum muscle strength. The usual adult maintenance dosage is 15 to 100 mg/day in three to four divided doses. Vital capacity measurements are evaluated during the periods of dosage adjustment.

The initial daily dosage for children is based on the calculation of 0.3 mg/kg of body weight, and that dosage is divided for administration three to four times per day. The maintenance dosage for children is based on 1.5 mg/kg/day, and that dosage is divided for administration three to four times/day.

The skeletal muscle effects that are produced by the drug persist for four to eight hours. The drug is less frequently employed than pyridostigmine or neostigmine because there is a narrow margin of safety between the onset of adverse effects and the occurrence of a serious cholinergic crisis.

Neostigmine (PROSTIGMIN)

Therapy Considerations. The drug provides a direct cholinemimetic effect on skeletal muscle in addition to its anticholinesterase action. *Neostigmine bromide* is administered orally and *neostigmine methylsulfate* is given by subcutaneous, intramuscular, or intravenous injection. The oral drug has a slower action onset, longer duration of action, and more uniform effect than the parenteral drug. It can be administered intravenously for myasthenia gravis diagnostic tests, but edrophonium is the preferred drug for that purpose.

The usual initial oral dosage for adults is 15 mg three times per day. The daily dosage may be increased at intervals of one or more days until the maximum muscular strength is attained. The maintenance dosage is 15 to 375 mg/day. The initial oral dosage for children is calculated on the basis of 0.33 mg/kg of body weight, and that dosage may be given six times daily. The usual initial dosage is 7.5 to 15 mg every four hours.

The parenteral dosage is approximately one thirtieth of the oral dosage. The usual parenteral dosage is 0.5 to 2.5 mg. Atropine sulfate often is given (i.e., 0.6 to 1.2 mg) when intravenous dosages above that range are administered. The atropine is given to counteract the cholinergic effects on the cardiac, gastrointestinal, and urinary tract tissues. Neonates with myasthenia gravis may receive neostigmine subcutaneously at a dosage of 100 to 200 mcg or an intramuscular dosage based on the calculation of 30 mcg/kg of body weight. Those parenteral doses may be given every two to four hours. When therapy is to be terminated, the daily dosage is reduced gradually.

Neostigmine methylsulfate may also be given to increase muscle contraction and relieve postoperative distention of the intestines or urine retention. A dosage of 0.25 to 0.5 mg is administered by subcutaneous or intramuscular injection at four-to-six-hour intervals for a period of two to three days. A catheter may be inserted into the rectum to facilitate the expulsion of flatus when the drug is given to increase peristalsis in postoperative patients. The peristaltic activity usually is evident within 10 to 30 minutes after the drug injection. The patient is catheterized when urinary retention is unrelieved by voiding within a period of one hour.

Pyridostigmine Bromide (MESTINON, REGONOL)

Therapy Considerations. Like neostigmine, pyridostigmine has a direct cholinomimetic effect on skeletal muscles in addition to its anticholinesterase activity. The drug is administered orally or by subcutaneous, intramuscular, or intraveneous injection. The usual initial daily oral adult dosage is 600 mg, which may be divided for administration three to four times per day. That dosage may be increased at intervals of two or more days until the maximum muscular strength is attained. The maintenance dosage is 60 mg to 1.5 gm/day. The initial daily oral dosage for children is calculated on the basis of 7 mg/kg of body weight, and that dosage is divided for administration five to six times per day.

The parenteral dosage of pyridostigmine is approximately one thirtieth of the oral dosage. The usual parenteral dosage of 2 mg is given at two-to-three-hour intervals. Atropine sulfate (i.e., 0.6 to 1.2 mg) is given concurrently with larger intravenous doses of the drug, and the patient is observed for evidence of excess cholinergic effects. Neonates with symptoms of myasthenia gravis are given the drug at a dosage of 5 mg orally every four to six hours or 50 to 150 mcg/kg of body weight intramuscularly every four to six hours.

The drug is available as an extended-release tablet that is used at bedtime by adults. Use of the drug provides anticholinesterase activity over an 8-to-12-hour period. When persons require a nighttime dosage of the drug, use of the extended-release tablet averts the dependency on an alarm clock awakening to take the regularly scheduled dosage during the hours of sleep.

The oral drug provides an onset of action in 30 to 45 minutes and that action persists for three to six hours. The drug effects are evident within two to five minutes after intravenous administration of the drug, and the increase in muscle strength persists for two to three hours. The onset of action occurs within 15 minutes after the drug is administered intramuscularly. Pyridostigmine crosses the placental barrier when it is taken in large doses. The drug is more rapidly metabolized and excreted in patients who have severe myasthenia gravis than in persons with a milder form of the disease.

Physostigmine Salicylate (ANTILIRIUM)

Therapy Considerations. The drug is an anticholinesterase agent that is employed primarily for short-term therapy to stimulate peristalsis in patients with postoperative bowel atony. It is also used to reverse the anticholinergic effects of preanesthetic doses of atropine sulfate or scopolamine hydrobromide that have produced adverse effects (i.e., delirium). When the drug is used to reverse the effects of those anticholinergic drugs, it is administered by intramuscular or intravenous injection at a dosage twice that of the anticholinergic drug. The intramuscular dosage for children is calculated on the basis of 50 mcg/kg of body weight when the drug is used to reverse anticholinergic drug effects.

The usual adult dosage is 0.5 to 2 mg intramuscularly or intravenously when the drug is used to stimulate peristalsis. A catheter is usually placed in the rectum to facilitate removal of flatus when the drug is given to patients with intestinal muscle atony in the postoperative period.

The onset of action occurs within three to eight minutes after the drug is injected. That action persists for one-half hour to five hours. The drug crosses the blood-brain barrier.

Cholinergic Agents

BETHANECHOL CHLORIDE

Action Mode

Bethanechol chloride (MICTROL, MYOTONACHOL, URECHOLINE) is the only cholinergic drug currently employed for treatment of postoperative or postpartum urine retention or neurogenic atony of the bladder. The drug acts primarily by directly stimulating the cholinergic receptors, and that action increases the frequency and duration of the smooth muscle fiber contraction. The action of bethanechol increases the peristaltic waves in the gastrointestinal tract and ureters and increases the contraction of the bladder detrusor muscle. The drug also produces increased pancreatic and gastrointestinal secretions.

Therapy Considerations

The drug is administered when the stomach is empty to avoid nausea or vomiting. The oral dosage is 30 to 120 mg/day and the dosage is divided for administration three to four times per day. The drug effect usually is seen in 60 to 90 minutes, and that effect persists for 60 minutes.

The adult dosage for subcutaneous administration is 5 mg; that dosage may be given at 15-to-30-minute intervals until the desired increase in muscle activity is evident. The drug dosage for adults who have urine retention associated with a chronic neurogenic bladder is 7.5 to 10 mg every four hours. The residual urine measurements provide the guidelines for dosage adjustments and for the duration of therapy. Oral therapy is usually started when the residual urine volume is below the pretreatment level.

Adverse Effects

Oral administration of the drug seldom produces adverse effects. When the drug is administered subcutaneously at high dosages, the adverse effects include abdominal cramps, flushing of the skin, sweating, lacrimation, salivation, malaise, headache, diarrhea, nausea, vomiting, bronchial constriction, belching, voiding urgency, and miosis.

Skeletal Muscle Relaxants

The drugs that act at central nervous system sites to produce skeletal muscle relaxation are *baclofen, carisoprodol, chlorphenesin, carbamate, chlorzoxazone, metaxalone, methocarbamol,* and *cyclobenzaprine. Dantrolene* acts directly on the skeletal muscles. Some of the antianxiety drugs (i.e., diazepam) also have muscle relaxant properties, and they are frequently employed for the treatment of persons who have muscle spasticity associated with muscle strain. Rest of the affected muscles, physical therapy, and analgesics are part of the total therapeutic plan for the person with muscle injury or spasm.

CENTRALLY ACTING MUSCLE RELAXANTS

The drugs are central nervous system depressants that have sedative and skeletal muscle relaxant properties. The muscle relaxant effects of the drugs are minimal when they are administered orally, and they are considered to provide relief of the discomfort associated with muscle spasm or strain by modifying the central perception of pain.

Baclofen

The drug is a muscle relaxant that is employed for the treatment of spasticity associated with disorders of the spinal cord (i.e., multiple sclerosis). The drug is an analog of the inhibitory neurotransmitter *gamma-aminobutyric acid* (GABA), but the precise mechanism of its action is unknown. It decreases flexor muscle spasticity by inhibiting monosynaptic and polysynaptic reflexes at the spinal level.

The initial dosage usually is 15 mg/day (Table 27–2), and increments of 15 mg are made at four-day intervals. The drug is rapidly absorbed after oral administration. Baclofen has a short plasma half-life (about 3 to 4 hours), and more than 80% of the unchanged drug is eliminated in the urine within 24 hours.

The most frequent adverse effects are drowsiness, insomnia, rashes, pruritus, dizziness, and weakness. The relief of spasticity, required by the patient with multiple sclerosis to walk or maintain a standing position, may produce problems with coordination. At the termination of therapy, the dosage is decreased gradually to avoid

Table 27–2.
Dosage of Selected Skeletal Muscle Relaxants

Drug	Route	Usual Therapeutic Dosage		
		Adult Daily Dosage	Child Daily Dosage	Number Divided Doses
Baclofen (Lioresal)	Oral	15–80 mg	—	3
Carisoprodol (Rela, Soma)	Oral	1.4 gm	25 mg/kg BW	4
Chlorphenesin carbamate (Maolate)	Oral	1.2–2.4 gm	—	4
Chlorzoxazone (Paraflex)	Oral	1–2.25 gm	20 mg/kg BW	3–4
Cyclobenzoprine (Flexeril)	Oral	20–40 mg	—	3
Dantrolene (Dantrium)	Oral	0.025–4 gm	13 mg/kg BW	4
Metaxalone (Skelaxin)	Oral	2.4–3.2 gm	—	3–4
Methocarbamol (Robaxin)	Oral	4–8 gm	60 mg/kg BW	4
	IM	1.5 gm	Same	3–4
	IV	1–3 gm	15 mg/kg BW	3–4

— Dosage not established.

the problems with auditory and visual hallucinations, anxiety, and tachycardia that occur within 12 to 30 hours after abrupt withdrawal of the drug. Patients should be cautioned against interrupting or discontinuing the drug therapy.

Carisoprodol

The drug is usually taken by adults or children three times a day, and a fourth dose is taken at bedtime (Table 27–2). The onset of action occurs within one-half hour, and the duration of action is four to six hours. The drug has a half-life of about eight hours. Carisoprodol is metabolized in the liver and the metabolites are excreted in the urine. The drug crosses the placenta and is secreted in the milk of nursing mothers in concentrations two to four times the maternal plasma levels.

The most frequent adverse effects are drowsiness and dizziness. The drug may also produce vertigo, tremor, irritability, headache, syncope, and insomnia. It occasionally produces allergic reactions after 24 hours of therapy (i.e., skin rash, erythema multiforme, pruritus, urticaria, eosinophilia). Anaphylaxis rarely occurs. Idiosyncratic reactions also may appear after 24 hours of therapy (i.e., extreme weakness, transient quadriplegia, dizziness, ataxia, temporary loss of vision, diplopia, dysarthria, agitation, euphoria, confusion, and disorientation). The idiosyncratic reactions usually subside within several hours. The drugs occasionally produces gastrointestinal disturbances (i.e., nausea, vomiting, hiccups, increased peristalsis, epigastric discomfort) and cardiovascular effects (i.e., tachycardia, postural hypotension, facial flushing).

Chlorphenesin Carbamate

The drug is taken orally four times per day for a maximum period of eight weeks (Table 27–2). The maximum plasma levels occur within one to three hours after the drug is taken orally. The drug has a plasma half-life of 2.3 to 5.1 hours. It is partly metabolized, and the unchanged drug and the metabolites are rapidly excreted in the urine.

The drug frequently produces drowsiness and dizziness. It occasionally produces confusion, weakness, nausea, epigastric distress, and paradoxic stimulation (i.e., agitation, insomnia, nervousness, headache). It rarely produces allergic reactions.

Chlorzoxazone

The drug is administered orally to adults and children three to four times per day (Table 27–2). The tablets may be crushed and mixed with milk, fruit juice, or puréed food when children or adults have difficulty swallowing the tablets. The onset of action occurs within one hour, and that action persists for three to four hours. The elimination half-life of the drug is about 66 minutes. The urine of persons taking the drug contains an *aminophenol* metabolite that produces an orange to purple-red discoloration when the urine is exposed to air.

The drug frequently produces drowsiness and dizziness. Light headedness, malaise, and headache also may occur. Chlorzoxazone also produces gastrointestinal disturbances (i.e., anorexia, nausea, vomiting, heartburn, abdominal distress, constipation, diarrhea). Allergic reactions rarely appear.

Metaxalone

The oral drug is taken by adults three to four times per day (Table 27–2). The onset of action occurs within one hour after the drug is taken and that action persists for four to six hours. The drug has a plasma half-life of two to three hours. Metaxalone is metabolized in the liver and the metabolites are excreted in the urine.

False-positive results are obtained when the tests for glycosuria are performed with cupric sulfate reagents (Benedict's Qualitative Solution, CLINITEST, Fehling's Solution). The glucose oxidase regents (CLINITIX, DIASTIX, TES-TAPE) should be used for urine testing.

The most frequent adverse effects are nausea,

drowsiness, and dizziness. The drug may also produce headache, nervousness, confusion, irritability, anorexia, dry mouth, vomiting, and urine retention. The allergic reactions that occur occasionally are skin rash and pruritus.

Methocarbamol

The drug is usually administered orally. It can be administered by intramuscular or intravenous injection when patients are unable to take the oral tablets (Table 27–2). The drug is irritating to the tissues and should be given deep into the intramuscular tissues or into a large vein to prevent pain and induration.

The oral drug is well absorbed and the onset of action occurs within 30 minutes after the drug is taken. Methocarbamol has a plasma half-life of 0.9 to 2.2 hours. The drug is metabolized in the liver. The drug crosses the placenta. The metabolites are excreted in the urine.

The most frequent adverse effects are drowsiness, dizziness, and lightheadedness. Blurred vision, headache, fever, and nausea can occur when the drug is administered orally or parenterally. Parenteral administration may also produce a metallic taste in the mouth, nystagmus, diplopia, flushing, vertigo, muscular incoordination, syncope, hypotension, and bradycardia. The allergic reactions that occasionally occur include urticaria, pruritus, skin rash and eruptions, nasal congestion, and conjunctivitis.

Cyclobenzaprine Hydrochloride

The drug is administered orally to a maximum daily dosage of 60 mg (Table 27–2). Cyclobenzaprine is employed primarily for treatment of muscle spasm that is associated with acute, painful musculoskeletal conditions. The usual course of therapy is two to three weeks, and that period of treatment provides relief of the pain, tenderness, and limitation of motion and functional abilities that usually accompany muscle spasms. The reduction in tonic somatic motor activity is provided by the action of the drug on the neural pathways of the brainstem.

The oral drug is well absorbed from the intestinal tract. Cyclobenzaprine has a plasma half-life of one to three days. It is extensively metabolized and the conjugates are excreted in the urine.

The most frequent adverse effects are drowsiness, dry mouth, and dizziness. The drug less frequently produces an increased heart rate, weakness, dyspepsia, paresthesias, unpleasant taste in the mouth, blurred vision, and insomnia.

High doses of the drug may produce temporary confusion, disturbed concentration, transient visual hallucinations, agitation, hyperactive reflexes, muscle rigidity, vomiting, and hyperpyrexia. Toxic dosages may produce drowsiness, hypothermia, tachycardia, cardiac rhythm disturbances, dilated pupils, convulsions, severe hypotension, stupor, and coma.

The drug is related to the tricyclic antidepressants, and the concurrent use of a monoamine oxidase inhibitor may produce a hyperpyretic crisis and convulsions. The drug enhances the sedative effects of other central nervous system depressants. The anticholinergic properties may increase the effects of belladonna alkaloids and other drugs with anticholinergic effects. The drug may also block the antihypertensive action of guanethidine.

PERIPHERALLY ACTING MUSCLE RELAXANTS

Dantrolene Sodium

Dantrolene sodium is the only direct muscle relaxant in common use for treatment of patients with muscle spasticity associated with central nervous system disorders (i.e., multiple sclerosis, cerebral palsy, spinal cord injury, stroke). The drug is a derivative of hydantoin.

Action Mode. Dantrolene is thought to act directly on the muscle fibers to reduce the release of calcium ions from the sarcoplasmic reticulum. That action decreases the muscle contraction in response to stimulation. There is a reduction in the muscle spasticity that is associated with direct stimulation of the efferent neural stimuli from the synaptic reflex pathways of the spinal cord.

Therapy Considerations.   The drug is administered orally to adults or children four times per day (Table 27–2). Only about 35 percent of the oral dosage of the drug is absorbed from the gastrointestinal tract. The therapeutic effects of the drug may occur within one week after therapy is initiated (i.e., a decrease in reflex muscle contraction, hyperreflexia, clonus, muscle stiffness, spasticity, and involuntary muscle movements).

Peak plasma drug concentrations are attained approximately five hours after the drug is taken. The plasma half-life of the drug is 8.7 hours in adults and 7.3 hours in children. The drug is metabolized in the liver and the metabolites are excreted in the urine.

Adverse Effects.   The most frequent adverse effect is muscle weakness. During the initial four days of therapy, the drug may produce drowsiness, dizziness, lightheadedness, diarrhea, nausea, malaise, and fatigue. The dosage is reduced when there is diarrhea or weakness associated with severe apathy. Therapy may be discontinued when diarrhea persists. Severe constipation, which occasionally occurs, often causes marked abdominal distention. Other adverse effects that occasionally occur are neurologic or emotional problems (i.e., speech disturbances, headache, visual disturbances, alterations of taste, depression, confusion, nervousness, insomnia, visual and auditory hallucinations), urinary tract problems (i.e., frequency, incontinence, nocturia, urine retention), tachycardia, blood pressure variations, phlebitis, and allergic reactions (i.e., phototoxicity, pruritus, urticaria). Prolonged use of the drug (i.e., > three months) may cause growth depression and reversible hepatotoxicity. Although the incidence of hepatotoxicity is relatively low, the nurse should be alert for evidence of the toxic effects (i.e., weakness, dizziness, fever, headache, drowsiness, nausea, vomiting, and diarrhea).

NURSING INTERVENTION

The absence of smoothly coordinated muscle movements interferes with many of the activities of daily living and makes each task a major chore for the individual. The muscle spasms associated with acute muscle strain lead to splinting of the injured muscles. The use of alternate muscle groups to accomplish necessary tasks places a strain on the muscles involved in the compensatory movements.

The drugs employed for relief of acute musculoskeletal conditions generally have central nervous system depressant effects that contribute to the relief of muscle spasm. The person should be cautioned to avoid hazardous tasks that could jeopardize safety when drowsiness occurs (i.e., driving a motor vehicle, operating machinery). Essential activities can be timed to avoid the peak periods of the sedative effects. The person should also be cautioned against exceeding the prescribed dosage of the drugs. The intense pain of acute muscle strain, coupled with the decreased judgment associated with central nervous system depression, can contribute to automatism and the potential hazard of unintentional overdosage.

The muscle relaxants are used with a planned program of muscle rest, carefully planned and limited exercises of the involved muscles, and warm baths or soaks that increase the blood supply to the affected muscle groups. Acute muscle strain is self-limiting, and at the termination of a two-to-four-week period, some improvement is predictable. Complete pain-free mobility may require gradual exercise-induced muscle building over a prolonged period of time.

The central nervous system–induced muscle spasms that are associated with cerebral palsy, multiple sclerosis, or parkinsonism are chronic problems that consistently interfere with the person's ability to control musculoskeletal function. The use of drugs to reduce muscle spasms may allow the person to increase the periods of assisted ambulation or to perform other desired tasks. During therapy, the person who has spasms of the muscles takes longer to perform activities of daily living than persons without muscle dysfunction. The goals for the person's participation in self-care, the time that is allowed for accomplishment of those tasks, and the assistance provided are dependent on the person's functional limitations.

The person's motivation to participate in activities that allow the attainment of short-term goals is a primary factor in the therapy plan. When the nurse provides assistance judiciously, the person's satisfaction with accomplishment of the task often raises the level of motivation. It frequently is difficult for the nurse to stand by while the person struggles to perform simple tasks (i.e., eating a meal), but the activity is important to the physical and psychologic health of the individual.

It is important for the nurse to consider the contributions that the patient can make to the preplanning of tasks that must be accomplished. Participation in the preplanning process allows the person to make judgments about capabilities and usually increases commitment to the completion of the activity. For example, the patient can be encouraged to select foods that can be managed with the least amount of difficulty or to plan the scheduling of muscle exercises at a time when functional abilities are greatest.

The nurse, physical therapist, and patient usually collaborate in the planning of consistent and progressive exercises to maintain and build muscle strength. Each contact with the patient provides an opportunity for the nurse to assess the effectiveness of the therapy plan and to provide the patient with reinforcement for the efforts that are made during activities.

Assessing Readiness for Self-Care

Patients who are incapable of performing activities of daily living independently require consistent assistance and supervision to assure that their basic needs are met and that therapy is continued. It is particularly important for the person with severe myasthenia gravis to be supervised and assisted with the conduct of the drug therapy plan. In the preplanning for posthospital care, the patient and a family member or a close associate must be counseled about the effects of the drugs and the implications of excess or deficiency of medication. Emphasis must be placed on the importance of accuracy in time and dosage of the medications, the importance of avoiding undue fatigue, and the recognition and treatment of *cholinergic crisis* or *anticholinergic crisis* (myasthenic crisis).

Complete return of muscle strength is not obtained with the use of the drugs, and the patient should be cautioned against increasing the dosage to obtain greater return of function. The specific discussion of factors that indicate that additional drug is required usually needs to be reiterated to assure that the patient is ready to assess changes in respiratory patterns and evidence of increased muscle weakness (i.e., difficulty in swallowing, increased ptosis). The high level of fatigue that exists before medication is taken may make it difficult for the person to obtain the required dosage unless assistance is available. In the absence of neuromuscular transmission, the person is incapable of calling out or of using the muscles to make a banging noise on the walls or floor to call attention to the need for assistance, and respiratory arrest is a potential hazard.

The respiratory depressions that occur with excess drug (cholinergic crisis) and deficient circulating drug (anticholinergic crisis) are similar. It is important for the patient and the person who will be responsible for posthospital care to be knowledgeable about the differences between the two crisis situations. The excess parasympathetic nerve activity that is present in cholinergic crisis produces small pupils, twitching of the muscles of the tongue, lips, or shoulder, excessive salivation, abdominal cramps, diarrhea, nausea, and excessive sweating in addition to difficulty in breathing, coughing, or swallowing. Anticholinergic crisis represents an inadequate amount of acetylcholine activity, and the pupils are normal or large, the muscles of the jaw are weak, the person has difficulty holding the head erect, there is increased ptosis, and the voice is nasal in addition to the difficulty with breathing, coughing, and swallowing. The patient is unable to treat the situation; it is necessary for a responsible person to be prepared to administer atropine sulfate when cholinergic crisis occurs or to administer the prescribed drug when the person's status indicates that there is inadequate acetylcholine available to maintain muscle function.

Review Guides

1. Explain the relationship between the central nervous system effects of levodopa and the improvement in muscle rigidity and sialorrhea in the person who has parkinsonism.
2. Outline the factors that would be included when explaining to the patient with parkinsonism the effects of the combination tablets that contain levodopa and carbidopa.
3. Explain why it is important trat the patient maintain a record of the drug taken to assure that a dose of amantadine hydrochloride is not omitted.
4. Ouline the assessments that would indicate that the dosage of levodopa should be reduced.
5. Explain the planned therapeutic outcomes of therapy with biperiden hydrochloride when it is employed for treatment of a patient with parkinsonism.
6. Describe the use of edrophonium chloride for diagnostic testing of a person who has a tentative diagnosis of myasthenia gravis.
7. Outline a plan for nursing care when the patient with myasthenia gravis is receiving pyridostigmine bromide.
8. Outline the nursing measures that would be employed when bethanechol chloride is administered to a postoperative patient.
9. Describe the symptoms of overdosage that may appear when the person is taking cyclobenzaprine hydrochloride for spasms of the back muscles.
10. Outline the factors that would be included when counseling the person with multiple sclerosis about the use of dantrolene sodium.

Additional Readings

Abramsky, Oded; Aharonov, Aharon; Teitelbaum, Dvora; and Fuchs, Sara: Myasthenia gravis and acetylcholine receptor. *Arch. Neurol.,* **32:**684, October, 1975.

Appel, Stanley H.; Almon, Richard R.; and Levy, Nelson: Acetylcholine receptor antibodies in myasthenia gravis. *N. Engl. J. Med.,* **293:**760, October 9, 1975.

Axelrod, Julius: Neurotransmitters. *Sci. Am.,* **230:** 58, June, 1974.

Bianchine, Joseph R.: Drug therapy: parkinsonism. *N. Engl. J. Med.,* **295:**814, October 7, 1976.

Carenzi, Angelo; Gillin, J. Cristan; Guidotti, Allesandro; Schwartz, Michael A.; Trabucchi, Marco; and Wyatt, Richard J.: Dopamine-sensitive adenyl cyclase in human caudate nucleus. *Arch. Gen. Psychiatry,* **32:**1056, August, 1975.

Celesin, Gastrone G., and Wanamaker, William M.: L-dopa-carbidopa: combined therapy for the treatment of Parkinson's disease. *Dis. Nerv. Syst.,* **37:** 123, March, 1976.

Cohen, Carolyn: The protein switch of muscle contraction. *Sci. Am.,* **233:**36, November, 1975.

Cotzias, George C.; Papavasiliou, Paul S.; Tolosa, Edwards S.; Mendez, Jorge S.; and Bell-Midura, Margaret: Treatment of parkinsonism with aporphines: possible role of growth hormone. *N. Engl. J. Med.,* **294:**567, March 11, 1976.

DiMascio, Alberto; Bernardo, Diosdado L.; Greenblatt, David J.; and Marder, Joseph E.: A controlled trial of amantadine in drug-induced extra-pyramidal disorders. *Arch. Gen. Psychiatry,* **33:** 599, May, 1976.

Doughty, Barbara, and Crozier, Julie: Understanding neurotransmitters and related drugs. *Can. Nurse,* **72:**39, August, 1976.

Fann, W. E.; Lake, C. R.; and Richman, B. W.: Drug-induced parkinsonism: a re-evaluation. *Dis. Nerv. Syst.,* **36:**91, February, 1975.

Fischbach, Frances Talaska: Easing adjustment to Parkinson's disease. *Am. J. Nurs.,* **78:**66, January, 1978.

Galdi, Albert P.: Essentials in the management of myasthenia gravis. *Am. Fam. Physician,* **17:**95, June, 1978.

Granacher, Robert P.: Physostigmine treatment of delirium induced by anticholinergics. *Am. Fam. Physician,* **13:**99, May, 1976.

Granacher, Robert P., and Baldessarini, Ross J.: Physostigmine. *Arch. Gen. Psychiatry,* **32:**375, March, 1975.

Greer, Melvin: How to achieve maximum benefit for the patient with Parkinson's disease. *Geriatrics,* **31:**89, April, 1976.

Hughes, John H.; Freimer, Earl H.; and Mantis, J. Kelly: Tetanus. *Am. Fam. Physician,* **13:**76, March, 1976.

Iverson, Leslie L.: Dopamine receptors in the brain. *Science,* **188:**1084, June 13, 1975.

Jus, A.; Pineau, R.; Lachance, R.; Pelchat, G.; Jus, K.; Pires, P.; and Villeneuve, R.: Epidemiology of tardive dyskinesia. Part 1. *Dis. Nerv. Syst.,* **37:** 210, April, 1976.

Khanna, Om P.: A new pharmacologic approach to the non-emptying bladder. *Am. Fam. Physician,* **17:** 162, May, 1968.

Klawans, Harold L.; Goetz, Christopher; and Bergen, Donna: Levodopa-induced myoclonus. *Arch. Neurol.,* **32:**331, May, 1975.

Langan, Rebecca J., and Cotzias, George C.: Do's and don'ts for the patient on levodopa therapy. *Am. J. Nurs.,* **76:**917, June, 1976.

Layzer, Robert B.: Remedial neuromuscular disorders. *Primary Care,* **2:**235, June, 1975.

Lester, Henry A.: The response to acetylcholine. *Sci. Am.,* **236:**106, February, 1977.

Ludin S.; Uden, D.; and Hanson, R.: Dantrolene-associated hepatitis. *Drug Intelligence Clin. Pharm.,* **11:**278, May, 1977.

McFarland, H. Richard: Treating parkinsonism in the era of levodopa. *Am. Fam. Physician,* **12:**99, September, 1975.

Martin, William E.; Tolosa, Eduardo S.; Loewenson, Ruth B.; Lee, Myoung C.; Resch, Joseph A.; and Baker, Abe B.: The effects of combining carbidopa with levodopa for Parkinson's disease. *Geriatrics,* **30:**39, December, 1975.

Murray, John M., and Weber, Annemarie: The cooperative action of muscle proteins. *Sci. Am.,* **230:**58, February, 1974.

Rayfield, Elliot J.; George, David T.; Eichner, Harvey L.; and Hsu, T. H.: L-dopa stimulation of glucagon secretion in man. *N. Engl. J. Med.,* **293:**589, September 18, 1975.

Stackhouse, Joan: Myasthenia gravis. *Am. J. Nurs.,* **73:**1544, September, 1973.

Teychenne, Paul F.; Calne, Donald B.; Lewis, Peter J.; and Findlay, Leslie J.: Interactions of levodopa with inhibitors of monoamine oxidase and L-aromatic amino acid decarboxylase. *Clin. Pharmacol. Ther.,* **18:**273, September, 1975.

Tinker, John H., and Wehner, Robert J.: Postoperative recovery and the neuromuscular junction. *Am. J. Nurs.,* **74:**74, January, 1974.

VanWinkle, W. B.: Calcium release from skeletal muscle sarcoplasmic reticulum: site of action of dantrolene sodium? *Science,* **193:**1130, September 17, 1976.

Walker, Jonathan E.: Clinical use of levodopa and amantadine in Parkinson's disease. *Clin. Med.,* **82:**27, March, 1975.

Weinman, Robert L.: Disorders of movement: a mercifully short primer. *Dis. Nerv. Syst.,* **36:**84, February, 1975.

Widroe, Harvey J., and Heisler, Stephen: Treatment of tardive dyskinesia. *Dis. Nerv. Syst.,* **37:**162, March, 1976.

Winkelman, Arnold C.: Update on drug treatment of parkinsonism. *Am. Fam. Physician,* **16:**118, July, 1977.

28

Surgical Anesthesia

Modern anesthesia represents a highly sophisticated balancing of several agents to provide the sedation, analgesia, muscle relaxation, and anesthesia required for operations of varying seriousness and complexity. The anesthesiologist's decision to employ particular agents is based on the status of the patient, the specific surgical procedure to be performed, and the duration of the surgery. Throughout the operative period, the anesthetist monitors the physiologic status of the individual and utilizes drugs and other supportive therapies to maintain physiologic equilibrium in the anesthetized patient.

PREOPERATIVE PREPARATION OF THE PATIENT

Preparation of the patient for the surgical experience is a team effort that requires the expertise of the physician, nurses, and anesthetist. Other health team members are involved selectively in complex major surgical procedures, (i.e., chest physical therapist, technicians with specialized skills in the use of particular equipment).

Collaboration between the nurse and physician is essential to the planning of preoperative and postoperative care of the patient. The anesthetist and the physician collaborate in the planning of the surgical procedure. Each of the professionals assumes responsibility for informing the patient about particular aspects of the surgical experience.

The physician discusses the planned surgical procedures, the risks involved, and the expected outcomes of the procedure with the patient and members of the immediate family. Signed operative permission must be obtained before the surgical procedure can be performed. The permission can be signed by the patient, a guardian, or a member of the immediate family when the patient is incapable of giving informed consent before surgery.

It is a useful practice for the nurse to accompany the physician during the explanation of surgery because patients often need clarification or additional information about specific points that remain unclear to them after the initial discussion. There are times when the patient's questions relate to such factors as the risks and outcomes of surgery, and the nurse relays those concerns to the physician for further clarification.

In most instances, patients seek reiteration of varying aspects of the discussion with the physician. The nurse who has participated in the discourse can amplify the relevant information to assure that the patient has a clear concept of the planned surgery.

The anesthetist audits the data in the clinical record and examines the patient before making the final decision about the anesthetic agents that will be employed. During the anesthetist's visit, patients have an opportunity to identify with the person who will be "putting them to sleep" before the surgery. The anesthetist utilizes the contact time to discuss the planned anesthesia methodology with the patient.

The intensity of the nurses' preoperative counseling about deep breathing, coughing, leg exercises, and other preparation of the patient for the postoperative experience is influenced by the type of surgery and the anesthetic agents that will be employed during the surgery. An accurate concept of the experiences that the patient predictably will encounter during the pre- and postanesthesia period is essential to the nurse who prepares the patient for those experiences. The data in this chapter will focus on the information about anesthetic agents that will influence nursing intervention in the pre- and postoperative periods.

An anticholinergic agent (i.e., atropine sulfate) and a narcotic analgesic are usually prescribed by the anesthetist to be given "on call" or one-half hour before the patient is transferred to the operating suite. The premedication assures that the patient will have minimal mucus secretions and will be relaxed, slightly euphoric, and drowsy at the time of arrival at the anesthesia induction area.

The individualized plan for balanced anesthesia may involve the concurrent or sequential use of many agents. For example, the relaxation of the muscles of the thoracic cage that is required for lung surgery can be provided by intravenous administration of a neuromuscular-blocking agent. Varying types of vapors and gases also may be administered with oxygen to provide anesthesia during the surgery. When abdominal surgery is to be performed, muscle relaxation can be provided by injection of a local anesthetic into the spinal fluid. An ultrashort-acting barbiturate may be infused intravenously, after the abdominal anesthesia level is established, to provide general anesthesia during the surgical procedure.

Neuromuscular Blocking Agents

The muscle relaxants employed as adjuncts to anesthetic agents during surgery include the nondepolarizing agents *gallamine triethiodide, metocurine iodide, pancuronium bromide,* and *tubocurarine chloride* and the depolarizing agents *decamethonium bromide* and *succinylcholine chloride.* Although the nondepolarizing agents and the depolarizing agents act at the motor end plate by a different mechanism in blocking the muscular response to stimulation by acetylcholine, both groups provide the muscle relaxation required for selected surgical procedures (i.e., orthopedic or thoracic surgery). The drugs are usually given as a continuous intravenous infusion that is regulated by the anesthetist to maintain the desired level of muscle relaxation during surgery.

In addition to their use as adjuncts to anesthesia, the muscle relaxants are employed to prevent the sudden, convulsive muscle movements that occur during electroconvulsive therapy of patients with mental depression. The drugs are also used selectively for the treatment of persons on controlled respiratory assistors to decrease the voluntary respirations that interfere with the automatic ventilation cycle.

Action Mode

The *nondepolarizing agents* have a high affinity for the acetylcholine receptors at the motor end plate of the myoneural junction. The agents compete with acetylcholine and block its access to the receptors. That interference with acetylcholine activity inhibits muscle depolarization, and there is a consequent decrease in the tone and contraction of the muscles.

The *depolarizing agents* also have a high affinity for the acetylcholine receptors. They act as agonists at the receptors and stimulate depolarization and conduction of the muscle action potential. The drugs are more resistant than acetylcholine to the effects of acetylcholinesterase and produce a more prolonged period of muscle depolarization. In the first phase of their depolarizing activity, the drugs produce sustained contractions and muscle fasciculations. Patients occasionally have residual muscle pain in the postoperative period when they have received a depolarizing agent. Continued infusion of the drug produces a second phase with poorly sustained muscle contraction that somewhat resembles the status of the muscles when nondepolarizing agents are administered.

Therapy Considerations

The anesthetist may start the intravenous infusion of the neuromuscular-blocking agent before the anesthetic agents are given or after the induction of general anesthesia. The first signs of muscle paralysis appear within one to two minutes after the intravenous infusion commences, and maximal effects generally occur within one to six minutes.

The small muscle groups that control the fine, rapid movements of the eyes, face, and neck are affected almost immediately after intravenous infusion of the neuromuscular-blocking agents is begun. The anesthetist usually sprays the oropharyngeal tissues with a local anesthetic and inserts an endotracheal tube immediately after the infusion is started when extensive muscle relaxation is planned during the operative procedure. Manual or mechanical artificial ventilation is instituted as soon as the endotracheal tube is in place. The progressive neuromuscular-blocking action of the drug paralyzes the muscles of the limbs, abdomen, and chest. The diaphragm

and the intercostal muscles are the last to be affected. During the recovery process, the muscle responses return in a sequence that is the reverse of that occurring during the induction process. Approximately 3 percent of the patients who receive the neuromuscular-blocking agents have a short period of hiccups when the effects of the drug are terminated. The hiccups are considered to be associated with the resumption of normal diaphragmatic activity at the termination of the drug therapy. With the exception of pancuronium, the neuromuscular-blocking agents cause the release of histamine, which causes a fall in blood pressure.

Nondepolarizing Agents

Gallamine triethiodide (FLAXEDIL) also has a parasympatholytic effect on the vagus nerve, which causes tachycardia. Hypertension occurs occasionally. The muscle relaxation reaches a maximum level within three minutes after the intravenous infusion is started. The effects generally persist for 15 to 20 minutes after therapy is terminated.

Metocurine iodine (METUBINE) provides a maximum effect within three to five minutes after the intravenous infusion is started. The muscular relaxation persists for 15 to 90 minutes after the drug therapy is terminated.

Pancuronium bromide (PAVULON) has a direct blocking effect on the cardiac acetylcholine receptors, in addition to its action at the motor end plate, which produces a slight tachycardia when the drug is administered at therapeutic dosages. The muscle relaxation is attained within two to three minutes after the intravenous infusion commences, and the effects generally subside 35 to 45 minutes after the infusion is terminated.

Tubocurarine chloride (TUBARINE) has histamine-releasing and ganglionic-blocking properties. Muscle relaxation occurs within five minutes after the intravenous infusion is started. The effects persist for 20 to 30 minutes after the infusion is terminated.

Depolarizing Agents

Decamethonium bromide (SYNCURINE) also has minimal histamine-releasing properties. Muscle relaxation occurs within one to three minutes and reaches a peak four to eight minutes after the intravenous infusion is started. The effect persists for 15 to 20 minutes after the infusion is terminated.

Succinylcholine chloride (ANECTINE, QUELICIN, SUCOSTRIN, SUX-CERT) is the drug most frequently employed for neuromuscular blockade during surgical procedures. Muscle relaxation occurs within one minute. The duration of the drug action is two to three minutes when a single dose is given. There may be residual effect for a period of ten minutes after the infusion is terminated. Although succinylcholine has a more rapid onset of action than the other neuromuscular-blocking agents, it is more rapidly degraded by the enzyme *pseudocholinesterase*. The drug is usually given as a continuous intravenous infusion. The enzyme inhibitor *hexafluorenium bromide* (MYLAXEN) is usually administered intravenously concurrently with succinylcholine to prevent its enzymatic degradation and prolong its duration of action.

Intravenously Administered Anesthetics

ULTRASHORT-ACTING BARBITURATES

The drugs provide a rapid action of short duration that is useful when basal anesthesia is required for intrusive diagnostic, minor surgical, or obstetric procedures. The hypnotic effect of *thiopental sodium* (PENTOTHAL), which is representative of the group of drugs, has popularized it as being "truth serum." *Methohexital sodium* (BREVITAL) and *thiamylal sodium* (SURITAL) are also employed for induction of short-term general anesthesia.

Premedication of the patient with atropine sulfate averts the parasympathetic nerve–induced sensitivity of the laryngeal reflexes that causes spastic adduction of the vocal cords when the drugs are administered intravenously. The barbiturates have a high lipoid affinity and rapidly move to the highly vascular lipid-containing cerebrocortical tissues.

The patient usually is asked to slowly count backward from 100 when the infusion is started. Within 20 to 60 seconds the oral counting ceases and the person is asleep. The depth of anesthesia is controlled by the dosage of the drug that is infused, and that dosage in turn is dependent on the level required for conduction of the planned procedure. The short period of the anesthetic effect can be prolonged by continuous intravenous infusion of the drug during the procedure. The patient awakens within 10 to 30 minutes after the drug infusion is terminated unless additional anesthetic agents are given.

The postanesthesia recovery period is generally smooth and rapid. Methohexital has the shortest duration of action, and recovery from anesthesia is more rapid than with the other ultrashort-acting barbiturates. Nausea and vomiting seldom occur when the drugs are administered to persons who have fasted before receiving the barbiturate. There have been a few reports of laryngospasm and shivering in the postanesthesia period.

KETAMINE

The drug (KETALAR, KETAJECT) is administered by intramuscular or intravenous injection. Ketamine induces a cataleptic state, and the patient appears to be awake but dissociated from activity in the environment. The drug action on central nervous system tissues aborts the pain response. The patient also has postanesthesia amnesia for events that occurred during the procedure.

The drug is used for intrusive diagnostic or minor surgical procedures and for the debridement of tissue or changing of dressings in extensively burned patients. It is also used as an alternate drug for induction of anesthesia when patients cannot be given an ultrashort-acting barbiturate.

Adults frequently have psychic disturbances in the immediate postanesthesia period (i.e., disturbing dreams, excitement, disorientation, delirium, hallucinations). The drug can produce vomiting, hypersalivation, lacrimation, or shivering in the postanesthesia period. The drug also has a cardiac-stimulating effect. It has a cocaine-like activity that produces tachycardia and increased cardiac output by elevating blood norepinephrine levels.

Inhalation Anesthesia

The inhaled anesthetics are gases or liquids with volatile vapors that enter the circulation from the alveoli. The circulating anesthetic travels to muscle and adipose tissues throughout the body. Its accumulation in the lipid tissues of the cerebral cortex provides the anesthetic action. The tissues gradually release the anesthetic into the circulation, and the agents are metabolized in the liver. The metabolites are excreted by the kidneys. Obese patients may have a slightly more delayed and prolonged anesthetic effect because the anesthetics are distributed into a greater volume and are more slowly released from the larger amount of adipose tissues.

The quantity of inhalation anesthetics currently administered during extensive major surgical procedures is markedly less than that given when the agents were first introduced. For example, during thoracic surgery the patient can be protected from pain and discomfort by the balanced use of a strong, or narcotic, analgesic; a neuromuscular-blocking agent; intravenous thiopental sodium during the initial induction period; and administration of an inhalant anesthetic during the period when the viscera are being manipulated. The electrical equipment employed for administration of the gas or vapor automatically controls the patient's respiratory cycles during the time that the anesthetic and oxygen mixture is being given. The balanced anesthesia plan provides adequate muscle relaxation, and the patient has less postanesthetic central nervous system depression than that occurring when pain control and muscle relaxation were dependent on the use of a single general anesthetic.

The *stages of anesthesia* follow a predictable sequence, but the intensity and duration of each stage varies with the type of anesthetic agent administered:

Stage I: Euphoria, gradual loss of consciousness.

Stage II: Hyperexcitement, thrashing of the extremities, attempts to manually remove the anesthesia mask or evasive side-to-side movements of the head, hyperactivity of the blinking and swallowing reflexes, dilation of the pupils.

Stage III: Depression of the corneal reflex and the pupillary response to light, decreased muscle tone, absence of voluntary muscle control.

Stage IV: Medullary paralysis, death.

POSTANESTHESIA SURVEILLANCE

During the postanesthesia period, recovery normally occurs in a sequence that is the reverse of the induction stages, and the intensity and duration of the stages are also affected by the types of anesthetic agents employed during the surgical procedure. For example, during stage II of general anesthesia induction, the patient's extremities and head are restrained to prevent self-injury and allow continued administration of the anesthetic. The period of hyperexcitability is more marked when a single anesthetic agent (i.e., ether) is used for induction, and it may pass almost unnoticed when the previously described balanced anesthesia is employed. During the postanesthesia period, the patient must also be

Table 28–1.

Problems Commonly Occurring Following the Administration of Inhalation Anesthetics

Anesthetic Agent	Postanesthesia Problems
Anesthetic Gas	
Cyclopropane	Hypotension, depressed respiratory rate, nausea, vomiting, headache, ventricular arrhythmias, occasionally delirium
Ethylene	Prolonged wound seepage, prolonged clotting time
Nitrous oxide	Short-term euphoria (laughing, crying)
Liquid with Volatile Vapor	
Ether	Copious secretions, nausea, vomiting, transient hyperglycemia, decreased urine output, decreased intestinal motility
Ethyl chloride	Muscle spasms, arrhythmias, hepatotoxicity
Enflurane (ethrane)	Convulsions, shivering
Halothane (fluothane)	Shallow and quiet respirations, shivering, hepatotoxicity, hyperpyrexia
Methoxyflurane (penthrane)	High-urine-output syndrome with a duration of 2 to 3 days (decreased concentration of urine in the distal tubules, intense thirst), hepatotoxicity, nausea, vomiting, prolonged analgesia, drowsiness
Trichloroethylene E (trilene)	Rapid respirations, bradycardia, ventricular arrhythmias
Vinyl ether	Copious secretions, nephrotoxicity, hepatotoxicity

protected against injury when the anesthesia lightens to the stage II level. Patients usually are emerging from stage I at the time that the surgical dressing is applied to the incision.

The residual effects of the central nervous system depressants remain evident when the person is moved to the recovery room. The patient is under the direct surveillance of the anesthetist until the cardiovascular, respiratory, and central nervous system assessments indicate that the patient is recovering from the effects of the anesthetic agents.

Nurses become the primary caretakers in the recovery room. They assess the physiologic status continually and provide for the comfort and safety of the patient until the vital signs are stable and the patient is transferred to the unit.

Predictable problems can occur in the postanesthesia period when anesthetic gases or vapors have been administered to the patient (Table 28–1). Some patients have shallow respirations as a consequence of the central nervous system depressant effects of the anesthetics. The direct drying effect of the inhaled gases and oxygen on the respiratory tract tissues increases the viscosity of mucus, and the secretions are more difficult to raise with coughing. Periodic deep breathing, coughing, and sighing are essential activities in the early postoperative period because they promote gas exchange, increase lung compliance, and facilitate the raising of mucus secretions from the tracheobronchial tree. The patient who has practiced deep breathing and coughing during the preoperative period and understands the rationale for those activities is less resistive to performing the procedures during the immediate postanesthesia period.

Local Anesthetics

Action Mode

The local anesthetics can block conduction through sensory, motor, and autonomic nerve fibers. The drugs are thought to compete with calcium ions for binding sites on the neural membranes, and that action decreases the membrane permeability to sodium ions. The action of the local anesthetics inhibits depolarization of the nerves and propagation of the action potential.

Topical Anesthesia

Local anesthetics may be applied directly to tissues (i.e., ethyl chloride), but they are more frequently ingredients of ointments, lotions, or solutions designed specifically for use at a particular topical site (i.e., eye, ear, nose, oral mucosa, perineum, hemorrhoids, or skin). The preparations provide relief of pain when the drug penetrates to the fine pain fibers that are close to the application site. The following listing of local anesthetics represents the drugs most commonly applied topically for the relief of pain:

Benoxinate hydrochloride (DORSACAINE)
Benzocaine or ethyl aminobenzoate (AMERICAINE, AEROCAINE, SOLARCAINE)
Butamben picrate (BUTESIN)
Cocaine
Cyclomethycaine sulfate (SURFACAINE)
Dibucaine hydrochloride (NUPERCAINE) *
Dimethisoquin hydrochloride (QUOTANE)
Diperodon (DIOTHANE)
Dyclonine hydrochloride (DYCLONE)
Ethyl chloride
Hexylcaine hydrochloride (CYCLAINE) †
Lidocaine hydrochloride (CAPPICAINE, L-CAINE, LIDA-MANTEL, SERACAINE, XYLOCAINE) †
Piperocaine hydrochloride (METYCAINE) †

* Also used for spinal anesthesia.
† Also used for nerve block.

Pramoxine hydrochloride (TRONOTHANE)
Proparacaine hydrochloride (ALCAINE, OPHTHETIC, OPHTHAINE)
Tetracaine hydrochloride (BUFOPTO ANACEL, PONTOCAINE) †

The local sensory and motor nerve block allows unintentional trauma of the anesthetized tissues. For example, when an anesthetic mouthwash or gargle is used (i.e., viscous lidocaine solution), biting of the inside of the cheek can occur when chewing food, and the injury may go unnoticed until termination of the anesthetic effect. The use of a similar preparation as a gargle for the relief of pain in oropharyngeal tissues desensitizes the uvula and peritonsillar pillars that normally stimulate the gag reflex. Oral fluids and foods should be withheld until the gag reflex returns.

Local or Infiltration Anesthesia

Local anesthetics are injected into the intradermal, subcutaneous, or submucosal tissues to provide a circumscribed area of anesthesia. Infiltration of the drug across the pathway of the nerves provides a local nerve block that is useful for such procedures as suturing of a laceration or extraction of teeth. The small nerves are more susceptible than large nerves to the effects of local anesthetics, and a weak drug solution is used to provide a rapid effect of short duration.

The addition of epinephrine to the anesthetic causes vasoconstriction in the localized area and prolongs the action of the anesthetic by slowing its absorption from the tissues. Penetration of a local anesthetic into the extracellular space is retarded by the unusually low pH of the fluids that is associated with severe inflammation or infection, and the drug produces a less effective level of anesthesia.

Regional Nerve Blocks

The local anesthetic can be injected at a perineural site distant from the desired anesthetic area to provide a wider area of anesthesia. The drug may be injected into the nerve trunk or ganglia, or it may be injected adjacent to the nerve pathway and allowed to infiltrate through the nerve sheath. Peripheral nerve blocks (i.e., brachial plexus, intercostal, paracervical, pudendal, or ulnar nerve block) may be performed to decrease intractable pain or to provide an anesthetic field for selected surgical procedures. The following listing includes the local anesthetics commonly employed for nerve blocks:

Bupivacaine hydrochloride (MARCAINE)
Chloroprocaine hydrochloride (NESACAINE, NESACAINE-CE)
Dehydrated alcohol
Etidocaine hydrochloride (DURANEST)
Lidocaine hydrochloride (XYLOCAINE)
Mepivacaine hydrochloride (CARBOCAINE)
Prilocaine hydrochloride (CITANEST)
Procaine hydrochloride (NOVOCAIN)

Spinal Nerve Blocks

Local anesthetics can be injected into the epidural space to block the paravertebral and peridural projections of the spinal nerves. The drugs can also be injected into the subarachnoid space to anesthetize the nerve roots that emerge from the spinal cord (Fig. 28–1). The action of the drugs blocks transmission in sensory, motor, and sympathetic nerves that are infiltrated by the local anesthetic.

The sympathetic nerves at the central sites are the first to be affected by infiltration of the drug. The sympathetic nerve block produces contraction of the bowel, relaxation of the sphincters of the gastrointestinal and urinary tract, and increased venous capacitance, which can cause hypotension. The vagus nerves are unaffected, and the pressure and visceral manipulation that occur during intrusive procedures can precipitate nausea and vomiting.

The local anesthetic slowly diffuses through the epidural space, and the peak anesthetic effect occurs in 15 to 30 minutes. The epineural membrane is the only diffusion barrier to nerve block when the drug is injected into the subarachnoid

space, and the onset of anesthesia occurs within 5 to 12 minutes. The site of injection and the strength of the local anesthetic solution are determined by the anesthetist on the basis of the planned surgical site and the predicted duration of the surgical procedure.

Subarachnoid Anesthetic Injection. The drug is given as a single injection into the subarachnoid fluid by insertion of a spinal needle into the space between the third and fourth lumbar vertebrae when upper abdominal sensory and motor nerve block is desired for surgery. The drug is given with a fine-gauge needle, and precautions are taken to avoid the leaking of cerebrospinal fluid, which contributes to the incidence of "spinal headache" in postoperative patients.

Dilution of the anesthetic with distilled water produces a hypobaric solution that gravitates in the cephalad direction. When a low spinal anesthesia is the desired anesthesia level, the drug is given as a hyperbaric solution by diluting it with dextrose, and that solution gravitates caudally. Tilting of the operating table is also used to control the gravitational movement of the drug in the cerebrospinal fluid.

The sensory nerves are blocked after the sympathetic nerves, and the motor nerves are the last to be affected. Recovery from the effects of the local anesthetics occurs in the reverse sequence to that of the induction period. The gradual upward block of the sensory nerves is tested by the anesthetist during the induction period. The patient is asked to describe whether the pinching of the skin on the abdomen causes sharp, dull, or no pain. The patient's response gives an indication of the level of anesthesia, and surgical skin preparation begins when sensory nerve block has reached the level desired for surgery.

Epidural Anesthetic Injection. The local anesthetic may be given as a single injection into the epidural space or it may be infused continuously during surgical or obstetric procedures. The drug provides anesthesia of the lower abdomen, perineum, and legs when it is injected into the intervertebral space at the junction of the fifth lumbar and the first sacral vertebrae. A more limited perineal anesthesia, or saddle block, is produced when the drug is injected into the epidural space at the level of the sacral hiatus (Fig. 28–1). A test dose of the drug may be given to assure that the injection has been made into the epidural rather than the subarachnoid space. When there is no evidence of sensory or motor anesthesia within a period of five minutes, the remainder of the drug is injected.

Toxicity. The local anesthetics are administered for spinal nerve blocks by a skilled anesthetist because excess dosage, rapid administration, or inadvertent intravascular injection of the drug can produce serious cardiovascular effects or central nervous system stimulation that is followed by life-threatening depression of the medullary centers. The excess drug blockage of inhibitory cortical synapses can produce convulsions.

Postanesthesia Surveillance. Adverse effects that may persist into the postanesthesia period

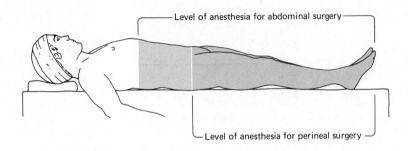

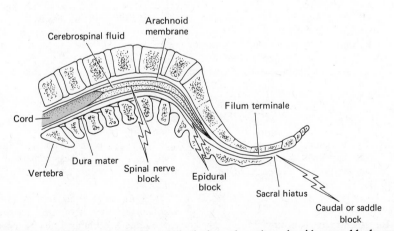

Fig. 28–1. Injection of a local anesthetic into the subarachnoid space blocks conduction in the spinal nerve roots. The anesthetic blocks sensory, motor, and autonomic nerve fibers up to the level of the diaphragm. Injection of a local anesthetic into the epidural space blocks conduction in the nerves that exit through the dura and provides a neural block in the lower abdomen, perineum, and legs. Caudal or saddle block provides anesthesia in the perineal area.

are related primarily to the inhibition of sympathetic nerves. The blocking of tonic constrictor impulses to the veins increases the vascular capacitance and allows the pooling of blood in the venous system. The consequent reduction in the return of venous blood to the heart decreases the cardiac output. The absence of sympathetic nerve–induced constriction of the arterioles causes peripheral vasodilation. The absence of the compensatory reflexes that normally maintain the circulating blood volume when cardiac output is reduced intensifies the level of hypotension. The low blood pressure can produce dizziness and syncope during position changes.

The return of motor and sensory nerve function can be mistakenly interpreted as a full return of neural function. Male patients often seek permission from the nurse to stand at the bedside to void in the urinal. That procedure can cause syncope associated with the decreased volume of circulating blood in cerebral tissues. Sudden position changes should be avoided until the cardiac rate and the blood pressure levels indicate that there is sympathetic tone in the vasculature.

Review Guides

1. Explain the primary differences in the action of tubocurarine and succinylcholine.
2. Outline the factors that would be included in the preoperative teaching of the patient when the anesthetist plans to administer gallamine triethiodide, thioamylal, and cyclopropane during surgery.
3. Outline the surveillance measures that would be used by the nurse during the postanesthesia period when the patient has received gallamine triethiodide, thioamylal, and cyclopropane.
4. Define the factors that would be included when describing the anesthesia experience to the patient who is to have ketamine during the changing of burn dressings in the operating room.
5. Outline the observations and nursing measures that would be included in the care plans for patients who have received the following general anesthetics:
   a. Ether
   b. Halothane
   c. Trichloroethylene
   d. Cyclopropane
6. Describe the rationale for administration of meperidine hydrochloride and atropine sulfate before administration of anesthetic agents.
7. Describe the similarities and differences in the effects of a local anesthetic that is injected into the epidural space and the subarachnoid space from the patient's point of view.
8. Describe the factors that would influence nursing care plans when the patient has a local anesthetic injected for blocking of the brachial plexus.

Additional Readings

Belfrage, Patrick; Berlin, Anita; Raabe, Nils; and Thalme, Bertil: Lumbar epidural analgesia with bupivacaine in labor. *Am. J. Obstet. Gynecol.,* **123**:839, December 15, 1975.

Carron, Harold: Relieving pain with nerve blocks. *Geriatrics,* **33**:49, April, 1978.

Ettinger, Bruce B., and McCart, Dorothy F.: Effects of drugs on the fetal heart rate during labor. *JOGN Nurs. (suppl.),* **5**:415, September/October, 1976.

Fehlau, Mary T.: Applying the nursing process to patient care in the operating room. *Nurs. Clin. North Am.,* **10**:617, December, 1975.

Grad, Rae Krohn, and Woodside, Jack: Obstetrical analgesics and anesthesia: methods of relief for the patient in labor. *Am. J. Nurs.,* **77**:242, February, 1977.

Greiss, Frank C., Jr.; Still, J. Gordon; and Anderson, Stephen G.: Effects of local anesthetic agents on the uterine vasculatures and myometrium. *Am. J. Obstet. Gynecol.,* **124**:889, April 15, 1976.

Knudsen, Kathleen: Play therapy: preparing the young child for surgery. *Nurs. Clin. North Am.,* **10**:679, December, 1975.

Laird, Mona: Techniques for teaching pre- and

postoperative patients. *Am. J. Nurs.,* **75:**1338, August, 1975.

Lyons, Mary Lou: What priority do you give preop teaching? *Nursing '77,* **7:**12, January, 1977.

McAllister, Roseanne G.: Obstetric anesthesia—a two-way street. *JOGN Nursing,* **5:**9, January/ February, 1976.

McConnell, Edwina A.: After surgery. *Nursing '77,* **7:**32, March, 1977.

Minckley, Barbara Blake: Physiologic hazards of position changes in the anesthetized patient. *Am. J. Nurs.,* **69:**2607, December, 1969.

Murray, Ruth L. E.: Assessment of psychologic stress in the surgical I.C.U. patient. *Nurs. Clin. North Am.,* **10:**69, March, 1975.

Poulton, Thomas J., and Mims, Grover R.: Periph-eral nerve blocks. *Am. Fam. Physician,* **16:**100, November, 1977.

Sangoul, Firooz; Fox, Gordon S.; and Houle, Germain L.: Effect of regional analgesia on maternal oxygen consumption during the first stage of labor. *Am. J. Obstet. Gynecol.,* **121:**1080, April 15, 1975.

Thomas, Jack; Long, Geoffrey; Moore, George; and Morgan, Denis: Plasma protein binding and placental transfer of bupivacaine. *Clin. Pharmacol. Ther.,* **19:**426, April, 1976.

Urban, Bruno J.: The current use of nerve blocks in the management of chronic pain. *Clin. Med.,* **82:** 27, May, 1975.

Wall, John J.: Axillary nerve blocks. *Am. Fam. Physician,* **11:**135, May, 1975.

VI
U N I T

Drugs Used to Maintain Nutritional Balance

29

Gastric Irritation and Vomiting

Gastric disturbances frequently occur in association with the use of drugs, acute illness, or stressful situations. Although those factors may cause a transient increase in gastric secretions and spasms of the stomach muscles that produce gastric distress, removal of the causative factor usually alleviates the symptoms. Persistent hypersecretion can produce erosion of the mucosal lining of the stomach and the persistent problems (i.e., pain, anorexia, nausea, food intolerances) associated with peptic ulcer.

Physiologic Correlations

The sight, smell, thought, or taste of food can provide the psychic stimulus at the cerebral cortex or the appetite center of the hypothalamus that initiates the digestive processes. The impulses from the brain centers are transmitted by the motor division of the parasympathetic nerves to the receptors in the gastric tissues. Acetylcholine is the neurotransmitter that activates the receptors in the stomach.

The parasympathetic or vagus nerves predominate over the sympathetic nerves in the control of digestion. The presence of food in the stomach stimulates the sensory divisions of the vagus nerves, and the impulses are transmitted to the brainstem. The efferent vagus motor impulses provide the stimulus for the increased motility and the secretion of enzymes that are required for the digestion of foods in the stomach.

GASTRIC SECRETIONS

The gastric glands secrete mucus, hydrochloric acid, pepsinogen, and small amounts of lipase and amylase. The tubular mucus-producing glands, which provide the viscid, alkaline protective coating for the gastric epithelium, are most abundant in the antral, cardiac, and pyloric areas of the stomach (Fig. 29–1). A dense barrier is provided by the mucus that adheres to the epithelium and protects the gastric lining from the proteolytic activity of *hydrochloric acid* and *pepsin.*

The gastric glands, which produce the secretions required for digestion, are located in the body and fundus of the stomach. The glands have parietal cells that secrete hydrochloric acid and chief cells that secrete *pepsinogen.* The inactive *pepsinogen* is converted in the stomach to the active enzyme pepsin in the presence of hydrochloric acid and previously activated pepsin. The proteolytic activity of pepsin is dependent on a gastric pH below 3.5; the presence of hydrochloric acid maintains the acidity required for digestion of proteins. Pepsin action is inhibited when the pH of the gastric content rises above 4.0.

The approximate daily volume of gastric secretions is 2000 ml. That figure represents the secretions that are produced as a consequence of neural and hormonal stimulation of the gastric glands. The vagus nerve directly stimulates the gastric glands. It also indirectly increases the production of digestive secretions by stimulating release of the hormone *gastrin.* The hormone is released into the bloodstream. Gastrin acts at the parietal cells to stimulate the secretion of hydrochloric acid and, to a lesser extent, the secretion of pepsinogen.

The presence of food distends the stomach, and that distention directly stimulates the release of gastrin from the mucosal glands. Gastrin release can also be precipitated by the presence of certain chemical substances in the gastric contents (i.e., caffeine, alcohol, partially digested proteins). The secretion of gastrin is blocked when the gastric content is down to pH 2.5 at the time it enters the duodenum.

The vagus nerve–induced release of glandular secretions and gastric motility is greater than that of gastrin, but the hormone stimulates the digestive processes over a longer period of time. Local myoenteric plexus reflexes also contribute to the motility of the stomach. The rhythmic churning contractions, which continually expose the gastric contents to the action of the digestive juices, gradually reduce the bulky food to chyme. The vagus nerve–induced relaxation of the pyloric sphincter allows the gastric contents to enter the duodenum.

Gastric emptying can be inhibited by the enterogastric reflex that depresses gastric motility and slows the production of gastric secretions. The reflex is stimulated when the duodenum is irritated or distended with food, or when its contents are acidic.

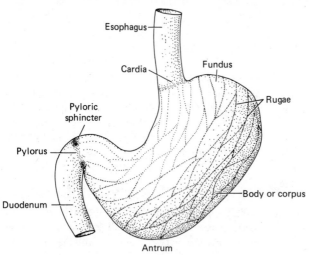

Fig. 29–1. Functional areas of the stomach.

Pathophysiologic Correlations

EXCESS GASTRIC SECRETIONS

Emotional or physiologic stress can produce sympathetic nerve impulses that affect gastric activity. The stimuli cause interdigestive production of hydrochloric acid and pepsin. The presence of those secretions in the absence of food allows their penetration of the mucus barrier and irritation of the mucosal lining of the stomach. The release of histamine (H_2) from the injured tissues provides a secondary stimulus to the secretion of hydrochloric acid and pepsinogen. Persistent or frequent stress-induced gastric activity can produce gastric erosion and peptic ulcer.

Transient vagus nerve–induced hypermotility and excess production of secretions can also cause gastric disturbances. The episodes may occur when the production of secretions is in excess of the amount required for the digestion of foods. The irritating effect of the secretions can cause gastric pain or a "burning sensation" between meals. The same gastric disturbances can occur when the person neglects to eat when the psychic stimulus that occurs with the thought, sight, or smell of food initiates the digestive processes. The epithelial protective coating of mucus can be altered chemically by drugs (i.e., corticosteroids, salicylates, phenylbutazone), and their action permits the proteolytic activity of pepsin to digest the gastric mucosa. The action of pepsin in the stomach and acidity of the duodenal content, which is produced by excess hydrochloric acid in the chyme, are considered to be the basis for the irritation and erosion that contribute to ulcerations.

VOMITING CENTER STIMULATION

Vomiting is a natural protective mechanism that occurs as a physiologic response to the ingestion of irritating substances. A common cause of vomiting is distention of the stomach by fluids or undigested foods. Afferent impulses from the stomach travel to the medullary vomiting centers, and the vagus nerve efferent motor impulses produce the changes that lead to evacuation of the stomach contents (Fig. 29–2).

The respiratory passages are protected from the entrance of vomitus by closure of the glottis. The soft palate also closes to occlude the nasopharynx. The descent of the diaphragm and the constriction of the abdominal muscles that occur concurrently with the constriction of the pyloric sphincter and relaxation of the cardiac sphincter provide the forceful compression that ejects the stomach contents upward through the esophagus.

Subthreshold impulses that arrive at the vomiting center produce nausea and its associated distressing autonomic responses (i.e., salivation, cold sweat, bradycardia, hypotension). The reflex swallowing that often occurs when a person is nauseated may produce gaseous distention of the stomach and precipitate vomiting. Lying supine sometimes reduces the pressure on the stomach and alleviates the nausea when the problem is secondary to gaseous distention.

CHEMORECEPTOR EMETIC TRIGGER ZONE STIMULATION

Direct pressure on the chemoreceptor emetic trigger zone of the medulla emits impulses that are transmitted to the adjacent vomiting centers. For example, increased intracranial pressure stimulates the chemoreceptor emetic trigger zone and precipitates projectile vomiting.

Persistent vomiting is often precipitated by the direct action of drugs (i.e., morphine, digitalis, apomorphine, antineoplastic drugs). Emetic substances that are liberated during uremia, infections, or radiation also produce persistent nausea or vomiting.

Disruption of the natural reciprocal responses of the paired vestibular systems of the inner ear may cause dizziness and nausea. When the position of the head or body stimulates the semicircular canal on one side of the head, the canal on the opposite side naturally responds with inhibitory impulses. Disruption in the natural

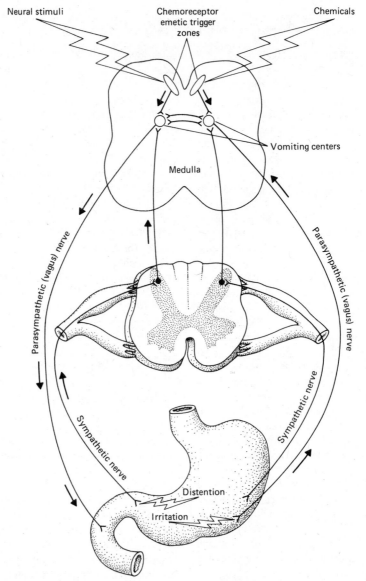

Fig. 29–2. Distention of the stomach or other abdominal viscera and irritation of the stomach stimulate the autonomic nerves that transmit impulses to the medulla vomiting center. The efferent parasympathetic motor impulses provide the musculature changes that produce vomiting. Chemical or neural stimuli at the chemoreceptor emetic trigger zones stimulate the nerves that conduct impulses to the vomiting center.

reciprocal movement of the perilymph initiates neural impulses that stimulate the chemoreceptor emetic trigger zone (Fig. 29–2). The transmission of those impulses to the vomiting center causes the nausea associated with the illusion of motion, or *vertigo*.

Gastric Antacids

DRUG THERAPY

The gastric antacids are commonly employed for treatment of persons with inflammation or ulcers in the stomach or duodenum. They are frequently used to minimize gastric irritation when the person is receiving drugs that cause thinning of the gastric mucosa (i.e., glucocorticoids). The antacids are also used when the person is receiving drugs that are weak acids (i.e., salicylates, phenylbutazone) to protect against their penetration of the gastric mucus barrier.

Gastric antacids are readily available as over-the-counter preparations. It is estimated that the public spends 16 million dollars a year to obtain relief from the "heartburn," nausea, and epigastric pain associated with irritation of the stomach and duodenum. There is evidence that the drugs contribute to the healing of gastric ulcers, but they appear to have little effect on the healing of duodenal ulcers.

Action Mode

The gastric antacids neutralize the hydrochloric acid and provide a protective coating on the epithelial lining of the stomach. The consistent frequent-interval administration of gastric antacids maintains the gastric pH at approximately 4.0. At that pH level there is reduced activity of the gastric enzyme pepsin, which is maximally active at pH 1.5 to 2.0. The gastric pepsin activity is adequate for the digestion of proteins in the diet.

Therapy Considerations

Most of the antacids in current use are combinations of aluminum, calcium, or magnesium salts that are poorly absorbed from the intestinal tract. Aluminum and calcium salts cause constipation, and combination with magnesium salts provides additional antacid and an osmotic effect that prevents constipation. Some persons have diarrhea during therapy with magnesium-containing antacids. Sodium bicarbonate reacts with gastric hydrochloric acid more rapidly than other antacids, but its high rate of absorption makes it undesirable for regular use.

The schedule for use of an antacid is usually one hour after meals and at bedtime when the drug is being employed for prevention or treatment of gastric or duodenal irritation. The duration of action is considered to be longer when the drug is taken one hour after eating than when it is taken at other between-meal intervals. During the acute phase of ulcer treatment, the drug may be prescribed for use at one-to-two-hour intervals. That schedule is usually modified after the initial phase of therapy.

In general, the liquid form of an antacid is more effective than the tablet form of the same antacid. Many people use the tablets during working hours and the liquid form when they are at home. One of the recurrent problems during therapy with gastric antacids is "taste fatigue." The person who takes the drug at frequent intervals each day reaches a point when the drug is unpalatable and the antacid grudgingly is taken. Some persons benefit from a change to another brand of the same drug because there are different flavors in the antacids that are produced by drug manufacturers.

Aluminum-Containing Preparations

Aluminum hydroxide is the most widely used gastric antacid. It is available as a liquid gel (AMPHOJEL, CREAMALIN) and as tablets. The drying process that is used for the preparation of the tablets is considered to decrease their effectiveness as gastric buffering agents. Aluminum hydroxide gel is available in combination with kaolin, *magnesium trisilicate* (TRISOGEL) or *magnesium hydroxide* (ALUDROX, MAALOX). *Magaldrate* (RIOPAN) is a chemical compound of aluminum and magnesium hydroxide. The low sodium content (0.7 mg/5ml) makes the drug useful for persons on a restricted sodium intake. Aluminum and magnesium hydroxides are also available in combination with the antiflatulent agent *simethicone* (GELUSIL, MYLANTA II, SIMECO).

The usual dosage for all forms of the liquid gel is 5 to 30 ml in one-half glass of water at two-to-four-hour intervals. One 300-mg tablet is approximately equivalent to 5 ml of gel. The tablets are chewed well before they are swallowed and may be taken with water or milk. The liquid drug may be administered as a continuous intragastric drip through a nasogastric tube in acute situations. The drug is diluted in two to three parts of water or milk and infused at a rate that provides approximately 40 ml of drug per hour.

Aluminum hydroxide combines with phosphate ions in the intestinal tract to form insoluble aluminum phosphate, and that compound is excreted with the feces. Aluminum hydroxide may be used therapeutically to bind phosphates in the intestine and prevent the formation of phosphate calculi in the kidneys or to increase the excretion of phosphates when the person has renal failure. The drug can cause hypophosphatemia or osteomalacia in persons who regularly take the drug over prolonged periods of time for control of gastric irritation.

Aluminum hydroxide complexes with the tetracyclines, and the absorption of the antibiotic is reduced when the drugs are employed concurrently. The drug may also interfere with the absorption of anticholinergic agents, barbiturates, digoxin, quinine, quinidine, and warfarin.

Aluminum phosphate has approximately one half the acid-neutralizing capacity of aluminum hydroxide. The initial dosage of the gel is 15 to 30 ml every two to four hours. The maintenance dosage is usually 15 to 30 ml after meals and at bedtime. The drug may be taken with milk or water.

Dihydroxyaluminum aminoacetate (ROBALATE) is the aluminum salt of the amino acid *glycine*. The usual adult dosage is 0.5 to 1 gm after meals and at bedtime. Higher dosages may be used in the treatment of peptic or duodenal ulcers (i.e., 1 to 2 gm). Dihydroxyaluminum aminoacetate has a faint, sweet taste. The drug is also available as *dihydroxyaluminum sodium carbonate* (ROLAIDS), as *aluminum carbonate gel,* basic (BASALJEL), and in combination with homatropine methylbromide and phenobarbital (ALZINOX COMPOUND).

Calcium-Containing Preparations

Precipitated calcium carbonate (DICARBOSIL, TUMS) tablets are used in a dosage of 1 gm with one-half glass of water four to six times a day. The drug reacts in the stomach to form calcium chloride, which reacts with the sodium bicarbonate in the intestinal tract to form sodium chloride and calcium carbonate. The sodium chloride and up to 30 percent of the ingested calcium are reabsorbed. The remaining calcium is excreted in the feces. The drug is the least expensive of the gastric antacids. Persons taking the drug often find its chalky taste unpalatable. Because there are indications that the incidence of calcium-containing renal stones is increased when patients take the drug concurrently with a high intake of milk products, the FDA Antacid Advisory Committee has recommended a maximum daily dosage limit of 8 gm of calcium carbonate.

Magnesium-Containing Preparations

Magnesium carbonate has a high hydrochloric acid–neutralizing capacity and is a common ingredient of antacid preparations. The usual dosage of the drug is 0.5 to 2 gm between meals, and the drug is taken with one-half glass of water.

Magnesium hydroxide, or milk of magnesia, is a relatively potent antacid although it is most commonly used at higher dosages as a cathartic. The antacid dosage is 5 to 10 ml between meals and at bedtime.

Magnesium oxide is used as an ingredient in antacid preparations. It is hydrolyzed to the hydroxide in water and has the same therapeutic effect as magnesium hydroxide preparations.

Magnesium trisilicate is available as tablets that are used in a dosage of 6.5 to 1 gm between meals. The drug reacts slowly with the hydrochloric acid in the stomach, and gastric emptying may occur before the action of the antacid is completed. The drug is most frequently used in combination with aluminum hydroxide gel. Magnesium trisilicate forms insoluble complexes with iron preparations, and that action interferes with the absorption of iron from the gastrointestinal tract.

Antisecretory-Antispasmodic Drugs

DRUG THERAPY

The drugs employed for control of digestive secretions and gastrointestinal motility include the *anticholinergic drugs, anticholinergic–local anesthetic drugs,* and *smooth muscle relaxants.* The drugs are employed as part of an overall plan that includes the use of antacids or sedatives, and modifications in diet and activity, for control of inflammation or ulceration in the stomach or duodenum.

Anticholinergic Drugs

The anticholinergic, or parasympatholytic, drugs are belladonna alkaloids and their derivatives or synthetic substitutes for the belladonna alkaloids. Atropine sulfate is the prototype, or primary example, of the group of drugs that decrease secretions and reduce the motility of the digestive tract.

Action Mode. The antisecretory-antispasmodic drugs are substances that are avidly taken up by the receptors at the parasympathetic nerve endings. The presence of the anticholinergic drug blocks the activity of acetylcholine at the receptors. Blocking of the activity of the parasympathetic neurotransmitter reduces the production of salivary, gastric, and pancreatic secretions and decreases the motility of the digestive tract. The desired therapeutic effect is attained when there is inhibition of secretions evident by some dryness of the mouth or blurred vision. The dosage is usually reduced slightly at that point to decrease the discomfort of the person taking the drugs.

Preparations Available. Tincture of belladonna leaf (Table 29–1) contains the alkaloids hyoscyamine and atropine in approximately 68 percent alcohol. The drug is also available as an extract. The initial dosage is 0.6 ml three times per day, and the drug is taken one-half hour before meals. The dosage is increased in increments of one drop (0.05 ml) each day until there is dryness of the mouth. A calibrated dropper is provided with the drug to allow accurate measurement of the dosage.

Atropine sulfate is initially administered at a dosage of 0.25 mg 30 minutes before meals. The adult dosage of atropine is the same when the drug is given orally, subcutaneously, intramuscularly, or intravenously. The drug is administered at four-to-six-hour intervals. The dosage for infants one year of age is 0.12 mg. The dosage for children two to four years of age is 0.18 mg, and that dosage may be increased in increments of 0.02 mg for each year of age when the drug is given to children over four years of age. The maximum dosage for children weighing 18 to 30 kg (40 to 66 lb) is 0.3 mg, and for children weighing 30 to 41 kg (66 to 90 lb) it is 0.4 mg. Children weighing more than 41 kg may receive the adult dose.

Atropine sulfate is commonly used to decrease gastrointestinal motility and reduce the production of secretions at the time of surgery. It is used topically in the eye to produce the mydriasis and cycloplegia required for selected ophthalmic

Table 29–1.

Adult Oral Dosage of Natural and Synthetic Belladonna Alkaloids

Drug	Adult Single Oral Dose
Belladonna Alkaloids	
Atropine sulfate	0.4–0.6 mg
Belladonna alkaloids	0.4–0.8 mg
Belladonna extract	10.8–21.6 mg
Belladonna leaf, tincture	0.3–1 ml
Scopolamine hydrobromide	0.4–0.8 mg
*Alkaloid Derivatives**	
Homatropine methylbromide	
(HOMAPIN)	2.5–10 mg
Methscopolamine bromide	
(PAMINE)	2.5–5 mg
*Synthetic Alkaloids**	
Anisotropine methylbromide	
(VALPIN)	50 mg
Clidinium bromide	
(QUARZAN)	2.5–5 mg
Diphemanil methylsulfate	
(PRANTAL)	100–200 mg
Glycopyrrolate (ROBINUL)	1–2 mg
Hexocyclium methylsulfate	
(TRAL)	25 mg
Isopropamide iodide	
(DARBID)	5–10 mg
Mepenzolate bromide (CANTIL)	25–50 mg
Methantheline bromide	
(BANTHINE)	50–100 mg
Oxyphenonium bromide	
(ANTRENYL)	5–10 mg
Propantheline bromide	
(PRO-BANTHINE)	7.5–30 mg
Tridihexethyl chloride	
(PATHILON)	25–50 mg

* Quaternary ammonium derivatives.

examinations and is also used as topical eye ointment in the treatment of iritis.

Scopolamine hydrobromide (Table 29–1) is given orally three to four times per day. It may also be given subcutaneously, intramuscularly, or intravenously for preanesthetic medication at a dosage of 0.3 to 0.6 mg. Scopolamine produces central nervous system depression and produces amnesia when used in combination with mor- phine sulfate or meperidine hydrochloride. It can produce delirium when administered alone to a patient who is in pain. The drug is a more potent but shorter-acting mydriatic and cycloplegic than atropine sulfate when it is applied topically to the eye.

Homatropine methylbromide (Table 29–1) is considered to be less toxic than the natural belladonna alkaloids. It is less active than the alkaloids at peripheral sites but has four times as potent ganglionic-blocking effects.

The drug is given three times per day before meals. Infants with pyloric stenosis may be given 0.3 mg of homatropine diluted in water four to six times per day before feedings.

Methscopolamine bromide (Table 29–1) is administered orally, intramuscularly, or subcutaneously. The parenteral dosage for adults is 0.25 to 1 mg every six to eight hours. The dosage for infants 6 to 12 months of age is 2 to 3 mg/day, and for infants less than three months of age it is 0.5 to 1 mg/day. The drug lacks the central action of scopolamine. It is less potent and longer acting than atropine.

Anisotropine methylbromide (Table 29–1) is administered three to four times per day before meals and at bedtime. The dosage for children has not been established. Persons taking the drug frequently complain of a loss of taste sense.

Clidinium bromide (Table 29–1) has antispasmodic and antisecretory effects that approach those of atropine. It also provides ganglionic-blocking action at higher doses.

Diphemanil methylsulfate (Table 29–1) is given every four to six hours between meals. The drug may be given subcutaneously or intramuscularly for the treatment of acute symptoms. The parenteral dosage for adults is calculated on the basis of 0.5 mg/kg of body weight (50 mg maximum dosage), and that dosage may be given four times per day.

Glycopyrrolate (Table 29–1) is administered to adults orally or by subcutaneous, intramuscular, or intravenous injection. The parenteral dosage is 0.1 to 0.2 mg three to four times per day. The drug may be given undiluted as an intravenous injection or may be diluted in a solution of dextrose in water for infusion. A large vein should be used for the infusion because the drug causes a burning sensation in small veins.

Hexocyclium methylsulfate (Table 29–1) is administered orally to adults four times per day. The 75-mg extended-release tablet (GRADUMET) may be used for nocturnal control of gastric discomfort.

Isopropamide iodide (Table 29–1) has a 12-hour duration of action. The oral dosage is taken two times per day at 12-hour intervals.

Mepenzolate bromide (Table 29–1) is taken orally before meals and at bedtime. The initial dosage of 25 mg is increased gradually until a satisfactory response is attained.

Methantheline bromide (Table 29–1) is administered orally four times per day. The maintenance dosage usually is one half the initial dose. Diluted solutions containing 50 mg of the drug may be administered by intramuscular or intravenous injection. The drug provides ganglionic-blocking effects that may cause impotence when it is taken at high dosage.

Oxyphenonium bromide (Table 29–1) is taken orally by adults four times per day. The drug may be given by subcutaneous or intramuscular injection at a dosage of 0.5 to 2 mg. The dosage for intravenous injection is one half of that dosage. The daily oral dosage for children six to twelve years of age is 15 mg and for infants it is 2 mg. The pediatric dosage is divided for administration four times per day. The drug is a more potent ganglionic-blocking agent than methantheline. It has less potent peripheral effects than atropine.

Propantheline bromide (Table 29–1) may be administered orally or by intramuscular or intravenous injection. The parenteral dosage for adults is 30 mg every six hours. The drug has more potent ganglionic-blocking and peripheral action than methantheline.

Tridihexethyl chloride (Table 29–1) may be administered orally, or by subcutaneous, intramuscular, or intravenous injection. The parenteral dosage for adults is 10 to 20 mg four times per day. Infants with colic may be given 1 to 5 mg before each feeding.

Adverse Effects. The primary adverse effects of the anticholinergic drugs are related to their suppression of parasympathetic nerve activity (i.e., dryness of the mouth and throat, anhidrosis, blurred vision associated with mydriasis and cycloplegia, dysuria, urine retention, constipation, and tachycardia). The mydriasis that occurs with parenteral administration of the drugs may precipitate acute glaucoma in persons who are predisposed to angle closure. Dermatologic reactions may also occur (i.e., scarlatiniform rash).

Excess cholinergic blockade can occur when the drugs are used concurrently with drugs having anticholinergic properties (i.e., phenothiazines, antihistamines, tricyclic antidepressants, quinidine, procainamide).

Large doses of the belladonna alkaloids and the nonquaternary agents may produce central nervous system stimulation (i.e., restlessness, tremor, irritability, disorientation, incoherent speech, delirium, hallucinations). The phase of excitement is followed by a gradual onset of central nervous system depression that can include fatal medullary paralysis. Short-acting barbiturates may be used to control the excitement phase of toxicity, and cardiopulmonary resuscitative measures are implemented during the central nervous system depression phase.

Large doses of the quaternary agents (Table 29–1) may produce ganglionic blockade manifested by orthostatic hypotension and impotence. The neuromuscular-blocking action of the drugs can produce respiratory arrest.

Anticholinergic–Local Anesthetic Drugs

The drugs block acetylcholine activity, and their local anesthetic property provides a direct depressant action on the smooth muscles of the digestive tract. The oral drugs should be swallowed without chewing to avoid the local anesthetic effects on the oral mucosa. The drugs include *dicyclomine hydrochloride, methixene hydrochloride, oxyphencyclimine hydrochloride,* and *thiphenamil hydrochloride.*

Preparations Available. Dicyclomine hydrochloride (BENTYL) is administered orally or by intramuscular injection to adults at a dosage of 10 to 20 mg. The oral drug is given to children at a dosage of 10 mg and to infants at a dosage of 5 mg three to four times per day. The adverse effects of the drug are euphoria, slight dizziness, and abdominal distention. Nausea and skin rash have also been reported.

Methixene hydrochloride (TREST) is administered orally to adults at a dosage of 1 to 2 mg three times per day. It has a stronger central nervous system–stimulating effect than does atropine and produces the adverse effects common to the anticholinergic drugs. Skin rashes have been reported during therapy with methixene.

Oxyphencyclimine hydrochloride (DARICON, SETROL, VIO-THENE) is administered orally to adults at a dosage of 5 to 20 mg two times per day. The drug is not given to children younger than 12 years of age. In addition to the adverse effects common to the anticholinergic drugs, oxyphencyclimine occasionally causes skin rashes.

Thiphenamil hydrochloride (TROCINATE) is administered orally to adults at a dosage of 200 to 400 mg four times per day. The drug infrequently produces dryness of the mouth and constipation. The dosage for children is not established.

Smooth Muscle Relaxants

The drugs provide relaxation of the smooth muscles of the gastrointestinal tract by their local anesthetic action. They have minimal effect on the production of secretions in the digestive tract. The only drug in current use is *adiphenine hydrochloride* (TRASENTINE), which is administered orally to adults at a dosage of 75 to 150 mg three to four times per day before meals. The adverse effects of the drug include tachycardia and nervous excitability.

Antisecretory Drugs

Histamine Inhibitor

Cimetidine (TAGAMET) recently was released by the Food and Drug Administration for treatment of patients with a duodenal ulcer or for pathologic hypersecretory conditions (i.e., mastocytosis, multiple endocrine adenomas, Zollinger-Ellison syndrome). The drug also is employed for prophylactic treatment of asymptomatic patients who are considered to be ulcer-prone because of drug therapy (i.e., glucocorticoids) or the physiologic stress associated with acute illness.

Action Mode. Cimetidine competitively inhibits the action of histamine at the histamine (H_2) receptor. The drug inhibits daytime and nocturnal basal gastric secretions that are stimulated by the presence of food or caffeine in the stomach or by the action of endogenous histamine or insulin.

Therapy Considerations. The drug is administered orally to adults at a dosage of 300 mg with meals and at bedtime. The concurrent administration of antacids is essential to the effectiveness of cimetidine. The drug may also be given at a dosage of 300 mg by intravenous injection at six-hour intervals or may be diluted for infusion over a 15-to-20-minute period.

The basal gastric acid secretion can be 90 to 100 percent inhibited for a four-hour period after a single dose of cimetidine is taken. Although healing of the ulcer may occur within one to two weeks after therapy is started, the planned treatment course is four to six weeks. Patients with ulcers should be cautioned to maintain the therapy plan without interruption because relapses have occurred with dosage reduction or abrupt termination of therapy.

Adverse Effects. Mild and transient diarrhea, muscular pain, dizziness, fever, and rash have been reported in about 1 percent of the patients taking the drug. Mild gynecomastia has been reported in a few patients. There have been reports of slurred speech, delirium, and hallucinations. Confusion commonly occurs in elderly patients taking the drug.

Antiemetics

DRUG THERAPY

The antiemetic drugs are relatively selective central nervous system depressants that raise the threshold for emesis at the medullary vomiting center and reduce the sensitivity of the chemoreceptor emetic trigger zone to chemical stimuli. Some of the antiemetic drugs decrease impulse transmission in the vestibular-cerebellar pathways and reduce the response of the chemoreceptor emetic trigger zone to those neural impulses. That combined action provides effective control of motion sickness and the vertigo associated with functional problems in the middle ear.

Vomiting is a distressing and exhausting experience for the individual. Persistent nausea or vomiting interferes with the intake of foods and causes the loss of large amounts of the sodium and chloride of the gastric secretions. Those electrolytes normally travel into the intestine and are reabsorbed, and their loss can cause hyponatremia and alkalosis. Intravenous fluids are usually administered to provide for replacement of the electrolytes until nausea or vomiting is controlled by the antiemetic drugs.

The drugs most commonly employed for control of emesis are the antihistamines *cyclizine, dimenhydrinate, hydroxyzine,* and *meclizine;* the phenothiazines *prochlorperazine, promethazine,* and *thiethylperazine;* and miscellaneous drugs, which include *benzquinamide, diphenidol, trimethobenzamide,* and *phosphorated carbohydrate solution.* All the antiemetics are more effective when they are administered prophylactically to prevent nausea or vomiting.

Antihistamines

The drugs have a depressant effect on the vestibular-cerebellar pathways, and they are useful for prevention and treatment of motion sickness, vertigo, labyrinthitis, and Meniere's syndrome. They are also employed for control of nausea or vomiting that occurs postoperatively or in association with febrile illness and with radiation or drug therapy.

Cyclizine. *Cyclizine hydrochloride* is administered orally, and *cyclizine lactate* is administered by intramuscular injection (Table 29–2). The drug is given before meals for the control of nausea or vomiting. It is taken one-half hour before motion sickness–inducing travel and three to four times per day when required for control of persistent nausea or vomiting. The parenteral route may be used for administration of the drug when the person is unable to take it orally.

The oral or parenteral dosage for children six to ten years of age is one-half of the adult dose and is divided for administration three to four times per day. The drug is not used for children younger than six years of age.

Adverse effects during therapy are uncommon. Drowsiness may occur when the drug is used at high dosage levels.

Dimenhydrinate. The drug (Table 29–2) is used primarily for prevention and treatment of motion sickness. The oral, rectal, or intramuscular dosage for children 8 to 12 years of age is 25 to 50 mg. The drug may be given up to three times per day to children. The use of the drug may mask ototoxic symptoms and lead to irreversible damage when it is given with ototoxic drugs.

Hydroxyzine. The drug (Table 29–2) is used for control of nausea and vomiting associated with most disease processes but is seldom used for treatment of patients with motion sickness. *Hydroxyzine pamoate* is administered orally, and

Table 29–2.
Adult Dosage of Antiemetic Drugs

Drug	Route	Single Dose (mg)	Daily Doses
Antihistamines			
Cyclizine (MAREZINE)	Oral	50	4–6
	IM	50	4–6
Dimenhydrinate (DRAMAMINE)	Oral	50–100	6
	Rectal	100	1–2
	IM	Same	6
	IV	Same	6
Hydroxyzine (ATARAX, VISTARIL)	Oral	25–100	3–4
	IM	Same	4–6
Meclizine (ANTIVERT, BONINE)	Oral	25–100	1
Phenothiazines			
Prochlorperazine (COMPAZINE)	Oral	5–30	3–4
	Rectal	25	2
	IM	5–30	6–8
	IV	Same	6–8
Promethazine (PHENERGAN)	Oral	25	1–3
Thiethylperazine (TORECAN)	Oral	10	1–3
	IM	Same	1–3
Miscellaneous			
Benzquinamide (EMETE-CON)	IM	50	6–8
	IV	25	1
Diphenidol (VONTROL)	Oral	25–50	6
	IM	20–40	6
	IV	20	2
Trimethobenzamide (TIGAN)	Oral	250	3–4
	Rectal	200	3–4
	IM	200	3–4

hydroxyzine hydrochloride is administered orally or by intramuscular injection.

The drug produces marked discomfort at the site of the injections. The adult intramuscular dose should be injected into the upper outer quadrant of the gluteal muscle or into the midlateral muscles of the thigh. Children with nausea or vomiting may be given an oral or an intramuscular dosage calculated on the basis of 1.1 mg/kg of body weight. The intramuscular injection should be given to children in the midlateral muscles of the thigh.

Adverse effects occur infrequently. The initial drowsiness usually disappears when therapy is continued.

Meclizine Hydrochloride. The drug (Table 29–2) is employed for control of nausea and vomiting associated with surgery, motion sickness, or chemical stimulation of the chemoreceptor emetic trigger zone. The long duration of action (8 to 24 hours) provides control of emesis without frequent use of the drug. The drug occasionally produces drowsiness and dryness of the mouth.

Phenothiazines

The drugs are frequently employed for short-term control of nausea or vomiting. They are often administered parenterally for the nausea and vomiting that occur during radiation therapy. Short-term use of the drugs decreases the incidence of the adverse effects that are common with long-term use of the phenothiazines. The drugs used for control of nausea and vomiting include *prochlorperazine, promethazine,* and *thiethylperazine.*

Prochlorperazine. The drug (Table 29–2) is used primarily for control of the severe nausea or vomiting caused by chemical stimulation of the chemoreceptor emetic trigger zone. The daily oral or rectal dosage for children over two years of age is based on the calculation of 0.4 mg/kg of body weight, and that dosage is divided for administration in one to three doses. The dosage for a single intramuscular injection for children is based on the calculation of 0.13 mg/kg of body weight. Sedation and hypotension may occur with the parenteral administration of the drug.

Promethazine Hydrochloride. The drug (Table 29–2) is effective in the control of chemical stimulation of the chemoreceptor emetic trigger zone. It is also effective in control of the nausea and vomiting associated with motion sickness. Children may be given a dosage of the drug calculated on the basis of 0.5 mg/kg of body weight. That dosage may be repeated in 8 to 12 hours when the nausea and vomiting persist. Sedation frequently occurs when a person receives promethazine.

Thiethylperazine Maleate. The drug (Table 29–2) is given to children over 12 years of age at the adult dosage. Children younger than 12 years of age are not given the drug because it frequently produces extrapyramidal effects in younger children. Drowsiness and dryness of the nose and mouth are the most common adverse effects. The drug may produce drowsiness or restlessness when it is given to patients during the postoperative period. It may be given to the patient as a deep intramuscular injection shortly before termination of anesthesia to prevent nausea or vomiting in the postoperative period.

Miscellaneous Drugs

Benzquinamide Hydrochloride. The drug (Table 29–2) is used primarily for the control of postoperative nausea and vomiting. The preparations currently available are for parenteral administration. The antiemetic effects occur within 15 minutes after the drug is administered. Oral dosages of 100 mg three to four times per day and rectal dosages of 100 to 200 mg two times per day are being used investigationally for treatment of nausea or vomiting. Drowsiness frequently occurs. The drug may also produce insomnia, restlessness, headache, excitement, or nervousness. Intravenous administration of benzquinamide may produce a sudden elevation in blood pressure and transient arrhythmias.

Diphenidol. The drug (Table 29–2) acts on the vomiting center and on the chemoreceptor emetic trigger zone to suppress vomiting. It is effective for the control of the nausea and vomiting caused by chemical or neural stimuli. The oral or rectal dosage for children is based on calculation of 0.88 mg/kg of body weight (maximum of 5.5 mg/kg/day), and the intramuscular dosage is based on 0.44 mg/kg (maximum of 3.3 mg/kg/day). The drug may be given to children at four-hour intervals. The drug may produce dryness of the mouth, nausea, indigestion, blurred vision, dizziness, drowsiness, malaise, headache, weakness, nervousness, skin rash, and urticaria. The drug is given to patients who are under supervision because it can produce hallucinations, confusion, and disorientation.

Trimethobenzamide Hydrochloride. The drug (Table 29–2) is used for control of nausea and vomiting related to labyrinthine excitability or motion sickness. It is also used for control of the emesis that occurs postoperatively. The oral or rectal dosage for children weighing 13 to 40 kg (30 to 90 lb) is 100 to 200 mg three to four times per day. The oral or rectal dosage for children weighing less than 13 kg is 100 mg three to four times per day.

The rectal suppositories contain benzocaine 2 percent to decrease the irritating effect of the drug on the tissues. The drug should be administered deep into the intramuscular tissues to avoid the pain, stinging, burning, redness, and swelling caused by the irritating effects of the drug. Hypotension may occur in postoperative patients who are given the drug by intramuscular injection.

Phosphorated Carbohydrate Solution (EMETROL).   The preparation is a hyperosmolar solution of levulose, dextrose, and orthophosphoric acid that is thought to act directly on the gastrointestinal tract. It is used for symptomatic relief of functional nausea or vomiting and vomiting of psychogenic origin. The solution is administered undiluted, and oral fluids are withheld for at least 15 minutes after the dose is taken. Adults are given 15 to 30 ml at 15-minute intervals until nausea or vomiting is controlled. Infants and children may be given 5 to 10 ml at 15-minute intervals.

NURSING INTERVENTION

Inflammation and ulceration of the stomach and duodenum are common health problems associated with the personality patterns of individuals who are highly competitive and with the stresses of modern living patterns. Strategy-planning or problem-solving luncheons, meals hurriedly eaten, and the skipping of breakfast and lunch are the common, disruptive patterns that interfere with the normal digestive processes.

The alertness required by a business-oriented luncheon can produce sympathetic nerve stimulation and a consequent decrease in gastrointestinal motility. The tense individual who eats heavily at the luncheon usually has uncomfortable abdominal distention later in the day. When social interactions during the meal interfere with eating, the person may have gastric pain as a consequence of the outpouring of secretions in excess of the amount required for digestion of the ingested foods.

Infrequent disruptions in eating patterns seldom produce significant adverse effects, but repetition of the insults to the gastrointestinal tract can cause injury to the epithelial lining of the stomach or duodenum.

Assessing Progress

Individuals with a primary irritation or ulceration of the upper digestive tract are usually treated on an ambulatory basis. The same problems may occur secondary to the stress of acute illness or as a consequence of drug therapy in hospitalized patients. Drugs that have a high potential for causing gastric irritation are often given with milk, meals, or a snack to reduce their contact with the gastric epithelium. An antacid may be administered at regular intervals between meals and at bedtime to reduce the stress or drug-induced irritation of the stomach.

Patients who are receiving frequent doses of a gastric antacid usually have the drug at the bedside to facilitate its administration by the nurse. In many instances, the drug may be taken independently by patients who are capable of using the drug on a regularly scheduled basis. Cold, fresh milk in a thermal pitcher may also be at the bedside of patients during the intensive period of ulcer therapy.

Gastric secretions are released during the rapid eye movement (REM) periods of sleep, and their presence in the empty stomach of a patient with an ulcer causes gnawing pain and nausea. The patient who wakens in distress can readily relieve the discomfort by taking the antacid when it is at the bedside.

Regularly scheduled observation of the patient allows early detection of gastritis or bleeding. Guaiac testing of all stools and vomitus allows determination of the presence of red blood cell products in the excreta before they can be detected visually. The release of larger quantities of blood is evident in changes in the coloration of the excreta (i.e., black, tarry stools, red or "coffee-ground" vomitus). Concurrent physical assessment for evidence of bleeding includes examination of the abdomen for distention, listening with a stethoscope for increased bowel sounds, and monitoring the pulse and blood pressure. The patient's statement of abdominal discomfort or pain may provide the initial subjective clue to the presence of gastrointestinal hemorrhage or the perforation of an ulcerated area.

Persons with gastrointestinal problems that are precipitated or intensified by stress may benefit from the nurse's assistance with the planning of measures that can reduce those stresses. Changes in favored living patterns are difficult for the person to accept. A description of the physiologic effects associated with stress may help the person to understand the need for change and to identify personal living patterns that can be modified. It is essential to discuss the effects of excessive amounts of irritating substances (i.e., alcohol, spices, coffee, tea) on the digestive tract tissues.

A variety of physiologic and psychologic factors contributed to gastric distress, nausea, and vomiting. For example, children often become nauseated and vomit after intravenous administration of antineoplastic drugs, which stimulate the chemoreceptor emetic trigger zone in the medulla. Antiemetics can be employed to control the drug-induced vomiting. During continued therapy, the children often become nauseated as soon as the intravenous equipment is brought to the bedside. Nurses find that the children have less nausea, which is psychic in origin, during the intravenous infusion when the equipment is placed out of the child's line of vision before and during infusion of the drug.

The patient's identification of factors that precipitate nausea often makes it possible to reduce the stimulus. In some instances, simply protecting the patient from the discussion, sight, or smell of food reduces nausea. When gastric acidity is causing nausea, it may be reduced if the person eats small amounts of nutritious foods at frequent intervals. For example, the nausea of early pregnancy can sometimes be controlled by decreasing the fat content of the diet and by the liberal eating of dry carbohydrates (i.e., unsalted popcorn or crackers).

Antiemetic drugs are most effective when administered prophylactically. Patients should be advised to take the drug 30 to 45 minutes before a known precipitating event (i.e., meals, motion sickness–inducing travel) to avert the discomfort and to allow the intake of nutrients essential to health. Antiemetic drug administration is essential to control persistent vomiting, which causes high losses of fluid and of the potassium, sodium, and chloride ions essential to the body's fluid and electrolyte balance.

The drowsiness produced by the antiemetic drugs is therapeutic for the person who is exhausted after episodes of vomiting. Ambulatory patients should be cautioned to avoid tasks that require mental alertness and coordination (i.e., driving a motor vehicle) when they are taking an antiemetic or an anticholinergic drug known to produce drowsiness or blurring of vision.

Review Guides

1. Describe the factors that would be included when counseling the patient with a gastric ulcer who is to take propantheline bromide and a gastric antacid containing aluminum and magnesium hydroxides with simethicone (GELUSIL).
2. Identify the observations that would be planned when the patient is admitted to the hospital with a diagnosis of duodenal ulcer.
3. Outline the areas that would receive greatest emphasis when taking the nursing history of a patient who is to be treated with a glucocorticoid and a gastric antacid.

4. Identify the factors that would be considered when planning the nursing care of a patient who is receiving promethazine hydrochloride during radiation therapy for control of persistent nausea and vomiting.

5. Describe the factors that would be included when counseling the patient who is to continue taking cimetidine and aluminum hydroxide gel for treatment of a duodenal ulcer after leaving the hospital.

6. Outline a plan for observation of the patient after administering the following drugs parenterally:
   a. Atropine sulfate
   b. Scopolamine hydrobromide
   c. Prochlorperazine
   d. Benzquinamide hydrochloride
   e. Hydroxyzine hydrochloride

Additional Readings

Black, Franklin O.: Vestibular causes of vertigo. *Geriatrics,* **30**:123, April, 1975.

Borland, James L.: Rational management of peptic ulcer disease. *Hosp. Pract.,* **11**:33, July, 1976.

Boyd, William P., Jr., and Boyce, H. Worth, Jr.: Diagnosis and management of duodenal ulcer disease. *Hosp. Med.,* **13**:68, July, 1977.

Brandborg, Lloyd L.: Peptic ulcer disease. *Primary Care,* **2**:109, March, 1975.

Brunner, Lillian S.: What to do (and what to teach your patient) about peptic ulcer. *Nursing 76,* **6**:27, November, 1976.

Facer, George W., and Maragos, Nicolas E.: The dizzy patient. *Postgrad. Med.,* **57**:73, May, 1975.

Gehringer, Gerald R.: Food poisoning: an update for an old problem. *Clin. Med.,* **83**:9, February, 1976.

Gibaldi, Milo, and Grundhofer, Barbara: Biopharmaceutic influences on the anticholinergic effects of proprantheline. *Clin. Pharmacol. Ther.* **18**:457, October, 1975.

Greenblatt, David J.; Shader, Richard I.; Harmatz, Jerold S.; Franke, Käte; and Koch-Weser, Jan: Influence of magnesium and aluminum hydroxide mixture on chlordiazepoxide absorption. *Clin. Pharmacol. Ther.,* **19**:234, February, 1976.

Holt, G. Richard, and Thomas, J. Regan: Vertigo. *Am. Fam. Physician,* **14**:84, October, 1976.

Isenberg, Jon I.: Therapy of peptic ulcer. *J.A.M.A.,* **233**:540, August 11, 1975.

Kaehny, William D.; Hegg, Arlene P.; and Alfrey, Allen C.: Gastrointestinal absorption of aluminum from aluminum-containing antacids. *N. Engl. J. Med.,* **296**:1389, June 16, 1977.

Kratzer, Joan B.: What to teach patients about duodenal ulcers. *Nursing 78,* **8**:54, January, 1978.

Longstreth, G. F.; Go, V.L.W.; and Malagelada, J.-R.: Cimetidine suppression of nocturnal gastric secretion in active duodenal ulcer. *N. Engl. J. Med.,* **294**:801, April 8, 1976.

Menguy, Rene: Gastric mucosal injury from common drugs. *Postgrad. Med.,* **63**:82, April, 1978.

Moody, Frank G.: Answers to questions on stress ulcer. *Hosp. Med.,* **13**:8, April, 1977.

Neeld, John B.; Allen, A. T.; Coleman, Elliott; Frederickson, Evan L.; and Goldberg, Leon I.: Cardiac rate and rhythm changes with atropine and methscopolamine. *Clin. Pharmacol. Ther.,* **17**:290, March, 1975.

Pearson, Bruce W.: The ear. *Postgrad. Med.,* **57**:50, May, 1975.

Rayford, Phillip L.; Miller, Thomas A.; and Thompson, James C.: Secretin, cholecystokinin and newer G-I hormones, part 1. *N. Engl. J. Med.,* **294**:1093, May 13, 1976.

Romankiewicz, John A.: Effects of antacids on gastrointestinal absorption of drugs. *Primary Care,* **3**:537, September, 1976.

Texter, E. Clinton, Jr.; Smart, Douglas F.; and Butler, Robert C.: Antacids. *Am. Fam. Physician,* **11**:111, April, 1975.

Walsh, John H.: Axioms on peptic ulcer disease. *Hosp. Med.,* **11**:44, November, 1976.

Wiele, Raymond L. Vande: Anorexia nervosa and the hypothalamus. *Hosp. Pract.,* **12**:45, December, 1977.

Wilson, Victor J.: The labyrinth, the brain, and posture. *Am. Scientist,* **63**:325, May–June, 1975.

Wyllie, J. H.: Histamine H_2-receptor antagonist. *Postgrad-Med.,* **63**:91, April, 1978.

30

Deficient Carbohydrate Assimilation

Diabetes mellitus, which is primarily a disorder of carbohydrate assimilation, is a common chronic health problem. It is generally described as the fifth leading cause of morbidity in the country. It is probable that many of the deaths attributed to other causes (i.e., heart disease, stroke) are consequences of the cardiovascular pathology produced by diabetes mellitus.

Physiologic Correlations

Ingested carbohydrates move across the intestinal mucosa as monosaccharides (i.e., glucose, fructose, galactose) and travel with the portal venous blood to the liver. Glucose is the primary product of the interconversion of the monosaccharides in the hepatic tissues. The initial phase of the metabolic pathway of glucose is its phosphorylation, which requires the activity of *glucokinase*, to form *glucose 6-phosphate* (Fig. 30–1). The glucose may be stored in the hepatic tissues as glycogen or may be utilized as an energy source.

GLYCOLYSIS

Several metabolic processes are involved in the splitting of the glucose molecules to provide the energy for the formation of adenosine triphosphate (ATP). The energy stored in ATP is released when the phosphate radical is split off during the formation of adenosine diphosphate (ADP). Each phosphate radical provides approximately 8000 calories that can be utilized to meet the energy needs of the cell.

The initial phase of glycolysis, which occurs in

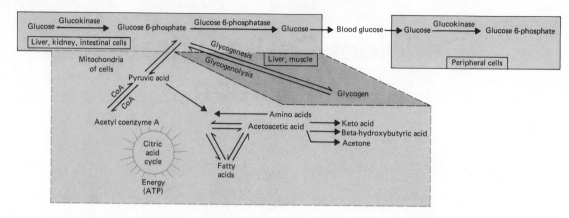

Fig. 30–1. Simplified diagram of the metabolic pathways of carbohydrates, fatty acids, and amino acids.

the mitochondria of the cells, is splitting of the glucose molecule to form two molecules of pyruvic acid. In the subsequent reversible metabolic processes, *coenzyme A* forms *acetyl coenzyme A* (acetyl Co-A) from pyruvic acid.

The primary pathway for energy production is the *citric acid,* or *tricarboxylic acid, cycle.* The acetyl portion of acetyl coenzyme A that enters the cycle is degraded to carbon dioxide and to the hydrogen ions, which provide the energy for formation of adenosine triphosphate.

The metabolism of fatty acids and some amino acids also leads to the formation of acetoacetic acid or acetyl coenzyme A. Those conversions are reversible processes that allow additional quantities of the acetyl molecule to enter the citric acid cycle. Some of the acetoacetic acid is metabolized, and that process releases ketones (keto acid, beta-hydroxybutyric acid, and acetone).

GLYCOGENOLYSIS

The stores of glycogen can be mobilized to meet the cellular requirements when glucose is unavailable. Glycogenolysis in the liver provides glucose that is released into the circulation. The metabolism of glycogen in muscle cells provides glucose that generally remains in the muscle and

is utilized to meet the energy needs of the fibers during periods of activity.

Glycogenolysis is accelerated by the action of the hormones *epinephrine* and *glucagon.* Epinephrine is released from the adrenal medulla in response to sympathetic nerve stimulation and promotes glycogenolysis in the liver and muscle tissues. Glucagon is released from the alpha cells of the pancreas when the blood glucose levels are low and it acts at liver tissues to promote the release of glucose. The hormones activate *adenyl cyclase* at the cell membrane. The enzyme stimulates the production of intracellular *cyclic adenosine-3′,5′-monophosphate* (cAMP), which activates the enzyme *phosphorylase* that is required for the breakdown of glycogen.

CELLULAR GLUCOSE ASSIMILATION

At cellular membranes, the large glucose molecules combine with a carrier that facilitates their diffusion to the intracellular fluids. The activity of insulin, which is released from the beta cells of the islets of Langerhans, is essential for transfer of glucose across the cellular membrane.

Insulin combines with the receptor proteins on the cell membrane and provides the stimulus for the facilitated diffusion of glucose. In the presence of insulin, the circulating glucose rapidly moves into the skeletal muscles, myocardium, visceral smooth muscles, and adipose tissues. The soluble intracellular glucose provides the nutrients that are oxidized for the formation of adenosine triphosphate.

It is estimated that 30 to 50 percent of the ingested carbohydrates are metabolized and stored in the body cells as triglycerides. The glycerol portion of those triglycerides can be utilized for energy when the cells are deprived of glucose.

Pathophysiologic Correlations

DIABETES MELLITUS

The chronic hyperglycemia that is present in the untreated person with diabetes mellitus may represent complete or partial dysfunction of the beta cells of the pancreatic islets of Langerhans. In the absence of endogenous insulin, the hormone must be administered in quantities sufficient to maintain cellular carbohydrate assimilation. Individuals who have some residual pancreatic function may receive oral hypoglycemic agents that stimulate the release of insulin from the remaining functional pancreatic cells.

Some drugs can precipitate a transient, reversible hyperglycemic state. For example, glucocorticoids accelerate glycogenolysis and the breakdown of fats and proteins for the formation of glucose (gluconeogenesis). During therapy with the drugs, patients sometimes have hyperglycemia and glycosuria.

Hyperglycemia

The physiologic problems caused by hyperglycemia are similar in persons with untreated diabetes and in diabetics who ingest carbohydrates in excess of the amounts appropriate for the insulin dosage taken. During strenuous exercise glucose can move into the muscles without the facilitating action of insulin, but other peripheral tissues are dependent on insulin activity at the cell membranes.

The high osmolality associated with the elevated circulating glucose levels causes movement of fluid from the cells and the interstitial fluids. The additional fluid in the vasculature increases

the output of urine (polyuria). When the blood glucose concentration is elevated above 180 mg/ 100 ml, the renal tubule urine glucose content exceeds the amount that can be reabsorbed and the urine glucose content is elevated.

Continued diuresis gradually intensifies the tissue dehydration, and the person drinks fluids excessively (polydipsia) to satisfy the continual thirst. Hunger, which primarily is associated with the deficiency of nutrients in the cells, is intensified by the osmotic movement of fluid from the gastrointestinal tract into the circulation. In addition to the high ingestion of foods (polyphagia), polyuria, and polydipsia that are associated with hyperglycemia, the dehydration of superficial tissues produces pruritus.

Diabetic Acidosis

The metabolism of triglycerides that are stored within the cells can provide the energy required for cellular function for short periods of time. During longer periods of glucose deprivation, adipose tissues provide the fatty acids that are utilized for energy. Many of the pathologic changes associated with the acceleration of atherosclerosis in persons with diabetes are a consequence of the chronic mobilization of fatty acids (i.e., hypertension, myocardial infarction, cataracts, nephropathy, retinopathy).

When the blood glucose levels are markedly elevated (i.e., above 300 mg/100 ml), the increased rate of hepatic lipolysis converts fatty acids to ketones to meet the cellular energy requirements. The high blood concentrations of ketones produce metabolic acidosis. Sodium combines with the strong ketoacids to facilitate their excretion in the urine, and the sodium losses from the serum intensify the metabolic acidosis.

The increased concentrations of hydrogen ions present in acidosis stimulate the medulla respiratory centers, and the person's breathing typically is rapid and deep (Kussmaul respirations). Exhalation of excess carbon dioxide decreases the bicarbonate content of the extracellular fluids. The exhalation of acetones is readily identified by the sweet odor of the person's breath. Coma generally occurs when the blood pH is below 7.0.

Diabetic acidosis is a medical emergency. High doses of insulin are administered intravenously. The repeated administration of insulin may be necessary until the acidotic state is reversed because the acidic plasma acts as an antagonist to insulin. The high blood levels of free fatty acids and ketones also interfere with glucose utilization. Therapeutic measures are employed to correct the dehydration and acidosis (i.e., intravenous sodium bicarbonate, sodium lactate) and to replace the potassium that rapidly moves with glucose from the extracellular fluid into the cells when insulin is administered.

Insulin

DRUG THERAPY

Insulin preparations, which are extracts from porcine or bovine pancreas, are similar to the hormone secreted by the beta cells of the pancreatic islets of Langerhans. Although the onset, peak, and duration of action of the preparations differ according to the additives (i.e., protamine, zinc) or the size of the protein molecules that delay their absorption from the injection site, the insulins have comparable physiologic effects.

The dosage of insulin is expressed in USP Units per milliliter. The hormone is standardized according to its ability to lower blood glucose levels of normal fasting rabbits as compared to the USP Insulin Reference Standard.

Action Mode

The use of insulin for replacement therapy in persons with diabetes mellitus increases the uptake of glucose into the liver and the skeletal muscles where it is utilized for the energy requirements of the tissues or stored as glycogen. The movement of glucose from the extracellular fluids to the intracellular fluids of adipose tissues, which is facilitated by insulin, increases triglyceride synthesis and stimulates lipogenesis. Hepatic glycolysis mobilizes the stores of glycogen when insulin is available to stimulate the activity of the glycolytic enzymes. Excess glucose is stored as glycogen in the muscles and liver. Insulin also increases the rate of protein synthesis in body tissues.

The administration of insulin is planned to maintain the metabolism and assimilation of carbohydrates, protein, and fats in quantities sufficient to meet the energy requirements of the body. One insulin unit promotes the metabolism of approximately 1.5 gm of glucose. An additional physiologic objective is storage of glycogen and fats that can be liberated to meet the requirements for added nutrients during periods of stress.

Therapy Considerations

Insulin is absorbed from the tissues at a predictable rate according to the particular type of preparation that is injected. Insulin-binding serum proteins develop in all persons who take insulin for a period of two to three months, and injected insulin is then absorbed from the tissues at a rate slightly lower than the initial absorption rate. In a few persons, the concentration of insulin-binding proteins is elevated enough to cause refractoriness that is described as *insulin resistance*.

Insulin dosages are planned to meet the individual needs of the person with diabetes. The preplanning includes a careful analysis of the living patterns of the individual to assure that the insulin dosage is as close as possible to that required by dietary intake, physical activity, and predictable stress periods in daily living patterns. Within the limits of predictability, the therapeutic regimen is planned to provide neither too much nor too little insulin in the circulation at any period of time.

Persons with diabetes may require a short-acting insulin in addition to dosages of an intermediate-acting or long-acting insulin (Table 30–1). *Insulin injection* can be mixed with all other insulins in the same syringe. *Insulin injection* can be mixed with *isophane insulin suspension* in any proportion without change in the activity of either insulin preparation. *Insulin injection* that is mixed with *insulin zinc suspension* at less than a 1:1 ratio retains the activity duration of each of the insulin preparations.

Mixing of *insulin injection* with *protamine zinc insulin suspension* is generally avoided because a ratio greater than 1:1 is required to prevent the binding of insulin injection to the excess protamine zinc insulin suspension. The binding that occurs at lower ratios produces total insulin activity similar to that of protamine zinc insulin

suspension alone. When the ratio of insulin injection to protamine zinc insulin suspension is 2:1, the mixture has insulin activity similar to that of isophane insulin suspension; at a ratio greater than 2:1, the mixture has insulin activity similar to that of insulin injection and isophane insulin suspension.

Insulin therapy is an essential aspect of the overall plan for control of hyperglycemia in persons with a deficiency of the endogenous hormone. The use of insulin improves the assimilation of nutrients and is considered to delay the onset of the cardiovascular complications that commonly occur in persons with diabetes mellitus.

Persons who have insulin-dependent diabetes should be counseled at the initiation of therapy to assure their readiness to implement the plans for dietary modification, regularly scheduled exercise, personal hygiene, and monitoring of changes in physiologic status that occur as a consequence of insufficient or excess circulating insulin or glucose. The comprehensiveness of the behavioral changes required for the control of the chronic health problem makes it necessary to plan personalized, individualized counseling. Dietary mod-

Table 30–1.
Insulin Activity Periods After Subcutaneous Injection

Insulin	Onset (hr)	Peak (hr)	Duration (hr)
Fast Acting			
Insulin injection (REGULAR ILETIN)	0.5–1	2–6	5–8
Prompt insulin zinc suspension (SEMILENTE)	0.5–1	3–9	12–16
Intermediate Acting			
Globin zinc insulin injection	1–4	6–10	12–18
Insulin zinc suspension (LENTE)	1–4	7–12	18–24
Isophane insulin suspension (NPH ILETIN)	1–2	7–12	18–24
Long Acting			
Extended insulin zinc suspension (ULTRALENTE)	4–8	10–30	34–46
Protamine zinc insulin suspension (PROTAMINE ZINC, PZI ILETIN)	1–8	12–24	30–36

ifications and the administration of insulin are usually difficult for the person to accept and require the greatest emphasis. Information about those aspects of the therapy should be presented in small, carefully planned learning packets until the necessary understanding and skills are acquired by the person (Fig. 30–1).

Insulin injection is an unmodified preparation. Other insulin preparations have additives, and the active ingredient is in the form of a precipitate in suspension. To assure that the person receives a dosage of the homogeneous mixture, the vial is gently inverted and rotated between the palms of the hands before the dosage is withdrawn. Shaking of the vial produces foam that enters the syringe when the insulin is withdrawn from the vial. The foam interferes with the accurate measurement of the dosage. Insulin should be stored in the refrigerator at temperatures between 2° to 28° C to assure that it is protected from extremes of temperature.

Each of the insulins is administered by subcutaneous injection. Although they can be administered intramuscularly, absorption of the drug is less consistent, and the injections frequently produce pain, hematoma, and sterile abscesses. Insulin injection is the only preparation that can be administered intravenously.

Fast-Acting Insulins

Insulin Injection. The hormone preparation is a clear, colorless solution that is usually administered by subcutaneous injection. It is the only form of insulin that can be administered intravenously. Insulin injection provides a rapid and relatively short duration of hypoglycemic activity. It is frequently used for the control of hyperglycemia as defined by the blood and urine glucose levels during the initial phases of insulin dosage adjustment or when a person with diabetes is acutely ill.

Insulin injection is frequently used to determine the initial daily dosage of an intermediate or long-acting insulin that is required to meet the needs of the individual. The dosage of insulin injection is adjusted to maintain the postprandial

blood glucose levels below 160 mg/100 ml. After control is achieved with insulin injection, the person may be transferred to an intermediate-acting insulin. The initial dosage of the intermediate-acting insulin is based on 75 to 80 percent of the established total daily dose of insulin injection. It is also used alone or with a longer-acting insulin during periods of stress (i.e., postoperatively) and acute infections or when diabetes is too labile to control with a longer-acting insulin preparation.

The usual initial dosage of insulin injection is 10 to 20 units 30 minutes before each meal and at bedtime. When insulin injection is employed for periodic hyperglycemia during the 24-hour period, it is usual for the dosage to be prescribed for administration in a dosage based on the urine tests of glucose and acetone content. That method of dosage determination is described as a sliding-scale dosage. The urine is tested for glucose and ketone bodies one-half hour before each meal and at bedtime, and insulin injection is given as prescribed according to the test reaction. For example, the prescription may provide instructions for the administration of insulin for varying glycosuria or acetone reactions in the following manner: 4+ test reaction, give 8 units of insulin; 3+ test reaction, give 4 units of insulin; 2+ or 1+, give no insulin; moderate to large quantity of ketone bodies, give 2 units of insulin injection.

Insulin injection may be administered intravenously for control of diabetic acidosis or coma. An initial dosage of 50 to 100 units may be given intravenously, and a similar dosage may be given subcutaneously after the blood glucose level has been determined. Subsequent dosages are based on evaluations of the blood glucose and ketone levels. Blood samples are taken at hourly intervals during the acute situation and at two-hour intervals when the person's status improves. The intravenous dosage for emergency treatment of children with severe diabetic acidosis is based on calculation of 40 to 60 units/M^2 of body surface area.

When the status of the patient and the blood values show improvement (i.e., blood glucose levels below 200 mg/100 ml, ketone levels below 50 mg/100 ml, negative acetone), dextrose may be infused intravenously to avert the hypoglycemia that can occur as a consequence of frequent intravenous administration of high dosages of insulin injection (i.e., 1 gm dextrose per one unit of insulin administered). Intravenously administered insulin is considered to become bound to plasma proteins or antibodies. When those proteins becomes saturated, the release of free insulin can cause a marked hypoglycemic reaction.

Prompt Insulin Zinc Suspension. The usual initial dosage of the drug is 10 to 20 units. One dose of insulin is given 30 minutes before breakfast, and a second dosage is usually given before the evening meal. Although the insulin preparation provides a fast action similar to that of insulin injection, it cannot be administered intravenously.

Intermediate-Acting Insulins

Globin Zinc Insulin Injection. The preparation of insulin is modified by the addition of zinc chloride and globin, which is obtained from beef blood. The usual initial dosage is 10 to 20 units. The insulin is given as a single dose one-half to one hour before breakfast. The dosage is usually increased in increments of 2 to 5 units/day. The person's response is carefully evaluated during the period of dosage adjustment.

Insulin Zinc Suspension. The preparation of insulin is modified by addition of zinc chloride. The usual initial dosage is 10 to 20 units. The insulin is given as a single dose one-half to one hour before breakfast. The dosage is usually increased in increments of 2 to 5 units/day. The person's response is carefully evaluated during the adjustment period.

Isophane Insulin Suspension. The preparation of insulin is modified by addition of zinc chloride and protamine, which is obtained from fish sperm. The usual initial dosage is 10 to 20 units. The insulin is given as a single dose 30 to 90 minutes before breakfast. When a second dose of the drug is required to control nocturnal glycosuria, two thirds of the daily dose is given before breakfast and one third is given 30 minutes before the evening meal. The daily dosage is increased in increments of 2 to 5 units/day until the maintenance dosage is determined.

Long-Acting Insulins

Extended Insulin Zinc Suspension. The preparation of insulin is modified by addition of zinc chloride in a manner that produces a crystalline precipitate. The usual initial dose is 7 to 20 units. The insulin is given as a single dose 30 to 90 minutes before breakfast.

Protamine Zinc Insulin Suspension. The insulin preparation is modified by addition of zinc chloride and protamine, which is obtained from the sperm of fish. The usual initial dosage is 7 to 20 units. The insulin is given as a single dose one-half to one hour before breakfast.

Adverse Effects

A hypoglycemic reaction, which occurs suddenly, is the most common and serious adverse effect. It occurs as a consequence of excess circulating insulin in relation to the endogenous supply of available glucose. It usually occurs when the amount of food intake is deficient or when strenuous exercise has induced rapid metabolism of available glucose. The behavioral and functional disturbances associated with the hypoglycemic reaction represent the responses of vital tissues to glucose deprivation. The hypoglycemic status is manifested as uncontrollable yawning, irritability, disorientation, and extreme excitement, which resembles a state of alcohol intoxication.

Increased peripheral norepinephrine and epinephrine activity produces the early warning signs of hypoglycemia, which include anxiety, tachycardia, palpitations, and muscle weakness. The skin is cool to touch, and beads of sweat collect on the skin surface as the catecholamine-induced vasconstriction progresses. The person is pale, sweating, and trembling.

Headache, nausea, and hunger are also characteristic of the hypoglycemic reaction. The person may experience numbness in the circumoral tissues, tingling in the fingers, blurred or double vision, and incoordination.

The brain primarily utilizes glucose to meet its energy requirements, and extreme insulin overdosage may produce psychic disturbances (i.e., aphasia, personality changes, maniacal behavior), tonic-clonic seizures, and unconsciousness. Prolonged, untreated hypoglycemia can produce brain damage. The intake of candy, a sugar cube, or orange juice reverses hypoglycemia within 15 to 45 minutes. Extreme insulin overdosage often requires administration of glucagon or glucose intravenously.

Insulin injections produce local reactions in approximately one fourth of the patients taking the drug. The reactions generally occur one to three weeks after therapy is instituted and gradually decrease within a few weeks when therapy is continued. The localized reactions include itching, redness, swelling, stinging, and warmth of the tissues in areas where the injections have been given.

Atrophy or hypertrophy of subcutaneous fat tissues may occur at the site of insulin injections. Atrophy occurs more frequently in women and children and hypertrophy occurs more frequently in men. Planned alternation of the injection sites reduces the incidence of the tissue disfiguration.

Newly diagnosed persons whose hyperglycemia is rapidly brought under control, or persons with long-term untreated diabetes, may have transient presbyopia or blurred vision. The transient visual disturbances are considered to result from the change in osmotic equilibrium between the lens and the ocular fields that is associated with rapid lowering of the blood glucose levels.

Generalized allergic reactions, which rarely occur, include urticaria, lymphadenopathy, angioedema, and anaphylaxis. The type of insulin preparation is changed when the allergic reactions appear because they represent sensitivity to the additives or to the insulin from a particular source (i.e., porcine, bovine).

Acute insulin resistance may develop in persons with diabetes during episodes of severe infections, surgical procedures, severe trauma, or emotional disturbances. The *Somogyi effect* is an uncommon insulin resistance phenomenon that occurs in persons who have received an overdose of insulin. The overdose produces hypoglycemia. Repeated insulin overdose (i.e., persistent inaccurate measurement of the insulin dosage) causes endogenous release of hormones (i.e., glucocorticoids, epinephrine) that antagonize the insulin and result in rebound hyperglycemia. A change in the type of insulin preparation usually alleviates the insulin resistance.

Interactions

The hypoglycemic action of insulin is potentiated by anabolic steroids, cyclophosphamide, monoamine oxidase inhibitors, guanethidine, and large doses of salicylates. The hypoglycemic effect of insulin is antagonized by thyroid, corticosteroids, dextrothyroxine, phenytoin, and epinephrine. The use of oral contraceptives may decrease glucose tolerance in diabetic females and increase their insulin requirements.

Glucagon

The drug is similar to the hormone liberated by the alpha cells of the pancreatic islets of Langerhans. Glucagon is a glycogenolytic hormone that elevates the blood glucose by activating the hepatic *adenyl cyclase,* which pomotes the formation of *cyclic adenosine-3',5'-mono-* *phosphate* (cAMP). The cAMP activates phosphorylase, which in turn promotes hepatic glycogenolysis. The endogenous secretion of glucagon is stimulated when the blood glucose is low or when the insulin content of the blood is elevated. Effectiveness of glucagon is dependent on the availability of hepatic glycogen stores, and it is effective only until those reserves are depleted.

The drug is used to mobilize the hepatic glycogen reserves in the emergency control of severe hypoglycemic reactions associated with high circulating levels of insulin. Parenteral administration of the drug produces a maximal effect within 30 minutes, and that effect persists for one to two hours.

The usual dosage of glucagon is 0.5 to 1 mg, and that dosage may be given by subcutaneous, intramuscular, or intravenous injection. The dose is repeated one to two times at 20-minute intervals when the comatose state of the person remains unchanged after the initial dosage is given. Intravenous dextrose is usually administered when the person does not respond to the initial dose of glucagon.

Oral Hypoglycemic Drugs

DRUG THERAPY

The oral hypoglycemic agents are employed for treatment of persons with insulin-independent diabetes (formerly called maturity-onset diabetes). The residual functional ability of the beta cells of the islets of the pancreas is essential to the activity of the drugs. The drugs produce degranulation of the beta cells of the pancreas, and the subsequent increased rate of insulin secretion from the islet cells lowers the blood glucose levels. An essential aspect of therapy is regulation of diet to assure the intake of nutritious foods that provide carbohydrate, protein, and fats in quantities calculated to meet the activity requirements of the individual.

The oral hypoglycemic agents are sulfonylurea derivatives that lack the antibacterial activity of the sulfonamides, which have a similar chemical structure. The oral hypoglycemics are *acetohexamide, chlorpropamide, tolazamide,* and *tolbutamide*. The primary difference between the sulfonylureas is their duration of action. The duration of hypoglycemic action of tolbutamide is 6 to 12 hours, that of tolazamide 16 hours, that of acetohexamide up to 24 hours, and that of chlorpropamide 60 hours.

Therapy Considerations

An initial one-week period of therapy is usually planned to determine the effectiveness of the balanced diet, activity, and the oral hypoglycemic drug in the control of hyperglycemia. When the

initial period of treatment shows a reduction in the blood glucose levels (i.e., <200 mg percent), reduction in glycosuria and ketonuria, and alleviation of the symptoms of pruritus, polyuria, polydipsia, and polyphagia, prolonged maintenance therapy is planned for the individual. Persons who are nonresponsive during the trial period require insulin therapy for consistent control of symptoms. The drugs are used infrequently with insulin for persons who have inadequate control of hyperglycemia with the oral hypoglycemic drug alone.

Adults who have been maintained on insulin at dosages less than 40 units/day sometimes have sufficient islet cell function to allow transfer to the use of an oral hypoglycemic drug. During the initial conversion period, the person usually continues to receive one half the insulin dosage concurrent with the oral hypoglycemic drug. The person's response is evaluated frequently during the transition period. The oral agent may be used without continuance of insulin therapy when the person has been maintained on less than 20 units of insulin per day.

The requirements for endogenous insulin are elevated during periods of stress or illness, and each person who receives an oral hypoglycemic drug should be counseled about the relationship between dietary intake, illness, and endogenous insulin requirements. The oral agents are used as long as they provide adequate endogenous insulin to maintain the blood glucose levels within normal limits. Insulin administration may be required during periods of illness or stress, and persons taking the oral agents should learn how to administer insulin subcutaneously.

Annual or semiannual drug-free periods may be planned to evaluate whether the person requires the hypoglycemic drug. Some individuals whose blood glucose levels are well regulated during therapy with an oral hypoglycemic drug and diet modification can maintain a normal blood glucose level with carefully managed diet. For those individuals, use of the drugs can be terminated.

Acetohexamide

Therapy Considerations. The drug (DYMELOR) is administered at a dosage of 0.25 to 1.5 gm/day. The initial dosage is usually at the lower level of the range (0.25 gm/day), and the drug is taken before breakfast. The dosage may be increased in increments of 0.25 to 0.5 gm at five-to-seven-day intervals until the blood glucose levels indicate that the dosage provides adequate endogenous insulin.

A loading dose schedule may be used at the initiation of therapy. For example, 1.5 gm may be given on day one, 1 gm on day two, and the maintenance dosage may be given after that period of time. Dosages of 1.5 gm/day may be divided for administration in the early morning and before the evening meal.

The oral drug is readily absorbed from the gastrointestinal tract. The metabolism of acetohexamide produces the active metabolite *hydroxyhexamide*, which is considered to contribute significantly to the 12-to-24-hour duration of hypoglycemic activity of the drug. Trace amounts of the unchanged drug and approximately 50 percent of the active metabolite are excreted in the urine within 24 hours.

Chlorpropamide

Therapy Considerations. The drug (DIABINESE) is administered at a dosage of 100 to 500 mg/day. The dosage is usually taken with breakfast but may be divided for use two times per day when persons have gastrointestinal disturbances when taking the single morning dose. The initial dosage may be 250 mg/day. The dosage may be increased in increments of 50 to 125 mg at three-to-five-day intervals until the maintenance dosage required for the control of hyperglycemia is determined.

The oral drug is well absorbed from the gastrointestinal tract. Plasma drug concentrations usually are at the peak level within two to four hours, and the hypoglycemic effect persists for 60 hours. The drug has a half-life of 36 hours. The serum drug concentrations reach a plateau after three or more days of therapy. There is little metabolism of chlorpropamide, and approximately 80 to 90 percent of the unchanged drug is excreted in the urine over a period of 96 hours.

Tolazamide

Therapy Considerations. The drug (TOLINASE) is administered at a dosage of 0.1 to 1 gm, and the dosage is taken daily with breakfast. Dosages of 500 mg or more per day may be divided for administration two times per day. Dosage increases usually are made in increments of 100 to 250 mg at four-to-six-day intervals.

The drug is more slowly absorbed from the gastrointestinal tract than other sulfonylureas. The onset of the hypoglycemic effect occurs in four to six hours and the hypoglycemic effect persists for 16 hours. The half-life of the drug is seven hours. The drug is extensively metabolized, and approximately 85 percent of the metabolites appear in the urine.

Tolbutamide

Therapy Considerations. The drug (ORINASE) is administered at a dosage of 0.5 to 3 gm/day. The drug is taken as a single dose with breakfast or in divided doses with meals.

Tolbutamide is readily absorbed from the gastrointestinal tract. Plasma drug concentrations are usually at their peak level within three hours. The maximal hypoglycemic effect persists for eight hours, and there is significant hypoglycemic activity for 12 hours. The plasma half-life of the drug is approximately four to six hours. The drug is metabolized in the liver, and the inactive metabolites are excreted in the urine within 24 hours.

Adverse Effects

Hypoglycemic reactions that can occur with use of the oral sulfonylurea drugs are rarely severe. The manifestations of hypoglycemia are similar to those that occur during the use of insulin.

The sulfonylurea drugs also produce gastrointestinal disturbances (i.e., anorexia, nausea, vomiting, epigastric distress, abdominal cramps, constipation, or diarrhea). Persons taking the oral hypoglycemics occasionally have an intolerance to alcohol. The oral hypoglycemic drugs can also produce neurologic symptoms (i.e., headache, weakness, paresthesias). Hypersensitivity reactions, which include jaundice and pancytopenia, and allergic reactions may also occur (i.e., pruritus, skin rash, low-grade fever, eosinophilia).

The mild leukopenia that occurs during therapy with the sulfonylureas usually reverses spontaneously when therapy is continued. The drugs occasionally produce thrombocytopenia and mild anemia. Those blood dyscrasias are readily reversible when therapy is discontinued. Hypothyroidism has occurred during prolonged therapy with the sulfonylurea drugs.

Interactions

The hypoglycemic effect of the drugs can be increased when the person concurrently receives insulin, sulfonamides, oxyphenbutazone, phenylbutazone, salicylates, probenecid, or monoamine oxidase inhibitors. The sulfonylureas may prolong the action of barbiturates and other sedatives. The thiazide diuretics interfere with the hypoglycemic effects, and an increase in the dosage of the sulfonylurea may be required when the drugs are employed concurrently. The inter-

action is considered to be associated with thiazide-induced hypokalemia, and the use of potassium supplements may avert the interaction.

NURSING INTERVENTION

The person with diabetes mellitus is more actively involved in the medical aspects of the therapy plan than most individuals with a chronic health problem. Long-term health maintenance requires that the person control the dietary intake of carbohydrates, proteins, and fats and make judgments about the requirements for insulin in relation to perceived physiologic changes.

The initial preparation of the patient for that role requires intensive counseling by the physician, nutritionist, and nurse. Because the person learns and gains reinforcement of that learning during contacts with each of the professionals, it is important that the preparation of the patient be a team effort. The collaboration of the professionals allows advancement of the therapy plan according to the learning progress of the patient. For example, the nutritionist primarily counsels the person about the dietary modifications that are indicated by the caloric allowance the physician has prescribed. After a nutrition history is taken, the plan for the distribution of carbohydrates, proteins, and fats is described to the patient. The nutritionist also instructs the person in the method for selecting and exchanging foods that are included on the exchange lists for meal planning.

When the patient is unable to eat a particular food at mealtime, the nurse has an opportunity to ascertain the person's ability to select a substitute food from the exchange lists to complete the planned nutrient intake for the meal. The person's ability independently to manage the substitution should be discussed with the nutritionist so additional counseling can be provided when it is required.

All of the counseling provided during the initial phases of the treatment plan is directed at assisting the patient to adapt to the requirements of the diabetic therapy regimen. Many of the hygienic measures that are provided by the nurse (i.e., special foot care) offer an opportunity to discuss the rationale for the measures and problems that are to be discussed promptly with the physician (i.e., lesions that are slow to heal). When the person is incapable of performing aspects of care, a responsible family member or close associate is instructed in the procedures.

Although there are clearly defined learning outcomes for all persons with diabetes, the progression of learning is highly individualized. It generally facilitates the person's learning when the nurse outlines the overall plan and actively involves the patient in establishing a schedule for attainment of short-term goals. For example, the insulin-dependent diabetic must learn to administer insulin. The steps of the procedure and the manipulation of the syringe and vial of insulin are complex behaviors for the learner. The nurse can define small learning packets, which are based on the individual's abilities, when assisting the person with attainment of the required skills (Fig. 30-2).

The patient who is to mix two types of insulin in one syringe may be able to manage the procedure for preparing the insulin suspension and the unmodified insulin injection after observing the nurse's preparation of the insulins. The nurse can provide the guidance that is required while the patient sterilizes the stoppers of the two vials, injects air into the vial of the insulin suspension, withdraws the needle and injects air into the vial of unmodified insulin injection, measures the dosage while aspirating the insulin from the vial, and finally aspirates the insulin suspension to the exact dosage. The patient usually expresses a sense of satisfaction when arriving at the point of gently rotating the syringe to mix the insulin suspension and the unmodified insulin injection. Some patients need smaller learning seg-

ments (i.e., withdrawing a single insulin preparation), and the nurse completes the dosage preparation for those patients.

The decision about injecting the prepared dosage is dependent on the person's level of readiness to take that final step. Many persons postpone that step for as long as possible. It is important that a specific target date and time be set for completion of that procedure to assure that the patient has adequate supervised practice and guidance in planning for rotation of injection sites.

Meal planning and the preparation of insulin and its injection are important skills, but the control of diabetes also involves exercise, urine testing, and the ability to recognize the signs of hyperglycemia and hypoglycemia. The patient who views urine testing as a means of validating the effectiveness of the insulin or oral hypoglycemic agent in controlling the blood glucose levels may more conscientiously do the urine tests. For example, the patient who is receiving an intermediate-acting insulin (i.e., isophane insulin suspension, or NPH insulin) should understand that the urine tests for glucose and acetone that are done before breakfast provide an assessment of the adequacy of the insulin in controlling glucose utilization over the 24-hour period after it is administered; the test before the evening meal provides an assessment of the effectiveness of the insulin during the daytime: and the prebedtime test provides an indicator of the effectiveness of the insulin in utilizing the foods eaten at the evening meal. The same specificity is meaningful when explaining the rationale for premeal and bedtime urine glucose and acetone testing to the patient who is receiving insulin injection or the daily urine glucose testing to the person who is receiving an oral hypoglycemic agent. The patients should also be instructed to maintain an ongoing account of the urine tests with the record of insulin dosages taken each day.

The booklets published for diabetics by the

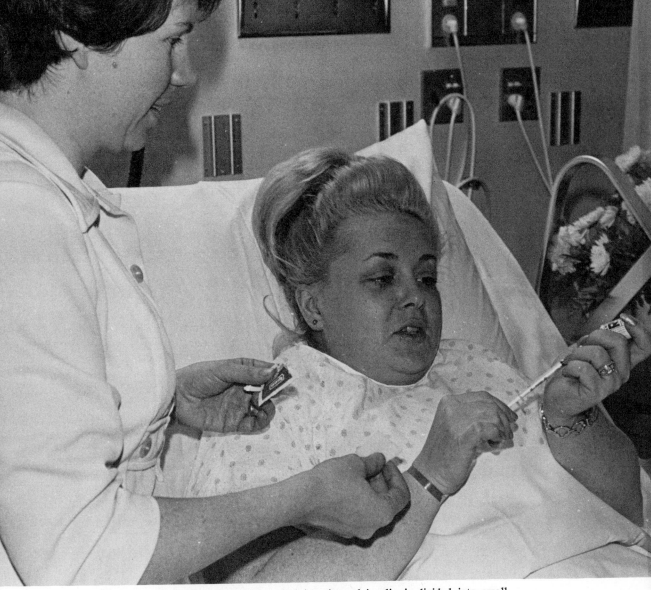

Fig. 30–2. The procedure for the administration of insulin is divided into small learning packets. The patient is supervised by the nurse during each step of the learning process. Instructions are provided as the patient measures the insulin dosage. (Courtesy, Lynn Hospital School of Nursing, Lynn, Massachusetts.)

American Diabetes Association or by drug manufacturers are useful aids when teaching patients about the therapy regimen. Although a few persons will seek extensive information about the disease and its control, most individuals benefit from simple, concise guides that are relevant to their personal care. It is useful to preview the material and to highlight (i.e., with marginal brackets, underlining) what is relevant to the individual's therapy plan.

The printed booklets outline the signs of

hyperglycemia and hypoglycemia, and the listing provides a useful guide for the patient when a reaction occurs. Most patients with diabetes mellitus can recall the signs of hyperglycemia and acidosis that were present at the time of their diagnosis. That experience provides a basis for discussing prevention, recognition, and treatment of hyperglycemia and acidosis. In addition to reinforcing the necessity of taking insulin regularly, the nurse should emphasize that the insulin dosage is to be taken as long as the urine is glucose positive even though the patient is nauseated or unable to eat. One half of the usual dosage of intermediate-acting insulin is taken and the physician is notified when the person is unable to eat for more than a few hours. An infection or illness increases the metabolic rate and mobilizes the endogenous sources of glucose. Those physiologic changes increase the insulin requirements.

Patients usually recall the early symptoms of hyperglycemia and acidosis (i.e., polyuria, polydipsia, polyphagia, pruritus; pain, numbness, or tingling of the extremities; visual disturbances; malaise; nervousness and irritability). Many persons also can recall some of the later symptoms of acidosis, which include extreme loss of appetite, nausea, vomiting, abdominal pain, extreme fatigue, weakness, sweet breath odor, air hunger, and increased sleepiness. Coma is a later manifestation of acidosis. It is important to review even those familiar symptoms to assure that the patient is prepared to recognize the problems and understand the importance of continued testing of each voiding for glucose and acetone content.

The person and a family member also should clearly understand the early warning signs of hypoglycemia, which are related to the increased endogenous epinephrine activity (i.e., irritability, weakness, nervousness, profuse sweating, trembling of the fingers and hands, headache, nausea, hunger). The later symptoms rapidly lead to unconsciousness (i.e., anxiousness, extreme excitement, mental confusion, bizarre behavior, blurred vision, perioral numbness or tingling, tachycardia, cold and moist skin, shallow respirations, drowsiness). The unconscious patient must have intravenous glucose to correct the hypoglycemic state.

The symptoms of hypoglycemia are less familiar to the patient and are given special emphasis. The reaction progresses rapidly unless glucose is ingested promptly. All patients with diabetes must understand the necessity for having an immediately available emergency supply of carbohydrate. The sugar can be utilized when a meal is unavoidably delayed or when strenuous exercise rapidly depletes the available endogenous glucose. Patients usually are instructed to take 2 teaspoonsful of sugar in orange juice or ginger ale, two lumps of sugar, or hard candy immediately. Persons who take a long-acting insulin should also take a longer-acting carbohydrate (i.e., a slice of bread, glass of milk). When the person has difficulty discriminating between hyperglycemia and hypoglycemia, which have some similar characteristics, he should take a rapid-acting glucose. A subsequent urine test can be used as a guide for insulin dosage when there is evidence of glycosuria.

Early instruction of the patient is important because it provides an opportunity for supervised practice and reinforcement of learning. Ongoing evaluation of the patient's therapeutic regimen provides an opportunity for the individual to discuss aspects of the plan that are unclear or problematic (Fig. 30–3). One of the most important outcomes of the nurse's periodic contact with the patient is communication of the nurse's belief that the person can manage the plan and maintain a normal living pattern. That psychologic reinforcement is the additive to factual information that the patient needs when learning to manage the chronic health problem.

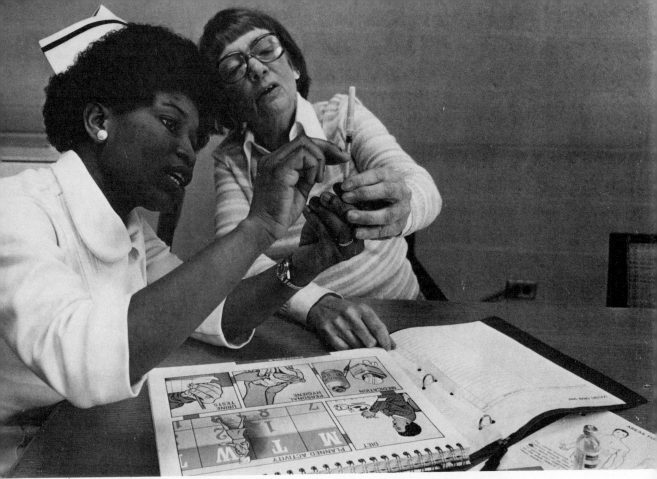

Fig. 30–3. The periodic counseling that is provided by the nurse helps the patient to understand the overall therapy plan and to resolve problems that occur during implementation of the plan. (Courtesy, Northeastern University College of Nursing, Boston.)

Review Guides

1. Describe the physiologic factors that produce hypoglycemia when the person is taking unmodified insulin injection.

2. Describe the physiologic factors that produce acidosis and contribute to the atherosclerotic changes in the untreated person with diabetes.

3. Identify briefly the relationship of exercise to the dosage of a long-acting insulin that is required by the patient.

4. Explain the differences between insulin injection, isophane insulin suspension, and protamine zinc insulin.

5. Outline the steps in the procedure for preparing the dosage of unmodified insulin injection and isophane insulin suspension in the same syringe.

6. Describe the rationale for use of unmodified insulin injection for the patient in diabetic acidosis.

7. Explain the rationale for rotation of the sites for injection of insulin.

8. Outline the primary differences between acetohexamide, chlorpropamide, tolazamide, and tolbutamide.

9. List the factors that would be included when counseling the person who is to receive an oral hypoglycemic agent for the control of insulin-independent diabetes.

Additional Readings

Askew, Gail B., and Letcher, Kenneth I.: Oral hypoglycemic agents: a little teaching makes therapy go a long way. *Nursing 75,* **5:**45, August, 1975.

Bierman, Edwin L.: The oral antidiabetic agents. *Am. Fam. Physician,* **13:**98, January, 1976.

Bruce, Glennda L.: The Somogyi phenomenon: insulin-induced posthypoglycemic hyperglycemia. *Heart Lung,* **7:**463, May–June, 1978.

Colwell, John A.: Use of oral agents in treating diabetes mellitus: a perspective. *Postgrad. Med.,* **59:**139, January, 1976.

Davies, Derek: Advances toward understanding diabetes mellitus. *Geriatrics,* **30:**79, November, 1975.

Felig, Philip: Combating diabetic ketoacidosis and other hyperglycemic-ketoacidotic syndromes. *Postgrad. Med.,* **59:**150, January, 1976.

Fletcher, H. Patrick: The oral antidiabetic drugs: pro and con. *Am. J. Nurs.,* **76:**596, April, 1976.

Forbath, Nicholas: Oral hypoglycemic agents. *Primary Care,* **4:**629, December, 1977.

Garber, Rita: The use of a standardized teaching program in diabetes education. *Nurs. Clin. North Am.,* **12:**375, September, 1977.

Gray, Gary M.: Carbohydrate digestion and absorption: role of the small intestine. *N. Engl. J. Med.,* **292:**1225, June 5, 1975.

Guthrie, Diane W.: Exercise, diets and insulin for children with diabetes. *Nursing 77,* **7:**48, February, 1977.

Halperin, Mitchell L.: Lactic acidosis and ketoacidosis: biochemical and clinical implications. *Can. Med. Assoc. J.,* **116:**1034, May 7, 1977.

Hayter, Jean: Fine points in diabetic care. *Am. J. Nurs.,* **76:**594, April, 1976.

Hofeldt, Fred D.; Adler, Robert A.; and Herman, Robert H.: Postprandial hypoglycemia. *J.A.M.A.,* **233:**1309, September 22, 1975.

Kennell, Carol: Outpatient management of the juvenile diabetic. *Pediatr. Nurs.,* **2:**19, November–December, 1976.

Levin, Marvin E.; Boisseau, Vincenza C.; and Avioli, Louis V.: Diabetes mellitus and bone mass in juvenile and adult-onset diabetes. *N. Engl. J. Med.,* **294:**241, January 29, 1976.

McConnell, Edwina A.: Meeting the special needs of diabetics facing surgery. *Nursing 76,* **6:**30, June, 1976.

McFarlane, Judith M.: The child with diabetes mellitus. *Pediatr. Nurs.,* **1:**6, October, 1975.

McGarry, J. Denis, and Foster, Daniel W.: Ketogenesis and its regulation. *Am. J. Med.,* **61:**9, July, 1976.

Moss, James M., and Tucker, H. St. George: New trends in the management of diabetic ketoacidosis. *Am. Fam. Physician,* **17:**111, February, 1978.

Owen, Oliver E.; Boden, Guenther; and Shuman, Charles R.: Managing insulin-dependent diabetic patients. *Postgrad. Med.,* **59:**127, January, 1976.

Petrokas, Judith C.: Common sense guidelines for controlling diabetes during illness. *Nursing 77,* **7:**36, December, 1977.

Reaven, Gerald M.; Bernstein, Robert; Davis, Bonnie; and Olefsky, Jerrold M.: Nonketotic diabetes mellitus: insulin deficiency or insulin resistance? *Am. J. Med.,* **60:**80, January, 1976.

Renshaw, Domeena C.: Impotence in diabetes. *Dis. Nerv. Syst.,* **36:**369, July, 1975.

Rigberg, Leon A.; Robinson, Morton J.; and Espiritu, Carmelita: Chlorpropamide-induced granulomas. *J.A.M.A.,* **235:**409, January 26, 1976.

Schumann, Delores: Assessing the diabetic. *Nursing 76,* **6:**62, March, 1976.

Shen, Shiao-Wei, and Bressler, Rubin: Drug therapy: clinical pharmacology of oral antidiabetic agents. *N. Engl. J. Med.,* **296:**493, March 3, 1977.

———: Drug therapy: oral antidiabetic agents. *N. Engl. J. Med.,* **296:**787, April 7, 1977.

Slater, Norma L.: Insulin reactions vs. ketoacidosis: guidelines for diagnosis and intervention. *Am. J. Nurs.,* **78:**875, May, 1978.

Suren, Jean V.: Education of the culturally and educationally deprived diabetic. *Nurs. Clin. North Am.,* **12:**427, September, 1977.

Thomas, Katherine P.: Diabetes mellitus in elderly persons. *Nurs. Clin. North Am.,* **11:**157, March, 1976.

Thompson, Robert G.: Juvenile-onset diabetes. *Primary Care,* **3:**551, September, 1976.

Wit, Karen: HHNH, a newly recognized syndrome to watch for. *Nursing 76,* **6:**66, February, 1976.

Wolfe, Lawrence: Insulin: paving the way to a new life. *Nursing 77,* **7:**38, November, 1977.

31

Abnormal Metabolic Activity

Physical and metabolic activity affects the endogenous rate of nutrient utilization. Sustained activity requires utilization of readily available nutrients and metabolism of fat and protein reserves to provide the energy for cellular processes. Ingestion of foods in excess of those that are required for energy production leads to storage of the superfluous nutrients in adipose tissues.

Physiologic Correlations

The iodide content from natural food sources (i.e., water, fish) or from the additives to foods (i.e., iodized table salt, white bread) provides the basic element required for synthesis of thyroid hormone. The hormone has a key role in the control of most metabolic processes.

THYROID HORMONE SYNTHESIS

The ingested iodides that enter the circulation are rapidly taken up by the thyroid tissues. The inorganic iodides are held in a concentrated state until they are oxidized to iodine. The uniting of iodine with tyrosine begins the process of thyroid hormone synthesis. The hormones *thyroxine* and *triiodothyronine* may be released into the circulation or incorporated with thyroglobin molecules in the follicles of the thyroid gland. The iodinated hormones are cleaved from the thyroglobulin and released from storage when the levels of circulating hormone are low. There is generally more thyroxine than triiodothyronine in the circulation, but the latter hormone has a more potent effect on metabolic processes.

THYROID-STIMULATING HORMONE

The structural integrity of the thyroid gland, the synthesis of thyroid hormones, and the release of the hormones from the gland are controlled by the activity of *thyroid-stimulating hormone* (TSH), which is secreted by the anterior pituitary gland. The release of *thyrotropin-releasing factor* from the hypothalamus provides the stimulus for pituitary secretion of TSH when the circulating levels of thyroid hormone are low. TSH is thought to act on thyroid tissues by stimulating the activity of *adenyl cyclase,* which increases the production of the intracellular cyclic *adenosine-3′,5′-monophosphate* (cAMP) that mediates the response to TSH stimulation.

CALCITONIN SECRETION

The parafollicular cells of the thyroid gland secrete *calcitonin,* which contributes to the calcium ion balance by reducing elevated serum calcium ion levels. The calcium content of the blood perfusing the thyroid gland provides the stimulus for release of calcitonin. The hormone acts primarily by inhibiting bone resorption. It is thought to interact with a specific receptor on the plasma membrane of osteoclasts to activate *adenyl cyclase.* The consequent increase in the activity of intracellular cAMP alters the transport of calcium and phosphate across the membranes of the osteoclasts. The hormone also promotes the renal excretion of calcium and phosphates by decreasing their tubular reabsorption.

PARATHYROID HORMONE ACTIVITY

Parathyroid hormone affects the absorption, utilization, and excretion of calcium and phosphates and enhances the activity of vitamin D. The primary action of the hormone is the stimulation of osteoclast formation to accelerate the release of calcium from bone. When the circulating levels of calcium ions are low, the parathyroid hormone–induced development of osteoclasts increases the resorption of bone, and there is a consequent elevation of the circulating levels of the cation. Osteoclasts have a limited period of activity before they become osteoblasts. The bone construction that occurs after the transition maintains the integrity of the skeletal structure.

Parathyroid hormone has a secondary effect at the renal proximal convoluted tubules that inhibits phosphate reabsorption and increases its excretion while it increases calcium ion reabsorption. The hormone also facilitates the renal conversion of vitamin D_3 to its active form, *1,25-dihydroxycholecalciferol,* which is required for the production of calcium-binding protein and the intestinal absorption of calcium. The increased activity of the vitamin accelerates the absorption of calcium and phosphate ions from the duodenum and proximal jejunum.

Pathophysiologic Correlations

HYPERTHYROIDISM

The elevated levels of circulating thyroid hormone that are released from hyperplastic thyroid tissues markedly accelerate the metabolic rate. The endogenous heat production causes heat intolerance and profuse perspiration; the metabolism of body proteins to meet cellular energy requirements causes extreme weight loss and muscular weakness; and the stimulation of the smooth muscle of the intestine produces diarrhea. The central nervous system manifestations of the high level of thyroid hormone activity include psychic disturbances, nervousness, insomnia, and tremor of the hands.

In addition to the direct effects of the increased metabolic activity, the increased thyroid hormone activity indirectly places demands on other endocrine glands. For example, the increased levels of circulating glucose require an increase in the pancreatic production of insulin, and the increased rate of glucocorticoid metabolism in hepatic tissues requires the adrenal glandular production of additional quantities of that hormone. Male patients with hyperthyroidism may be impotent, and female patients may have oligomenorrhea or amenorrhea.

The toxic symptoms persist until the activity of the thyroid tissue is decreased. Radioactive sodium iodide (I^{131}) is often employed to destroy hyperplastic thyroid tissue. The gland can also be removed surgically (thyroidectomy). Postoperative patients are observed carefully for evidence of the accelerated thyroid hormone activity that occurs as a consequence of release of the hormone into the circulation during the surgical procedure (i.e., delirium, hyperpyrexia, tachycardia, cardiac arrhythmias, extreme diaphoresis, shock, vomiting, dehydration). Hypothyroidism is often associated with therapies for the reduction of hyperplastic thyroid tissues.

HYPOTHYROIDISM

The manifestations of decreased circulating levels of thyroid hormone are the converse of those that appear during hyperthyroidism. Extreme somnolence, physical and mental sluggishness, bradycardia, decreased cardiac output, low blood volume, obesity, constipation, decreased libido, thinning of the hair, scaling of the skin, and huskiness of the voice characteristically are associated with hypothyroidism. Females may have excessive menstrual flow (menorrhagia) or frequent menstrual periods (polymenorrhea).

Myxedema

Severe, prolonged hypothyroidism produces a generalized edematous appearance. The collection of mucopolysaccharides is thought to be the pathogenesis of the interstitial collections of fluid. The interstitial fluid is evident primarily around the eyes as a fullness or "bagginess" of the tissues and in the generalized swelling of the facial tissues. The mucopolysaccharides gradually absorb

the interstitial fluid, and the formation of an interstitial gel increases the heaviness of the tissues. Atherosclerosis and arteriosclerosis are also accelerated in persons with hypothyroidism.

In the absence of thyroid hormone production the anterior pituitary gland secretes greater quantities of TSH. The subsequent deposits of large quantities of thyroglobulin in the follicles and enlargement of the thyroid tissue become evident in the thickening or widening of the neck. Thyroid hormone replacement gradually corrects the problem. Persons with hypothyroidism that is associated with a deficient intake of iodides usually have normal thyroid hormone levels when the iodide deficiency is corrected.

Cretinism

The congenital absence of a thyroid gland or deficient thyroid production in infants and children produces physical and mental growth retardation that is described as *cretinism*. The maternal blood provides the necessary thyroid hormones to the fetus in utero, and the residual activity of the hormone may mask the symptoms for a few weeks after the birth of the infant. The thyroid hormone deficiency initially is evident as sluggish movements and low muscle activity.

Thyroid hormone replacement is essential within a few months after birth to prevent permanent retardation of neuronal development in the brain. Skeletal growth is also retarded severely unless hormonal replacement is initiated and continued.

HYPERPARATHYROIDISM

Increased activity of parathyroid hormone produces continued osteoclastic activity that destroys bone tissues and elevates the concentrations of calcium in the extracellular fluids. The severe osteoclastic resorption may cause large cystic areas in the bone described as *osteitis fibrosa cystica*. The bones become fragile and can be broken with minimal trauma. The concurrent osteoblastic activity, which represents a compensatory attempt to maintain the structural integrity of the bones, produces a marked rise in the alkaline phosphatase in the body fluids.

A similar destruction of bones occurs when there is a deficiency in the circulating levels of calcitonin. In the absence of hormonal inhibition of osteoclastic activity, the bones become porous and fragile. That entity is described as Paget's disease, or *osteitis deformans*.

The hypercalcemia that is associated with excessive bone resorption can cause the formation of calcium phosphate stones in the alveoli of the lungs, tubules of the kidneys, thyroid gland, gastric mucosa, and walls of the arteries. Hypercalcemia also depresses central and peripheral neuromuscular transmission, which is evident in muscular weakness, constipation, or cardiac arrest during diastole.

HYPOPARATHYROIDISM

In the absence of parathyroid hormone, the production of osteoclasts is minimal. The plasma calcium ion levels become depressed when the resorption of bone is insufficient to provide the reserve stores to replace the cation. Severe hypocalcemia (i.e., < 6 to 7 mg/100 ml) produces tetany. When the levels of calcium remain low, the spasm of the sensitive laryngeal muscles can obstruct the airway and cause death. Intravenous administration of calcium is required to reverse the severe hypocalcemia.

Antithyroid Agents

The drugs employed for control of excess thyroid hormone production and the associated metabolic hyperactivity include *radioactive sodium iodide* (I^{131}) and the antithyroid drugs *strong iodine solution, sodium iodide solution, propylthiouracil, methimazole,* and *methylthiouracil.*

RADIOACTIVE SODIUM IODIDE

The radioactive sodium iodides that are employed for diagnostic studies of thyroid function and for the treatment of hyperthyroidism are chemically and physiologically similar to the naturally occurring iodide (I^{127}). Two weeks or more before the person is to have diagnostic tests of thyroid function, the ongoing drug therapy plan of the patient is carefully audited by the physician to determine whether the person is taking drugs that may interfere with uptake of the iodide solutions by the thyroid gland (i.e., antihistamines, antithyroid and thyroid drugs, corticotropin, corticosteroids, phenylbutazone, progesterone, salicylates, sulfonamides, sulfonylureas, testosterone, vitamin A). The person is instructed to abstain from eating or drinking fluids for eight hours before the testing period.

Radioactive sodium iodide (I^{125} or I^{131}) emits gamma particles that make it possible to trace the movement of radio-tagged iodide in the body. The agents are used for diagnostic studies, which include evaluation of the thyroid gland uptake, conversion, and release of iodine after oral or intravenous administration of the radioactive agent. The circulating inorganic iodide is absorbed avidly by the thyroid gland. The absorbed inorganic iodide is concentrated in the thyroid gland at the rate of approximately 2 percent per hour, and the gamma emissions from the gland initially can be detected within minutes after the drug is administered. The iodide is oxidized to iodine, which readily binds with tyrosine. That organic complex is the precursor for the synthesis of the thyroid hormones.

Radioactive uptake studies at the end of a 24-hour period provide data about the functional status of the thyroid gland. In hypothyroidism less than 10 percent of the radioactive iodide dosage is taken up by the gland. The uptake of more than 40 percent of the dose indicates hyperthyroidism. Conversion ratios, which are also measured 24 hours after the drug is administered, identify the rate at which the thyroid hormones are formed and released from the thyroid gland. A conversion of less than 20 percent of the plasma radioactive iodide to protein-bound iodine

(PBI) indicates a hypothyroid status, and conversion of more than 50 percent of the iodide indicates hyperthyroidism. After a 72-hour period, protein-bound iodine studies are evaluated. Generally a PBI that is greater than 0.27 percent of the radioactive iodide dose per liter of plasma is an indication of hyperthyroidism.

Radioactive sodium iodide (I^{131}) emits gamma particles that are traced during diagnostic studies and it also emits beta particles. The emission of beta particles with a 2-to-3-mm range of radioactivity allows use of the drug for therapeutic destruction of hyperplastic thyroid tissues. The use of radiation has markedly decreased the frequency of surgical thyroidectomies.

The radiation therapy infrequently produces transient gastritis with nausea and vomiting, inflammation of the salivary glands, and decreased leukocyte counts. There may be a transient exacerbation of toxic symptoms of hyperthyroidism or transient hypothyroidism. Permanent hypothyroidism occurs in approximately one third of the patients who receive therapeutic doses of the radioactive iodide for treatment of hyperthyroidism.

The ingested iodides are concentrated in the salivary glands and in the gastric mucosa. Those secretions enter the gastrointestinal tract, and the iodide is reabsorbed. Small quantities of the iodides can also be detected in nasal secretions, sweat, and the tissues of the oral cavity, trachea, female breasts, gallbladder, liver, and intestines. The iodides cross the placenta. Approximately 65 to 90 percent of the iodide is excreted in the urine in 24 hours. The measurement of the 24-hour urinary excretion of iodide provides an estimation of the functional status of the thyroid gland. Approximately 20 percent of an ingested dose appears in the milk of nursing mothers within 24 hours.

IODIDE SOLUTIONS

Strong Iodine Solution (LUGOL'S SOLUTION)

Sodium Iodide Solution

Action Mode. The drugs (Table 31–1) generally are employed for the involution of the thyroid gland and the reduction of hyperplasia when

Table 31–1.
Dosage of Drugs Used for Suppression or Replacement of Thyroid Hormone Activity

Drugs	Route	Usual Adult Daily Dosage	
		Initial Dosage	Maintenance Dosage
Antithyroid Agents			
Iodine solution, strong	Oral	0.3–0.9 ml	—
Methimazole (TAPAZOLE)	Oral	15–60 mg	5–15 mg
Methylthiouracil (METHIACIL,			
MURACIN)	Oral	200 mg	200 mg
Propylthiouracil	Oral	300–400 mg	100–300 mg
Sodium iodide solution (10%)	IV	1–3 gm	
Thyroid Replacement			
Dextrothyroxine sodium			
(CHOLOXIN)	Oral	1 mg	4–8 mg
Levothyroxine (LETTER,			
SYNTHROID)	Oral	0.025–0.1 mg	0.1–0.3 mg
Liothyronine (CYTOMEL)	Oral	12.5–25 mcg	75–100 mcg
Liotrix (EUTHROID, THYROLAR)	Oral	15–30 mg	
Thyroglobulin (PROLOID)	Oral	16–32 mg	32–190 mg
Thyroid, desiccated (THYRAR)	Oral	15–30 mg	60–180 mg

surgical removal of the thyroid gland is contemplated. The iodides reduce the vascularity of the gland. During therapy with the drugs there is an increase in the accumulation of colloids in the follicles and the thyroid gland becomes firm. The iodides also inhibit iodotyrosine synthesis and antagonize the thyrotropin and *cyclic adenosine-3',5'-monophosphate* (cAMP) stimulation of hormone synthesis. Those actions rapidly provide the reduction in the levels of circulating thyroid hormones that is vital in the treatment of persons with severe thyrotoxicosis. The decrease in metabolic activity may be evident within 24 hours. The drugs are employed primarily for short-term treatment of preoperative patients and for treatment of persons with thyrotoxicosis.

Therapy Considerations. The iodides are also employed in combination with other antithyroid drugs for treatment of persons with simple or colloidal goiter or exophthalmic goiter. Sodium iodide is usually given when parenteral therapy is required. The additive action of the combined drugs more rapidly produces a euthyroid state. The use of the iodides with another antithyroid agent prior to thyroidectomy reduces the high level of vascularity and friability of the gland produced by the antithyroid *thioamide derivatives*. The iodides are usually given three times per day in water after meals for seven to ten days before the date of the planned surgery.

Adverse Effects. Adverse effects infrequently occur during short-term use of the iodides. The symptoms of iodism, which occasionally occurs with use of the drugs, include a burning sensation or a brassy taste in the mouth, soreness of the gums, excess salivation, acute rhinitis, redness of the conjunctiva, edema of the eyelids, frontal headache, and gastric or respiratory irritation. Allergic reactions, which rarely occur, include acneiform rash, fever, jaundice, pruritus, angioedema, and serum sickness. Goiter with hypothyroidism has been reported in adults and in infants whose mothers have taken iodides for prolonged periods of time.

THIOAMIDE DERIVATIVES

Propylthiouracil

The drug (Table 31–1) is the prototype of the thioamide derivatives, which include *methimazole* and *methylthiouracil*, that are used as antithyroid agents. The drugs have similar chemical structures, actions, therapeutic indications, and adverse effects.

Action Mode. Propylthiouracil interferes with oxidation of iodide, which is an essential preliminary step in the formation of thyroid hormone. The stores of thyroglobulin in the thyroid gland maintain the plasma levels of circulating hormone for several days, and the decreased propylthiouracil-induced reduction in hormone synthesis becomes evident when the stored hormone is depleted.

Therapy Considerations. Propylthiouracil is readily absorbed from the gastrointestinal tract after it is taken orally. The rapid rate of its metabolism necessitates administration of the drug at eight-hour intervals during the 24-hour period. Approximately 35 percent of the unchanged drug and its metabolites are secreted in the urine in 24 hours. The drug is secreted in the milk of nursing mothers. Strong iodine solution is usually given concurrently with propylthiouracil for a period of seven to ten days preoperatively to counteract the increased friability and vascularity of the hyperplastic gland that are produced by propylthiouracil.

Prolonged conservative management of hyperthyroidism may involve concurrent administration of thyroid hormone or a synthetic hormone preparation with the antithyroid drug. The effective maintenance dosages are established by evaluations of the basal metabolic rate. Permanent remission occurs in 50 to 60 percent of the persons who are treated conservatively for a period of one year.

Adverse Effects. Agranulocytosis is the most serious adverse effect. Leukopenia and thrombocytopenia can also occur during therapy with propylthiouracil. Regularly scheduled evaluations of blood cell counts are planned throughout therapy. The person who is taking the drug should understand the rationale for the blood tests and the importance of informing the physician when there is evidence of unusual bleeding, fever, sore throat, or other infections.

The most common manifestation of the allergic reactions, which infrequently appear during therapy, is a mild skin rash or urticaria that often subsides spontaneously. Enlargement of the salivary glands or lymph nodes may also occur. Therapy is discontinued when severe skin rash or gland and node enlargement appears. Other adverse effects include gastrointestinal disturbances, hepatic damage, arthralgia, visual disturbances, headache, drowsiness, and vertigo. There have been reports of drug fever, lupus-like reaction, and hypoprothrombinemia during therapy with propylthiouracil.

Methimazole

The drug (Table 31–1) has actions, clinical uses, and adverse effects similar to those of propylthiouracil. The therapeutic effects appear more promptly, but the drug is somewhat less consistent in its action than propylthiouracil. There are indications that agranulocytosis occurs less frequently with the use of methimazole than with propylthiouracil.

Methylthiouracil

The drug (Table 31–1) is employed less frequently than propylthiouracil for preoperative or maintenance treatment of hyperthyroidism. Methylthiouracil is also considered to produce agranulocytosis and other adverse effects more frequently than propylthiouracil. Its use is usually reserved for those persons who cannot tolerate other antithyroid drugs.

Thyroid Preparations

DRUG THERAPY

Thyrotropin, which is a purified extract of bovine anterior pituitary glands, is the thyroid-stimulating hormone used for differential diagnosis between primary hypothyroidism and pituitary gland hypofunction–induced hypothyroidism. When the injection of 10 USP units of thyrotropin (THYTROPAR) produces stimulation of the thyroid gland, the pathology exists in the pituitary gland. Thyroid preparations are utilized for treatment of patients who have primary or secondary hypothyroidism.

Action Mode

The thyroid preparations have similar pharmacologic and therapeutic properties and produce physiologic responses comparable to those of the endogenous thyroid hormone. The hormones promote gluconeogenesis, increase the mobilization of glycogen stores and the utilization of carbohydrates, and stimulate the synthesis of proteins. Thyroid hormone also increases lipolysis thereby reducing the hepatic and serum levels of cholesterol. The stimulatory effect of thyroid on the energy transport mechanisms at the cellular level has a positive effect on most metabolic, growth, and developmental processes. The thyroid replacement preparations include *desiccated thyroid, dextrothyroxine sodium, thyroglobulin, levothyroxine sodium, liothyronine sodium,* and *liotrix* (Table 31–1).

Thyroid, Desiccated

Therapy Considerations. The thyroid preparation, which is obtained from animal sources, contains the levothyroxine, thyroglobulin, and small amounts of triiodothyronine that naturally are found in the thyroid gland. The orally administered drug has a slow onset of action. Thyroid is initially given at a lower dosage (Table 31–1), and the dosage is increased at one-to-three-week intervals when the person's response and laboratory tests of thyroid function indicate the need for additional thyroid hormone for maintenance of the normal metabolic activity levels. The maximum response to therapeutic dosages may not become apparent for a few weeks or months after initiation of therapy.

The thyroid hormone dosages for children increase with their ages, but the dosage per kilogram of body weight decreases as their weight increases. The initial dosage for children is 15 to 30 mg/day to avoid the onset of thyrotoxicosis, which can occur at higher dosage levels. The dosage generally is adjusted to maintain the serum protein-bound iodine (PBI) at 5 to 9 mcg/100 ml. Infants with cretinism may be given 45 to 60 mg/day when they are two to six months of age and 60 to 90 mg/day when they are six months to one year of age.

Adverse Effects. The adverse effects, which represent dosages in excess of those required for maintenance of normal physiologic processes, resemble the characteristic manifestations of hyperthyroidism. The adverse effects include tachycardia, cardiac arrhythmias, palpitation, anginal pain, elevated pulse and blood pressure, dyspnea, heat intolerance, hyperhidrosis, diarrhea, abdominal cramps, weight loss, vomiting, headache, nervousness, mental agitation, insomnia, and twitching or tremors of small muscle groups. The drug therapy is interrupted to allow reduction in the circulating hormone levels when adverse effects appear. Accelerated bone maturation in infants and children can occur when the maintenance dosage exceeds that required for development.

Thyroglobulin

The drug is the final purified product of the thyroid gland that is obtained from animal sources. Thyroglobulin contains levothyroxine and levotriiodothyronine and has the same biologic activity as thyroid. The drug is administered orally and has a slow onset of action. It is employed less frequently for therapy than desiccated thyroid, but it shares the actions, clinical indications, and adverse effects of that drug. Thyroglobulin (Table 31–2) is administered as a single daily oral dose. The dosage of the drug used for treatment of infants with cretinism is the same as that of thyroid.

Levothyroxine Sodium

The drug (Table 31–1) is a synthetic preparation of the principal hormone *thyroxine* (T_4) of the thyroid gland. It has a slower onset and a longer duration of action than liothyronine.

The drug can be administered orally or intravenously. The initial daily dosage is increased in increments of 50 to 100 mcg at intervals of one to four weeks until the desired response is attained. When oral therapy is not feasible, the drug may be given intravenously at a dosage of 0.2 to 0.4 mg. An additional dose of 0.1 to 0.2 mg may be given when the desired response is not obtained within 24 hours.

The maximum initial oral dosage for children is 50 mcg/day. The dosage is increased in increments of 25 to 50 mcg/day at one-to-four-week intervals. The dosage for infants with cretinism is usually 100 mcg/day.

Liothyronine Sodium

The drug (Table 31–1) is a synthetic preparation of the hormone triiodothyronine (T_3) with actions, clinical indications, and adverse effects similar to those of desiccated thyroid. The initial daily dosage for adults is increased gradually in increments of 5 to 10 mcg/day at one-to-two-week intervals until the desired response is attained.

The maximum initial dosage for elderly persons and children is 5 mcg/day. The maintenance dosage for children is determined by the gradual increases in increments of 5 mcg/day at one-to-two-week intervals. The increments are made at four-to-five-day intervals when liothyronine is employed for treatment of infants with cretinism.

Therapeutic effects of liothyronine appear earlier than with other thyroid preparations. Adverse effects may be evident within 24 to 72 hours when the drug dosage exceeds that required for maintenance of metabolic activity.

Dextrothyroxine Sodium

The drug (Table 31–2) is used selectively for treatment of patients with heart disease and hypothyroidism. Its use is limited to those patients who cannot tolerate other thyroid preparations.

Liotrix

The drug (Table 31–1) is a synthetic thyroid combination, which contains four parts of sodium levothyroxine and one part of sodium liothyronine. Liotrix is usually taken orally as a single daily dose on arising. Increments in the adult daily dosage are usually made at one-to-two-week intervals, and the increments for children are made at two-week intervals.

Drugs Affecting Bone Resorption

DRUG THERAPY

The primary functions of the parathyroid gland are regulation of calcium balance and utilization of the calcium ions for the building of bone. In the absence of adequate parathyroid function, *parathyroid hormone* is used to maintain the natural hormone activity, *calcitonin* is used to inhibit bone resorption, and *dihydrotachysterol* is used to maintain serum calcium levels. The selection of a particular agent for therapy is dependent on the total body calcium balance and the status of the skeletal structure.

Parathyroid Hormone

The preparation is a polypeptide product obtained from animal sources. The expense of the product and the occurrence of refractoriness after a few days of therapy limit the use of the drug. The action of the hormone on the bone, intestines, and kidneys in the maintenance of total body calcium levels is similar to that of the endogenous hormone. The hormone-induced stimulation of osteoclast formation controls the transfer of calcium to and from the bones and the circulating fluids. The concurrent osteoclastic and osteoblastic activity builds, shapes, and maintains the structure of the bony skeleton. The action of the hormone at proximal renal tubule sites increases the excretion of phosphates and decreases the excretion of calcium ions. The hormonal stimulus for the renal conversion of vitamin D_3 to its active form contributes to the increased vitamin-induced absorption of calcium in the intestinal tract. The action of the hormone maintains the calcium balance in persons with hypoparathyroidism.

Therapy Considerations. The drug is administered by intramuscular or intravenous injection. It is infrequently administered subcutaneously because moderate inflammation occurs at the injection site. The usual parenteral dosage for adults is 20 to 40 units every 12 hours. The parenteral dosage for infants with transient hypoparathyroidism is usually 25 to 50 units every 12 hours for one to three days. Dosages are adjusted to maintain the serum calcium levels at 9 to 12 mg/100 ml.

Parathyroid hormone may also be used for diagnosis of parathyroid gland function. The drug is administered as a slow intravenous infusion over a period of 15 minutes at a dosage of 200 to 300 units for the diagnosis of hypoparathyroidism. The urinary content of *cylic adenosine-3',5'-monophospate* (cAMP) is measured and compared to the predrug cAMP levels. When the person has hypoparathyroidism, the increased activity of parathyroid hormone at renal sites produces an elevation in the urine content of cAMP during the three-hour period after the drug is administered.

The injected drug is well absorbed from the

parenteral tissues. An elevation in the serum calcium levels is evident one hour after intravenous administration and within four hours after the drug is administered intramuscularly or subcutaneously. The peak serum calcium levels are attained in 12 to 18 hours. At the end of a 20-to-24-hour period the serum calcium levels return to the pretreatment levels. Parathyroid hormone has a plasma half-life of 20 minutes. The drug is metabolized in the liver, spleen, and kidneys, and the metabolites are excreted in the urine.

Adverse Effects. The most serious adverse effect is hypercalcemia. Frequent evaluations of the serum calcium levels are planned during therapy with parathyroid hormone to prevent the occurrence of marked hypercalcemia. Early symptoms of excess serum calcium levels include muscular weakness, ataxia, vertigo, tinnitus, lethargy, headache, exanthema, anorexia, nausea, vomiting, abdominal cramps, and diarrhea or constipation. When the serum calcium levels exceed 12 mg/100 ml, there may be evidence of serious cardiovascular effects (i.e., vasodilation, decreased blood pressure, bradycardia, cardiac arrhythmias, syncope, cardiac arrest). Therapy is interrupted immediately when there is evidence of hypercalcemia. The intake of fluids and the use of measures to accelerate the excretion of calcium (i.e., phosphate or sulfate laxatives, nonthiazide diuretics) rapidly return the calcium levels to the normal range.

Interactions. The concurrent use of thiazide diuretics can promote the hypercalcemic action of the hormone by interfering with secretion of calcium ions at renal tubule sites. Dactinomycin competitively inhibits the osteoblastic activity of parathyroid hormone. Concurrent administration of anticonvulsants interferes with hormone-induced excretion of phosphates in the urine.

Calcitonin

The drug (CALCIMAR) is a polypeptide hormone obtained from salmon. It is similar to the hormone released by the human thyroid gland in response to increased levels of calcium in the blood perfusing the gland.

Action Mode. The interaction of calcitonin at receptors on the plasma membrane of osteoclasts causes the intracellular accumulation of *cyclic adenosine-3',5'-monophosphate* (cAMP), and that action reduces the activity of the osteoclasts. The hormone inhibits osteoclast activity for a longer period of time than does the endogenous hormone. The drug action decreases bone resorption, and the circulating calcium becomes incorporated with phosphates on the bone matrix. Calcitonin is employed primarily for treatment of persons with Paget's disease of the bone (osteitis deformans).

Calcitonin decreases the renal tubular reabsorption of many electrolytes, and there is a consequent higher rate of their excretion (i.e., calcium, phosphate, sodium, magnesium, chloride, potassium). During therapy with calcitonin, there may be a decrease in the excretion of calcium in response to the lower circulating levels that occur when bone resorption is reduced.

Therapy Considerations. Calcitonin is administered by subcutaneous or intramuscular injection. Local inflammation occurs at the injection site in about 10 percent of the persons receiving the drug. The dosage of the drug is expressed in the international reference standard of the Medical Research Council (MRC) of Great Britain.

An intradermal test is done prior to therapy to determine sensitivity to the protein product. A test dose of 10 MRC units (0.05 ml) of the reconstituted drug is diluted to 1 ml by addition of 5 percent dextrose or 0.9 percent sodium chloride, and 0.1 ml of that solution is injected intracutaneously on the flexor surface of the forearm. The dosage of calcitonin is given when the reaction is negative 15 minutes after the injection.

The initial subcutaneously administered dosage of calcitonin for treatment of persons with Paget's disease is 100 MRC units/day. When there is evidence of improvement in the bone structure and serum calcium levels, the drug is usually given at a maintenance dosage of 50 to 100 MCR units three times per week.

The drug effect on serum calcium levels is evident almost immediately after intravenous injection and the effect persists for 12 hours. The effects are evident within 15 minutes after the drug is injected subcutaneously or intramuscularly. The effect on serum calcium levels reaches a peak in four hours and persists for 8 to 24 hours. The deposition of calcium on the bone matrix produces an improvement in its structure after several months of therapy. The drug is thought to be metabolized in the blood, peripheral tissues, and kidneys. The inactive metabolites are excreted in the urine. Approximately 2 percent of the persons receiving the drug have facial flushing.

Dihydrotachysterol

The drug (HYTAKEROL) is a synthetic preparation of vitamin D_2 that maintains the serum calcium levels in a manner similar to that of parathyroid hormone. Administration of the drug leads to increased intestinal absorption of calcium, and bone calcium is mobilized in the absence of parathyroid hormone or functional renal tissue.

Therapy Considerations. Dihydrotachysterol is administered orally in the treatment of hypocalcemia associated with hypoparathyroidism. The usual initial dosage for adults is 0.75 to 2.5 mg/day. A loading dose that is two to four times the maintenance dosage may be given for a period of four days to rapidly elevate the serum calcium levels and provide the calcium for integration into bone. The maintenance dosage is 0.2 to 2 mg/day. The particular dosages employed during long-term therapy are determined by the evaluations of serum calcium levels. Concurrent administration of calcium lactate or calcium gluconate, 10 to 15 gm, or an increase of the dietary calcium content is often planned during therapy with dihydrotachysterol.

The initial dosage for children is 0.8 to 2.4 mg/day. The usual maintenance dosage is 0.2 to 1 mg/day. The serum calcium levels are monitored throughout therapy with the drug to avoid the onset of hypercalcemia because the dosage that produces hypercalcemia is only slightly higher than the therapeutic dosage.

Anorexigenic Drugs

DRUG THERAPY

The anorexigenic agents are employed as adjuncts in treatment plans for obese persons. A well-balanced, nutritious, low-calorie diet is an essential aspect of initial and long-term programs for weight reduction. In addition to dietary counseling, effective treatment plans for the control of exogenously induced obesity include behavior modification counseling. Long-term programs for sustained weight control are usually dependent on reduction of the person's habitual intake of calories in excess of the amounts required by physical activity patterns.

The anorexigenic agents are extensively misused and abused drugs. They have been widely misused by persons seeking to combat fatigue when prolonged periods of wakefulness are desired. For example, the drugs are taken by athletes, students studying for an examination, or long-distance truck drivers to produce sustained periods of alertness. The drugs are also taken orally or by injection as "uppers" by drug abusers who attempt to balance the stimulant and depressant effects of the drugs they are taking. The anorexigenic drugs provide the desired mental stimulation that produces periods of wakefulness, but abstinence or abrupt withdrawal of the drug after prolonged or regular use produces withdrawal symptoms (i.e., depression, fatigue, psychoses).

The occurrence of psychologic and physical dependence and the potential for abuse of the drugs led to the legal restriction of their distribution. The drugs are subject to the controls of the Federal Controlled Substances Act of 1970 (Table 31–2). Their designation as drugs with a potential for abuse and for the production of psychologic or physiologic dependence limits the distribution of the drugs through legitimate channels, but illicit distribution of the drugs remains a problem.

The amphetamines, which are the oldest of the anorexigenics, provide central stimulatory effects that are also useful in the treatment of narcolepsy, mental depression, drug-induced respiratory depression (i.e., barbiturate intoxication), or the hyperkinetic syndrome in children. The amphetamine congeners and mazindol produce less central nervous system stimulation and are generally employed in preference to the amphetamines for treatment of obese persons.

Action Mode

The amphetamines are considered to contribute to weight reduction by their depressant effects on the lateral hypothalamic feeding centers. The amphetamines also release norepinephrine, which activates the neurons of the reticular arousal system in the brain. Those central actions reduce the desire for food and provide mental alertness and restlessness that produces a marked increase in physical activity. There may be an associated 15 percent increase in metabolic ac-

Table 31–2.
Drugs Used for Short-Term Control of Exogenous Obesity

Drug	Controlled Substances Schedule	Usual Adult Oral Dosage (mg)	Number of Doses Per Day
Mazindol (SANOREX)	III	1–2	1–3
Amphetamines			
Amphetamine sulfate (BENZEDRINE)	II	5–10	3
Dextroamphetamine hydrochloride (CURBAN, DARO, DEXEDRINE, OBOTAN)	II	5–10	3
Methamphetamine hydrochloride (DESOXYEPHEDRINE, DESOXYN, OBEDRIN-LA)	II	2.5–5	3
Amphetamine Congeners			
Benzphetamine hydrochloride (DIDREX)	III	25–50	1–3
Chlorphentermine hydrochloride (PRE-SATE)	III	65	1
Clortermine hydrochloride (VORANIL)	III	50	1
Diethylpropion hydrochloride (TENUATE, TEPANIL)	IV	25	3
Fenfluramine hydrochloride (PONDIMIN)	IV	20–40	3
Phendimetrazine tartrate (PLEGINE)	III	35	2–3
Phenmetrazine hydrochloride (PRELUDIN)	II	25	2–3
Phentermine hydrochloride (FASTIN, WILPO)	IV	8–37.5	1–3
Phentermine resin (IONAMIN)	IV	15–30	1

tivity in some persons, but the metabolic rate may remain unchanged in others who take the drugs.

The amphetamines have a direct action on the alpha-adrenergic receptors of the sympathetic nerves of the peripheral vasculature. They also have an indirect effect produced by the release of norepinephrine stores from the sympathetic nerve terminals to the effector organs. At therapeutic dosage levels, the drug-induced increase in norepinephrine activity produces peripheral vaso-constriction, and there is a consequent elevation in the systolic and diastolic blood pressure. The concurrent effect of the drugs on the beta-adrenergic receptors may increase the pulse pressure and produce bradycardia. The sympathomimetic activity of the amphetamines is similar to that of endogenous *norepinephrine,* but their onset of action is slower and the vasoconstriction is more prolonged.

The drugs decrease the acuity of the senses of smell and taste, and that effect contributes to the control of food intake. The sympathomimetic activity of larger doses of the drugs produces mydriasis, bronchodilation, contraction of the urinary bladder sphincter, and decreased gastro-intestinal motility.

Dextroamphetamine is generally preferred as an anorexigenic agent because it produces stronger central nervous system effects and less peripheral effects than amphetamine. Metham-phetamine hydrochloride produces central nervous system stimulation similar to that of amphetamine but has less peripheral effects than that drug.

The amphetamine congeners and mazindol (Table 31–2) provide central effects that aid in weight control with less central nervous system stimulation and peripheral vascular effects than the amphetamines. Fenfluramine, unlike other amphetamine congeners, frequently produces depression rather than stimulation of the central nervous system. Mazindol, which is chemically unrelated to the amphetamines, has pharma-cologic activity similar to that of the ampheta-mines. It is considered to provide an anorexigenic effect by facilitating electrical activity in the septal area of the limbic system.

Therapy Considerations

The anorexigenics, or "anorectics", are useful agents for short periods of therapy, but tolerance to the appetite suppressant effects generally oc-curs within a period of four to six weeks. Most of the drugs are taken orally one-half to one hour before meals three times per day. The last dose is taken at least six hours before bedtime to avoid the stimulatory effects that can interfere with sleep. The longer-acting drugs and the extended-release formulations are usually taken as a single midmorning dose.

The oral drugs are readily absorbed from the gastrointestinal tract. The absorbed drug is distributed in most body tissues, and the highest concentrations appear in the brain and in the cerebrospinal fluids. The anorexigenic drugs cross the placental barrier. The drugs are excreted primarily in the urine. When the tubular urine is alkaline (i.e., pH 8.0), the nonionized drug is readily reabsorbed in the tubules and only mini-mal amounts are excreted in the urine (i.e., 2 to 3 percent). Approximately 80 percent of the drug is excreted when the urine is at the normal acidic levels.

The amphetamines are given orally to hyper-kinetic children and parenterally to persons with acute barbiturate intoxication. *Amphetamine hydrochloride, amphetamine phosphate,* and *am-phetamine sulfate* are administered orally or parenterally. The oral dosage of amphetamine phosphate or sulfate for hyperkinetic children is 2.5 to 20 mg/day. The dosage of amphetamine is 20 to 50 mg when it is administered by intra-muscular or intravenous injection to adults with barbiturate intoxication. Doses of 50 to 100 mg may be given at 30-to-60-minute intervals until the person has regained consciousness. The drug is also available as amphetamine complex (BI-PHETAMINE), which is a resin complex of am-phetamine and dextroamphetamine in equal amounts.

Dextroamphetamine hydrochloride, dextroam-phetamine phosphate, dextroamphetamine sulfate, and *dextroamphetamine tannate* are given orally. A dosage of 2 to 15 mg/day is given to hyperkinetic children, and that dosage is divided for administration three times per day. The initial dosage of dextroamphetamine sulfate is 10 to 20 mg when the drug is given by intramuscular or intravenous injection to adults with barbiturate intoxication. The dosage may be repeated at 30-minute intervals until the person regains consciousness.

Methamphetamine hydrochloride is given at a dosage of 2.5 to 15 mg at bedtime when it is used for the treatment of children with enuresis. The initial intravenous dosage of 10 to 30 mg may be given at hourly intervals in the treatment of adults with barbiturate intoxication. The drug dosage is at the lower level of the range (10 mg/hr) when there is evidence of improvement in the person's state of consciousness.

Adverse Effects

The principal adverse effects of the anorexigenic drugs are manifestations of central nervous system stimulation (i.e., nervousness, insomnia, irritability, hyperverbalization, increased libido, dizziness, headache, increased motor activity, hyperexcitability). The effects of the drugs on the cardiovascular system may produce hypertension or hypotension, tachycardia, palpitations, cardiac arrhythmias, chilliness, pallor, or flushing. The drugs occasionally produce a metallic taste in the mouth and gastrointestinal disturbances (i.e., nausea, vomiting, abdominal cramps, diarrhea or constipation, dry mouth, anorexia). The drugs can also produce paradoxic depression or agitation in patients who receive them for the treatment of mental depression. The newborn infant may be agitated and hyperglycemic when the mother has taken an anorexigenic drug prior to delivery.

Toxicity

Abstinence or abrupt withdrawal of an anorexigenic drug produces a withdrawal syndrome in persons who are drug dependent as a consequence of prolonged use of the drug. The syndrome includes marked fatigue, depression, asthenia, tremors, and gastrointestinal disturbances. Fenfluramine withdrawal can produce severe mental depression. The initial symptoms are followed by persistent drowsiness and a prolonged period of sleep, which represent the unmasking of chronic fatigue as a consequence of the prolonged drug-induced insomnia. Psychotic reactions can also occur.

Although overdosage may produce severe adverse effects, the drugs have a relatively high therapeutic index, and death is seldom a direct consequence of an overdose of the anorexigenic drugs. Hyperpyrexia is a frequent sign of acute drug intoxication. The initial effects of overdosage include flushing or pallor, palpitations, labile pulse rate and blood pressure levels, extrasystoles, and heart block. When children take an overdosage, the drug may produce twisting, turning, and purposeless movements, mumbling, hyperactivity, hyperirritability, and tremulousness for a period of 12 hours after the toxic dose is ingested.

The toxic effects that occur from 36 to 48 hours after an overdose of the anorexigenic drugs include slurred speech, ataxia, tachypnea, confusion, delirium, and toxic psychoses (i.e., vivid visual and auditory hallucinations, panic, paranoid ideation, changes in affect in a person with a clear sensorium). The dose of the drug is excreted over a five-to-seven-day period, and the psychotic reaction gradually improves when the person abstains from taking additional doses of the drug. The treatment of toxicity includes acidification of the urine to increase the rate of drug excretion, administration of short-acting sedatives, treatment of shock, and symptomatic treatment.

Chronic abuse of the drugs produces emotional lability, loss of appetite, somnolence, mental impairment, and deterioration of social and occupational function. The chronic drug abuser characteristically shows chewing movements of the mouth, grinding of the teeth (bruxism), and persistent rubbing movements of the tongue along the inside of the lower lip that causes an irritation and subsequent breakdown in the tissues of the tongue and inner lips.

Review Guides

1. Outline the factors that should be included when describing the diagnostic test to the person who will receive radioactive sodium iodide (I^{125}).
2. Describe the assessments that would be appropriate when the patient is receiving strong iodine solution and propylthiouracil for treatment of hyperthyroidism.
3. Outline the factors that would be included when discussing therapy with desiccated thyroid with the parents of a child with cretinism.
4. Identify the primary differences between liothyronine and thyroglobulin.
5. Describe the planned therapeutic outcomes when the patient is receiving parathyroid hormone as compared to those occurring when the person is receiving calcitonin.
6. Outline the differences in the nursing intervention when the patient is receiving parathyroid hormone as compared with dihydrotachysterol.
7. Describe the assessments that would be appropriate when the person is receiving calcitonin for the treatment of osteitis.
8. Explain the rationale for gradual reduction of the dosage of amphetamines when the four-week period of therapy is to be terminated.
9. Outline the assessments that would be planned when the person enters the emergency room with probable amphetamine toxicity.

Additional Readings

Bergstrom, William: Calciferol deficiency here and now. *Am. J. Dis. Child.*, **129:**1137, October, 1975.

Burrow, Gerard N.: Therapeutic uses of thyroid hormone in euthyroid individuals. *Primary Care*, **2:**689, December, 1975.

Carlson, Harold E., and Hershman, Jerome M.: The hypothalamic-pituitary-thyroid axis. *Med. Clin. North Am.*, **59:**1045, September, 1975.

Charney, Evan; Goodman, Helen Chamblee; McBride, Margaret; Lyon, Barbara; and Pratt, Rosalie: Childhood antecedents of adult obesity. *N. Engl. J. Med.*, **295:**6, July 1, 1976.

Crile, George, Jr.: Diagnosis and management of thyroid cancer. *Hosp. Med.*, **13:**48, July, 1977.

Gillies, Dee Ann, and Alyn, Irene Barrett: Caring for patients with thyroid disorders: how good are your skills? *Nursing 77*, **7:**77, October, 1977.

Gilliland, Paul F.: Myxedema: recognition and treatment. *Postgrad. Med.*, **57:**61, January, 1975.

Gold, Donald D., Jr.: Psychologic factors associated with obesity. *Am. Fam. Physician*, **13:**87, June, 1976.

Gordon, John E.: Nutritional individuality. *Am. J. Dis. Child.*, **129:**422, April, 1975.

Griffiith, John D.; Nutt, John G.; and Janinski, Donald R.: A comparison of fenfluramine and amphetamine in man. *Clin. Pharmacol. Ther.*, **18:**563, November, 1975.

Hallal, Janice C.: Thyroid disorders. *Am. J. Nurs.*, **77:**417, March, 1977.

Ibarra, Jesse D.; Gilliland, Paul F.; Petty, F. C.;

Roberts, John W.; Peake, Robert L.; and Crile, George, Jr.: Treatment of hyperthyroidism. *Postgrad. Med.*, **57:**84, June, 1975.

Ingbar, Sidney H.: When to hospitalize with thyrotoxicosis. *Hosp. Pract.*, **10:**45, January, 1975.

Kreisberg, Robert A.: Phosphorus deficiency and hypophosphatemia. *Hosp. Pract.*, **12:**121, March, 1977.

McBeath, Andrew A.: The aging skeleton: osteoporosis and degenerative arthritis. *Postgrad. Med.*, **57:**171, June, 1975.

McConahey, William M.: Diagnosing and treating myxedema and myxedema coma. *Geriatrics*, **33:**61, March, 1978.

McConnell, Robert J.; Menendez, Carlos E.; Smith, Frank Rees; Henkin, Robert I.; and Rivlin, Richard S.: Defects of taste and smell in patients with hypothyroidism. *Am. J. Med.*, **59:**354, September, 1975.

Melehinger, David: Helping obese patients lose weight. *Primary Care*, **2:**547, December, 1975.

Mills, Lewis C.: Treatment of hypothyroidism. *Am. Fam. Physician*, **14:**170, November, 1976.

Morrow, Lewis B.: How thyroid disease presents in the elderly. *Geriatrics*, **33:**42, April, 1978.

Oreopoulos, D. G.; Husdan, H.; Harrison, J.; Meema, H. E.; McNeill, K. G.; Murray, T. M.; Ogilvie, R.; and Rapoport, A.: Metabolic balance studies in patients with Paget's disease receiving salmon calcitonin over long periods. *Can. Med. Assoc. J.*, **116:**851, April 23, 1977.

Pitkin, Roy M.: Calcium metabolism in pregnancy: a review. *Am. J. Obstet. Gynecol.,* **121:**724, March 1, 1975.

Ramey, James N., and Burrow, Gerald N.: Clinical uses of thyrotropin-releasing hormone. *Am. Fam. Physician,* **12:**93, July, 1975.

Refetoff, Samuel: Thyroid hormone therapy. *Med. Clin. North Am.,* **59:**1147, September, 1975.

Rivlin, Richard S.: Drug therapy: therapy of obesity with hormones. *N. Engl. J. Med.,* **292:**26, January 2, 1975.

Smith, David M., and Edmondson, James W.: Common adult osteopenic states: osteoporosis and osteomalacia. *Am. Fam. Physician,* **14:**160, November, 1976.

Sterling, Kenneth: Radioactive iodine therapy. *Med. Clin. North Am.,* **59:**1217, September, 1975.

Teitelbaum, Steven L.; Bone, J. Michael; Stein, Paul M.; Gilden, Jerome J.; Bates, Margaret; Boisseau, Vincenza C.: and Avioli, Louis V.: Calciferol in chronic renal insufficiency. *J.A.M.A.,* **235:**164, January 12, 1976.

Tripp, Alice: Hyper and hypocalcemia. *Am. J. Nurs.,* **76:**1142, July, 1976.

Urbanic, Robert C., and Mazzaferri, Ernest L.: Thyrotoxic crisis and myxedema coma. *Heart Lung,* **7:**435, May–June, 1978.

Vagenakis, Apostolos G., and Braverman, Lewis E.: Adverse effects of iodides on thyroid function. *Med. Clin. North Am.,* **59:**1075, September, 1975.

Wallach, Stanley: Paget's disease: a new treatment of an old disease. *Am. Fam. Physician,* **13:**78, January, 1976.

Wurtman, Richard J.: The effects of light on the human body. *Sci. Am.,* **233:**68, July, 1975.

Zeluff, George W.; Suki, Wadi N.; and Jackson, Daniel: Depletion of body phosphate—ubiquitous, subtle, dangerous. *Heart Lung,* **6:**519, May-June, 1977.

Pharmacology and Drug Therapy References

The books that are included in the following list present comprehensive information about varied aspects of drug therapy. Many of the references included in the listing provided useful information in the preparation of this text.

Albanese, Joseph A., and Bond, Thomas: *AMA Drug Evaluations,* 3rd ed. Publishing Sciences Groups, Inc., Littleton, Mass. 1977.

————: *APhA Drug Names.* American Pharmaceutical Association, Washington D.C., 1976.

————: *Drug Interactions: Basic Principles and Clinical Problems.* McGraw-Hill Book Co., Inc., New York, 1978.

Azarnoff, Daniel L. (ed.): *1977 Year Book of Drug Therapy.* Year Book Medical Publishers, Chicago, 1977.

Bassuk, Ellen L., and Schoonover, Stephen C.: *The Practitioner's Guide to Psychoactive Drugs.* Plenum Medical Book Co., New York, 1977.

Benet, Leslie Z. (ed.): *The Effects of Disease States on Drug Pharmokinetics.* American Pharmaceutical Association, Academy of Pharmaceutical Sciences, Washington, D.C., 1976.

Bevan, John A.: *Essentials of Pharmacology,* 2nd ed. Harper and Row Publishers, Inc., Hagerstown, Md., 1976.

Bourne, Peter G. (ed.): *A Treatment Manual for Acute Drug Abuse Emergencies.* Department of Health, Education, and Welfare, Rockville, Md., 1976.

Bowman, W. C., and Rand, M. J.: *Textbook of Pharmacology,* 2nd ed. J. B. Lippincott Co., Philadelphia, 1977.

Bradley, P. B., and Costa, E.: *Studies of Narcotic Drugs.* Pergamon Press, Elmsford, N.Y., 1976.

Clarke, Frank H.: *How Modern Medicines Are Developed.* Futura Publishing Co., Mt. Kisco, N.Y., 1977.

Dukes, M. N. G.: *Evaluations of Drug Interactions,* 2nd ed. American Pharmaceutical Association, Washington, D.C., 1976.

————: *Side Effects of Drugs Annual 1977.* Excerpta Medica, New York, 1977.

Garb, Solomon: *Undesirable Drug Interactions,* 2nd ed., 1974–75, revised ed. Springer Publishing Co., New York, 1974.

Goldstein, A.; Aronow, L.; and Kalman, S. M.: *Principles of Drug Action,* 2nd ed. John Wiley & Sons, Inc., New York, 1974.

Goodman, Louis S., and Gilman, Alfred (eds.): *The Pharmacological Basis of Therapeutics,* 5th ed. Macmillan Publishing Co., Inc., New York, 1975.

Goth, Andres: *Medical Pharmacology,* 8th ed. C. V. Mosby Co., St. Louis, 1976.

Gouveia, W. A.; Tognoni, G.; and van der Kleijn, E.: *Clinical Pharmacy and Clinical Pharmacology.* Elsevier North-Holland, New York, 1977.

Green, H. I., and Levy, M. H.: *Drug Misuse.* Marcel Dekker, Inc., New York, 1976.

Griffin, J. P., and D'Arcy, P. F.: *A Manual of Adverse Drug Interactions.* Year Book Medical Publishers, Chicago, 1976.

Griffiths, Mary E. (ed.): *Handbook of Nonprescription Drugs,* 5th ed. American Pharmaceutical Association, Washington, D.C., 1977.

————: *USAN and the USP Dictionary of Drug Names.* United States Pharmacopeial Convention, Inc., Rockville, Md., 1975.

Hansten, Philip D.: *Drug Interactions,* 3rd ed. Lea & Febiger, Philadelphia, 1975.

Hartshorn, Edward A.: *Handbook of Drug Interactions,* 3rd ed. Drug Intelligence Publications, Hamilton, Ill., 1976.

Jarvik, Murray E.: *Psychopharmacology in the Practice of Medicine.* Appleton-Century-Crofts, New York, 1977.

Kastrup, Erwin K., and Boyd, James R. (eds.): *Facts and Comparisons.* Facts and Comparisons, Inc., St. Louis, 1978.

Kline, Nathan S.; Alexander, Stewart F.; and Chamberlain, Amparo: *Psychotropic Drugs.* Van Nostrand Reinhold, New York, 1974.

Melmon, Kenneth L., and Morrelli, Howard F. (eds.): *Clinical Pharmacology,* 2nd ed. Macmillan Publishing Co., Inc., New York, 1978.

Meyers, Frederick H.; Jawetz, Ernest; and Goldstein, Alan: *Review of Medical Pharmacology,* 5th ed. Lange Medical Publications, Los Altos, Calif., 1976.

Miller, Russel R., and Greenblatt, David J. (eds.): *Drug Effects in Hospitalized Patients.* John Wiley & Sons, Inc., New York, 1976.

Miller, Russell R., and Greenblatt, David J.: *Drug Therapy Reviews,* vol. 1. Masson Publishing USA, Inc., New York, 1977.

Modell, Walter (ed.): *Drugs of Choice 1976–1977.* C. V. Mosby Co., St. Louis, 1976.

Modell, Walter; Schild, Heinz O.; and the late Wilson, Andrew: *Applied Pharmacology.* W. B. Saunders Co., Philadelphia, 1976.

Pradhan, S. N. (ed.); Dutta, S. N. (asst. ed.): *Drug Abuse.* C. V. Mosby Co., St. Louis, 1977.

Ralston, Susan E., and Hale, Marion: *Review and Application of Clinical Pharmacology.* J. B. Lippincott Co., Philadelphia, 1977.

Ray, Oakley S.: *Drugs, Society and Human Behavior.* C. V. Mosby Co., St. Louis, 1972.

Reilly, Mary Jo (ed.): *American Hospital Formulary Service,* vols. 1 and 2. American Society of Hospital Pharmacists, Washington, D.C., 1978.

Roe, Daphne A.: *Drug-Induced Nutritional Deficiencies.* AVI Publishing Co., Westport, Conn., 1976.

Sapira, Joseph D., and Cherubin, Charles E.: *Drug Abuse.* Excerpta Medica, New York, 1976.

Shirkey, Harry C. (ed.): *Pediatric Therapy,* 5th ed. C. V. Mosby Co., St. Louis, 1975.

Smith, D. L.: *Medication Guide for Patient Counseling.* Lea & Febiger, Philadelphia, 1977.

Swonger, Alvin K., and Constantine, Larry L.: *Drugs and Therapy.* Little, Brown & Co., Boston, 1976.

Usdin, Earl, and Forrest, Irene S.: *Psychotherapeutic Drugs,* part I, vol. 2. Marcel Dekker, Inc., New York, 1976.

Index*

---

* Tables are indicated by the page number followed by *t.*
Illustrations are indicated by page numbers in **boldface** type.